P9-BZQ-127

Reproductive Hazards of Industrial Chemicals

This work was funded by a grant from the Health and Safety Executive, U.K. Any conclusions drawn are those of the authors.

Reproductive Hazards of Industrial Chemicals

An evaluation of animal and human data

SUSAN M. BARLOW AND FRANK M. SULLIVAN

Department of Pharmacology
Guy's Hospital Medical School
University of London

1982

ACADEMIC PRESS

A Subsidiary of Harcourt Brace Jovanovich, Publishers

London · New York
Paris · San Diego · San Francisco
São Paulo · Sydney · Tokyo · Toronto

ACADEMIC PRESS INC. (LONDON) LTD.
24/28 Oval Road
London NW1

United States Edition published by
ACADEMIC PRESS INC.
111 Fifth Avenue
New York, New York 10003

British Library Cataloguing in Publication Data

Barlow, S. M.
Reproductive hazards of industrial chemicals.
1. Human reproduction 2. Chemicals—Toxicology
I. Title II. Sullivan, F. M.
616.6 QP251

Library of Congress Catalog Card Number: 82–71008

ISBN: 0–12–078960–4

Phototypeset by Latimer Trend & Company Ltd, Plymouth
Printed in Great Britain by
St Edmundsbury Press

Preface

Reproductive hazards from industrial chemical exposure is one of the fastest growing areas of concern in toxicology today. This is not yet matched however, by any substantial body of reliable evidence that would permit some assessment of the extent of the potential problem. This information gap extends from inadequate or non-existent animal toxicology studies right through to the absence of epidemiological studies on humans exposed to the majority of industrial chemicals. Most human evidence has come as a result of industrial or environmental accidents with gross over-exposure. Thus, even with chemicals such as lead, organic mercury, chlordecone, dibromochloropropane (DBCP), and organo-chlorine compounds known to affect human reproduction, the evidence is inadequate to assess the effects of low levels of exposure.

We were invited by the U.K. Health and Safety Executive to collect and review the available evidence on the reproductive toxicity of approximately 50 industrial chemicals chosen from the Threshold Limit Values (TLV) list because of their general interest or widespread use. It was hoped that such a review would show the range and types of information available on industrial chemicals and possibly indicate the size of the potential reproductive hazard. We took it upon ourselves to exclude a few substances such as inorganic lead about which a great deal of easily obtained information is already available. We also added some others such as DBCP which we knew had already presented a reproductive hazard to exposed workers. This was to illustrate the value and limitations of animal studies for prediction of human hazards and to demonstrate the value of epidemiological studies in workers exposed not only in the production of such substances but also in their subsequent use. This book therefore obviously cannot be regarded as a catalogue of all of the potentially hazardous chemicals, but is a detailed review of all the available evidence on some out of many thousands of such chemicals. However, it includes many substances with widespread use as solvents and intermediates and with environmental impact as pollutants, and we hope will be of interest and value to those concerned with industrial health and hygiene and environmental pollution in its widest sense.

Each chemical has been reviewed using the same general format. First animal studies on relevant pharmacology and toxicology, endocrine and gonadal effects have been described. This is followed by animal data on fertility and pregnancy including teratogenicity, multigeneration, postnatal and behavioural teratology studies where available. In the mutagenicity sections only studies on mammalian cells *in vitro* and *in vivo* have been reviewed. Carcinogenicity studies have only been very briefly covered by reference to the excellent International Agency for Research on Cancer (I.A.R.C.) World Health Organization (W.H.O.) monographs unless specific data on transplacental carcinogenicity studies were found. The animal studies are followed by reports of human studies following the same general format where possible. Each review ends with a brief summary and our evaluation of the potential hazard to reproduction. A section on reproductive outcome by occupational groups has also been included. In this, the individual chemical or chemicals responsible for the effects may not have been identified, but they indicate the need for further work to attempt to do so.

We are grateful to our numerous colleagues, library assistants and secretarial friends for their help in producing this book and to the Health and Safety Executive for funding the project which turned out to be a much bigger job than any of us had imagined.

June 1982

S. M. BARLOW
F. M. SULLIVAN

Contents

Each of the following compounds is arranged in a standard format comprising animal studies, human studies and a summary and evaluation. Animal and human studies are subdivided into sections on pharmacology and toxicology, endocrine and gonadal effects, fertility, pregnancy, mutagenicity and carcinogenicity.

PART 1
Scientific background to testing and recognition of reproductive hazards

Reproductive hazards

HISTORICAL PERSPECTIVES

The first systematic reports linking reproductive effects to an industrial chemical were on lead toxicity and were published towards the end of the nineteenth century, culminating at the turn of the century in the banning of women from work in many of the heavy lead-using trades. Unusually high rates of infertility, spontaneous abortion, stillbirth, neonatal death, macrocephaly and convulsions in offspring were recorded in lead working communities in many different parts of Europe (reviewed by Rom, 1976). The reports suggested that both male and female reproductive capacity were affected, with adverse reproductive outcomes both in women lead workers themselves and in women who were married to men working in the pottery, printing and white lead trades. In retrospect, it is difficult to assess to what extent the effects seen in the wives of male lead workers may have been due to direct exposure to lead brought home on the husband's workclothes and to generally raised levels in the environment close to heavy lead-using industries, or were the consequences of male reproductive malfunction. However, more recent evidence suggests that at blood lead levels commonly found in male lead workers there is a deterioration in sperm count, sperm motility and sperm morphology (Lancranjan *et al.*, 1975), though the effects on reproductive outcome of these changes, if any, are not known. Despite this early history of the effects of lead on workers, the issue of reproductive hazards in the work place was largely neglected in ensuing years, apart from the measures that were taken to protect pregnant women from excessive radiation exposure (NCRP, 1971) and occasional references to possible hazards for women newly entered into the chemical industry during wartime (U.S. Department of Labor, 1942; Baetjer, 1946). Even the explosion in research on the causation of birth defects that occurred following the thalidomide disaster in the 1960s did not generally encompass the notion that industrial chemicals might also be teratogenic. In the 1970s, however, reports (reviewed by Koos and Longo, 1976) began to appear from Minamata and Niigata in Japan of the birth of children with severe neurological abnormalities in communities living round waters that had been heavily contaminated with mercury discharged in industrial effluent. The mercury, as methylmercury, was present in high concentrations in fish which formed the staple diet of much of the local population. Many adults succumbed to chronic methylmercury poisoning and 6% of all births in the Minamata area were affected. This disaster also emphasized that the developing embryo and fetus might be particularly susceptible to environmental chemicals, a number of affected children being born to apparently symptomless mothers. The explosion at the chemical plant in Seveso, Italy, in 1976, also had a worldwide impact on the public; the release of a cloud of dioxin, a highly toxic and teratogenic by-product from trichlorophenol manufacture, over a wide area inhabited by some 2000 people brought into sharp focus the possibility that industrial chemicals might have a serious reproductive impact beyond just to those occupationally exposed.

Also in the 1970s, two other incidents, both involving men engaged in the manufacture of pesticides (chlordecone and dibromochloropropane) in the U.S.A., further extended awareness of reproductive hazards into the area of male infertility (see page 00). The suggestion that men exposed to vinyl chloride monomer had an increased risk of fathering a child with a central nervous system malformation (see page 00) further broadened the perspective beyond just the need to protect the pregnant woman and the fetus from exposure to hazardous chemicals, though curiously, it was women who were banned from working with vinyl chloride monomer in the U.S.A. on the basis of animal data showing that it was a transplacental carcinogen. More recently, epidemiological studies have suggested there may well be a link between parental occupation and childhood cancer (see page 00), with most studies to date focussing on the role of the occupation of the father.

Thus, the investigation of potential reproductive hazards from industrial chemicals should encompass preconceptional exposure of males and females as well as pregnancy and exposure of infants during lactation. Ascertainment of effects should extend from reproductive cycles, sexual behaviour, fertility, pregnancy and birth events, right through to late-manifesting defects in the offspring such as mental retardation or cancer. A more detailed consideration of ways in which chemicals may interfere with reproductive function is given below.

THE RANGE OF POSSIBLE REPRODUCTIVE HAZARDS OF INDUSTRIAL CHEMICALS

Libido and potency

Sexual behaviour may be affected by changes in libido or potency and these are most likely to occur with agents that interfere with hormone secretion or have a central or a peripheral action on the nervous system. Libido and potency may also be affected secondarily to general debilitation from other toxic effects or may be psychogenic in origin, and care must be taken in human studies to rule out these possibilities before ascribing effects to any specific reproductive toxicity of the chemical. Alterations in libido and potency can occur in both males and females. Where females are affected it may well be masked in human studies looking only at indices of fertility and pregnancy outcome but may be revealed in animal studies where display of proceptive behaviour by the female is important for successful mating to take place.

Fertility

True infertility may result from a primary effect on ova or sperm or on the reproductive tract preventing fertilization. Apparent infertility may result from failure of the fertilized ovum to implant, or from early spontaneous abortion that passes unrecognized. In females, ovulation may not occur if there is interference with the cyclical release of the gonadotrophic hormones, luteinizing hormone (LH) and follicle stimulating hormone (FSH), from the pituitary gland, which is under the control of the hypothalamus and higher centres in the brain and feedback from ovarian hormones. Alternatively, ovulation may be prevented if direct toxicity to the ovary renders it unresponsive to the pituitary hormones. If defective or "blighted" ova are released then fertilization by sperm may not occur. Successful implantation of the fertilized ovum is critically dependent on normal timing of cyclical ovarian hormone secretion which brings the endometrial lining of the uterus into a receptive condition just at the time when the blastocyst arrives in the uterus after a journey of several days through the Fallopian tubes. Interference with pituitary and/or ovarian hormone secretion, particularly in the second half of the oestrous or menstrual cycle following ovulation, can render the uterus unreceptive, even if successful fertilization has been achieved.

Menstruation

Disturbances of the hypothalamic-pituitary-ovarian axis with alterations in hormone release patterns may manifest themselves as alterations in menstrual bleeding in women and primates. Similar changes can be detected by suitable investigative techniques in the oestrous cycle in rodents. For this reason, menstrual histories may be an important indicator of effects on sex hormone levels and may thus indicate a potential for reproductive toxicity.

Sperm

In males, reduction in sperm number (oligospermia) or reduced motility, or an increased proportion of sperm with abnormal morphology may individually or additively diminish fertilizing capacity. Although the consequences of complete absence of sperm (azoospermia) are predictable, the fertility of males with oligospermia is unpredictable. It is generally assumed however that men with a sperm count of less than 20 million per ml of semen are unlikely to be fertile. Alterations in sperm morphology and semen chemistry are areas where even less is known in terms of their reproductive consequences. Sperm with grossly abnormal morphology are generally less likely to fertilize an egg than normal sperm, but they may do so occasionally. Similarly, sperm with less visually obvious defects, including genetic damage, may also be fertile. However, not even the background frequency for such events in the general population is known.

Mutations

Chemicals causing chromosome damage (breaks, rearrangements, single gene mutations etc.) are more likely to affect males than females when exposure occurs during adulthood; in males the production of sperm in adult life is continuous, and repeated cell divisions during the sperm cycle maximize the opportunities for chemical attack on the chromosomes. On the other hand, once removed from exposure to the damaging agent then recovery of normal sperm production can occur in weeks, provided the stem cell spermatogonia are not affected. In females, the full complement of ova develop during fetal life, thus they are more resistant to genetic damage in adulthood. Should damage occur to the fetal germ cells, however, effects may be carried through to adult life and become evident when reproduction begins.

Where there is chromosome damage to either ovum or sperm, but fertilization takes place, then the embryo is frequently aborted. In humans, more than 50% of spontaneous abortions have chromosome defects. In mammals, genetic changes incompatible with survival of the embryo are termed dominant lethal mutations and in such cases the dead embryo will be aborted or resorbed. Some genetic changes, however, may be compatible with survival of the fetus to term. Such offspring may be born with congenital structural, biochemical or behavioural abnormalities. To assess the true frequency of such events, long-term follow-up is necessary since some late-manifesting abnormalities, such as impairment of intellectual function, may not be obvious at birth. If there is damage to the fetal germ cells the effects may pass undetected until reproductive life begins, or, in the case of recessive mutational changes, may not become apparent for several generations.

Pregnancy

Damage to the developing fetus through exposure of the pregnant woman to chemicals is often, incorrectly, thought to be the only hazard to reproduction. The possible effects of such exposure range through abortion, stillbirth, neonatal death, growth retardation, malformation, functional deficit and behavioural changes, to development of cancer in the offspring. The effects produced will depend on the time and severity of exposure and the type of chemical to which the mother is exposed, and may result either from a direct effect of the chemical on the embryo and fetus or indirectly from toxicity in the mother.

Cancer induction

Chemicals that induce cancer with gestational exposure are known as transplacental carcinogens. Only one such agent, the drug, diethylstilboestrol, has been identified with certainty in humans. Animal studies however have shown that the majority of carcinogens can act transplacentally, and that often the fetus is more sensitive to the carcinogenic effect than adults. Certainly, the presence of tumours in some children at birth suggests that the latent period between initiation of processes leading to disordered cell division and the appearance of a tumour may well be shorter in early life than in adulthood.

Postnatal development

Finally, the exposure of infants to environmental chemicals during early postnatal life, either in the air, brought home on the workclothes of the parents or via the breast milk, may cause developmental defects or death. Developmental toxicity may be similar to adult toxicity or may differ, as for example with chemicals acting on the central nervous system. In the human infant, brain development continues after birth for about the first 2 years of life. Interference with brain development occurring postnatally may thus result in permanent deficits, whereas exposure of the adult might produce only transient effects on the central nervous system.

It is clear that the safety assessment of industrial chemicals should include effects on both males and females from preconceptional and postconceptional exposure. From the survey of the literature on selected industrial chemicals which follows it is evident that examples may be found of chemicals that affect many of the various aspects of reproductive function discussed above. In our opinion, reproductive toxicity from industrial chemicals is likely to be rare, but where it does occur it may be the most sensitive indicator of toxicity and will be of considerable importance to those who are affected.

References

Baetjer, A. (1946). Women in Industry. W. B. Saunders, Philadelphia and London.

Koos, B. J. and Longo, L. D. (1976). Mercury toxicity in the pregnant woman, fetus and newborn infant. *American Journal of Obstetrics and Gynecology* **126**, 390–409.

Lancranjan, I., Popescu, H. I., Găvănescu, O., Klepsch, I. and Serbănescu, M. (1975). Reproductive ability of workmen occupationally exposed to lead. *Archives of Environmental Health* **30**, 396–401.

National Council on Radiation Protection and Measurements. (1971). Occupational exposure of fertile women, NCRP Report No. 39.

Rom, W. N. (1976). Effects of lead on the female and reproduction: a review. *The Mount Sinai Journal of Medicine* **43**, 542–552.

U.S. Department of Labor. (1942). Standards for maternity care and employment of mothers in industry. *Journal of the American Medical Association* **120**, 55–56.

Reproductive toxicity testing in animals

Tests for reproductive toxicity can be divided into two main categories—single generation studies and multigeneration studies. The single generation studies were primarily devised for testing safety of new drugs following the thalidomide disaster, whereas multigeneration studies were primarily devised to test the safety of food additives and unintentional food additives such as pesticides and packing material residues. The majority of investigations of chemicals of industrial interest have been carried out using one or other of these basic tests without great consideration being given to whether these may be the most satisfactory model for workers exposed occupationally or populations exposed via environmental pollution.

SINGLE GENERATION STUDIES

The most widely used basic protocol for single generation studies is that originally published by the U.S. Food and Drug Administration (FDA, 1966) for safety testing of new drugs. Basically this comprises three parts illustrated below:

Treatment periods

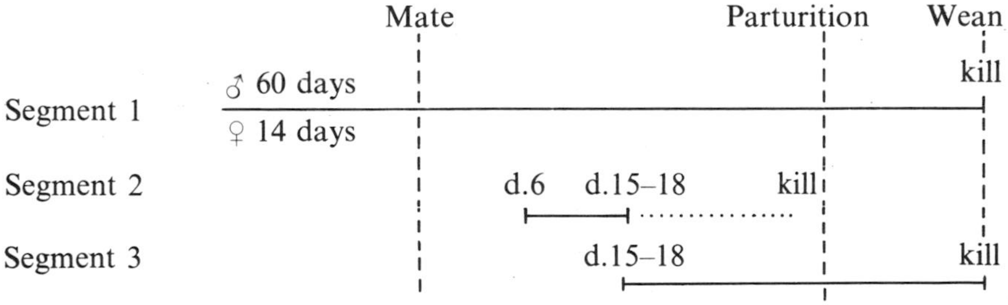

		Mate		Parturition	Wean
Segment 1	♂ 60 days ♀ 14 days				kill
Segment 2			d.6 d.15–18	kill	
Segment 3			d.15–18		kill

SEGMENT 1 STUDIES

This is essentially a fertility study, usually carried out in rats in which young males are treated for about 60 days to cover the major period of spermatogenesis and mature females are treated for 14 days to cover about 3 oestrous cycles. They are then mated together and the pregnant females allowed to deliver the young spontaneously and rear them to weaning at 21 days. The males are treated with the test compound until the end of the mating period and the females are treated throughout the whole test from before mating until weaning. Usually 3 dose levels plus controls are used for the test and in theory it gives a general overall view of the effects of the test compound on each stage of reproduction covering both males and females and effects on the offspring during lactation. For compounds which produce no effects up to very high doses this may be a satisfactory result. However, when effects are observed it is often very difficult to define exactly what aspect of reproduction has been affected. For example, if the females fail to become pregnant it may be due to action on the male or female or both. If the females become pregnant but have a high resorption rate due to embryonic or fetal death, this may be an effect on the dam interrupting the maintenance of pregnancy, on the embryo as a direct toxic effect, or even on the father as a dominant lethal mutagenic effect. Likewise if poor post-natal survival is observed, this may be an effect on maternal rearing behaviour or lactation, a toxic effect on the pups which may receive the compound via the milk or later directly from the food if the test compound is given by that method, or even an effect on the father (see Soyka and Joffe, 1980). This seems an attractive test at first sight, however when a compound produces a positive effect, so many sub-tests have to be carried out to analyse the site of action that many workers prefer a variant of the test in which treated males are mated with untreated females and *vice versa*, but even then, quite extensive analysis of positive effects is necessary.

SEGMENT 2 STUDIES

This is generally referred to as the "teratology test". Pregnant females are treated during the period of embryogenesis with the test compound, viz. days 6–15 or 16 in mice and rats or days 6–18 in rabbits. In the hamster, which is used much less frequently, embryogenesis is very condensed and the test compound need only be given on days 8–9. The dams are killed one day prior to expected delivery and the fetuses quickly removed and examined for viability, weight and the presence or absence of any morphological defects i.e. congenital abnormalities. Usually 3 doses of compound plus controls are used in this segment and usually the top dose can be higher than that used in the fertility segment since the animals are already pregnant at the start of the test and the general malaise produced by a toxic dose and which might interfere with mating behaviour, is not a limiting factor. The reason for killing the dams in order to obtain the fetuses by Caesarian section for examination and not allowing spontaneous delivery to take place, is because dams may kill or eat malformed offspring and offspring found dead may have been born dead or killed or neglected by the dam. It is for these reasons that fertility tests or multigeneration studies are not satisfactory substitutes for a teratology test.

SEGMENT 3 STUDIES

This is the peri-post-natal test and is designed primarily to test the effect of substances on parturition and in the post-natal period. The compound is administered, usually at 3 dose levels plus control during the last one-third of pregnancy, or from the end of the teratology segment, through parturition and up to weaning. It is unlikely that this segment by itself would be of much value in the study of chemicals of industrial interest.

VARIATIONS IN THE ABOVE PROTOCOL

Many variations on the above protocols have been used and provided certain basic requirements are retained, each design has advantages and disadvantages. It is, in practice, impossible to test every possible combination of events and the best compromise for each individual situation has to be chosen. The above protocol, as mentioned, was designed primarily for drug testing where a woman may receive high doses of a substance after she has become pregnant and possibly only for a short period of time—days or weeks. With industrial chemicals, chronic exposure to low concentrations for prolonged periods before and during pregnancy may be more common. Very few animal studies, however, take this into account and the majority of teratology tests at least tend to follow the "drug" protocols, with short periods of exposure to maximum tolerated doses. There are two major differences between short and long term exposure to chemicals which may affect the result of reproduction tests. The first depends on the pharmacokinetics or toxicokinetics of the test substance. If the substance is highly lipid soluble, and not metabolized to any high degree, like for example the organohalides, then cumulation in the tissues may occur over prolonged periods, so that adverse effects may result from exposure to lower levels than would be predicted from the acute toxicity. This could clearly affect the assessment of the minimal effective toxic exposure level.

The second important factor depends on the activity of the parent compound relative to the activity of the metabolites. If the metabolites are more toxic than the parent compound, then with chronic exposure there will be more time for metabolites to accumulate, or if enzyme induction occurs, as is common with polychlorinated biphenyls and with many pesticides, the blood levels of metabolites may increase dramatically with duration of exposure. Thus quite different minimal effective levels may be determined in acute and chronic studies. Depending on relative toxicity of the metabolites and their toxicokinetics, misleadingly high or low levels of toxicity may be determined using the traditional short exposure protocols. Very little work in this area using industrial chemicals has been carried out.

FERTILITY STUDIES IN MALES

Protocols for fertility studies in males have been less extensively studied than those for females. The basic designs for fertility studies in males are essentially similar to those which are used for dominant lethal tests. The important feature of a male fertility test is that it should be conducted in such a manner that effects on any part of the spermatogenic cycle would be detected. Spermatogenesis is a process in which the basic male germ cells in the testis, the spermatogonia, divide by mitotic division to produce daughter cells which in turn also divide by mitotic and later meiotic division and mature through a succession of cell types, the spermatocytes, spermatids and finally spermatozoa. The spermatozoa, or sperm, then pass from the testes through the epididymis where they undergo a maturation process and acquire fertilizing ability, and are finally stored. The whole process takes from about 8 weeks in mice to 10 weeks in rats and man. Chemicals can affect any one or several stages of spermatogenesis and the effect observed depends on the stages affected. Thus if a substance affected mature sperm only, then exposure would result in immediate infertility which would persist for the duration of the exposure, but fertility would be expected to return within a few days of cessation of exposure. At the other extreme, if a substance prevented division of spermatogonia only, then no effect would be observed for the first 2 months or so after initial exposure while the already divided cells continued their development through the stages of spermatogenesis. A period of infertility would then follow however which would persist for at least a further 10 weeks after cessation of long term exposure, while new sperm were being formed. In practice, division of spermatogonial cells may remain inhibited for many months following exposure to some compounds such as cytotoxic drugs (MacLeod and Gold, 1951) and recovery of fertility may not occur until 2–3 years after cessation of exposure. The most serious effect is seen if there is actual loss of the spermatogonial stem cells. Following dibromochloropropane (DBCP) exposure for example, biopsy examination of the testes of some of the workers revealed absence of stem cells. If such absence is in fact complete, then fertility would never be expected to return.

Some of the exposed workers were still infertile more than 5 years after removal from exposure, so the prognosis must be poor.

The standard drug testing protocols, referred to under Segment 1 studies, involve treatment of male rodents for 60 days prior to mating. This covers the majority of spermatogenesis and in practice is sufficient to detect compounds with antifertility action at any stage of spermatogenesis. For adequate testing of industrial compounds, where long-term low level exposure is more common, more prolonged animal exposure may be necessary to detect cumulative effects at the spermatogonial stage.

MULTIGENERATION STUDIES

The most commonly used protocol for multigeneration studies has been that used by the U.S., F.D.A. for the testing of food additives (Fitzhugh, 1968). Essentially this involves treatment of young males and females for about 2 months. These are then mated and allowed to produce two litters (F1a and F1b). The offspring of the first litter are killed and examined at weaning, but some of the offspring of the second litter are selected to form the parents of the next generation. These selected offspring are reared to maturity and allowed to produce two litters (F2a and F2b), the second of which is reared to produce the third generation (F3a and F3b). At the end of the study, the F3b offspring are killed and subjected to dctailed examination of the tissues, including histology. The basic design is shown below:

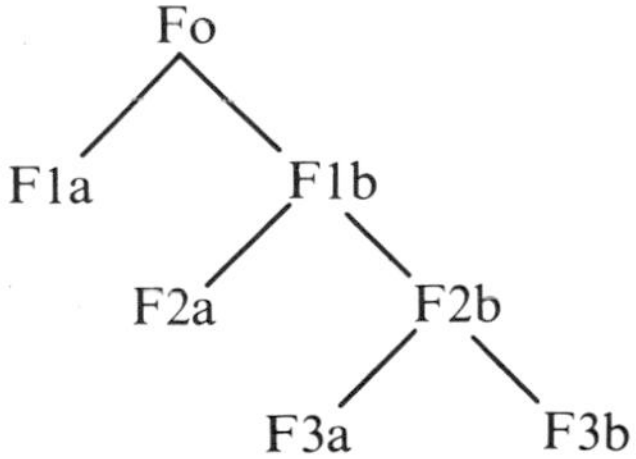

Treatment, usually at 3 dose levels, is normally given in the diet and continues throughout the whole study from the start of the Fo to the killing of the F3b. This type of study will detect chronic effects of substances, usually given at relatively low doses compared with the acute toxic dose. Effects on fertility, pregnancy, parturition, lactation, growth and development may be detected. In particular effects of chemicals on the developing gonads and on fertility of the offspring may be detected. The test is obviously a long and expensive one to perform and may take up to 2 years to complete. There has been considerable debate as to whether such a prolonged study is in fact necessary to detect potential adverse effects of substances and whether effects would in practice be observed at the third generation which would not already be obvious by the second generation (see, F.D.A., 1970). There has been agreement at the Tripartite Meetings of governmental regulatory authorities (i.e. between U.S.A., Canada and the U.K.—Fairweather, personal communication) that instead of the 3 generation 2 litter study described above, a 2 generation 2 litter study should be acceptable. The above designs are regarded as satisfactory for food additives, etc., to which the population at large may be exposed throughout a life-time. Whether such rigorous testing is required for the majority of industrial chemicals is open to question; though it could be of value with industrial compounds causing widespread pollution, such as heavy metals, PCBs, etc. The EEC 6th Amendment on dangerous substances (Council Directive, 1979), lists multigeneration tests (e.g. 3 generation studies) as required at level 2 (i.e. over 1000 tonnes annually or 5000 tonnes total) only if an effect on fertility has previously been seen at level 1.

Several variations have been described of the above protocols in an attempt to reduce the size of the experiments involved. For example, the U.S.A. Environmental Protection Agency has suggested a 2 generation 1 litter test as an alternative. Insufficient work has been done on these tests however to define the most satisfactory design. One advantage of having 2 litters per generation is that in the event of a slight effect being observed, it is easier to determine if this is compound related or whether it is due to some random spontaneous variation. Experience with these multigeneration studies where substances have been given by inhalation, as may be appropriate for industrial chemicals, is seriously lacking.

INTERPRETATION OF ANIMAL EXPERIMENTS AND EXTRAPOLATION TO HUMANS

For those inexperienced in interpreting animal reproductive toxicity data, there are a number of questions of particular interest in relation to industrial chemical exposure, which may or may not be relevant when dealing with drugs, food additives or pesticides. Some of these will be considered briefly.

WHAT TYPES OF REPRODUCTIVE TOXIC HAZARD MAY BE PREDICTED FROM ANIMAL EXPERIMENTS?

It is clear from the review of the animal and human data provided later, that animal models do have good predictive value for man. For example, it can be seen from Table 1 that substances which affect menstrual cycles in women also affect menstrual cycles in monkeys and oestrous cycles in rodents. Since the sex hormones involved in the cycles in all these species are the same, this is not too surprising. However, the higher neuronal control of the cycles does vary very widely between species, for example some species like sheep are only seasonal breeders, and some species like rabbits do not ovulate spontaneously but only after coitus. Thus care must be taken not to imagine that all effects on cyclicity in animals will be reflected by changes in the menstrual cycle in humans.

Effects on fertility in rodents also seem to be a good indicator for effects in humans, and most work on contraceptive agents in man stems from original studies in rodents. In particular, agents causing toxic damage to the testis in animals seem to have a similar effect in humans. The effects of dibromochloropropane were first observed in rodent studies and prognosticated precisely the effects in man (see Table 1).

One of the many complications in the interpretation of the animal data on fertility relates to effects of toxic doses on the sexual behaviour of the animals. There are obvious differences in behaviour between animals and humans and care has to be taken not to misinterpret animal results. It is probable however that substances which specifically depress sexual activity in rodents may well also suppress libido in humans.

The predictive value of animal experiments for effects in pregnancy however is more complex. The physiology of pregnancy in rodents and humans has many important differences. For example, pituitary function is essential for the whole of the first half of pregnancy in rodents, but, once conception has occurred, it is not required for maintenance of pregnancy in humans. Ovarian function is essential for the whole of pregnancy in rodents but only for the first 2–3 months in humans. Thus chemicals given in toxic doses may alter physiological mechanisms in animals so as to cause abortions (or resorptions) but which may have no effect at all in humans. When effects are observed on pregnancy in animals it is sometimes possible by analysis of the mode of action of the substance, to predict whether this would be likely to be hazardous in humans (see Sullivan, 1976).

The prediction of teratogenic effects in humans from animal studies presents special problems, and some of these are dealt with below. Finally, the prediction of transplacental carcinogenicity from animal studies would seem to be as good as prediction of direct carcinogenicity. Most adult animal carcinogens also act as transplacental carcinogens (Tomatis, 1974). The only major difference between rodents and humans seems to be in the stage of fetal development at which sensitivity to transplacental carcinogens develops. This is towards the end of pregnancy in the rat but would probably be earlier in

TABLE 1
Some examples of reproductive toxic effects common to animals and humans

Compound	Effect in animals	Effect in humans
Benzene	Oestrous cycle disturbance—rat	Menstrual disorders (?)
PCB	Prolonged oestrous cycle—rat Prolonged menstrual cycle—monkey	Menstrual disorders (?)
Styrene	Oestrous cycle disturbance—rat	Menstrual disorders (?)
Chlordecone	Testicular atrophy, decreased fertility—mouse, rat, rabbit	Decreased sperm count and motility, abnormal morphology
Chloroprene	Testicular damage, decreased sperm count, dominant lethal mutations—mouse, rat, cat	Decreased libido, impotence, decreased sperm count, motility, abnormal morphology. Increased abortion in wives (?)
DBCP	Testicular atrophy, decreased fertility, dominant lethal mutations—rat, rabbit	Testicular atrophy, decreased sperm count, decreased fertility
Arsenic	Embryolethal, teratogenic—mouse, hamster, rat	Low birth weight, spontaneous abortions (?)
Carbon monoxide	Fetotoxic, low birth weight, poor postnatal development and brain damage—rodent, rabbit, sheep, pig, monkey	Fetotoxic, low birth weight, fetal brain damage
PCB	Low birth weight, high peri- and postnatal mortality, poor postnatal growth, skin discoloration—mouse, rat, rabbit, pig, dog, monkey	Low birth weight, high postnatal mortality, skin discoloration

humans, and seems to relate to the development in the fetus and placenta of the activating enzymes needed to metabolize the chemical into the proximate carcinogen (Sullivan, 1980).

IF A COMPOUND PRODUCES CONGENITAL ABNORMALITIES WHEN GIVEN TO PREGNANT ANIMALS SHOULD IT BE REGARDED AS A POTENTIAL TERATOGEN FOR HUMANS?

There is insufficient data on well established teratogens in man to answer this question with complete certainty. Furthermore, new drugs and other chemicals which are found to be highly teratogenic in animal toxicity studies are not normally administered to humans so that the predictive value of the current animal studies will always be difficult to measure. There is, however, fairly general agreement among teratologists that not every substance which adversely affects pregnancy in animals will also do so in man. For example, aspirin is often used as a positive control teratogen in rodents, yet several large epidemiological studies have failed to demonstrate that it is teratogenic in man. If large doses of chemicals are given to pregnant animals then one or more of the following effects are commonly observed:

i. Embryolethality.
ii. Retardation of ossification and reduced fetal weight.
iii. Increase in congenital anomalies.
iv. Increase in non-specific congenital malformations.
v. Increase in specific congenital malformations.

The significance of each of these will be briefly discussed.

Embryolethality

It is obvious that if sufficiently high doses of chemicals are administered to pregnant animals ultimately either the fetus or the mother will die. If the dam is sufficiently ill following toxic doses of chemicals it is likely that the delicate hormonal balance necessary for the maintenance of pregnancy will be upset resulting in fetal death. Thus if embryolethality occurs at doses which are toxic or near lethal to the dam then this is not regarded as a specific or important fetal effect. However, if embryolethality is observed at doses which are clearly not toxic to the dam, then it would be regarded as a potentially important reproductive toxic effect. Death of the embryo or fetus is usually followed by resorption of the tissues in rats and mice, and either by resorption or abortion in rabbits. Abortion in rats and mice is rare.

Retardation of ossification and reduced fetal weight

These are very commonly observed in teratology studies. If they are only observed at doses which produce some toxicity or stress in the dams, and especially when food and/or water intake is reduced, then they are not normally regarded as specific embryotoxic effects. In the absence of effects on the dam and with normal length of gestation, retarded growth and ossification are regarded as significant. In cases of doubt, observation of the offspring postnatally will show whether catch-up occurs. Failure to thrive postnatally may require crossfostering of offspring to untreated dams to control for lactational defects as well.

Increase in congenital anomalies

Anomalies are usually defined as variations in the skeleton or soft tissues which are relatively uncommon in controls but which do not seem detrimental to the offspring. Examples are extra ribs, or dilated renal pelvis. There is wide variation between workers in the definition of an anomaly as opposed to a malformation, so that no hard and fast rules apply and it is important that all anomalies observed are listed in detail so that the reader can decide on their possible importance. An interesting review of the control incidences of anomalies in various species has been published (Palmer, 1977). There is no agreement among teratologists on the importance of an observed increase in incidence of anomalies following chemical treatment. Some workers feel that this may be an important and sensitive test for teratogens (Berry and Germain, 1975) since many teratogens increase the anomaly incidence. They argue that the chemical may be acting on a polygenic system to cause expression of a latent defect which might otherwise not appear. The majority of workers however feel that small increases in the incidence of anomalies are so commonly observed in teratology experiments, and the variation even between control groups examined in the same laboratory at different times is so large, that these changes are not usually regarded as of toxicological significance in the absence of other effects.

Increase in non-specific congenital malformations

Although there are marked species and strain differences, around 1–2% of all control fetuses may be expected to have serious malformations which would affect the survival of the offspring. It is a common observation that with many chemicals at very high doses, toxic to the dam, there may be a small increase of 2–3 fold in the number of malformed fetuses. If no specific pattern is observed in these malformations, then they may be secondary to the toxic effects on the dam, and most workers do not regard these as of toxicological significance.

Increase in specific congenital malformations
If a chemical induces an increase in the incidence of specific malformations, this may indicate a direct teratogenic effect on the fetus. This is particularly so if the effect observed is rare in controls, and if it is produced at doses well below those toxic to the dam. Such compounds would usually be regarded as potential teratogens for humans, unless investigation of the mode of action of the compound in animals revealed a mechanism which would make such an effect unlikely in the human. For example, in some strains of mice it is very easy to induce cleft palate in a high proportion of the offspring. This may relate to a stress induced increase in adrenocortical hormone release. It is known that mice and rabbits are sensitive to cleft palate induction by corticosteroids but man is not. Therefore the single observation of increase in cleft palate in mice following chemical administration is not necessarily a sign of teratogenic potential. Likewise it is important that certain signs of developmental delay such as dilated cerebral ventricles, enlarged renal pelvis, reduced occipital bones etc. should not be misinterpreted as malformations.

IF A COMPOUND IS TERATOGENIC IN ANIMALS, CAN A "NO EFFECT LEVEL" BE DETERMINED?

Unlike carcinogens for which no threshold is assumed to exist, the majority of teratologists believe that thresholds do exist for teratogens. The concept for teratogens is however more complex than for carcinogens, since not only are single events at the cellular level important, but the actual final production of a congenital abnormality involves the interaction of the genetic background, the presence of the teratogen in relation to the timing of embryological development, the gross morphology of the surrounding tissues as well as the size of the dose of teratogen. The term multifactorial has been used to describe this interaction between genetic and environmental factors in the determination of thresholds for teratogens. This can be illustrated by the action of agents causing cleft palate. Closure of the palate involves a critical balance between the size of the palatal shelves, the distance between them which depends on the width of the head and the time at which the shelves move up into the horizontal plane to fuse. If this balance is upset either by altered tissue growth or delay in movement of the shelves, closure of the palate may never occur. (See Fraser, 1976 for a detailed discussion of some of the threshold concepts in teratology.)

There are several reasons why thresholds are thought to exist for teratogens. It is empirically observed in most animal studies that abnormalities may be observed above a critical dose but not below. There are several theoretical reasons to account for such an effect. At early stages of development the embryonic cells have the ability to reprogramme so that if some cells are destroyed by chemical action, other cells can fulfil their function. There also seems in later stages of development to be considerable redundancy of cells in the developing embryo which are later removed by cell death. It would seem that if some cells are killed by chemical toxicity, these redundant cells can substitute. The embryo also has considerable capacity to repair damage not only at the DNA level, but also by increased rate of cell growth so that quite extreme damage to the embryo may be undetectable by term. Furthermore, some teratogens act indirectly by affecting the mother and not directly on the fetus. In this case, at low doses, the homeostatic mechanisms of the mother may compensate for the effects and so prevent any adverse effect on the fetus.

It thus seems very likely that substances may be teratogenic at high doses but not teratogenic at lower doses. In determination of the "No Effect Level" it is clear that the size of the experimental groups is important. Since it is common to use group sizes of only about 20 animals in teratology experiments, application of some safety factor or alternatively much larger group sizes may be necessary. The intergroup variation between controls in both rats and mice is very large so that several replicates of studies may sometimes be necessary and even then, studies involving 200–300 rats or mice per group may be necessary to detect even a 10% increase in embryolethality (Nelson and Holson, 1978).

IF A COMPOUND IS TERATOGENIC IN SOME SPECIES BUT NOT IN OTHERS, HOW DOES THIS AFFECT HAZARD ASSESSMENT FOR MAN?

The various problems discussed in the interpretation of teratologic experiments apply equally to the comparison of species differences in response to suspected teratogens. If differences are found between species then sometimes it is possible to define the reason for this. For example there may be differences in the toxicokinetics (absorption, distribution, metabolism or excretion rates) which could be of importance. It may be that a teratogenic metabolite can be identified which is produced in some species but not others. There may be differences in protein binding and placental transfer, though the placental barrier does not in practice differ very much between the commonly used species. Where any specific factor can be defined this may indicate whether the affected species are better or worse predictors of hazard for humans.

Several authors have compared the value of different species as predictors of teratogenic hazard for humans. A recent review of the literature by the U.S., F.D.A. (1980) looked at the animal data on 38 compounds (unspecified) for which there are reports of birth defects in humans. All, except one, had a positive study in at least one animal species, with 80% positive in more than one species. Positive responses were observed 85% of the time in the mouse, 80% in the rat, 60% in the rabbit, 45% in the hamster, and 30% in the monkey. Of the less commonly used species on which only a few compounds have been tested, there were nevertheless over 80% positive responses in dogs, pigs, cows and cats. On the other hand, of 165 compounds not known to be teratogens in humans, 28% were negative in all animal species and 50% negative in multiple species, but 41% positive in more than one species. No positive effects were found for these compounds 80% of the time in monkeys, 70% for the rabbit, 50% for the rat and 35% for the mouse and hamster. Thus the predictive power of animal studies for positive teratogens in humans would seem rather better than for non-teratogens. All of the above discussion however is subject to the very important reservation that in general the human data is likely to be even less reliable than the animal data, i.e. very few of the 38 reported positive compounds have been adequately studied to be classed as definite human teratogens and probably even fewer of those "not reported as teratogenic in humans" have been adequately so confirmed by large epidemiological studies. The conclusion of the U.S., F.D.A. is that positive animal studies are at least suggestive of potential human response and that positive results in multiple species may increase their predictive value. No single species can be defined as predicting more accurately than others, and differences between the test species and humans have to be taken into account, where such information exists, in evaluating the relevance of particular tests for humans.

References

Berry, C. L. and Germain, J. P. (1975). Polygenic models in teratological testing. *In* "Teratology—Trends and Applications", pp. 83–102. (Eds. Berry, C. L. and Poswillo, D. E.). Springer-Verlag, Berlin.

Council Directive of EEC. (1979). Sixth amendment to directive 67/548/EEC on the approximation of the laws, regulations and administrative provisions relating to the classification, packaging and labelling of dangerous substances (79/831/EEC). *Official Journal of the European Communities* No. L 259/10–28, 15th October 1979.

Fitzhugh, O. G. (1968). Reproduction tests. *In* "Modern Trends in Toxicology", Volume 1, pp. 75–85. (Eds. Boyland, E. and Goulding, R.). Butterworths, London.

Food and Drug Administration Advisory Committee on Protocols for Safety Evaluations. (1970). Panel on Reproduction Report on Reproduction Studies in the Safety Evaluation of Food Additives and Pesticide Residues. *Toxicology and Applied Pharmacology* **16**, 264–296.

Fraser, F. C. (1976). The multifactorial/threshold concept—uses and misuses. *Teratology* **14** (3), 267–280.

MacLeod, J. and Gold, R. C. (1951). The male factor in fertility and infertility. II. Spermatozoon counts in 1,000 men of known fertility and 1,000 cases of infertile marriage. *Journal of Urology* **66**, 436–449.

Nelson, C. J. and Holson, J. F. (1978). Statistical analysis of teratologic data: problems and advancements. *Journal of Environmental Pathology and Toxicology* **2**, 187–199.

Palmer, A. K. (1977). Incidence of sporadic malformations, anomalies and variations in random bred laboratory animals. *In* "Methods in Prenatal Toxicology", pp. 52–59. (Eds. Neubert, D., Merker, H.-J. and Kwasigroch, T. E.). Georg Thieme Publishers, Stuttgart.

Soyka, L. F. and Joffe, J. M. (1980). Male mediated drug effects on offspring. *In* "Drug and Chemical Risks to the Fetus and Newborn", pp. 49–66. (Eds. Schwartz, R. H. and Yaffe, S. J.). Alan R. Liss, New York.

Sullivan, F. M. (1976). Effects of drugs on fetal development. *In* "Fetal Physiology and Medicine", pp. 43–58. (Eds. Beard, R. W. and Nathanielsz, P. W.). W. B. Saunders, London.

Sullivan, F. M. (1980). Teratogenic and other reproductive toxic aspects of polycyclic aromatic hydrocarbon exposure. *VDI-Berichte* Nr. **358**, 351–356.

Tomatis, L. (1974). Role of prenatal events in determining cancer risks. *In* "Modern Trends in Toxicology", Volume 2, pp. 163–178. (Eds. Boyland, E. and Goulding, R.). Butterworths, London.

U.S. Food and Drug Administration. (1966). Guidelines for reproduction studies for safety evaluation of drugs for human use.

U.S. Food and Drug Administration. (1980). Federal Register **45**, (205), 69823–69824.

Assessment of reproductive effects in humans

MULTIPLE EXPOSURES

A major problem in assessing human evidence on reproductive toxicity is that in cases of occupational exposure or exposure to general environmental pollutants it is often difficult to identify the causal agent since there is usually exposure to a number of different chemicals. Incidents such as that of chlordecone (Kepone) toxicity, where Kepone was the only agent manufactured in the factory concerned, are rare; farm workers, for example, may be exposed to a number of pesticides and herbicides; laboratory and hospital workers to a number of chemicals and perhaps also to radiation; smelter workers to a number of heavy metals, and residential areas with heavy environmental pollution may have clusters of different industries with potentially hazardous emissions.

Multiple exposures pose not only the problem of identifying the toxic chemical responsible but also the problem of interaction between chemicals in expression of toxic effects. Combinations of agents may give rise to entirely new toxic effects not seen with any of the agents alone or may synergise to produce toxicity at much lower levels than would be caused by any agent alone.

EXPOSURE LEVELS

A number of epidemiological surveys where the major chemical exposure(s) have been identified are included in the present review under the appropriate chemical headings, but it is frequently not possible, except by weight of evidence, to attribute the adverse effects observed to the chemical concerned, due to poor control of many other potentially confounding variables (see "Selection of controls"). Other epidemiological studies relate reproductive outcome to occupational groupings for which chemical exposures are not ascertained, or are too numerous to be given, or may not be relevant to the effects observed. These studies have been reviewed separately (see Reproductive hazards associated with different occupational groups, page 32). Even where the predominant chemicals are known, data on exposure levels are frequently lacking or inadequate due to infrequent sampling or too few sampling points within a workplace. The limitations of current monitoring techniques must be taken into account when assessing the reliability of exposure data where given.

SELECTION OF CONTROLS

One of the most problematic areas in epidemiology is selection of appropriate controls. For studies of pregnancy outcome, for example, matching of subjects and controls for age, parity, nutritional and socioeconomic status, smoking and alcohol habits, etc., is crucial. Many studies are inadequately reported in these respects or use clearly inappropriate controls, such as factory workers compared with office workers. At the other end of the spectrum, there are studies where matching of exposed and control groups is very close, but where controls may also be exposed to a potential reproductive hazard, thus masking effects in the exposed group. This might occur in comparisons of arsenic workers with lead worker controls, or plastics workers with rubber worker controls.

BACKGROUND INCIDENCE OF EVENTS

Some types of reproductive disturbance, such as infertility, menstrual disorders and spontaneous abortions, are very common in the population as a whole and little significance can be attached to single case reports or other anecdotal evidence of such occurrences in connection with occupational exposure to chemicals. However, small clusters of such events occurring in one place may draw attention to a potential reproductive hazard. This was the case with dibromochloropropane, where the workers themselves discovered in casual conversation that several of them were infertile. Similarly, Espir *et al.* (1970), reporting 4 cases of impotence in farm workers from a single estate who were exposed to a variety of herbicides and pesticides, noted that isolated cases of impotence are unlikely to arouse suspicion of a toxic cause, and it was only because 3 of the men attended the same general practitioner that any causal connection with occupation was made.

There are also problems in detection where the background incidence of events is very low, if the chemical concerned only has a small effect. For example, to detect a doubling in frequency of a congenital malformation such as anencephaly, with a background spontaneous incidence of one in 1000 live births, a total of 23,000 live births to exposed persons would need to be studied. Even then, there would still be a 5% chance of missing a genuine effect. Clearly, few studies will be of sufficient size to exclude the possibility of such small effects.

RELIABILITY OF ASCERTAINMENT

Some aspects of reproduction cannot be reliably assessed. Examples are early abortion which may pass unnoticed, say as a slightly late, heavy period; libido and potency which may vary widely in subjective assessments or may be subject to bias with prior knowledge of a possible problem in the workforce; and late manifesting congenital abnormalities such as heart defects which are poorly reported. Other aspects of reproductive function, however, can be assessed reliably in careful studies, such as sperm count, menstruation, numbers of live and still births, birth weight, infant survival and malformations.

INTERPRETATION OF FINDINGS

The implications of some findings may be clear. For example, an increased incidence of infertility or congenital malformations in offspring has clear implications for removal of the causal agent(s). However, for other indices, such as reductions in sperm count or motility in the absence of fertility data, menstrual cycle disturbances, or increased frequency of chromosome aberrations in offspring, in the absence of data on the health effects, if any, of such changes, few conclusions may be drawn on whether they pose a reproductive hazard. Further research in this area is needed to follow-up such affected persons and relate these indices to subsequent health and reproductive capacity.

EXPOSURE IN THE BREAST MILK

Exposure of the nursing infant to industrial chemicals in the breast milk may, in some instances, be more hazardous than *in utero* exposure or exposure of adults. Of those compounds so far investigated, almost all foreign compounds that appear in the blood of a lactating woman also appear in the breast milk. Physico-chemical factors which may influence the quantities transferred into breast milk have been reviewed by Giacoia and Catz (1979); they include molecular weight, degree of ionization, pH difference between plasma and milk, relative fat:water solubility, binding to plasma and milk proteins, and blood flow to the mammary glands. Isolated measurements of chemicals in breast milk are of little value except to indicate whether or not the chemical under consideration can pass into the milk. Quantitative determination of exposure of the infant can only be made from serial measurements in breast milk relative to known exposures in the woman, and this has rarely been done for industrial chemicals.

However, some classes of industrial compounds, particularly those which are fat-soluble and water-insoluble, are known to pass into the breast milk in significant quantities. Examples are the organohalides and for some of these, such as polychlorinated or polybrominated biphenyls, which are not broken down and persist in the body for very long periods of time, excretion via the breast milk may be the only major route of elimination from the body. Other industrial chemicals known to be selectively concentrated in the breast milk include pesticides such as chlordecone (Kepone), heptachlor epoxide, mirex, chlordane, aldrin, dieldrin, DDT and its metabolites and the antifungal agent hexachlorobenzene.

For a number of these substances known to be concentrated in the breast milk, the World Health Organisation and the U.S. Food and Drug Administration (FDA) have set regulatory or "allowable" levels for daily intake. However, as can be seen from Table 2 below, nursing infants may actually be exposed to higher levels than these acceptable daily intakes (ADIs).

TABLE 2
Intakes of some organohalides from breast milk (taken from Rogan *et al.*, 1980)

Substance	Typical levels in human breast milk	FDA action level for cows milk[a]	ADI	Daily intake of breast-fed baby[b]
Dieldrin	1–6 ppb	7·5 ppb	0·1 μg kg^{-1}	0·8 μg kg^{-1}
Heptachlor epoxide	8–30 ppb	7·5 ppb	0·5 μg kg^{-1}	4 μg kg^{-1}
PCB	40–100 ppb	62·5 ppb	1·0 μg kg^{-1}	14 μg kg^{-1}
DDT (including metabolites)	50–200 ppb	50·0 ppb	5·0 μg kg^{-1}	28 μg kg^{-1}

[a] Level at which FDA would order removal from market.
[b] Intake for 5 kg baby, 700 ml milk per day, based on high values given.

In the setting of ADIs there is usually a 100 to 1000 times safety margin for adults and so the intake of the nursing infant may not be toxic. However, babies may be more susceptible to toxic effects and poisoning of nursing infants who were not exposed *in utero*, sometimes resulting in death, has been recorded following accidental exposure of lactating women to high concentrations of hexachlorobenzene, polychlorinated biphenyls and organic mercury compounds (see Council on Environmental Quality, 1981, and present review). A single case of obstructive jaundice has also been recorded in an infant exposed to dry-cleaning agent, tetrachloroethylene, in the breast milk (see present review).

In general, there have been very few investigations of the concentrations of industrial chemicals in breast milk of women occupationally exposed, except in the U.S.S.R. where clinics and nurseries attached to large factories enable lactating women to continue working and to be readily accessible for such studies. With the increasing proportion of women returning to the workforce soon after childbirth, more information in this area is urgently required.

References

Council on Environmental Quality, U.S.A. (1981). Chemical Hazards to Reproduction. Prepared by Clement Associates, Inc. Available from Superintendent of Documents, U.S. Government Printing Office, Washington, D.C. 20402.

Espir, M. L., Hall, J. W., Shirreffs, J. G. and Stevens, D. L. (1970). Impotence in farm workers using toxic chemicals. *British Medical Journal* **1**, 423–425.

Giacoia, G. P. and Catz, C. S. (1979). Drugs and pollutants in breast milk. *Clinics in Perinatology* **6** (1), 181–196.

Rogan, W. G., Bagniewska, A. and Damstra, T. (1980). Pollutants in breast milk. *New England Journal of Medicine* **302**, (26), 1450–1453.

Mutagenicity testing*

PREDICTIVE VALUE

Evaluation of the mutagenicity of industrial chemicals may be carried out in a number of different ways involving both *in vitro* and *in vivo* testing in bacterial systems, animals and humans. The value of the short-term *in vitro* tests is that they indicate the potential mutagenicity of a compound, while the mammalian *in vivo* tests can assist in risk evaluation by taking into account absorption, distribution of the parent compound and its metabolites, species differences, etc.

Mutagenicity tests are now widely accepted by regulatory agencies as being of some value for prediction of carcinogenic potential. However, the relationship between mutagenic effects in bacterial or somatic cells and mutagenicity in germ cells is very poorly defined as yet. The majority of animal tests utilize somatic rather than germ cells and in human testing, only somatic cells can be used unless gonadal biopsy is performed. The presence of an additional Y chromosome, indicative of chromosomal non-disjunction, can be detected in mature spermatozoa treated with fluorescent dye (the YFF test). Extra Y chromosomes are indicated by the presence of more than one fluorescent spot in spermatozoa. However, the likelihood of such sperm fertilizing on ovum and resulting in an XYY conceptus is not known. Neither does this method enable any of the other 22 chromosomes in the sperm to be examined. Thus little is known about the mutagenicity of industrial chemicals in germ cells and it is not known whether germ cells are more, or less susceptible to mutagens than somatic cells. However, the fact that in the adult male reproductive system spermatogenesis involves the continual division of cells by mitosis and meiosis, may render the male germ cell more susceptible to mutagens than somatic cells generally. In the female, meiosis and most mitoses of the germ cells occur in fetal life and so the most vulnerable period for mutagenesis is likely to be at this stage rather than in adult life. However, it should also be pointed out that transient exposure to a germ cell mutagen in the adult male, provided the stem cell spermatogonia are not affected, will cause only temporary effects which disappear as new spermatozoa are formed

* Here used in its broadest sense to include clastogenic (chromosome-breaking) effects as well as the narrower definition of mutation as a single gene event.

from unexposed cells, whereas in the female, mutagenic changes in the ova occurring in fetal life will persist into adulthood. The capacity of genetically altered spermatozoa or ova to fertilize or be fertilized may well be reduced but there is sufficient evidence from animal and human data that fertilization can and does occur.

SIGNIFICANCE OF MUTAGENIC CHANGES FOR REPRODUCTION

If spermatozoa or ova with chromosome damage are fertile, or there is direct exposure of the developing embryo and fetus to a mutagen, then a variety of outcomes is possible. Intrauterine death of the embryo or fetus is the most likely outcome for certain types of chromosome abnormalities but structural and functional damage to the offspring compatible with life may also occur. Dead embryos and fetuses are generally aborted (or resorbed in the case of rodents), and live, damaged embryos and fetuses may also be aborted. In humans, about 50% of spontaneous abortuses are found to have chromosomal abnormalities, thus the sensitivity of this measure for detecting industrial mutagens is somewhat diminished unless large surveys are undertaken. Mutations may result in congenital abnormalities recognizable at birth or late manifesting defects or cancer. With selective damage to the germ cells of the embryo and fetus inducing recessive gene mutations, then effects may not become apparent until subsequent generations in the form of infertility, increased intrauterine deaths or malformation of offspring.

IN VITRO TESTING AND METABOLISM

For a number of industrial compounds it is known that it is not the compound itself which is mutagenic, but a reactive intermediate formed from the parent compound after oxidation by mixed function oxidases located in microsomes. Thus, mutagenicity testing of industrial chemicals *in vitro* should include provision for metabolic activation as well as testing of the parent compound. Metabolic studies in mammals, with analysis of distribution and excretion of the parent compound and its metabolites can also be a useful adjunct to prediction and evaluation of mutagenic potential. Methods for testing substances for mutagenic activity *in vitro* and *in vivo* have been described in detail by Kilbey *et al.* (1977) and will not be reviewed here.

HUMAN TESTING

Methods

Systems for assessing the mutagenic potential of industrial chemicals in humans are based on *in vitro* culture of phytohaemagglutinin-stimulated peripheral lymphocytes, cultured fibroblasts derived from various tissues, or, more rarely, bone marrow biopsies. Comparisons may be made between cells from exposed and unexposed workers or healthy cells may be exposed to the test agent *in vitro*. T-lymphocyte cells taken from exposed workers are indicative of damage occurring in the previous year since they are long-lived and rarely undergo mitosis *in vivo*, but will do so when stimulated by phytohaemagglutinin *in vitro*. Bone marrow cells undergo frequent spontaneous divisions and are therefore more indicative of recent damage, though formation of viable abnormal cell clones in the past may also be detected.

Types of abnormality

Classification of groups of chromosome abnormalities into different categories may vary from study to study but the definitions of the individual abnormalities should not. The most frequent abnormality is a chromatid break, defined as a clear discontinuity of the chromatin material in a single chromatid with an obvious non-alignment of the distal fragment. An isochromatid break is a break occurring at the same locus in both chromatids of the chromosome with a distal displacement of the double fragment. Since repair of one of the chromatids in an isochromatid break may occur during incubation where 2 or 3 cell divisions can occur in 72h, chromatid and isochromatid breaks are generally scored together. Chromatid gaps are defined as a discontinuity of the chromatin material without displacement of the distal fragment. Such gaps are often recorded but not generally included in the overall frequency of chromosome abnormalities since their mutagenic significance, if any, is not known. The third class of chromosomal abnormalities is structural rearrangements including dicentric chromosomes, ring chromosomes or translocation figures. The incidence of polyploidy (3 or more sets of the haploid number of chromosomes) may also be assessed.

Translocation figures include exchange of chromatin material between homologous pairs of chromatids and between non-homologous chromosomes, sometimes involving more than two chromosomes. Sister-chromatid exchange (SCE) is employed as a more sensitive indicator of cytogenetic damage. *In vivo*, SCEs only remain in lymphocytes for 1–2 weeks after induction and so fluctuating exposure to mutagens may confound results. *In vitro*, the frequency of SCE may be increased by compounds which do not otherwise cause obvious chromosomal changes, but conversely, not all agents known to induce chromosomal aberrations also increase the frequency of SCE and the predictive value of this test remains to be evaluated.

Acentric fragments, dicentric and ring chromosomes are unstable changes and the cells affected generally die after one or two mitotic divisions. Translocations, deletions and inversions of chromatids are more stable and may persist unless eliminated by the immune system of the body, but they require more sophisticated methods to detect them than do the unstable changes. Thus the most potentially hazardous changes as far as reproduction is concerned, i.e. the stable changes which may persist and be passed on through the germ cells, are the most difficult to detect.

Interpretation of results

The difficulties in interpretation of results from human cell cultures include the known induction of chromatid breaks *in vitro* by non-specific factors such as constituents of the culture medium, pH, temperature changes, stage of the cell cycle and the fixation treatment of the cells. However, there is some evidence that non-specific factors induce randomly distributed abnormalities, whereas specific chemical mutagens induce non-randomly distributed changes (Funes-Cravioto *et al.*, 1974).

Chromosome aberrations also increase with age, recent viral infection, drug and radiation exposure, and may be influenced by smoking, so there must be careful matching of exposed and control subjects, and knowledge of the background "spontaneous" incidence of chromosomal changes in the population under study is advantageous.

References

Funes-Cravioto, F., Yakovienko, K. N., Kuleshov, N. P. and Zhurkov, V. S. (1974). Localization of chemically induced breaks in chromosomes of human leucocytes. *Mutation Research* **23**, 87–105.

Kilbey, B. J., Legator, M., Nichols, W. and Ramel, C. (Eds.). (1977). *In* "Handbook of Mutagenicity Test Procedures". Elsevier Scientific Publishing Co., Amsterdam.

Reproductive hazards associated with different occupational groups

SPONTANEOUS ABORTIONS

Hemminki *et al.* (1980e) have analysed spontaneous abortions from the Hospital Discharge Registry of the National Board of Health, Finland, in relation to women's occupation. Information on a total of 11,731 spontaneous abortions involving hospital treatment in 1973–1975 was available. In broad occupational categories there was a significant increase in risk of spontaneous abortion in agricultural, industrial and construction workers and a significant decrease in risk in book-keeping and office occupations and in service trades (includes housewives). The patients in the Registry were then classified in more detail into about 600 occupations and the frequency of spontaneous abortions analysed in each occupation. The occupations with increased risk of spontaneous abortion are given in Table 3. The same data was also analysed with respect to age and social class (Hemminki *et al.*, 1980d) and both were found to be significant variables. Since, in the analysis by occupation, there was no control for these variables, nor for parity, alcohol or smoking habits, the significant increase in risk of spontaneous abortion found in certain occupational groups (some involving physical stress, some involving chemical exposure) can only be taken as pointers towards possible causal relationships.

In a similar study, Hemminki *et al.* (1980a) have analysed spontaneous abortions in Finnish chemical workers in 1973–1976, linking information on specific occupation from the files of the Union of Chemical Workers with spontaneous abortion records from the Hospital Discharge Registry of the National Board of Health. A total of 52 abortions were recorded among chemical workers giving a significantly increased spontaneous abortion rate (spontaneous abortions/pregnancies × 100) of 8·50% compared with 5·52% for Finnish women as a whole and also significantly higher compared with the rate of 5·8% in industry and construction trades workers. When grouped by 5 year age groups, numbers in each group were small but the risk was most pronounced in the age group 15–19 years. With analysis by branch of employment, again numbers were small, but some types of workers were particularly at risk (see Table 3 for details). This type of analysis cannot distinguish between chemical exposure and other occupationally related

TABLE 3
Finnish studies on women's occupations with a significantly increased risk of spontaneous abortion compared with overall rates

Author(s) and type of study	Occupations
Hemminki *et al.*, 1980e All workers	Machine shop workers; shoe seamstresses and gluers; plastic workers; food processors; weavers; water, gas and sewage plant operators; motor vehicle and tram drivers; radiotherapists; nurses; sports trainers; farmers; gardeners; farm hands; cooks; laundry workers
Hemminki *et al.*, 1980a Chemical workers	Plastic industry; styrene production and use; viscose rayon industry
Hemminki *et al.*, 1980c Metal workers	Radio and television production section of electronics industry

factors, such as nutrition, socio-economic status, etc. However, since the risk of spontaneous abortion was higher for chemical workers than women employed in industry or construction trades it suggests that chemical rather than socioeconomic factors might be causally related to the risk.

In an analysis of spontaneous abortions among women employed in the Finnish metal industry in 1973–1976, Hemminki *et al.* (1980c) linked information from the files of the Union of Metal Workers with records from the Hospital Discharge Registry of the National Board of Health. A total of 195 spontaneous abortions were recorded among metal workers. The overall rate of spontaneous abortions was not significantly increased compared with Finnish women as a whole, but it was significantly increased in the radio and television production section of the electronics industry and further analysis of this sub-group indicated women working in soldering were over-represented. In an age-standardized analysis, the rate of spontaneous abortions was significantly increased after joining the Union of Metal Workers compared with the rate before joining and this was particularly marked in electronics workers. This particular analysis suggests that the increased risk of spontaneous abortion may well be causally related to work factors, as opposed to other, such as social and cultural factors.

Strandberg *et al.* (1978) have reported an increased risk of spontaneous abortion amongst women employed in a Swedish county hospital laboratory who were "exposed" to laboratory work. In the "exposed" group 8/24 pregnancies aborted compared with 9/47 in controls also employed in the laboratory but not doing laboratory work (presumably administrative personnel). However, the crude risk ratio of 1·7 was not particularly high ($p < 0.05$) and the accuracy of the data may be in doubt since it was obtained from the women by questionnaire and covered pregnancies over a large period from 1943–1977.

MALFORMATIONS AND PERINATAL DEATHS

Baltzar *et al.* (1979) have ascertained outcome of pregnancy in a 1% sample (30,048 infants) of all Swedish women employed in hospitals (doctors, nurses, laboratory assistants) in 1973–1975 and who worked during the major part of their pregnancy. Comparison with delivery records of all births in Sweden over the same time period, with data adjusted for maternal age and parity, showed a significant increase in perinatal deaths in 1973 but not in 1974 or 1975. The overall perinatal deaths in 1973–1975 was 412 compared with an expected number of 378 ($p = 0.09$). Malformations, adjusted for distribution between delivery units, were not significantly increased (observed:expected 1551:1491, $p = 0.12$).

Meirik *et al.* (1979) have reported on malformations and perinatal deaths in pregnancies of women working in Uppsala University laboratories in 1972–1977. Data obtained from central registers were corrected for maternal age, parity and distribution between delivery units. Of a total of 322 deliveries identified, 245 had worked in laboratories during the relevant pregnancy and 65 had not. Comparison of perinatal deaths with expected numbers calculated from all deliveries in the delivery units in question showed no increase in either group (working or not working in laboratories). However, there was a significant increase in malformation rate, especially serious malformations, in those working in laboratories during pregnancy (observed:expected 29:17, $p < 0.01$). The authors noted an unusually high incidence of 4 cases of anal or oesophageal atresia or stenosis, the normal frequency of such diagnosis being 1 in 1000 in Sweden.

Erickson *et al.* (1978) have noted an increased frequency of omphalocoele or gastroschisis amongst offspring of women printing workers in a birth defects monitoring programme in the Atlanta area, U.S.A. Occupational data was collected on the parents of 989 babies born with certain congenital malformations. Of these, 4 of the mothers worked in printing and 3 of these gave birth to children with omphalocoele or gastroschisis, while one had multiple anomalies. Printing workers appeared 37 times more frequently in the category of omphalocoele or gastroschisis than in other defect categories.

Hemminki *et al.* (1980b) have analysed associations between maternal and paternal occupation and congenital malformation using the Finnish Register of Congenital Malformations. This is a case-referant register including central nervous system (CNS), oral cleft and musculoskeletal malformations. Referents are the births previous to the cases in the same maternity welfare district, matched for time and place of birth. A total of 3300 pairs collected between 1967 and 1977 were analysed and odds ratios for different occupations calculated. No statistically significant effects were found in relation to paternal occupation, but increased odds ratios were found for some maternal occupations; women working in industrial and construction occupations had more children with CNS and musculoskeletal malformations with odd ratios of 1·57 ($p<0{\cdot}01$) and 1·31 ($p<0{\cdot}05$) respectively, and women in transport and communication occupations had more children with oral clefts with an odds ratio of 1·94 ($p<0{\cdot}05$). When these occupational groups were broken down into more specific occupations, those with increased odds ratios were telephone operators and teachers (oral clefts), and gardeners and women in the food industry and unspecific factory work (musculoskeletal malformations). In a later publication, Hemminki *et al.* (1981) have further analysed the data on women in industry, construction, transport and communication occupations to control for 22 possible confounding factors such as characteristics of the mother and of the child and of the family (maternal age, previous obstetric history, socioeconomic status, smoking, etc.), maternal illness in the first trimester of pregnancy, and maternal medication and X-ray exposure. Several of these variables were found to be significant confounding factors, but after controlling for these factors using multivariate analysis there were still significant associations between CNS malformations and oral clefts and maternal occupation in industry, or construction, transport and communication work (odds ratios 1·98, $p<0{\cdot}001$, and 1·38, $p<0{\cdot}05$ for CNS and oral cleft malformations respectively). This analysis indicates there may be a causal relationship between some occupational factors and congenital malformations.

CANCER IN THE OFFSPRING

Fabia and Thuy (1974) studied the occupation of the father at the time of birth for a series of 386 children who died of malignant disease before 5 years of age in Quebec, Canada, during 1965–1970. Cases were traced from death certificates, hospital insurance data and hospital records, data on fathers' occupation, residence, maternal and paternal age from birth certificates. Controls were children not dying of malignant disease whose birth registration immediately preceded and followed that of each case. Comparison of cases and controls revealed a significant excess of fathers in hydrocarbon-related occupations among cases, with a relative risk of 2·1 ($p<0{\cdot}0001$). Excesses for cases were mainly among motor-vehicle mechanics, machinists, miners and painters. There were no significant differences between cases and controls with regard to geographical distribution of residence, maternal or paternal age.

The results of the above Canadian study prompted a similar investigation in Finland by Hakulinen *et al.* (1976). The series comprised 1409 cases of childhood cancer reported to the Finnish Cancer Registry in 1959–1968, of which information on the fathers' occupation was available for 852 cases. The Registry covers the whole country and is thought to contain all cases diagnosed. Controls were taken as the child whose date of birth immediately preceded that of each case and who was born in the same maternity welfare district, thus cases and controls were matched for age, season of birth and place of residence. Occupation of the father was obtained from antenatal records taken in the first trimester of pregnancy. Relative risk ratios were calculated for 3 different occupational categories of motor-vehicle mechanics, machinists and miners (group I), painters, dyers and printers (group II) and motor-vehicle drivers (group III). Cases diagnosed up to 5 years of age and cases diagnosed up to 15 years of age were analysed separately. No significant increases in risk ratios could be found for any group nor for motor-vehicle mechanics alone (the group characterized by a high risk in all main tumour categories in the Canadian study). However, they were unable to exclude the risk ratio of 2·1, obtained in the Canadian study, for children of groups I and II under 5 years of age (risk ratio 1·10, 95% confidence limits 0·42–2·9).

Zack *et al.* (1980) have carried out a further survey of childhood cancer and paternal occupational exposure to hydrocarbons. A total of 296 cases were selected from children less than 16 years of age with cancer attending the Texas Children's Hospital Research Haematology Clinic in Houston, Texas, U.S.A. in 1976–1977. Controls were 283 children without cancer seen at the clinic during the same interval, siblings of the parents of the case group matched by age and number of children (413 uncles) and 228 neighbourhood adults selected by the parents of the cases from families with children of about the same number and ages as their own. Information on race, sex, age, educational status, marital status, relationship to the child, residence history and job history of the parents was obtained by face-to-face or telephone interviews. No association was found within the specific hydrocarbon-related occupations previously identified in the Canadian study as high-risk (i.e. motor-vehicle mechanics, service station attendants, machinists, miners, painters, dyers and cleaners), nor when a broader definition of hydrocarbon-related occupations was used, nor when divided into petroleum and chemical industries.

One major difference between the positive Canadian study and the negative Finnish and American studies is that in the former study only cases of death from cancer under 5 years of age were used, whereas in the latter studies cases diagnosed or diagnosed and undergoing treatment up to 15 or 16 years of age were used. Thus it is possible that paternal hydrocarbon-related occupations may be associated with early onset, rapidly fatal disease or associated with early death due to lack of medical care rather than overall tumour incidence. Alternatively, if hydrocarbon-related occupations are only associated with certain types of tumours then differences between the studies in percentage distribution of cancer type might explain the differences between them. Finally, the smaller sample size in the American study may not have been large enough to detect an effect the size of that observed in the Canadian study. Thus further studies are needed to clarify this issue.

One further study relevant to hydrocarbon exposure of the father and childhood cancer has been located. Kantor *et al.* (1979) carried out a case-control study of 149 children with Wilms's tumour who were reported to the Connecticut Tumour Registry, U.S.A. between 1935 and 1973. Controls without cancer were selected from the Connecticut State Health Department files of birth certificates and matched with cases for sex, race, and year of birth. Occupations of the fathers at the time of the child's birth were ascertained from birth certificates for cases and controls. For fathers in hydrocarbon-related occupations there was an increased relative risk of 2·4 of having a child with Wilms's tumour and this excess was largely due to occupations where there was exposure to petrol and its combustion products, i.e. driver, motor vehicle mechanic and service station attendant. The relative risk was highest in lead-related occupations (odds ratio 3·7), i.e. driver, motor vehicle mechanic, service station attendant, welder, solderer, metallurgist and scrap metal worker. Wilms's tumour was chosen since it is usually diagnosed before 4 years of age and thus factors operating around the time of conception, pregnancy and birth may be important in its aetiology. In the studies reviewed above there were insufficient cases of Wilms's tumour for separate analysis.

Hemminki *et al.* (1980e) have analysed data on parental occupation and childhood cancer for cases on the Finnish Cancer Registry, which covers all cases diagnosed before 15 years of age, between 1959 and 1975. Information was available on the mother's occupation for 1592 cases and 2234 controls (children not having cancer born immediately before or after the cases, from the same maternity welfare district). A significantly increased risk was observed of 1·20 ($p<0{\cdot}05$) for women living on farms (e.g. farmers' wives, not agricultural workers themselves) and of 2·39 ($p<0{\cdot}05$) for women in the food industry, shown to be due mainly to bakers who had a relative risk of 2·62 ($p<0{\cdot}05$). Information was available on the fathers' occupation for 1558 cases and 2163 controls. A significantly increased risk of 1·26 ($p<0{\cdot}05$) was found for men in agriculture and forestry, due mainly to farmers who had a relative risk of 1·27 ($p<0{\cdot}05$), and of 1·25 ($p<0{\cdot}05$) for motor vehicle drivers.

GENE MUTATIONS IN OFFSPRING

Funes-Cravioto *et al.* (1977) have studied the incidence of chromosome aberrations in cultured lymphocytes from children of female laboratory workers who had worked during the relevant pregnancy. When compared with control children, an increase in chromatid and isochromatid breaks was found in 14 children aged 4–11 years of 11 women laboratory workers and an increased incidence of sister-chromatid exchange was found in 4 children of 2 of the women workers. The women were exposed to one or more of chloroform, toluene, benzene, cyclohexane, diethyl ether, isooctane, methanol, or xylene, and they too showed increased incidence of chromosome aberrations and sister-chromatid exchange, in comparison with controls. This study suggests genetic changes may be passed on to the offspring but further studies are required to confirm this possibility.

References

Baltzar, B., Ericson, E. and Kallen, B. (1979). Pregnancy outcome among women working in Swedish hospitals. *New England Journal of Medicine* **300** (11), 627–628.

Erickson, J. D., Cochran, W. M. and Anderson, C. E. (1978). Birth defects and printing. *Lancet* **i**, 385.

Fabia, J. and Thuy, T. D. (1974). Occupation of father at time of birth of children dying of malignant diseases. *British Journal of Preventive and Social Medicine* **28**, 98–100.

Funes-Cravioto, F., Kolmodin-Hedman, B., Lindsten, J., Nordenskjöld, M., Zapata-Gayon, C., Lambert, B., Norberg, E., Olin, R. and Swensson, Å. (1977). Chromosome aberrations and sister-chromatid exchange in workers in chemical laboratories and a rotoprinting factory and in children of women laboratory workers. *Lancet* **ii**, 322–325.

Hakulinen, T., Salonen, T. and Teppo, L. (1976). Cancer in the offspring of fathers in hydro-carbon-related occupations. *British Journal of Preventative and Social Medicine* **30**, 138–140.

Hemminki, K., Franssila, E. and Vainio, H. (1980a). Spontaneous abortions among female chemical workers in Finland. *International Archives of Occupational and Environmental Health* **45**, 123–126.

Hemminki, K., Mutanen, P., Luoma, K. and Saloniemi, I. (1980b). Congenital malformations by the parental occupation in Finland. *International Archives of Occupational and Environmental Health* **46**, (2), 93–98.

Hemminki, K., Niemi, M.-L., Koskinen, K. and Vainio, H. (1980c). Spontaneous abortions among women employed in the metal industry in Finland. *International Archives of Occupational and Environmental Health* **47**, 53–60.

Hemminki, K., Niemi, M.-L., Saloniemi, I., Vainio, H. and Hemminki, E. (1980d). Spontaneous abortions by occupation and social class in Finland. *International Journal of Epidemiology* **9**, (2), 149–153.

Hemminki, K., Saloniemi, I., Luoma, K., Salonen, T., Partanen, T., Vainio, H. and Hemminki, E. (1980e). Transplacental carcinogens and mutagens: childhood cancer, malformations and abortions as risk indicators. *Journal of Toxicology and Environmental Health* **6**, (5–6), 1115–1127.

Hemminki, K., Mutanen, P., Saloniemi, I. and Luoma, K. (1981). Congenital malformations and maternal occupation in Finland: multivariate analysis. *Journal of Epidemiology and Community Health* **35**, (1), 5–10.

Kantor, A. F., McCrea Curnen, M. G., Meigs, J. W. and Flannery, J. T. (1979). Occupations of fathers of patients with Wilms's tumour. *Journal of Epidemiology and Community Health* **33**, 253–256.

Meirik, O., Kallen, B., Gauffin, U. and Ericson, A. (1979). Major malformations in infants born of women who worked in laboratories while pregnant. *Lancet* **ii**, 91.

Strandberg, M., Sandback, K., Axelson, O. and Sundell, L. (1978). Spontaneous abortions among women in hospital laboratory. *Lancet* **i**, 384–385.

Zack, M., Cannon, S., Loyd, D., Heath, C. W., Falletta, J. M., Jones, B., Housworth, J. and Crowley, S. (1980). Cancer in children of parents exposed to hydrocarbon-related industries and occupations. *American Journal of Epidemiology* **111**, (3), 329–336.

Conclusion

It is clear, from both experiments in animals and epidemiological studies in humans that industrial chemicals do have the potential to cause reproductive toxicity, affecting all possible aspects. There are undoubtedly problems in detecting such effects both from the wide baseline variability in such aspects as libido, potency and menstrual cycle disorders, and also from the technical difficulty of assessing infertility and detecting early abortions. However these problems should not deter investigators from attempting to carry out studies on exposed groups of workers. Certain parameters can be measured reliably provided that a reasonable degree of cooperation is received. For example records of menstruation, and semen examination for sperm counts, morphology and motility have been successfully used. Hormone levels in blood can be measured, records of live births, still births, birth weight, infant survival and congenital malformations are available. One of the major problems in conducting such studies is the choice of a satisfactory control group and baseline data on all of these aspects in the normal healthy working population are lacking. In the review of compounds which follows, a wide range of effects on exposed workers have been reported and although very few of these reports can withstand critical assessment by present day standards of epidemiology, nevertheless they do indicate the need for confirmation or denial by further work. Examples of these effects and some of the chemical substances implicated, although often at generally toxic doses are given below. In very few of these examples is a causal relationship firmly established.

EFFECTS REPORTED IN MALE WORKERS

Decreased libido and impotence
Chloroprene, manganese, organic lead, inorganic mercury, toluene diisocyanate, vinyl chloride.

Testicular damage or infertility
Chlordecone (Kepone), chloroprene, dibromochloropropane, organic lead.

EFFECTS REPORTED IN FEMALE WORKERS

Menstrual and other gynaecological disorders
Aniline, benzene, chloroprene, formaldehyde, inorganic mercury, polychlorinated biphenyls (PCB), styrene, toluene.

Abortions or infertility
Anaesthetic gases, aniline, arsenic, benzene, ethylene oxide, formaldehyde, lead.

Decreased fetal growth, low birth weight or poor survival
Carbon monoxide, formaldehyde, PCB, toluene, vinyl chloride.

Teratogenic effects
Organic mercury

Maternal death related to pregnancy
Beryllium, benzene.

EFFECTS REPORTED IN ANIMAL STUDIES BUT WITH NO HUMAN EVIDENCE

The following review also shows that a number of chemicals have produced reproductive toxic effects in animals, usually only in rodents but sometimes in other species too. Where these occurred only at high toxic doses they may be of no significance at all as indicators of hazard to humans. However, for many of the substances, marked species differences have been shown to exist and for none of them is there any adequate human evidence to allow risk assessment. Examples of such effects and the chemicals implicated are:

Testicular damage or reduced male fertility
Benzene, benzo(a)pyrene, boron, cadmium, epichlorohydrin, ethylene dibromide, polybrominated biphenyl (PBB).

Fetotoxic or embryolethal effects
Chloroform, dichloromethane, ethylene dichloride, ethylene oxide, inorganic mercury, nitrogen dioxide, PBB, selenium, tetrachloroethylene, thallium, trichloroethylene, vinylidine chloride, xylene.

Teratogenic effects
Arsenic, benzo(a)pyrene, chlorodifluoromethane, chloroprene, monomethyl formamide, acrylonitrile, methyl ethyl ketone, tellurium, vinyl chloride.

Transplacental carcinogenesis
Arsenic, benzo(a)pyrene, vinyl chloride.

Finally, for about 6% of the chemicals reviewed, viz., o-dichlorobenzene, dioxane and o-toluidine, no reproductive toxicity data were available in either animals or humans. It is very likely considering the method of choice of compounds for review (see Preface), that the proportion of totally uninvestigated compounds is much greater than 6% and of course the majority of chemical substances do not even have TLV values allocated. With the introduction virtually world-wide of legislation on toxicity testing of industrial chemicals, like the EEC 6th Amendment and Toxic Substances Control Act in the U.S.A., it is hoped that this gap in our knowledge will gradually be filled.

PART 2
Review of compounds

Background to the review of compounds

THE LITERATURE SEARCH

A number of computer-based data retrieval systems are available for location of literature on occupational and industrial hazards and environmental pollution. These include Toxline, Medline, Excerpta Medica, Biosis, CACon/CASIA and the Congressional Information Service. For the present review we initially compared retrieval rates on Medline and Toxline for 11 specific industrial chemicals using keywords relevant to reproduction in male and female animals and humans (see Table 4 below).

TABLE 4
Comparison of Toxline versus Medline for retrieval of relevant papers

Chemical	Toxline		Medline		Medline relevant
	Retrieved	Relevant	Retrieved	Relevant	Toxline Missed
Acrylonitrile	48	12	2	2	0
Aniline	388	39	13	6	5
Beryllium	95	22	13	4	0
Carbon monoxide	624	93	403	52	5
Chlorodifluoromethane	56	8	14	0	0
Nitrogen dioxide	276	14	28	4	2
Ozone	264	24	42	10	1
Styrene	256	50	81	20	2
Vinyl chloride	347	52	56	20	0
Vinylidene chloride	88	15	2	2	0
Xylene	126	14	7	5	1

As can be seen from Table 4, many more relevant papers emerged from Toxline than Medline, though a greater proportion of total references retrieved on Toxline were not relevant. Overall on Toxline, the proportion of relevant references ranged from 0·8–45% of references retrieved (average 15%). Retrieval of relevant references was poorest where the compound also had medical as well as industrial uses (e.g. chloroform, ethylene oxide, formaldehyde, trichloroethylene). For example, because "sterility/steril" was used as a keyword, the use of ethylene oxide as a sterilizing agent for equipment resulted in a large number of irrelevant retrievals. It can also be seen from Table 4 that, with the exception of aniline and carbon monoxide, none or only a very few of the relevant references picked up by Medline were missed by Toxline. Slightly more were missed by Toxline in the case of aniline because it is used as an investigative tool for liver function and thus appears frequently in the medical literature, and in the case of carbon monoxide, more references to smoking in pregnancy were retrieved from Medline, some of which were relevant to the review. Thus for the majority of industrial chemicals the Toxline data bases provide more satisfactory retrieval of relevant material, albeit at the expense of also including more redundant material than does Medline. However, where it is known that a chemical may also have medical implications (other than toxicity) or is a general environmental pollutant, then a Medline search may provide additional useful material. In the present review of 48 industrial chemicals, entities or related groups of compounds, 15 were searched on both Toxline and Medline and 33 on Toxline alone. All compounds were also hand searched using Teratology Lookout up to the end of 1980.

Copies of relevant papers were obtained and relevant citations quoted in these papers were also obtained. Review articles, monographs and books were also scanned. Towards the end of this process, it was rare to come across entirely new material and so it is hoped that this review is relatively comprehensive. Toxline searches contained material published up to early 1980 and important papers containing relevant new material which have come to our notice subsequently have been added up to the end of 1980. All foreign language papers without English abstracts and the majority of those with English abstracts were fully translated by the Translation Service of the Health and Safety Executive. In some cases translations were already available through the U.S. National Translations Center. Occasionally, where the English abstract only has been used this is stated in the text.

We also wrote to companies in the U.K. and U.S.A. involved in the manufacture of some of the compounds to ask if they had any animal or human toxicology data pertinent to our review. With one or two exceptions, the response was disappointing. None offered human data other than that already published, and presumably, in most instances, no attempt has been made to collect such data.

Some companies have published animal reproductive toxicity data in the scientific literature, most notably Dow Chemical Company, U.S.A., but in general it is rare for such information to be available. Unpublished information was made available to us from Haskell Laboratory, Du Pont,

U.S.A., B.P. Ltd., U.K. and one industry consortium, the Chemical Manufacturers Association (formerly Manufacturing Chemists Association), U.S.A. Responses from other companies ranged from no reply, replies to the effect that no studies had been carried out (most frequent response), or replies that relevant studies had been carried out but that the information could not be released.

CRITERIA FOR ACCEPTABLE METHODOLOGY IN ANIMAL STUDIES

In reviewing the teratology testing of industrial chemicals certain methodological criteria were applied to each study. If these were met then the study has been stated to be acceptable in the text. Studies with unacceptable methodology have also been reviewed but unsatisfactory aspects are pointed out in the text. Criteria for acceptability were as follows:

1. Species used stated.
2. Precise dating of the first day of pregnancy.*
3. Treatment period (not necessarily the whole of embryogenesis) stated.*
4. Precise information on dosage, route of administration and, for inhalational studies, daily duration of exposure given.
5. Numbers of animals per treatment group stated and preferably 10 or more dams per group.
6. Appropriate control group(s) (untreated, vehicle-treated, pair-fed, air-exposed in similar chambers for inhalational studies, etc.) run concurrently.
7. Maternal body weight monitored and toxic effects on the dams recorded.
8. Fetuses all removed by Caesarian section on the same day of pregnancy.
9. Embryonic and fetal resorption sites counted.
10. Corpora lutea counted if treatment began before implantation to estimate pre-implantation losses. (Note, these counts cannot be accurately done in the mouse.)
11. Fetuses weighed.
12. Gross external examination of all fetuses.
13. Some fetuses, usually $\frac{1}{3}$–$\frac{1}{2}$, examined internally for soft tissue defects by dissection or by the Wilson slicing technique.
14. Remaining fetuses examined for skeletal defects after Alizarin staining or by X-ray (suitable only for larger fetuses such as the rabbit).

* In the review, treatment periods given are exactly as stated by the authors, so will vary, depending on whether the first day of pregnancy is designated day 0 or day 1.

15. All defects including skeletal and soft tissue anomalies or variants, recorded, as well as major congenital malformations.
16. Results presented so that numbers of affected fetuses can be ascertained and preferably also the numbers of affected litters.
17. It should be clear whether in statistical analysis, n = number of dams or number of fetuses in any treatment group. (For discussion of relative advantages and disadvantages of these different approaches see Teratology **9**, 257–262 and **10**, 301–302, 1974).

Whilst the majority of studies met most of these criteria, it was not always possible to ascertain whether this was the case, due to inadequate presentation of methodological details. This applied particularly to studies appearing in abstract only and to the Russian literature. Many Russian teratology studies follow guidelines published by the Institute of Hygiene and Occupational Disease, Academy of Medical Science, U.S.S.R. entitled "Methods for experimental research to establish the action thresholds of industrial toxins for the generative (reproductive) function, Moscow, 1969" by I. V. Sanotsky, V. N. Fomenko, L. S. Salnikova *et al.* It has not been possible to obtain a copy of these guidelines. It should also be noted that Russian authors may offer interpretations of their data which are not acceptable to other teratologists; all statistically significant results ($p < 0{\cdot}05$) are often accorded equal importance, despite wide variability between control groups and/or absence of dose-response relationship. The lowest level producing a statistically significant effect is often used in estimating the no-effect level, sometimes despite evidence from the same experiment that several higher dose level groups were without effect. In our evaluation of the data we have given emphasis to biological as well as statistical significance for estimation of no-effect levels, taking into account such factors as methodological acceptability, control variability, dose-response relationships, maternal toxicity, severity of the effects and replication in different studies. Nevertheless, we feel it is important that the Russian literature is not ignored since on occasions it is the only source of information on the reproductive toxicity of particular industrial chemicals. Furthermore, in animal studies, Russian workers may run more comprehensive investigations of maternal toxicity, which has provided much of the information available to date on the effects of industrial chemicals on the pregnant animal itself (as opposed to the fetus) and offering more insight into the way in which functional changes in the mother may indirectly affect the embryo and fetus.

Generally only data from experiments in mammalian species have been included in the review. For teratogenic screening we do not regard the chick embryo as a relevant model since it is unusually susceptible to physical or chemical disturbances and it lacks the maternal and placental factors which are often important determinants of embryonic and fetal disorders. However, on occasions, toxic effects on avian species have been included, for example in the review of chlordecone, where effects on sex hormones pertinent to mammalian reproduction have been recorded.

MUTAGENICITY

Mutagenicity studies have not been reviewed comprehensively unless these involved mammalian studies on reproductive function such as dominant lethal tests, or have involved studies on people occupationally exposed. In general, other information has been taken from the IARC monographs.

CARCINOGENICITY

All data on carcinogenicity, except for transplacental carcinogenicity, has been taken directly from the IARC monograph summaries where available, and the information given is that of the IARC.

Bibliography and further reading

Hunt, V. R. (1975). Occupational health problems of pregnant women: a report and recommendations for the Office of the Secretary, (Order No. SA-5304–75). Department of Health, Education and Welfare, U.S.A.

Hricko, A. and Brunt, M. (1976). Working for your life: a woman's guide to job health hazards. Labour Occupational Health Program and Public Citizen's Health Research Group, U.S.A.

Bingham, E. (Ed.). (1977). Women and the workplace: Proceedings of a conference, June 17–19, 1976 Washington, D.C., U.S.A. Society for Occupational and Environmental Health.

George, A. (1976). Health risks for women at work—a review. Advisory Council on the Status of Women, Ottawa, Canada.

Hunt, V. R. (1977). The health of women at work—a bibliography. Occasional Papers No. 2, Program on Women, Northwestern University, Illinois, U.S.A.

American College of Obstetricians and Gynecologists (1978). Comprehensive bibliography on pregnancy and work. U.S. Department of Health, Education and Welfare, NIOSH, Maryland, U.S.A.

Strobino, B., Kline, J. and Stein, Z. (1978). Chemical and physical exposures of parents: effects on human reproduction and offspring. *Journal of early human development* **1** (4), 371–399.

Sullivan, F. M. and Barlow, S. M. (1979). Congenital malformations and other reproductive hazards from environmental chemicals. *Proceedings of the Royal Society B*, **205**, 91–110.

Hunt, V. R. (1979). Work and the health of women. CRC Press, Inc. Florida, U.S.A.

Neubert, D., Bass, R., Bedürftig, A. and Kreft, R. (1979). Evaluation of the teratogenic activity of various agents to which human beings are frequently exposed. Commission of the European Communities.

Council on Environmental Quality (1981). Chemical hazards to human reproduction. U.S. Government Printing Office, Washington, D.C., U.S.A.

1. Acrylonitrile

TECHNICAL DATA

Formula	$CH_2{=}CHCN$
CAS registry number	107–13–1
Chemical abstracts name	2-propenenitrile
Synonyms	AN; cyanoethylene; propenenitrile; VCN; vinyl cyanide.
Uses	Manufacture of acrylic fibres; in the plastics, surface coatings and adhesives industries; intermediate in the synthesis of antioxidants, pharmaceuticals, dyes, surface-active agents, etc., in organic synthesis to introduce a cyanoethyl group; modifier for natural polymers; pesticide fumigant for stored grain.
TLV	2 ppm

ANIMAL STUDIES

A. RELEVANT PHARMACOLOGY AND TOXICOLOGY

No relevant data found.

B. ENDOCRINE AND GONADAL EFFECTS

No relevant data found.

C. FERTILITY

No relevant data found.

D. PREGNANCY

The effects of acrylonitrile given orally or by inhalation have been examined in a large, well-conducted study in rats by Murray *et al.* (1978). Groups of 29–43 animals were given 0, 10, 25 or 65 mg/kg/day orally by gavage, or exposed to 0, 40 or 80 ppm acrylonitrile by inhalation for 6 h/day, on days 6–15 of pregnancy. Significant maternal toxicity was seen in the 65 mg/kg, 40 and 80 ppm groups, with reduced weight gain during the dosing period and, in the 65 mg/kg group, increased liver weight at term. In the 65 mg/kg group, complete resorption of some litters shortly after implantation, significant reductions in fetal body weight and crown-rump length, a significant increase in minor skeletal variants (delayed ossification, split sternebrae) and a significant increase in total malformations were seen. In particular, the incidence of short tail, associated in some fetuses with short trunk, missing vertebrae and anteriorly displaced ovaries, was significantly increased to 4% compared with 0·2% in controls. At 25 mg/kg and 80 ppm a lower, but non-significant, incidence of the same malformation was noted (0·6% and 0·5% respectively). No other adverse effects were seen in any of the treatment groups.

In this large study, significant embryonic and fetal toxicity and teratogenicity were observed only in the group given 65 mg/kg/day orally where maternal toxicity was also evident. However, the authors comment that it is unlikely that the malformations can be attributed to maternal toxicity alone since there was no apparent correlation between the degree of toxicity seen in the individual dams and the occurrence of malformations in their offspring. Furthermore, the specific malformation of short tail etc. has not increased in other studies in their laboratory where the dams have been stressed to an even greater degree.

Conclusion

From this one study, it may be tentatively concluded that 10 mg/kg/day orally and 40 ppm by inhalation are without effect and that doses above these may be both embryotoxic and teratogenic. However, further studies are required to confirm these data.

E. MUTAGENICITY

Acrylonitrile is mutagenic in the Ames test with metabolic activation, but not without activation (Milvy and Wolff, 1977; Venitt, 1978; De Meester *et al.*, 1978). No other relevant mutagenicity studies have been found.

F. CARCINOGENICITY

IARC Monograph Vol. 19 (1979) summarized studies in the rat showing acrylonitrile is carcinogenic in the rat after oral or inhalational administration. It should therefore be considered as a potential transplacental carcinogen, but there are no studies on this aspect of toxicity.

HUMAN STUDIES

A. RELEVANT PHARMACOLOGY AND TOXICOLOGY

No relevant data found.

B. ENDOCRINE AND GONADAL EFFECTS

No relevant data found.

C. FERTILITY

No relevant data found.

D. PREGNANCY

No relevant data found.

E. MUTAGENICITY

Thiess and Fleig (1978) examined lymphocyte cultures from 18 male workers, aged 37–59 years, who had been exposed to acrylonitrile for an average of 15·4 years (range 12–21 years). Prior to 1963 the environmental exposure levels were unknown. Between 1963–1974 the exposure level was reported to be about 5 ppm on average with occasional higher levels. From 1975–1977 the monthly average monitored level was 1·5 ppm, but occasional levels were higher than this. They examined 100 lymphocytes in metaphase from each subject and compared with results with those from 18 unexposed workers, age-matched as controls. No difference was found in the number of chromosomal aberrations, including or excluding gaps. The percentage of cells with chromosomal aberrations, excluding gaps, was 1·8 ± 1·3 compared with 2·0 ± 1·6 in exposed and controls respectively. Including gaps and isogaps the respective percentages were 5·5 ± 2·5 and 5·1 ± 2·4.

Although no effect was found in this study the authors refer to a Du Pont, U.S.A. preliminary report which found an increased incidence of cancer among workers exposed to acrylonitrile at a Du Pont textile fibres plant.

F. CARCINOGENICITY

IARC Monograph Vol. 19 (1979) reported on one epidemiological study of workers occupationally exposed to acrylonitrile in one U.S. textile fibre plant, which showed an increased risk of cancer morbidity and mortality of the lung and large intestine.

SUMMARY AND EVALUATION

EXPERIMENTAL STUDIES

No studies on fertility, endocrine or gonadal effects were found.

There is evidence from one study in rats that it was embryotoxic and teratogenic at 65 mg/kg orally, a dose which also produced maternal toxicity. Non-significant increases in the same type of malformation were observed at 25 mg/kg orally and 80 ppm by inhalation. No adverse effects were observed at 10 mg/kg orally or 40 ppm by inhalation.

It is mutagenic in bacterial systems with activation.

It is carcinogenic in rats but no data are available on transplacental carcinogenicity.

HUMAN STUDIES

No studies were found on endocrine or gonadal effects, or of effects on fertility or pregnancy. One study on lymphocytes from exposed workers showed no mutagenic effects. There is one study suggesting a carcinogenic risk in exposed workers.

EVALUATION

There is limited evidence that acrylonitrile is embryotoxic and teratogenic in the rat at maternally toxic doses.

In view of the limited animal data and the absence of any human reproductive data no evaluation can be made.

References

De Meester, C., Poncelet, F., Roberfroid, M. and Mercier, M. (1978). Mutagenic activity of acrylonitrile. A preliminary study. *Archives Internationales de physiologie et de Biochemie* **86**, (2), 418–419.

IARC Monographs on the Evaluation of the Carcinogenic Risk of Chemicals to Humans: Some monomers, plastics and synthetic elastomers, and acrolein (1979). Volume 19. Lyon, France.

Milvy, P. and Wolff, M. (1977). Mutagenic studies with acrylonitrile. *Mutation Research* **18**, (3/4), 271–278.

Murray, F. J., Schwetz, B. A., Nitschke, K. D., John, J. A., Norris, J. M. and Gehring, P. J. (1978). Teratogenicity of acrylonitrile given to rats by gavage or inhalation. *Food and Cosmetic Toxicology* **16**, (6), 547–551.

Thiess, A. M. and Fleig, I. (1978). Analysis of chromosomes of workers exposed to acrylonitrile. *Archives of Toxicology* **41**, 149–152.

Venitt, S. (1978). Letter to the editor. *Mutation Research* **57**, (1), 107–113.

2. Aniline

TECHNICAL DATA

Formula	(benzene ring with NH_2)
CAS registry number	62–53–3
Chemical abstracts name	Benzenamine
Synonyms	Aminobenzene, aminophen, aniline oil, benzenamine, blue oil.
Uses	Manufactured dyes, medicinals, resins, varnishes, perfumes, shoe blacks; vulcanizing rubber; as solvent. Hydrochloride used in manufacture of intermediates, aniline black and other dyes, in dyeing fabrics or wood black.
TLV	2 ppm (skin)

ANIMAL STUDIES

A. RELEVANT PHARMACOLOGY AND TOXICOLOGY

Sex differences in the hepatic metabolism of aniline by aniline hydroxylase using *in vitro* preparations of liver microsomes have been investigated in rats (reviewed by Pence and Schneil, 1979). Some have found no differences, while others have reported decreased metabolism in female rats of certain strains. The hormonal basis for these differences is indicated by experiments showing hepatic aniline hydroxylase activity may be decreased in male rats by lowering androgen levels or treating with 17β-oestradiol, and increased in females by treating with testosterone.

In vitro experiments by Feuer and Kardish (1975) and Gut *et al.* (1976) have shown a further decrease in hepatic aniline hydroxylase activity in pregnant rats in comparison with non-pregnant females, dependent on the level of progesterone metabolites. However, such experiments take no account of possible placental metabolism nor of increases in total liver weight during pregnancy, and *in vivo* experiments have shown no significant changes in the rate of aniline metabolism in the pregnant rat compared with the non-pregnant rat (Gut *et al.*, 1976).

Placental transfer of aniline has been studied in late pregnancy in rats by Maickel and Snodgrass (1973). It is highly lipid soluble and readily crosses into the fetus, reaching fetal:maternal plasma ratios of >1 within 1 h of s.c. injection into the dam. Tissue ratios are <1, and the half-life of around 1·5 h is similar in maternal and fetal blood.

B. ENDOCRINE AND GONADAL EFFECTS

No relevant data found.

C. FERTILITY

No relevant data found.

D. PREGNANCY

No relevant data found.

E. MUTAGENICITY

Garner and Nutman (1977) have shown aniline and p-hydroxyaniline to be negative in Ames tests, with and without metabolic activation. Two studies found negative results with aniline in Chinese hamster cells *in vitro* as assessed by chromosome breaks (Ishidate and Odashima, 1977; Abe and Sasaki, 1977) but a positive result was obtained in one of these studies (Abe and Sasaki, 1977) when assessed by sister-chromatid exchange counts. The authors were very cautious about the interpretation of this and felt it required confirmation.

F. CARCINOGENICITY

IARC Monograph Vol. 4 (1974) stated that at that time there was no adequate data to indicate that aniline is carcinogenic in animals.

HUMAN STUDIES

A. RELEVANT PHARMACOLOGY AND TOXICOLOGY

No relevant data found.

B. ENDOCRINE AND GONADAL EFFECTS

Podluzhnyi (1979) states that the proportion of women employed in factories in the aniline dye industry in W. Urals, U.S.S.R., is 49–59% of the total workforce. A team consisting of a gynaecologist, therapist, neuropathologist, dermatologist and a hygienist conducted examinations and interviews on 1264 women, i.e. 84·5% of the total number of women employed in the main and auxiliary workshops. Of these, 82% worked in organics production (organic dyes, intermediates, aniline and its derivatives, etc.). A multiple cohort selection system was used taking account of age (25–39 years), married state, length of time employed in the given capacity (not <5 years), production process (organic, non-organic, auxiliary, i.e. servicing, transport, packaging, heating, etc.). The control group consisted of workers in the factory management departments, housing and community departments, creches and playground staff, who had never worked in chemical production. There was an overall relationship between total amount of illness and type of work performed—highest in women in main workshops and lowest in those in management and similar positions. The 5 main causes of incapacity for work were diseases of the respiratory, digestive, cardiovascular and skeletomuscular systems and urogenital organs. Detailed analyses (not given) showed that the sickness patterns related to the type and nature of the work performed. A major factor reviewed in the paper related to the nutrition of the women and a direct relationship between nutrition and malfunction or diseases of the sex organs was found. Women who had a well-balanced diet and with regular meals 3–4 times per day had significantly less disturbances of the menstrual cycle, abortions and inflammatory disease of the sex organs than those who did not. There were no differences in pre-cancerous changes in the uterus or malposition of the uterus. The incidence of gynaecological disease was highest in women who had both poor nutrition *and* who worked in certain specific jobs. The highest incidences were among women working on production of organic dyes and intermediates, employed as machine operators, packers, chemical equipment repairers and laboratory workers. The commonest disorder reported was disturbance of menstrual and ovarian function in 48% of women in organic production compared with the overall factory incidence of 26% and only 3% of controls. The incidence of gynaecological problems was further analysed for women in the organic dye production area (the highest incidence area) with regard to nutrition, level of education, material and housing conditions, exact occupation and length of work service. Important factors were precise occupation, length of time employed and nutrition.

Problems in the interpretation of this paper are that few technical details are given. No indication is given of the number of women in each group other than that, of the 1264 women examined, 81·9% (1035) were employed in organic production, so that the numbers in the other groups must have been much fewer. No indication is given of the size of the control group or of the variability of response in the various groups. No description is given of the details of the gynaecological disorders, how they were assessed or how severe they were. No indication is given of the regression with time of exposure or the variability of the actual nutritive factors. There was also no indication of the actual environmental levels of aniline or the other intermediates so that the specific causes of the observed effects cannot be defined.

C. FERTILITY

No relevant data found.

D. PREGNANCY

In one study (Podluzhnyi, 1979) of women working in the aniline dye industry (see Section B. for details), an increase in abortion rate was reported. The incidence however was highest in women working in a low exposure area where high physical exertion was required. Their abortion rate was 23% compared with 14% in the factory overall. Since no other details were given, evaluation of this study in relation to the effects of aniline is impossible.

One of the well known toxic effects of aniline is anoxia and cyanosis due to the formation of methaemoglobin. Methaemoglobin is a normal constituent of human blood with a mean of 0·09 g% and a range of 0–0·5 g%. Cyanosis occurs at levels of 1·5 g% or over. The importance of low levels of methaemoglobin in human pregnancy is uncertain but Schmitz (1961) found slightly (but not significantly) higher levels of methaemoglobin in women who aborted or threatened to abort in the first trimester. Cattle fed on forage high in nitrate, which also induces methaemoglobinaemia, may abort as a result. It has been known since 1886 (Rayner, 1886) that babies are especially sensitive to this toxic effect of aniline and may become cyanosed if nappies stamped with aniline dyes are used without prior laundering. This may be partly related to the enhanced percutaneous absorption of substances, especially in low birth weight babies (Nachman, 1970) and partly due to the impaired ability of the newborn to reduce methaemoglobin (Ross and Desforges, 1959).

Aniline is normally metabolized by p-hydroxylation and there is ample evidence that the enzymes necessary for this are already present in human fetal liver, but not placenta, by 6–7 weeks gestation (Pelkonen, 1977; Pelkonen and Kärki, 1973) and by other fetal tissues—adrenal, kidneys and placenta by 8–22 weeks (Juchau and Pedersen, 1973; Pelkonen *et al.*, 1973; Juchau *et al.*, 1973; Rane *et al.*, 1973; Pelkonen, 1973; Rane and Ackermann, 1972). This seems to be earlier than in the fetus in many species, in which the enzymes are not present in significant amounts until later in pregnancy (Rane and Ackermann, 1972). As well as p-hydroxylation, human fetal liver can also N-oxygenate aniline to produce phenylhydroxylamine and coincidentally methaemoglobin (Rane and Ackermann, 1972). This is of toxicological significance since the fetus has a low ability to reduce methaemoglobin.

E. MUTAGENICITY

No relevant information found.

F. CARCINOGENICITY

IARC Monograph Vol. 4 (1974) stated that the weight of epidemiological evidence available at that time suggests that aniline is not a human bladder carcinogen.

SUMMARY AND EVALUATION

EXPERIMENTAL STUDIES

Aniline readily crosses the placenta in rats. No studies were found on endocrine or gonadal effects, or of effects on fertility or pregnancy.

Mutagenicity studies in bacterial and mammalian cells were negative. There are no adequate data on carcinogenicity in animals and no data on transplacental carcinogenicity were found.

HUMAN STUDIES

An epidemiological study of women employed in the aniline dye industry showed a high incidence of menstrual and ovarian disorders, related to precise occupation, duration of employment and nutrition. An increased abortion rate was also observed but was highest in low exposure areas where physical exertion was required.

No studies were found on fertility, or pregnancy outcome other than abortion. No reports on mutagenicity were available. The weight of evidence suggests that it is not a bladder carcinogen.

EVALUATION

The animal evidence is inadequate for evaluation of reproductive toxic effects. Due to lack of exposure data and inadequate control data, the single human study is inadequate to assess the effects of aniline. Attention is drawn to the particular sensitivity of babies to methaemoglobinaemia induced by exposure to small amounts of aniline dye.

References

Abe, S. and Sasaki, M. (1977). Chromosome aberrations and sister chromatid exchanges in Chinese hamster cells exposed to various chemicals. *Journal of the National Cancer Institute* **58**, (6), 1635–1640.

Feuer, G. and Kardish, R. (1975). Hormonal regulation of drug metabolism during pregnancy. *International Journal of Clinical Pharmacology and Biopharmacy* **11**, (4), 366–374.

Garner, R. C. and Nutman, C. A. (1977). Testing of some azo dyes and their reduction products for mutagenicity using Salmonella typhimurium TA 1538. *Mutation Research* **44**, (1), 9–19.

Gut, I., Becker, B. A. and Gutova, M. (1976). Effect of pregnancy on hepatic microsomal drug metabolism in rabbits and rats. *Archives of Toxicology* **35**, 41–47.

IARC Monographs on the Evaluation of Carcinogenic Risk of Chemicals to Man: Some aromatic amines, hydrazine and related substances, N-nitroso compounds and miscellaneous alkylating agents (1974). Volume 4, Lyon, France.

Ishidate, M. and Odashima, S. (1977). Chromosome tests with 134 compounds on Chinese hamster cells in vitro—a screening for chemical carcinogens. *Mutation Research* **48**, (3/4), 337–354.

Juchau, M. R. and Pedersen, M. G. (1973). Drug biotransformation reactions in the human fetal adrenal gland. *Life Sciences* **12**, (2), 193–204.

Juchau, M. R., Pedersen, M. G., Fantel, A. G., Shepard, T. H. (1973). Drug metabolism by placenta. *Clinical Pharmacology and Therapeutics* **14**, (4), 673–679.

Maickel, R. P. and Snodgrass, W. R. (1973). Physicochemical factors in maternal-fetal distribution of drugs. *Toxicology and Applied Pharmacology* **26**, 218–230.

Nachman, R. L. (1970). Low birth weight related to toxicity. *Journal of Pediatrics* **76**, (2), 327–328.

Pelkonen, O. (1973). Drug metabolism and drug-induced spectral interactions in human fetal liver microsomes. *Biochemical Pharmacology* **22**, 2357–2364.

Pelkonen, O. (1977). Formation of toxic intermediates in fetal tissues. *In* "Biological Reactive Intermediates. Formation, Toxicity, and Inactivation". (Eds. Jollow, D. *et al.*). Proceedings of an International Conference, Turku, Finland, July 1975. Plenum, New York.

Pelkonen, O., Kaltiala, E. H., Larmi, T. K. I. and Kärki, N. T. (1973). Comparison of activities of drug-metabolizing enzymes in human fetal and adult livers. *Clinical Pharmacology and Therapeutics* **14**, (5), 840–846.

Pelkonen, O. and Kärki, N. T. (1973). 3,4-Benzpyrene and aniline are hydroxylated by human fetal liver but not by placenta at 6–7 weeks of fetal age. *Biochemical Pharmacology* **22**, 1538–1540.

Pence, D. H. and Schnell, R. C. (1979). Sex-related differences in biotransformation of aniline hydroxylase in Sprague-Dawley rats. *Pharmacology* **18**, (1), 52–56.

Podluzhnyi, P. A. (1979). Importance of the nutrition factor in the comprehensive social hygiene study of the health of female workers in the chemical industry. *Gigiena I Sanitariya* (1), 44–47.

Rane, A. and Ackermann, E. (1972). Metabolism of ethylmorphine and aniline in human fetal liver. *Clinical Pharmacology and Therapeutics* **13**, (5), 663–670.

Rane, A., Sjoqvist, F. and Orrenius, S. (1973). Drugs and fetal metabolism. *Clinical Pharmacology and Therapy* **14**, (4), 666–672.

Rayner, W. (1886). Cyanosis in newly born children caused by aniline marking ink. *British Medical Journal* **1**, 294.

Ross, J. D. and Desforges, J. F. (1959). Reduction of methemoglobin by erythrocytes from cord blood: further evidence of deficient enzyme activity in the newborn period. *Paediatrics* **23**, 718–726.

Schmitz, J. T. (1961). Methemoglobinemia—a cause of abortions? *Obstetrics and Gynecology* **17**, 413–415.

3. Arsenic and its Compounds

TECHNICAL DATA

(a) *Arsenic*

Formula	As
CAS registry number	7440–38–2
Chemical abstracts name	Arsenic
Synonyms	Arsen; arsenic black; gray arsenic; metallic arsenic.

(b) *Arsenic compounds* (Reviewed by IARC)

Formula	CAS registry number	Chemical abstracts name
$C_6H_4NH_2.AsO(OH)_2$	98–50–0	Arsanilic acid
As_2O_5	1303–28–2	Arsenic pentoxide
As_2S_3	1303–33–9	Arsenic sulphide
As_2O_3	1327–53–3	Arsenic trioxide
AsH_3	7784–42–1	Arsine
$Ca_3(AsO_4)_2$	7778–44–1	Calcium arsenate
$(CH_3)_2AsO(OH)$	75–60–5	Dimethylarsinic acid
P_6HAsO_4	7784–40–9	Lead arsenate
$CH_3AsO(ONa)_2$	144–21–8	Methanearsonic acid, disodium salt
$CH_3AsO(OH)ONa$	2163–80–6	Methanearsonic acid, monosodium salt
KH_2AsO_4	7784–41–0	Potassium arsenate
$KH(AsO_2)_2$	10124–50–2	Potassium arsenite
Na_3AsO_4	7631–89–2	Sodium arsenate
$NaAsO_2$	7784–46–5	Sodium arsenite
$(CH_3)_2AsO(ONa)$	124–65–2	Sodium cacodylate

Uses	In metallurgy for hardening copper, lead, alloys; manufacture of certain types of glass; pigment production; insecticides, fungicides, rodent poison.
TLV	0·2 mg/m^3 (as arsenic).

ANIMAL STUDIES

A. RELEVANT PHARMACOLOGY AND TOXICOLOGY

Schroeder *et al.* (1968) have fed male and female rats 5 ppm sodium arsenite in the drinking water from weaning until death. Apart from a significant increase in heart weight and serum cholesterol levels in the males in comparison with controls, not seen in the females, there were no sex differences in response to this dose. It should be noted that despite large tissue accumulations of arsenite, it was remarkably non-toxic at this dose level in terms of growth rate and survival of either sex. Kiyono *et al.* (1974) have found no sex differences in the lethality of arsenic trioxide given orally in doses of 5–10 mg/kg/day to rats from 1–21 days of age.

Placental transfer of organic arsenicals has been shown by Underhill and Amatruda (1923) to be very low in the rabbit and cat following i.v. administration to the mother; large amounts are stored in the placenta, however, and others have shown increasing transfer in the rabbit as pregnancy progresses (see review by Ferm, 1977). Placental transfer of inorganic arsenic salts has been shown in the rodent species mouse, rat and hamster.

Matsumoto *et al.* (1975) have given sodium arsenite orally during pregnancy (dose and timing not stated). They noted transfer of small amounts to the fetus and prolonged retention in fetal tissues. In the rat, Burk (1977) has noted transfer of radiolabelled sodium arsenate, after injection on day 10 of pregnancy. Twenty-four and 48 h after injection maternal blood radioactivity levels were high, reflecting the known binding of arsenic to haemoglobin in rat erythrocytes. Embryos had low but detectable ^{74}As counts and placental levels increased between 24 and 48 h suggesting sequestration of arsenic. Tanaka (1976) has shown placental transfer of arsenic when given orally as arsenic trioxide or arsenite on days 1–20 of pregnancy in the rat. Placental levels were higher than fetal levels on day 21, and in the fetus liver levels were quite high but brain levels low. Antidotes such as dimercaprol, thioctic acid and ascorbic acid given orally to the dam at the same time as arsenite decreased fetal levels except in the liver and brain. Morris *et al.* (1938) have shown a dose-related transfer of arsenic to the fetus in rats fed on a diet containing arsenic trioxide from 21 days of age through to breeding and subsequently.

Hanlon and Ferm (1977) have shown placental transfer of radiolabelled sodium arsenate in the hamster following i.v. injection on day 8 of pregnancy. The dams were killed 24 or 96 h after injection. Tissue concentrations of arsenate were similar in embryo and maternal blood at 24 h and high concentrations were found in the allantoic placenta. By 96 h after injection maternal blood, liver, placenta and embryonic levels had fallen by 77–91%. These data suggest there is rapid equilibration between maternal and embryonic compartments and fairly rapid elimination of arsenate from the body. Maternal and embryonic tissue distribution following trace or teratogenic doses of arsenate was identical.

Morris *et al.* (1938) have compared arsenic levels in newborn and 15-day-old rats nursed by dams fed on a diet containing arsenic trioxide before pregnancy and during pregnancy and lactation to see if arsenic is transferred in the milk. There was no difference in total body levels between newborns and 15-day-old pups, suggesting that if arsenic is transferred then it is rapidly excreted. Alternatively, if it is not transferred, levels accumulated in fetal life are retained.

Arsenic is known to be present in cow's milk (Kroger, 1973), normally at a concentration of 0·05–0·07 mg/kg. Kroger has noted, however, that after World War II, when use of arsenical pesticides reached a peak, milk concentrations as high as 0·2 mg/kg were found.

B. ENDOCRINE AND GONADAL EFFECTS

Bencko *et al.* (1968) have exposed hairless mice to arsenic in the drinking water at doses of 5 or 50 ppm (5 or 50 mg As/1), given as arsenic trioxide, for 256 days. At 5 mg/1 pathological changes were seen in the skin, liver, kidneys and spleen, but not the testes. At 50 mg/1 more extensive pathology was seen in the above mentioned organs and the germinal epithelium of the testes was also degenerating markedly.

Treu *et al.* (1974) have investigated sexual behaviour, semen quality and fertility in boars during an outbreak of poisoning due to arsanilic acid normally used to cure swine dysentery. During the acute phase 7/16 boars died and all showed signs of gross toxicity including vomiting, blindness, paresis and balance disturbance. Thirty-one days after the outbreak, 5 boars appeared clinically normal and 4 still showed ataxia of the rear limbs. Beginning on the eleventh day after the outbreak, boars showing little or no poisoning symptoms at this time had normal sexual behaviour (ejaculation within 10 min of placing with a dummy sow) after 2–7 days with the fading away of clinical symptoms. But 3 boars with more marked clinical signs of toxicity showed adverse effects on sexual behaviour long after other signs of toxicity disappeared; one boar produced semen for the first time on day 28 and another on day 49 after the outbreak. The third boar showed poor libido for more than 120 days and did not again accept the dummy sow. In 4 of the 9 surviving boars semen quality was within the normal expected range in terms of volume, appearance, pH, sperm count, motility and morphology, but with sperm preservation, motility was reduced up to 40 days after poisoning. Two boars developed orchitis, and epididymitis preceded deficient semen quality, and 2 boars showed low sperm counts, low motility and increased morphological abnormalities of sperm at 35 and 65 days after poisoning, in the absence of any disturbance of sexual behaviour or other clinical signs of toxicity. It is suggested that the disturbances in sexual behaviour may have been due to central and peripheral nerve damage known to occur with arsenic poisoning, but the effects on semen quality are more likely to be a direct effect of arsenic on the testes and/or epididymides. When semen samples were used in artificial inseminations, 3/5 boars had normal fertility whilst 2 showed a 10% reduction in fertility.

C. FERTILITY

The adverse effects on fertility of an outbreak of arsanilic acid poisoning in boars have been detailed in section B. After recovery from acute clinical signs of poisoning, fertility in boars with normal sexual behaviour was normal or only 10% reduced, but a number of animals never regained normal sexual behaviour or testicular function and were thus incapable of fertilizing sows.

Nadeenko *et al.* (1978) have carried out a fertility test on female rats given 0·0025 mg/kg orally in the drinking water for 7 months including during pregnancy. The pre-mating exposure period was not stated. There was no mention of any effect on fertility, but post-implantation losses were significantly increased from 24% in controls to 38%. Pre-implantation losses, implants/dam, fetal weight, placental weight and skeletal development were unaffected. Isolated cases of dilatation of the cerebral ventricles, renal pelvis and bladder were seen in arsenic-exposed fetuses but not in controls.

Morris *et al.* (1938) have carried out 2-generation fertility tests on groups of 9 male and female rats fed on a diet containing arsenic trioxide at a level of 26·8 or 215 mg As/kg of diet. The first parent generation were started on the diet at weaning age and pair-mated to other treated or control partners at 90–110 days of age They were kept on the diet, except for brief 5-day mating periods, during the production and rearing of 4 litters. The F_2 generation were taken from the second litters which were kept on the same diet as their parents from weaning age and allowed to produce one litter. There were no effects on fertility, pups/litter, postnatal mortality or weaning weights of any of the offspring in any of the treatment groups.

Dominant lethal studies on arsenic have been carried out. Gencik *et al.* (1977) gave 0·25 or 1 mg/kg arsenic orally to male mice, but no dominant lethal effects were seen when they were mated with control females. Šrám (1976) has shown potentiation of the dominant lethal effects of tris (1-aziridinyl) phosphine oxide (TEPA) with sodium arsenite in the mouse. Males were given 10 or 100 mg As/1 as sodium arsenite in the drinking water for 8 weeks. They were then given a single mutagenic dose of TEPA. Neither dose of arsenic alone had significant dominant lethal activity, but the highest dose of 100 mg As/1 potentiated the dominant lethal effect of TEPA. Similar results were obtained when males were exposed for 4 generations, 8 weeks/generation to arsenic followed by TEPA injection. The explanation of such potentiation may be that arsenic blocks the normal mechanisms for repair of damaged chromosomes, thus unmasking the full extent of TEPA-induced damage.

Conclusion

Exposure to arsenic at low doses does not appear to affect fertility in male or female rats and shows no dominant lethal activity of its own in the mouse. However, it may potentiate the dominant lethality of other compounds, and as yet, no fertility tests have been done on exposure to high doses of arsenic.

D. PREGNANCY

Hamster

The first demonstration of the teratogenicity of inorganic arsenic salts in mammals was by Ferm and Carpenter (1968) in the hamster. Administration of 20 mg/kg sodium arsenate by i.v. injection in 18 hamsters on day 8 of pregnancy caused 35% resorptions compared with 4·4% in controls, and 43% malformations, mainly exencephaly, compared with none in controls. A lower dose of 5 mg/kg was without effect, and a higher dose, 40 mg/kg, killed all the embryos. In a later study by the same group, these results were confirmed using 20 mg/kg sodium arsenate and the full spectrum of malformations noted as exencephaly, encephalocoele, cleft palate, microphthalmia and ear malformations, with exencephaly predominating (Holmberg and Ferm, 1969). Further observations on the hamster using i.v. injections of sodium arsenate (Ferm *et al.*, 1971) showed that with injection at a given time on day 8 resorption rates increased with increasing doses between 15 and 25 mg/kg, but that the later on day 8 the injection was given the lower the resorption rate. Malformation rates remained similar throughout day 8 but the spectrum of malformations varied with time of injection, as might be expected in the hamster where organogenesis is compressed into a short period on days 8–9 of gestation. In addition to exencephaly and encephalocoele, genito-urinary malformations were also seen and rib malformations were prominent with injections late on day 8 of pregnancy. Eighty to 90% of surviving embryos were malformed after treatment at any time on day 8.

Ferm and Kilham (1977) have shown that minimally teratogenic levels of arsenic (10 mg/kg sodium arsenate i.p.) and hyperthermia (50–60 min in a 40°C incubator) have a synergistic effect on malformation rates when applied together. Malformation rates of 1·6% with arsenate alone or 6% with hyperthermia alone were increased to 50% when both were applied. The explanation for this synergism is not known.

Holmberg and Ferm (1969) have shown that arsenate-induced embryolethality and teratogenicity in the hamster can be markedly reduced by simultaneous injection of sodium selenite, which is not itself teratogenic in the hamster. Metabolic interactions between selenium and arsenic are known and may account for the protective effects observed.

It should be noted that in none of these studies in the hamster was full teratological evaluation carried out. Only external abnormalities and rib abnormalities (visible through the translucent skin) were ascertained.

Mouse

Hood and co-workers have carried out a series of studies in the mouse with full teratological evaluation of external, soft tissue and skeletal development. Hood and Bishop (1972) gave groups of 8–10 mice i.p. injections of 25 or 45 mg/kg sodium arsenate on one of days 6–12 of pregnancy. The lower dose was without effect. The higher dose was described as "barely sublethal" to the dam, but no details of maternal toxicity were given. Thirty-six to 78% of implants were resorbed or dead when examined on day 18 of gestation, and a number of litters were completely resorbed after treatment on any day except 7. Fetal weight was significantly reduced after treatment on all days except day 12 when resorption rate was highest and none of the survivors malformed. After treatment on days 7–11, 8–63% of fetuses were malformed, with the highest abnormality rate on day 9. A very wide spectrum of external, internal soft tissue and skeletal malformations were seen, with exencephaly, hydrocephaly, exophthalmos, fused and forked ribs being the most common. The embryolethality and teratogenicity of i.p. sodium arsenate may be markedly reduced by simultaneous s.c. administration of a non-teratogenic dose of 2,3-dimercaptopropanol (BAL) which is known to reduce the general toxicity of arsenic (Hood and Pike, 1972).

Hood (1972) has also shown that arsenite is embryolethal and teratogenic in the mouse. Injection of 10 or 12 mg/kg sodium arsenite on one of days 7–12 of pregnancy caused death of some dams, 20–100% resorptions, significant reductions in fetal weight (except on day 12), and malformations after injections on days 8, 9 and 10. The spectrum of malformations seen was very similar to that induced by arsenate (Hood and Bishop, 1972).

Hood *et al.* (1978) have compared the teratogenicity of oral versus i.p. routes with sodium arsenate in the mouse after administration on one of days 7–15 of pregnancy. Maternal toxicity of 120 mg/kg orally was similar to that of 40 mg/kg i.p., but i.p. treatment affected resorption and malformation rates to a much greater extent than the oral route; malformations were seen in 0·6–5% of fetuses exposed via the oral route on days 7–11 of pregnancy, compared with a frequency of 3·7–30·6% in those exposed via the i.p. route on days 7–10. Single oral doses up to 100 mg/kg were without effect, and doses of 60 mg/kg orally on 3 consecutive days between 7 and 15 were without effect. The authors speculated that slower absorption into the blood stream and/or increased methylation of arsenate, reducing its toxicity, may account for the lower reproductive toxicity of orally administered arsenate compared with injection.

Matsumoto *et al.* (1973) have also given sodium arsenate orally by gavage in doses of 0, 10, 20 and 40 mg/kg on days 9–11 of pregnancy in the mouse. Fetuses were examined externally for malformations and for skeletal defects only. At 40 mg/kg there were significant decreases in fetal and placental weight and marked increases in resorptions and fetal deaths. Malformations (bent tail, open eyelids and cleft palate) occurred in 6% and 4% of fetuses from the 10 and 40 mg/kg groups respectively. Retarded ossification showed a dose-related increase. These results differ from those of Hood *et al.* (1977) in that higher embryolethality and teratogenicity were seen at a much lower oral dose, but the study is reported in abstract only and no further details are given to permit proper comparison of the 2 studies.

Hood *et al.* (1979) have also investigated the teratogenicity of chromated copper arsenate (35% arsenic pentoxide), which is used as a wood preservative. Neither oral administration in the mouse, nor dermal application in the rabbit had any embryotoxic or fetotoxic effects.

Rat

Beaudoin has investigated the teratogenicity of arsenic in the rat. Initially he reported (Beaudoin, 1973) lack of teratogenicity of sodium arsenate given as a single i.p. injection on day 8 of pregnancy in doses of 20–50 mg/kg. At 50 mg/kg all litters were resorbed, and at 40 mg/kg, 50% were resorbed but only 3% of survivors malformed. At 20 and 30 mg/kg, 1% were resorbed and none malformed. This study, however, was published in abstract only, and later, in a full study, Beaudoin (1974) reported sodium arsenate was teratogenic in the rat when given i.p. at doses around 30 mg/kg. Groups of

4–14 rats were given single i.p. injections of 20, 30 or 40 mg/kg on one of days 7–12 of pregnancy. A group of 29 rats served as controls. Acceptable teratological methods were used. Maternal toxicity was not mentioned. Fetal weight was reduced in all groups given 30 or 40 mg/kg and the difference between treated and control groups was significant after injection on days 8, 9 and 11. With 20 mg/kg, increased resorption rates were not seen but after injection of this dose on days 9 and 10, 39% and 16% of survivors respectively were malformed. At 30 and 40 mg/kg there was a dose-related increase in resorptions and malformations on all days, with a peak effect on day 9 when resorptions were 59% and 91% and malformations of survivors 89% and 100% in 30 and 40 mg/kg groups respectively. As in the hamster and the mouse, there was a wide variety of malformations in the rats, principally eye defects and exencephaly peaking on day 9, with gonadal and renal agenesis peaking on day 10. Subcutaneous haemorrhage, rib and vertebral defects were also very common.

Burk and Beaudoin (1977), in a detailed study of the developmental origin of arsenate-induced renal agenesis in the rat, confirmed the above findings of dose-related effects on fetal weight, resorptions and malformations, with i.p. injections of 30, 40 and 50 mg/kg of sodium arsenate on day 9, 10 or 11 of pregnancy, except that in this study the resorption rates were generally lower than before, and gonadal agenesis was not seen. The primary defect leading to renal agenesis was found to be retardation in growth of the mesonephric duct.

Hood *et al.* (1977) have summarized an unpublished study by Kimmel and Fowler showing no adverse effects on the offspring of administration of 30 or 90 ppm sodium arsenite or sodium arsenate in the drinking water throughout pregnancy in the rat.

Sheep

James *et al.* (1966) gave potassium arsenate to ewes orally in doses of 0·75 or 0·50 mg/kg/day for 18–147 days starting on the first day of pregnancy. One ewe given 0·75 mg/kg developed signs of toxicity (blackened gums) after 18 days and dosing was discontinued. At term a normal but small-for-dates lamb was born. The other 3 ewes given 0·5 mg/kg/day for 45, 140 or 147 days all gave birth to lambs of normal size and appearance.

Conclusion

Sodium arsenate has been shown to be highly embryolethal and teratogenic in 3 species of rodent, the hamster, mouse and rat, as has sodium arsenite in the one species it has been tested in, the mouse. In none of these studies is any mention made of maternal toxicity, so it is not known if adverse effects occur in the embryo and fetus at doses causing no maternal toxicity. However, three considerations suggest that arsenic may be a particularly potent teratogen.

First, there is a very rapid transition from absence of effects to 100% resorption or malformation of survivors over very small dose ranges in the hamster, mouse and rat. Secondly, in the rat, high malformation rates (up to 40%) with doses causing no embryolethality have been observed. Thirdly, a very wide spectrum of malformations has been seen suggesting it is a general teratogen capable of affecting all organ systems. In the mouse, rat and hamster the same variety of malformations have been seen with the exception of genitourinary malformations in the mouse and vertebral defects in the hamster, though in the latter case it should be noted that the vertebrae have not been properly examined in any study with the hamster.

The mechanism of action of arsenic salts as teratogens is not known. Arsenite interacts with sulphhydryl (-SH) groups and arsenate uncouples oxidative phosphorylation and interferes with phosphorus metabolism. Both these metabolic effects could potentially interfere with development at multiple sites. It has been suggested that arsenate may be teratogenic after conversion to arsenite, and certainly in the mouse, arsenite is teratogenic at lower doses than arsenate. However, the 2 salts differ somewhat in the ratio of embryolethal to teratogenic effects, and there is as yet no convincing evidence of the conversion to arsenite in all species.

E. MUTAGENICITY

IARC Monograph Vol. 23 (1980) reported that evidence on arsenic and its compounds in bacterial mutagenicity tests were inconclusive.

Šrám (1976), who showed arsenite potentiation of TEPA-induced dominant lethal mutations (see section C), has also shown arsenite potentiation of TEPA-induced chromosome aberrations in dividing bone marrow cells of mice. Sodium arsenite was given in the drinking water at doses of 10 or 100 mg/1 for 8 weeks, then a single mutagenic dose of TEPA was given. As in the dominant lethal test, 100 mg/1 but not 10 mg/1 of sodium arsenite potentiated the mutagenicity of TEPA alone, though arsenite by itself was not mutagenic.

F. CARCINOGENICITY

IARC Monograph Vol. 23 (1980) reports that there is inadequate evidence for the carcinogenicity of arsenic compounds in animals. It is one of the few known examples of a proven carcinogen in humans which has not been confirmed in animal experiments.

Transplacental carcinogenicity

Osswald and Goerttler (1971) have shown that arsenic is a transplacental carcinogen in the mouse. Mice were injected s.c. with 0·5 mg As/kg/day, given as the "sodium salt", throughout pregnancy. The dams were allowed to litter out and the offspring left untreated or given s.c. injections of 0·5 mg As/kg 20 times when "young". Litter size at birth was reduced to around 7 in As-treated litters compared with 10–12 pups/litter in controls. Average life expectancy was also reduced in the offspring exposed prenatally only to arsenic. The incidence of leukaemia over 2 years in the study was significantly increased from 0–8% in controls to 16–20% in prenatally exposed mice and was further enhanced to 42% in those exposed both prenatally and postnatally. The exposed dams showed a 46% incidence of leukaemia. Thus there is evidence from this study that arsenic is a transplacental carcinogen.

HUMAN STUDIES

A. RELEVANT PHARMACOLOGY AND TOXICOLOGY

Arsenic is a non-essential trace element normally present in the body and is transferred across the placenta into the fetus in humans. In the general population, levels in maternal blood, cord blood and placenta are very low; Creason *et al.* (1976), measuring 19 trace elements in these tissues in groups of 25 normal pregnancies from 8 different geographical areas, found arsenic was below detectable levels in many instances. In a later study from the same group (Kagey *et al.*, 1977) a more sensitive method capable of detecting 0·0002 μg/ml was used for maternal-fetal tissue samples obtained at delivery from 101 normal pregnancies in women living in 2 U.S. cities with low (Charlotte, North Carolina) or high (Birmingham, Alabama) air pollution levels. Maternal blood, cord blood and placental arsenic levels were independent of age, race, smoking history and city. Maternal and cord blood levels were similar within individuals, showing that arsenic is readily transferred across the placenta; blood levels ranged from $0{\cdot}2–37{\cdot}5 \times 10^{-3}$ μg/ml and placental levels from $0{\cdot}2–24{\cdot}0 \times 10^{-3}$ μg/ml. Mean placental levels were lower than blood levels in those living in the low air pollution area, whilst placental levels were higher than blood levels in those in the high pollution area.

In areas where arsenic contamination is found, placental levels may be quite high. Thieme *et al.* (1977) measured placental concentrations at delivery in women from industrial and rural areas in Germany. In the industrial areas of Essen and Munich, placental levels were $\leqslant 0{\cdot}02$ μg/g, but in the rural areas of Bayer, Wald and Altöttung, where there was thought to be widespread application of arsenic-containing plant pesticides, placental levels were around 0·12 μg/g.

Organic arsenicals readily cross the placenta in humans and this has formed the basis for successful antenatal treatment of congenital syphilis in the fetus by administration of arsphenamine to syphilitic pregnant women (Underhill and Amatruda, 1923). Symptom-free infants were born to women still with clinical signs of syphilis after arsphenamine treatment in pregnancy, suggesting that there might be accumulation of arsenic in the placenta which could be slowly released into the fetal circulation to destroy the spirochaetes. Eastman (1931) measured placental arsenic levels in 21 patients at delivery who had received antenatal arsphenamine or neoarsphenamine therapy. Placental levels in 10 of the women averaged 71 μg/100 g. In the remaining 11 cases, the placentae were divided into fetal and maternal portions; levels in the fetal portion averaged 92 μg/100 g and in the maternal portion 36 μg/100 g. This study confirmed that there was accumulation of arsenic on the fetal side and showed retention of arsenic in the placenta for up to 15 days after the last treatment was given.

Arsenic may also appear in the breast-milk in women; Morris *et al.* (1938) reported "it has been well established that it is transferred to the milk after arsenic medication", though no references to the original data are given.

B. ENDOCRINE AND GONADAL FUNCTION

No relevant data found.

C. FERTILITY

No relevant data found.

D. PREGNANCY AND THE NEONATAL PERIOD

Scanlon (1972) in a review of fetal hazards from environmental pollution with arsenic commented that since it is a potent inhibitor of —SH-containing enzymes, the expected fetal toxicity would be stillbirth or abortion. However, there is very little data on the effects of arsenic in pregnancy in women.

Lugo *et al.* (1969) have reported on a single case of newborn death following maternal ingestion of an arsenic-containing rodent poison. A 17-year-old woman, at 30 weeks' gestation, was admitted to hospital with acute renal failure 24 h after ingesting approximately 30 ml of arsenic trioxide with total elemental arsenic of 1·32%. Immediately after ingesting the poison, she developed abdominal pain and vomiting. On admission she was treated with 150 mg dimercaprol (BAL). Three days after admission she went into labour and delivered a live infant weighing 1·1 kg with a one-minute Apgar score of 4. The mother underwent haemodialysis and eventually recovered. The infant, however, had progressive respiratory distress and died at 11 h of age. A qualitative test for plasma arsenic in the infant before death was negative. At autopsy, besides the expected organ immaturity, generalised petechial haemorrhages and hyaline membrane disease, there was strikingly severe intra-alveolar pulmonary haemorrhage and high organ contents of arsenic; levels of arsenic trioxide/100 g wet tissue were 0·74 mg (liver), 0·150 mg (kidneys) and 0·0218 mg (brain), compared with normal levels in adult tissue reported at autopsy of 0·0050 mg (liver), 0·0048 mg (kidney) and 0·0048 mg (brain). Whilst most of the findings in this case may be attributed to the infant's immaturity at birth, arsenic may have played a role in the intra-alveolar haemorrhage and contributed to the death, and tissue levels in the infant were very high. Lugo *et al.* (1969) also mention a similar case of maternal ingestion of inorganic arsenic reported in 1928 by Barral, which resulted in both maternal and fetal death (no further details available).

Nordström and co-workers have carried out epidemiological studies in 4 populations living at different distances from a smelter in Rönnskär, northern Sweden and in female employees at the smelter. The smelting materials are of complex composition with a high content of arsenic and the smelter emits a number of potentially toxic substances including arsenic, lead and sulphur dioxide. In their first study, based on data collected in 1975–1976, Nordström *et al.* (1978a) found a significant reduction in birth weight in the offspring of the smelter employees and in the 2 small industrial populations living close to the smelter; average birth weight in 323 births to female employees was 3·39 kg, compared with 3·46 kg for 2700 births in a control area (Umeå) approximately 100 km from the smelter ($p<0·05$), or 3·49 kg ($p<0·01$) or 3·47 kg ($p<0·05$) in 2 areas more than 10 km from the smelter. In the 2 areas less than 10 km from the smelter, average birth weights were 3·39 kg and 3·41 kg, significantly lower than in the control area or the other 2 areas more than 10 km from the smelter ($p<0·001$–$0·05$). Distributions of parities within the groups were similar and so could not account for the differences observed. When pregnancy order was analysed separately, it was found that overall decreases in birth weight for all pregnancies were largely due to an effect in third pregnancies and above, whereas in controls birth weight increased with increasing parity. Employees were subdivided into factory, administration and laboratory workers; those in the laboratory area were less affected than factory or administration workers, but all 3 groups showed the decrease in birth weight with third pregnancies and above. Gestational age was not ascertained and it is not known if the observed effects were a direct effect of smelter emissions on fetal growth, a shortening of gestation, or other variables in the 6 populations such as smoking, maternal stress, socio-economic status, etc. The possible role of arsenic itself is even more difficult to ascertain, though the highest incidence of problems in the employees does suggest some factor related to the smelter itself.

Nordström *et al.* (1978b) have also reported on the frequency of spontaneous abortions amongst the same 4 population groups living at different distances from the Rönnskär smelter. From the files of the Department of Obstetrics and Gynaecology of the Skellefteå Hospital, data was obtained on all pregnancies of women born in 1930 or later, who attended the clinic and who were living in any of the 4 designated areas. There were records on a total of 4427 pregnancies. The overall incidence of spontaneous abortion ascertained from the records was highest in the area closest to the smelter (11·0%) and lowest in the area furthest away (7·6%, $p<0{\cdot}005$), with the other 2 areas in between having intermediate rates (9·2% and 7·6%). In the area nearest the smelter, there was also a significantly higher frequency of spontaneous abortions in first pregnancies (10·1%) compared with rates for the first pregnancies in the other 3 areas (6·3%, 7·3%, and in the area furthest away, 5·1%). In the area closest to the smelter, there were also significantly more women ($p<0{\cdot}025$) with a history of one or more abortions only and no normal pregnancies (2·6%) compared with the other 3 areas (1·23%, 1·71% and in the area furthest away, 0·91%). There are considerable methodological difficulties in the collection of this kind of data, including non-ascertainment of early non-hospitalized abortions and discrimination between spontaneous and induced abortions. There has also been an increase in ascertained spontaneous abortions over time in Sweden as a whole, increasing from 6% to 14% over the past 50 years, so matching over time would be important but it is not clear if this was done. Finally, there is the confounding factor of differing socio-economic backgrounds in the 4 areas examined and there was no matching for this variable. The authors considered, however, that the most probable explanation for their findings was pollution from the smelter, causing genetic damage resulting in an increased incidence of spontaneous abortions. The genetic damage could be to either male or female. In the absence of study of the female employees at the smelter, the data is less convincing than that of their birth weight study. It is also not known how many of the residents, particularly in the area nearest the smelter, were also employees at the smelter. In another study from the same group (Nordenson *et al.*, 1978) direct evidence of genetic damage in employees at the smelter was obtained (see section E for details).

Effects on neonates and children

In 1955 in Japan, an outbreak of arsenic poisoning occurred amongst infants, mostly under 12 months of age, who consumed powdered milk contaminated with arsenic (reviewed by Tsuchiya, 1977, original papers not seen by us). The Japanese Ministry of Health and Welfare in 1956 announced that there had been a total of 12,131 victims including 130 fatalities. At the time of the outbreak it was estimated the powdered milk contained 21–34 μg As/g and that total daily ingestion by the infants was 2·5–4·6 mg, depending on age (i.e. amount consumed). The principal acute symptoms were fever, diarrhoea, vomiting and anorexia, with swelling of the liver. Symptoms of the peripheral or central nervous systems were not common. However, one investigator (Hamamoto) noted encephalopathy with convulsions in 4/61 acute cases examined. Two other investigators (Ohira and Aoyama) reported abnormal EEG findings in 12% and findings suspicious of abnormality in 36% of a sample of 33 infants fed the contaminated milk, compared with rates of 4% and 21% for abnormal and suspicious findings in 48 breast-fed controls. These differences were said to be significant but involved very small numbers (only 4 cases and 2 controls were definitely abnormal). The possibility, however, of some long-term effects on the brain of arsenic exposure in infancy must be considered. A study by Yuwasa published in 1971 (reviewed by Tsuchiya, 1977) reported a higher prevalence of epilepsy among the children poisoned by the milk powder in infancy than in controls, and 13 years after the incident a group of nurses, school teachers and medical students visited the families of survivors and reported that residual effects (unspecified) did exist. A follow-up study by university researchers and physicians 14 years after the incident noted a great number of symptoms (unspecified) in the children who it was alleged had been poisoned, but records were incomplete over the 14 years and parental reporting of whether poisoning had or had not occurred was known to be inaccurate.

Three features of the Japanese baby-milk incident are important to note since they have not previously been associated with acute arsenic poisoning in adults or children, viz. abnormal EEG findings, late onset of epilepsy and chronic encephalopathy. They suggest that poisoning in early infancy may have more far-reaching consequences on brain development for survivors than poisoning in later childhood or adulthood, in which the peripheral rather than the central nervous system is affected.

This possibility of long-term effects on the brain is particularly worrying when taken in conjunction with measurements showing high arsenic uptake in young children compared with adults living in heavily polluted areas. Zaldívar (1977) has reported severe symptoms of chronic arsenic poisoning in children 0–15 years of age compared with adult or senile patients living in the city of Autofagasta, Northern Chile, an area of endemic poisoning due to arsenic-polluted drinking water. This was probably due to higher ingestion of arsenic in young children. Daily intake was estimated from a dietary survey of fluid intake; in the 0–10 year age group (median 1·7 years) intake averaged 0·063 mg/kg body weight/day and prevalence of symptoms was 7·3/1000; in older age groups intake was 0·02 mg/kg/day or less, declining with age, and prevalence rates were 2·0/1000 or less, also declining with age.

Milham (1978) had studied urinary arsenic levels in children living around a large copper smelter in Tacoma, Washington, U.S.A., emitting around 1000 pounds of As/day. Hair and urinary arsenic levels decreased with increasing distance of residence from the smelter and urinary levels varied with the level of activity of the smelter. Normal urinary arsenic levels were given as 14 μg/l. Urinary levels in children attending a school within 300 yards of the smelter complex, sampled between 1972 and 1976, averaged 35–114 μg/l, the highest levels being well into the range seen in smelter workers. Pre-school children in the same area, however, had average values of 270 μg/l in 1972 and 122 μg/l in 1976, (arsenic emissions from the smelter were halved over the study period) suggesting that it is the very young child who may be most at risk from arsenic exposure.

E. MUTAGENICITY

Severe chromosome damage has been observed in cell cultures of human lymphocytes from healthy persons, exposed to arsenic *in vitro*. Petres and Hundeiker (1968) showed mitotic inhibition and "chromosome pulverization" after exposure of lymphocytes in culture to 10^{-6} and $0{\cdot}5 \times 10^{-6}$ g of sodium arsenate (Petres *et al.*, 1977). Paton and Allison (1972) have also shown a significant increase in the incidence of chromatid breaks in cultures of human leucocytes or fibroblasts exposed *in vitro* to "sub-toxic" concentrations ($2{\cdot}9 \times 10^{-9}$ to $5{\cdot}8 \times 10^{-8}$ M) of sodium arsenite but not sodium arsenate. At effective doses of sodium arsenite, 20–60% of cells examined in metaphase had chromatid breaks.

Petres *et al.* (1970, 1977) have also carried out cytogenetic studies on lymphocytes from people exposed for therapeutic reasons or occupationally to arsenic. It is likely that the 34 exposed subjects in their earlier 1970 paper are included in the 62 subjects in the later 1977 paper. Only the latter results will be considered. The 62 arsenic-exposed subjects were attending the Dermatological Clinic of the University of Freiburg (i.Br.), Germany. Thirty-one had a history of extensive arsenic contact (unspecified) and in some cases the last contact was as much as 30 years before the study examination. Fourteen were psoriasis patients with therapeutic arsenical exposure and 17 were vine growers with occupational exposure to arsenic-containing pesticides. All showed typical arsenic hyperkeratoses on the palms of their hands and soles of their feet and several had already had arsenic-induced skin carcinomas excised. Controls comprised 14 psoriasis patients not exposed to arsenic and 17 healthy volunteers without traceable history of arsenic contact. No other details of personal or medical history of test subjects or controls were given, except for mean age (61·5 years in the arsenic-exposed groups, 51·2 years in controls) and sex ratio (female:male ratio 1:6·1 in the arsenic-exposed group, 1:1·2 in controls). The matching on these variables is poor and it is not known if there was any matching for history of drugs, infections, etc. It is not stated whether the cells were read blind or how many cells/subject were read. The frequency of chromosome aberrations was significantly increased in the arsenic-exposed group; 215 aberrations were seen in a total of 1121 mitoses, compared with 28 aberrations in 1247 control mitoses. Abnormalities seen at a higher frequency included secondary constrictions, achromatic lesions, gaps, chromatid breaks, acentric fragments and dicentric chromosomes. Results for the different sub-groups of arsenic-exposed subjects were not given separately, but the authors stated that frequent aberrations were seen even in those patients with an interval of decades since their last exposure. This suggests that initial damage to primary cells did not kill them, and they survived to form a stem cell population for pathological cells produced for years after.

Studies of chromosome aberrations in 39 workers (sex not specified) employed at the Rönnskär smelter in northern Sweden (see section D for description) were published in preliminary form (Beckman *et al.*, 1977) and as a full study (Nordenson *et al.*, 1978). For comparison, a series of apparently healthy males from Umeå, around 100 km away from the smelter, were also examined (matching procedures, if any, not described). Lymphocyte cultures were prepared and read blind according to WHO recommendations and in most cases 100 cells in metaphase were analysed for each person. For the smelter employees, data on duration of employment, urinary arsenic level, age and smoking habits were collected. They were divided into high (18 persons), medium (11 persons) and low (4 persons) exposure groups and a newly employed group (6 persons), based on the type and duration of work with arsenic compounds, nasal septum perforation and "arsenic burns". Mean age in the high exposure group was 54 years and that in the other 3 groups 31–33 years. Urinary arsenic levels were 290, 386 and 167 μg/l in high, medium and low exposure groups, the high mean in the medium exposure group being largely due to extreme values in one individual. The overall incidence of aberrations (gaps, chromatid aberrations, chromosome aberrations) in all 39 employees was significantly higher in comparison with the control population ($p<0{\cdot}001$), as was the frequency of each of the 3 types of aberration. In controls, most of the aberrations were gaps, the biological significance of which is not known, whereas in the employees relatively more aberrations were of the chromosomal type. There was no correlation between frequency of all aberrations and estimated degree of arsenic exposure, but frequency in the low exposure group (19 aberrations in 400 cells) was significantly lower than that in medium (101 in 1100 cells) or high (165 in 2006 cells) exposure groups. There were large individual variations within exposure groups and the individual with the highest frequency of aberrations had been exposed to arsenic, selenium and lead, all of which may be mutagenic. Although arsenic was one of the principal pollutants encountered in the smelter it was not the only one (see section D) and no air sampling measurements are mentioned. It is thus difficult to draw firm conclusions from this study, particularly as age may have confounded the findings in the high exposure group, but this and the studies of Petres and co-workers mentioned previously do indicate the need for further, more rigorous, studies to be carried out.

There is evidence from experimental studies on bacteria that arsenic compounds may act as cocarcinogens by inhibiting DNA repair (quoted by Beckman *et al.*, 1977), and Nordenson *et al.* (1978) have suggested that chromosome aberrations may be caused by other agents in the environment (e.g. smoking), whilst arsenic simply prevents their repair.

F. CARCINOGENICITY

IARC Monograph Vol. 23 (1980) reports that there is sufficient evidence that inorganic arsenic compounds are skin and lung carcinogens in humans. The data suggesting an increased risk for cancer at other sites were considered inadequate for evaluation.

SUMMARY AND EVALUATION

EXPERIMENTAL STUDIES

Studies in rodents and rabbits have shown that arsenic crosses the placenta and high tissue levels may be produced in the liver and placenta. Transfer to the milk also occurs. Arsenic does not appear to exert any specific toxic effect on the testes except at doses producing other signs of severe poisoning. A small study on rats fed continuously on diet containing up to 215 mg/kg diet of arsenic showed no adverse effects on fertility in either males or females. It has no dominant lethal activity when given alone but there is some evidence that it may potentiate the effects of other mutagens.

Sodium arsenate and to a lesser extent, sodium arsenite, are both embryolethal and teratogenic in rodents. A wide range of malformations has been produced suggesting that they may be able to affect development of many organ systems. Furthermore, teratogenic effects have been observed in rats at doses causing no embryolethality. No comment was made regarding maternal toxicity in these studies.

Data are inadequate to assess the mutagenicity and carcinogenicity of arsenic to animals, although it has been shown to induce leukaemia in mice exposed prenatally.

HUMAN STUDIES

Arsenic has been shown to cross the placenta in humans producing similar maternal and fetal blood levels, though some accumulation in the placenta may occur. No studies were found on effects on the gonads or on fertility. There is little evidence about the effects of arsenic in pregnancy but higher incidences of spontaneous abortion and low birth weight babies have been reported in those working in, or living close to a smelter emitting arsenic along with other pollutants. There are several studies which suggest that very young children may be especially sensitive to the toxicity of arsenic. They tend to show higher tissue levels than adults similarly exposed, and long term brain damage may be a feature of poisoning in infants.

There is limited evidence that arsenic may be mutagenic in people exposed either therapeutically or occupationally to arsenic with effects persisting for many years. Inorganic arsenic compounds are carcinogenic to the skin and lungs in humans. The data regarding other sites is inadequate for evaluation.

EVALUATION

There is sufficient evidence that arsenic is teratogenic when administered parenterally to rodents. Evidence following oral administration is inadequate for assessment. Attention is drawn to the lack of adequate data on mutagenicity and carcinogenicity in animals. The human data is inadequate for evaluation but the suggested adverse effects on pregnancy and in the young as well as the carcinogenic action indicate the need for further studies.

References

Beaudoin, A. R. (1973). Lack of teratogenic action of sodium arsenate in rats. *Teratology* **7**, (3), A–12.

Beaudoin, A. R. (1974). Teratogenicity of sodium arsenate in rats. *Teratology* **10**, 153–158.

Beckman, G., Beckman, L. and Nordenson, I. (1977). Chromosome aberrations in workers exposed to arsenic. *Environmental Health Perspectives* **19**, 145–146.

Bencko, V., Nejedly, K. and Somora, J. (1968). Histological picture of several organs after long-term peroral administration of arsenic to hairless mice. *Ceskoslovenska Hygiena* **13**, (6), 344–347.

Burk, D. T. (1977). Inorganic arsenic: placental transfer and effect on embryogenesis of the urogenital system of the rat. *Dissertation Abstracts International B*, **37**, 4805–4806.

Burk, D. and Beaudoin, A. R. (1977). Arsenate-induced renal agenesis in rats. *Teratology* **16**, (3), 247–259.

Creason, J. P., Svendsgaard, D., Bumgarner, J., Pinkerton, C. and Hinners, T. (1976). Maternal-fetal tissue levels of 16 trace elements in 8 selected continental United States communities. *Trace Substances in Environmental Health* **10**, 53–62.

Eastman, N. J. (1931). The arsenic content of the human placenta following arsphenamine therapy. *American Journal of Gynecology and Obstetrics* **21**, 60–64.

Ferm, V. H. (1977). Arsenic as a teratogenic agent. *Environmental Health Perspectives* **19**, 215–217.

Ferm, V. H. and Carpenter, S. J. (1968). Malformations induced by sodium arsenate. *Journal of Reproduction and Fertility* **17**, 199–201.

Ferm, V. H. and Kilham, L. (1977). Synergistic teratogenic effects of arsenic and hyperthermia in hamsters. *Environmental Research* **14**, 483–486.

Ferm, V. H., Saxon, A. and Smith, B. M. (1971). The teratogenic profile of sodium arsenate in the golden hamster. *Archives of Environmental Health* **22**, 557–560.

Gencik, A., Szokolayova, J. and Cerey, K. (1977). Dominant lethal test after peroral administration of arsenic. *Bratislavska Lekarska Listy* **67**, (2), 179–187.

Hanlon, D. P. and Ferm, V. H. (1977). Placental permeability of arsenate ion during early embryogenesis in the hamster. *Experientia* **33**, (9), 1221–1222.

Holmberg, R. E. and Ferm, V. H. (1969). Interrelationships of selenium, cadmium and arsenic in mammalian teratogenesis. *Archives of Environmental Health* **18**, 873–877.

Hood, R. D. (1972). Effects of sodium arsenate on fetal development. *Bulletin of Environmental Contamination and Toxicology* **7**, (4), 216–222.

Hood, R. D., Baxley, M. N. and Harrison, W. P. (1979). Evaluation of chromated copper arsenate (CCA) for teratogenicity. *Teratology* **19**, (2), 31A.

Hood, R. D. and Bishop, S. L. (1972). Teratogenic effects of sodium arsenate in mice. *Archives of Environmental Health* **24**, 62–65.

Hood, R. D. and Pike, C. T. (1972). BAL alleviation of arsenate-induced teratogenesis in mice. *Teratology* **6**, 235–238.

Hood, R. D., Thacker, G. T. and Patterson, B. L. (1977). Effects in the mouse and rat of prenatal exposure to arsenic. *Environmental Health Perspectives* **19**, 219–222.

Hood, R. D., Thacker, G. T., Patterson, B. L. and Szczech, G. M. (1978). Prenatal effects of oral versus intraperitoneal sodium arsenate in mice. *Journal of Environmental Pathology and Toxicology* **1**, (6), 857–864.

IARC Monographs on the Evaluation of the Carcinogenic Risk of Chemicals to Humans: Some metals and metallic compounds (1980). Vol. 23. Lyon, France.

James, L. F., Lazav, V. A. and Binns, W. (1966). Effects of sublethal doses of certain minerals on pregnant ewes and fetal development. *American Journal of Veterinary Research* **27**, (116), 132–135.

Kagey, B. T., Bumgarner, J. E. and Creason, J. P. (1977). Arsenic levels in maternal-fetal tissue sets. *Trace Substances in Environmental Health* **11**, 252–256.

Kiyono, S., Hasui, K., Takasu, K. and Seo, M. (1974). Toxic effect of arsenic trioxide in infant rats. *Journal-Physiological Society of Japan* **36**, 253–254.

Kroger, M. (1973). Chemical contaminants in milk. *Milchwissenschaft* **28**, 753–757.
Lugo, G., Cassady, G. and Palmisano, P. (1969). Acute maternal arsenic intoxication with fetal death. *American Journal of Diseases of Children* **117**, 328–330.
Matsumoto, N., Iijima, S. and Katsunuma, H. (1975). Fetal body burden of chemicals and its effect on fetal growth. *Congenital Anomalies* **15**, (4), 245–246.
Matsumoto, N., Okino, T., Katsunuma, H. and Iijima, S. (1973). Effects of Na-arsenate on the growth and development of the foetal mice. *Teratology* **8**, (1), 98.
Milham, S. (1978). Industrial toxins and the community. DHEW Publication (NIOSH) **78–168**, 262–270.
Morris, H. P., Lang, E. P., Morris, H. J. and Grant, R. L. (1938). The growth and reproduction of rats fed diets containing lead acetate and arsenic trioxide and the lead and arsenic content of newborn and suckling rats. *Journal of Pharmacology and Experimental Therapeutics* **64**, 420–448.
Nadeenko, V. G., Lenchenko, V. G., Genkina, S. B. and Arkhipenko, T. A. (1978). The influence of tungsten, molybdenum, copper and arsenic on the intrauterine development of the fetus. *Farmakologiya I Toksikologiya* **41**, (5), 620–623.
Nordenson, I., Beckman, G., Beckman, L. and Nordström, S. (1978). Occupational and environmental risks in and around a smelter in northern Sweden. II. Chromosomal aberrations in workers exposed to arsenic. *Hereditas* **88**, 47–50.
Nordström, S., Beckman, L. and Nordenson, I. (1978a). Occupational and environmental risks in and around a smelter in northern Sweden. I. Variations in birth weight. *Hereditas* **88**, 43–46.
Nordström, S., Beckman, L. and Nordenson, I. (1978b). Occupational and environmental risks in and around a smelter in northern Sweden. III. Frequencies of spontaneous abortion. *Hereditas* **88**, 51–54.
Osswald, H. and Goerttler, K. (1971). Arsenic-induced leucoses in mice after diaplacental and postnatal application. *Verhandlungen-Deutschen Gesellschaft fur Pathologie* **55**, 289–293.
Paton, G. R. and Allison, A. C. (1972). Chromosome damage in human cell cultures induced by metal salts. *Mutation Research* **16**, (3), 332–336.
Petres, J., Baron, D. and Hagedorn, M. (1977). Effects of arsenic cell metabolism and cell proliferation: Cytogenic and biochemical studies. *Environmental Health Perspectives* **19**, 223–227.
Petres, J. and Hundeiker, M. (1968). Chromosome pulverization induced in vitro in cell cultures by sodium diarsenate. *Archiv fur klinische und experimentelle Dermatologie* **231**, 366–370.
Petres, J., Schmidt-Ullrich, K. and Wolf, U. (1970). An investigation into chromosomal aberrations in human lymphocytes after chronic arsenic exposure. *Deutsche Medizinische Wochenschrift* **95**, (2), 79–80.
Scanlon, J. (1972). Human fetal hazards from environmental pollution with certain non-essential trace elements. *Clinical Pediatrics* **11**, (3), 135–141.
Schroeder, H. A., Kanisawa, M., Frost, D. V. and Mitchener, M. (1968). Germanium, tin and arsenic in rats: effects on growth, survival, pathological lesions and life span. *Journal of Nutrition* **96**, 37–45.
Šrám, R. J. (1976). Relationship between acute and chronic exposures in mutagenicity studies in mice. *Mutation Research* **41**, 25–42.
Tanaka, I. (1976). Studies on arsenic metabolism (XVII). Studies of placental transfer and antidotes and diets on placental transfer. *Folia Pharmacologica Japonica* **72**, 673–687.

Thieme, R., Schramel, P. and Kurz, E. (1977). Die Spurenelementkonzentration der menschlichen Plazenta in stark kontaminiertter Umwelt. *Geburtshilfe und Frauenheilkunde* **37**, (9), 756–761.

Treu, H., Hillmann, H. and Bollwahn, W. (1974). Semen quality and sexual behaviour in boars following arsanilic acid poisoning. *Deutsch Tierarztliche Wochenschrift* **81**, (10), 225–229.

Tsuchiya, K. (1977). Various effects of arsenic in Japan depending on type of exposure. *Environmental Health Perspectives* **19**, 35–42.

Underhill, F. P. and Amatruda, F. G. (1923). The transmission of arsenic from mother to fetus. *Journal of the American Medical Association* **81**, (23–26), 2009–2112.

Zaldívar, R. (1977). Ecological investigations on arsenic dietary intake and endemic chronic poisoning in man: dose response curve. *Zentralblatt fur Bakteriologie B*, **164**, 485–491.

4. Benzene

TECHNICAL DATA

Formula	(benzene ring)
CAS registry number	71–43–2
Chemical abstracts name	Benzene
Synonyms	Benzin;* benzine;* benzol; benzole; benzolene; bicarburet of hydrogen; carbon oil; coal naphtha; cyclohexatriene; motor benzol; phene; phenyl hydride; mineral naphtha; pyrobenzol; pyrobenzole.
Uses	Manufacture of medicinal chemicals, dyes and many other organic compounds, artificial leather, linoleum, oil cloth, airplane dopes, varnishes, lacquers; as solvent for waxes, resins, oil, etc.
TLV	10 ppm

ANIMAL STUDIES

A. RELEVANT PHARMACOLOGY AND TOXICOLOGY

The metabolism of benzene in humans and animals has been reviewed by Rusch *et al.* (1977) and is essentially similar in those species studied in detail, viz. mouse, rat, rabbit and man; some benzene is exhaled unchanged and the rest oxidized mainly in the liver to phenol, catechol, quinol and hydroxyquinol, which are excreted free in the urine or as conjugates with glucuronides or ethereal sulphates. Benzene itself is responsible for the acute

* These two names are no longer used for benzene. They have been used for many years to describe a low-boiling petroleum fraction predominantly containing aliphatic hydrocarbons.

toxicity on the central nervous system. Chronic toxicity, resulting from much lower levels of exposure, appears to depend on the level and duration of exposure to benzene metabolites. There is, however, some conflicting evidence on whether the haematopoietic toxicity is due to benzene itself or its metabolites, but the bulk of evidence points to the latter being responsible (Rickert *et al.*, 1979). Tissue distribution of benzene and its metabolites may vary with different routes of administration, but highest retention is in the fat, kidney and bone marrow.

There may be a sex difference in the haematopoietic toxicity of benzene in animals, as in human; an increased susceptibility to benzene has been reported in female rats and rabbits (Leong, 1977; Sato *et al.*, 1975). However, it has been suggested that sex differences in the rat and rabbit may be due solely to the influence of female hormones which affect the leukocyte count (in the rat the count is decreased during oestrus) (Leong, 1977), and one group has failed to find any sex differences in decreased erythrocyte or leukocyte counts following benzene exposure in the rabbit (Desoille *et al.*, 1962). In the rat, it has been suggested that the sex difference, if it exists, may be due to increased drug metabolizing capacity of the hepatic microsomal enzyme system in the male, and hence faster elimination of the total dose, whereas in the human the increased susceptibility of females appears to be due to the higher fat content in the body retaining benzene (Sato *et al.*, 1974, 1975).

Desoille *et al.* (1963, 1965, 1967) have studied the effect of pregnancy on the haematopoietic toxicity of benzene. In the rabbit, pregnancy enhances the leukopenic effect of benzene whereas in the rat it seemingly protects the animal from leukopenia, and in the guinea pig pregnancy has no influence at all on benzene-induced leukopenia.

There have been no studies on placental transfer of benzene, but in view of its high fat solubility and low molecular weight, it seems likely that transfer to the fetus would occur fairly readily.

B. ENDOCRINE AND GONADAL EFFECTS

Males

Wolf *et al.* (1956) have reported changes in testicular weight and histology following exposure to benzene by inhalation in the rat, guinea pig and rabbit. In all 3 species exposure to 80 or 88 ppm for 7 h/day, 5 days/week for 30–40 weeks caused increased testicular weight and/or histopathological changes in the testes described as degeneration of the seminiferous epithelium. These levels also caused one or more of the following changes; increased spleen weight, kidney, blood or bone marrow pathology and growth depression. No later studies have been found on testicular effects.

Females

Avilova and Ulanova (1975) have studied the effect of benzene on the oestrous cycle. Adult female rats were exposed to 1·6 or 9·4 ppm (5 or 30 mg/m^3) benzene by inhalation for 4 months. In the fourth month of exposure there was a significant increase in the duration of oestrus in the 9·4 ppm group to a mean of 1·46 days, compared with 1·15 days in controls. In the 1·6 ppm group total cycle length was significantly decreased to 4·80 days compared with 5·32 days in controls. Exposure of juvenile females, 1·5–2 months of age, to 1·6 ppm reduced the number of rhythmically cycling rats by the third month of exposure. The absence of any consistent or dose-related effects requires confirmation of a specific effect on the oestrous cycle in further experiments.

C. FERTILITY

Males

There have been no studies on the effect of benzene on male fertility with the exception of a dominant lethal study. Dean (1978) has reported on a negative dominant lethal study by Lyon in the male rat following i.p. injection of 0·5 ml benzene/kg (no further details available, original not seen by us).

Females

Avilova and Ulanova (1975) exposed groups of 22–30 female juvenile rats aged 1·5–2 months, and adult rats aged 4 months, to 0, 1·6 or 9·4 ppm (5 or 30 mg/m^3) benzene for 4 months. During the exposure period some small, but inconsistent, changes in the oestrous cycle were apparent (see section B). At the end of the exposure period they were mated to untreated males. There were no significant effects on the number of pregnancies, implants/dam or resorptions/dam. There was a tendency towards increased pre-implantation losses in all benzene-exposed groups in comparison with controls, but this reached significance only in the adult females exposed to 1·6 ppm and not in those exposed to 9·4 ppm. Fetuses from adult females exposed to 9·4 ppm had more haemorrhages than controls and were significantly heavier. In view of the wide variations in control and treated body weights, the latter finding may be of no biological significance, particularly since they have also observed a significant decrease in body weight of offspring from dams exposed to 9·4 ppm at one month of age. They also noted that offspring of juveniles exposed to 9·4 ppm had a high postnatal mortality of 38% compared with 16% in controls.

Gofmekler (1968) has shown that continuous exposure of female rats to 210 ppm (670 mg/m^3) benzene for 10–15 days before placing with a male, during the mating period, and thereafter, completely prevented pregnancy.

However, it is not known if this was due to failure to mate, infertility, or early pre-implantation losses of fertilized ova. With lower exposures of 0·3–20 ppm (1–63·3 mg/m^3) before mating and throughout pregnancy, normal numbers carried to term, but data given on outcome of pregnancy is inadequate to assess whether there was any effect on intrauterine mortality.

Batra and co-workers have carried out a series of studies on the effects of painting mouse ovaries directly with benzene. Ten to 15 days after painting the ovaries, the mice were mated with untreated litter mates. In comparison with controls, benzene-treated females produced fewer litters (Batra, 1966), had a high incidence (73%) of abnormal cleavage and death of blastocysts on days 1–3 of pregnancy (Solomon and Batra, 1964), and 8–20% incidence of abnormalities at birth, principally haemorrhages and tail defects in the newborns, which persisted through at least 4 generations (Sridharan *et al.*, 1963), small litter size at birth and high preweaning mortality of 58% in the F_1 generation (Batra, 1966), and possibly an increased incidence of tumours in the F_1 generation (Batra, 1959). Extensive histological changes were seen in the ovaries after painting with benzene, apparent as haemorrhagic areas 8 days after painting, with destruction of ovaries at 30 days and an increase in atretic follicles at 3 months (Batra, 1966). The relevance of this mode of administration to the inhalational and dermal routes normally encountered in industry may be questioned. However, haemorrhages in offspring have been observed following inhalational exposure to benzene during pregnancy, and these experiments do illustrate the potential of benzene for causing mutagenic changes in the germ cells.

D. PREGNANCY

Mouse

Watanabe and Yoshida (1970) were the first to claim teratogenic effects of benzene after administration during organogenesis only. Acceptable teratological methods were used except that there was no control group. Groups of 15 mice were given single s.c. injections of 3 ml benzene/kg on one of days 11–15 of pregnancy. This dose caused marked leukopenia lasting 24–48 h but had no effect on body weight in the dams. Litter size ranged from an average of 6·5–8·5 in the 4 treatment groups. Malformations were seen in most treated groups; cleft palate occurred in 5·5% of fetuses exposed on day 13 and in 1·0% of fetuses exposed on day 14 and agnathia or micrognathia was seen in 0·9%, 2·4% and 1·0% of fetuses exposed on days 11, 13 and 14 respectively. Extra 14th ribs were seen in 10–16% of fetuses in all treated groups. Fetuses from 5 dams treated on day 15 had no malformations but 24% had extra 14th ribs. In the absence of any control data it is not known if these represent significant increases in malformation and anomaly rates. Extra 14th rib(s), for example, can be a common skeletal variant in some strains of mice and rats.

Matsumoto *et al.* (1975) have given groups of 8–11 mice s.c. injections of 0, 2 or 4 ml of benzene/kg on days 8 and 9 or 12 and 13 of pregnancy. Fetuses were examined externally and for skeletal defects only; internal soft tissues were not examined. They claim that fetal weight was significantly decreased in both groups given 4 ml/kg and placental weight significantly reduced in those given 4 ml/kg on days 12 and 13 of pregnancy. However, reworking of the data shows p values of $>0{\cdot}4$ in all cases. Sporadic malformations (cleft palate and open eye) did not differ significantly between treated and control groups, neither did the incidence of dead or resorbed embryos and fetuses. A small degree of retarded ossification was seen in fetuses from dams given 4 ml/kg.

Nawrot and Staples (1979) have investigated the effects of oral administration by gavage of 0·3, 0·5 or 1·0 ml/kg on days 6–15 of pregnancy or 1·0 ml/kg on days 12–15 of pregnancy in the mouse. After dosing on days 6–15, 0·5 and 1·0 ml/kg caused some maternal mortality and embryolethality. Fetal weight was significantly reduced at all 3 dose levels but no increase in malformations was seen. There were similar findings after dosing on days 12–15, except that resorptions occurred later in gestation. The study is reported in abstract only and no further details are given.

There has been one study on benzene exposure by inhalation in the mouse. Murray *et al.* (1979) exposed groups of 35–37 mice to 0 or 500 ppm benzene for 7 h/day on days 6–15 of pregnancy. Acceptable teratological methods were used. There was no evidence of maternal toxicity. There were no effects on implants/dam, live fetuses/dam, resorptions/dam or malformation rates. Fetal body weight was significantly reduced and delayed ossification significantly increased in fetuses from the benzene group.

Iwanaga *et al.* (1970) have shown an increased postnatal susceptibility to benzene toxicity in mice exposed prenatally to benzene by injection of the dams with 4 ml benzene/kg on day 9 or 12 of gestation. At 10 weeks of age, the offspring were injected with 5 daily doses of 0·1 ml benzene/kg, and the effects on erythrocytes, leukocytes, body weight, thymus and spleen were more marked than in non-prenatally exposed controls.

Rat

Desoille *et al.* (1965) report absence of any effect of s.c. injection of 0·1 g/kg of a solution of benzene in olive oil throughout pregnancy in the rat on the length of pregnancy, maternal body weight, average litter size or neonatal mortality rate.

There have been several inhalational studies on benzene in the rat. In an unpublished study by Hazelton Laboratories America Inc., summarized by Murray *et al.* (1979), teratogenic effects were observed at 500 ppm; rats were exposed to 0, 10, 50 or 500 ppm benzene for 7 h/day on days 6–15 of pregnancy, and a low incidence of exencephaly, kinked ribs and abnormal ossification of the forepaws was noted at 500 ppm. In another unpublished study by Litton Bionetics Inc., U.S.A., quoted by Murray *et al.* (1979), no teratogenicity but increased embryolethality was seen after exposure to 10 or 40 ppm for 6 h/day on days 6–15 of pregnancy in the rat.

Hudák and Ungváry (1978) exposed groups of 19–26 rats to 0 or 313 ppm (1000 mg/m^3) benzene for 24 h/day on days 9–14 of pregnancy. Acceptable teratological methods were used. There was no maternal mortality but maternal weight gain was significantly reduced. There were no significant effects on live fetuses/dam, resorbed or dead fetuses/dam or malformation rate. Mean fetal weight was significantly reduced and retarded ossification, abnormal fusion of sternebrae and extra ribs were all significantly increased in the benzene-exposed group.

Green *et al.* (1978) exposed groups of 14–18 rats to 100, 300 or 2200 ppm benzene for 6 h/day on days 6–15 of pregnancy, each benzene-exposed group having a concurrent 0 ppm control group. Maternal weight gain was significantly reduced in the 2200 ppm group, but not at lower exposure levels. There were no significant effects on implants/dam, live fetuses/dam, resorptions/dam or malformation rates. There was a significant 10% reduction in fetal weight in the 2200 ppm benzene group, and skeletal anomalies were sporadically increased in benzene-exposed groups (missing sternebrae at 100 ppm, delayed ossification of sternebrae in female offspring only at 300 ppm and 2200 ppm, and missing sternebrae at 2200 ppm). The authors suggest the preponderance of affected female fetuses is in accordance with other observations on the increased susceptibility of females to benzene toxicity (see section A). In addition they observed a non-significant low incidence of haemorrhages in all 3 benzene-exposed groups which were not seen at all in control fetuses.

Gofmekler (1968) has exposed groups of 10–12 rats to 0·3–20 ppm (1–63·3 mg/m^3) benzene for 10–15 days before mating and throughout pregnancy. The rats were allowed to litter out. From the data presented it is not clear whether litter size was affected. Newborn body weight was not affected. Relative organ weights were significantly different from controls in a number of instances but there were no clear dose-response relationships except perhaps for elevated kidney and spleen weights at the 2 top exposure levels of 17·7 and 20 ppm. The data is generally unconvincing with sporadic, non-dose-related significant differences in one direction at lower dose levels and in the opposite direction at the higher levels. Analysis of ascorbic acid, nucleic acid and DNA levels in offspring and their dams exposed to 0·3–20 ppm benzene (Gofmekler *et al.*, 1968) again showed sporadic, non-dose-related differences in some tissues, which are probably of no biological significance. In particular, total nucleic acid and DNA levels in the brains of the offspring were unaffected. The age of the offspring is not stated; in the text they are variously described as "embryos", "fetuses" and "young"; however, it may well be that they were the same newborns as in the previously described experiment.

Rabbit

Desoille *et al.* (1963) report absence of any effect of s.c. injections of 0·25 ml/kg/day of a 40% benzene solution throughout pregnancy in the rabbit on length of gestation, abortion rate, neonatal mortality and anomaly rate (none seen).

Murray *et al.* (1979) have carried out a full teratology study on inhaled benzene in the rabbit. Groups of 20 does were exposed to 0 or 500 ppm benzene for 7 h/day on days 6–18 of pregnancy. Acceptable teratological methods were used. There were no signs of maternal toxicity but food and water consumption was increased in the benzene-exposed group towards the end of the exposure period. There were no significant effects on implants/dam, live fetuses/dam, resorptions/dam, fetal body weight or malformation rate. The proportion of fetuses with lumbar spurs or extra 13th ribs was significantly decreased in the benzene-exposed group, compared with controls.

Guinea-pig

Desoille *et al.* (1967) have reported absence of any effect of s.c. injections of 0·1 g/kg of a 40% benzene solution throughout pregnancy in the guinea-pig on maternal body weight, length of gestation, number of offspring, offspring body weight or neonatal mortality.

Conclusion

Remarkably consistent findings on benzene's effects during pregnancy in the mouse, rat and rabbit have emerged. Embryolethal and teratogenic effects are not seen even at maternally toxic doses, but significant fetotoxicity in terms of reduced body weight, sometimes accompanied by increases in skeletal variants and delayed ossification, is seen at doses which are not necessarily toxic to the dam. Three isolated reports of embryolethality and teratogenicity (low incidence only) after benzene exposure in pregnancy in the rat and mouse are impossible to assess since no control data are published for any of these studies. The absence of any such effects in a large number of adequately conducted studies reported in full suggests these observations may be of no biological significance. The role that benzene-induced maternal anaemia may play in any adverse effect on the offspring is not known.

E. MUTAGENICITY

Benzene has been shown to be without mutagenic effects in microbial systems such as the Ames test or host-mediated assay (reviewed by Dean, 1978).

A number of workers have examined the effects of benzene on dividing bone marrow cells. Dean (1969) gave male and female rats a single s.c. injection of 0·5 or 1·0 ml benzene/kg and examined bone marrow cells 24 h and 8 days after injection. At 0·5 ml/kg male but not female rats showed increased chromosome aberrations after 24 h (polyploid mitoses, chromatid gaps and breaks). At 1·0 ml/kg both sexes showed increased aberrations at 24 h. In controls, 1–2% of cells had aberrations, whereas in treated groups 5–13% of cells had aberrations. By 8 days after injection, chromosome damage was not evident, perhaps because damaged cells were incapable of division. Similar effects of increased aberrations at 24 h but not at 8 days were seen in cultured rat lymphocyte preparations.

Philip and Jensen (1970) also found a significant increase in chromosome damage (solely chromatid aberrations) in dividing bone marrow cells of male and female rats at 12 and 24 h, but not 36 h, after s.c. injection of 2 ml benzene/kg. In benzene-injected rats 9–27% of cells were damaged compared with 1·2% in controls.

Lyapkalo (1973) has reported a 57% incidence of chromosome aberrations in dividing bone marrow cells of rats injected s.c. with 1 g benzene/kg for 12 days, and Dobrokhotov (1972) has found increased damage after injection of 0·2 g/kg day. Dobrokhotov and Enikeev (1977) have also reported chromosome damage to dividing bone marrow cells during a 4 months chronic inhalation study where rats were exposed to 94 ppm (300 mg/m^3). One month after the end of exposure, chromosome aberrations were less frequent but still significantly increased in comparison with controls.

Dean (1978) has reported on studies by Lyon (original paper not seen by us) in the rat showing increased chromosome and chromatid aberrations in dividing bone marrow cells up to 8 days after an i.p. injection of 0·5 ml benzene/kg. By 70 days after the injection, there was still an increase in aberrations in the benzene group but the difference was no longer significant between treated and control groups. Benzene given as 2 i.p. doses of 0·05 and 0·25 ml/kg on successive days was positive in the micronucleus test in the rat, but 0·025 ml/kg × 2 had no effect.

In the rabbit, Kissling and Speck (1971) have shown that s.c. injections of 0·2 ml/kg/day for 18 weeks increased chromosome aberrations (mainly chromatid gaps and breaks) in dividing bone marrow cells from 6% in controls to 58%. Sixty days after stopping the injections, 36% of cells still showed aberrations.

These studies show a clear mutagenic effect of benzene which may persist for some time after dosing has stopped. The relevance of these studies to possible benzene-induced leukaemia in man is clear, but their relevance to reproductive toxicity is not yet known. It will be recalled, however, that benzene applied to the ovary caused adverse effects in the offspring transmitted through at least 4 generations (see section C). It remains to be seen whether indirect exposure of the germ cells to benzene, by inhalation, absorption or ingestion, affects chromosomes.

F. CARCINOGENICITY

IARC Monograph Vol. 7 (1974) reported that up to that time benzene had only been tested in mice by s.c. injection and skin application. The data reported did not permit any conclusion to be drawn on its carcinogenicity. A more recent evaluation however (IARC Monograph Vol. 29, 1982 in press) reviewing further evidence in mice and rats concluded that there is limited evidence of carcinogenicity of benzene in experimental animals.

HUMAN STUDIES

A. RELEVANT PHARMACOLOGY AND TOXICOLOGY

It has been widely believed that women are more susceptible than men to benzene poisoning; between 1897 and 1930 a number of largely descriptive studies were published (reviewed by Hunt, 1979) noting the particular problems in women exposed to benzene of vaginal bleeding and haemorrhagic complications of pregnancy, alongside the other usual symptoms of purpuric skin spots and bleeding from the nose and gingiva. The occurrence of vaginal bleeding in chronic benzene poisoning, it was noted at that time, was frequently associated with progression to severe and often fatal complications of the poisoning.

Later workers have attempted to investigate the mechanism(s) underlying the increased female susceptibility to benzene reported for both animals (see Animal Studies, section A) and humans. Sato *et al.* (1975) have suggested that there is slower elimination of benzene in women than in men, due to the storage of benzene in the larger body fat content in women. In their study, 5 male and 5 female volunteers, aged 21–24 years, inhaled 25 ppm benzene for 2 h through a breathing mask. Blood concentrations during inhalation were always higher in the males than in the females, but after cessation of inhalation blood and end-tidal air concentrations decayed faster in the males than females, so that by 4 h blood concentrations were higher in females than in males. The authors suggest that the lower blood levels in females during inhalation were not due to lower absorption of benzene, but due to the greater distribution volume (in the fat) in females than in males. They mention that a higher uptake rate for benzene in women than in men has been reported by Nomiyama and Nomiyama (original paper not seen by us) and, since there is no sex difference in the air-blood partition coefficient for benzene, this difference in uptake rate must be due to the difference in volume of distribution. In humans, there is little evidence of the large sex differences, seen for example in the rat, in metabolizing enzyme activity, to account for the difference in elimination rate. Thus females may be more susceptible to benzene poisoning because of higher uptake and longer persistence in the body than in males for any given exposure level.

Placental transfer of benzene in the human has been demonstrated. Dowty *et al.* (1976) collected 11 paired samples of maternal and cord blood at delivery in 11 normal, uneventful pregnancies. All infants were normal except for one with lumbosacral meningo-myelocoele and all were of normal weight. Many volatile, low molecular-weight compounds were detected in maternal and cord blood including halogenated hydrocarbons, plastic components and food preservatives. Benzene, carbon tetrachloride and chloroform were present in cord blood in amounts equal to or greater than maternal blood. This indicates that benzene crosses the placenta.

B. ENDOCRINE AND GONADAL EFFECTS

Early studies reviewed by Hunt (1979), mentioning the progression of chronic benzene poisoning to severe anaemia, with bleeding from the nose, gums and vagina in women, have already been mentioned in section A. Hunt also refers to a report by L. Selling (Johns Hopkins *Hospital Bulletin* **21**, 33, 1910, original not seen by us) on the short-lived use of benzene as a therapeutic drug for the treatment of leukaemia, administered orally in gelatin capsules, in doses of 3–5 g. This "therapy" generally resulted in death from chronic benzene poisoning before the final stages of leukaemia, and was clearly associated with menorrhagia.

In a more recent study, Michon (1965) has investigated the menstrual cycle in 500 women, aged from 20–40 years, working in a Polish factory producing leather and rubber shoes and exposed to benzene, toluene and xylene, which it was said were within permissible levels of 31 ppm for benzene, 67 ppm for toluene and 58 ppm for xylene.

Controls were 100 women in the same plant but not exposed to these solvents. Menstrual disturbances occurring more frequently in women exposed to the aromatic hydrocarbons were prolonged and/or heavy bleeding rather than any alteration in the length of the cycle (abstract only seen by us).

Mikhailova *et al.* (1971) have also reported an increased incidence of menstrual cycle disorders in women employed in a workshop where there was a "high concentration" of benzene and its homologues. Nine different categories of worker were studied and in the benzene-exposed group a total of 260 women were examined, of average age 37 years and average duration of employment in that job of 9 years. Menstrual cycle disturbances were reported in 18·5% of those exposed to benzene. However, the frequency of such disorders was higher in other groups, e.g. women exposed to lead (29·5%), mercury (26·8%), noise (22·2%), vibrations (40·0%) or shocks (53·8%). In other groups it was slightly lower, e.g. shop workers (10·8%), women engaged in physical labour (15·7%) and women exposed to superphosphate (16·9%). The incidence of other gynaecological disorders in the benzene-exposed group was, for inflammation of the uterus and tubes 9·3% (other groups 5·4–18·4%), for diseases of the cervix and vagina 6·1% (others 3·8–17·2%), for prolapse of the uterus and vagina 2·3% (others 0·8–11·8%). No information is given about their methods for ascertainment of the information on gynaecological disorders and no details are given about the nature of the menstrual disturbances. The frequency of the latter did not appear to be particularly high in comparison with the other groups of workers studied but more information would be needed to properly evaluate this study.

Mukhametova and Vozovaya (1972) have studied menstrual function in female gluing operatives in a mechanical-rubber product factory, exposed to petroleum and chlorinated hydrocarbons, particularly dichloroethane and methylene chloride. Since petroleum is a major source of benzene exposure, this study is considered for convenience in this section. Exposure levels in the air were not given but were stated to be for petroleum "as a rule within or lower than the maximum permissible levels" and for chlorinated hydrocarbons, "in 58·5% of the tests did not exceed the maximum permissible level, but in 41·5% they were 1·2–2·4 times higher". Apart from exposure by inhalation there was additional exposure through skin contact with these substances. The women were studied by "detailed interrogation" using a team including an obstetrician, gynaecologist, a therapist and a haemopathologist. A total of 360 exposed women aged 20–40 years were studied. Of these, 39·2% had worked on production for up to 3 years, 37·2% for 3–5 years and 23·6% for more than 6 years. They were compared with 616 women workers similar in age but with no contact with the chemical substances concerned. No further details about the control group were given. Gynaecological disorders were found in 54·2% of the exposed group compared with 33·1% of controls. In the exposed group these broke down into menstrual disorders (26·1%), inflammation of the sexual organs (24·2%), prolapse of the uterus and vagina

(1·7%), infantilism (1·1%) and benign tumours of the genitalia (0·6%). In controls menstrual disorders occurred in 15·2% of the group compared with 26·1% of the exposed group; hyper-polymenorrhoea (undefined) was found 3 times more often in the exposed group (10·6%) compared with controls (3·2%); acyclical disturbances (undefined) were found in 6·1% of the exposed group but only in 1·9% of controls. There was a direct relationship between disturbances of the menstrual cycle and length of service. Other gynaecological disorders were found most frequently in those who had worked on production for more than 5 years. The differences between exposed and control groups for disturbances of menstrual function were stated to be significant, but in the absence of any precise definitions for the disorders discussed, this study is difficult to evaluate. It is also not possible to assess the relative contribution of benzene and the chlorinated hydrocarbons to the changes in menstrual function observed.

C. FERTILITY

Mukhametova and Vozovaya (1972) also reported on fertility in the study discussed in detail in section B. Of the 360 female gluing operatives exposed to petroleum and chlorinated hydrocarbons, it was stated that 88·8% were sexually active and 91·1% had had one or more pregnancies. No comparable figures were given for the 616 controls. The incidence of infertility (undefined) was similar in the 2 groups, 2·9% in the gluing operatives and 2·4% in controls. The average number of pregnancies/woman from the time they had worked in the factories was 2·8 for both groups.

There have been no studies traceable on the effects of benzene on male fertility.

D. PREGNANCY

The study of Mukhametova and Vozovaya (1972), discussed in detail in section B, also included analysis of the records of 510 pregnant women and their previous childbearing history. Of these, 250 were gluers, exposed to petroleum and chlorinated hydrocarbons and 260 were from the control group. Abortion (mostly induced) was the outcome of the majority of pregnancies in both groups; only 25·8% of pregnancies in the gluing operatives and 30·3% in controls resulted in normal childbirth. However, there was a significant difference in the incidence of spontaneous abortions and premature births (figures for these 2 not given separately); in the gluing operatives 17·2% of pregnancies ended in this manner compared with 4·9% in controls.

Comparing the reproductive histories of gluing operatives before and after they started work at the factory showed a 3·4 fold increase in spontaneous abortions and a 3·7 fold increase in premature births, the frequency of premature births increasing with duration of employment in the factory, whereas in the control group of workers there was a marked reduction (figures not given) in those 2 types of event after starting work in the factory. In the gluers pregnancy and birth complications were recorded in 35·6% of all pregnancies compared with 15·5% in controls; these comprised mainly "late toxicoses" (? toxaemia) in 16·8% of gluers compared with 8·4% of controls, premature births in 11·2% of gluers compared with 4·2% of controls, and threatened abortion in 4·0% of gluers compared with 1·5% of controls. It should be noted that these latter figures for premature births, when taken in conjunction with the earlier combined figures for spontaneous abortion and premature births imply very low spontaneous abortion rates of 5·0% for gluers and 0·7% for controls. The accuracy of the above data may therefore be in some doubt, though the figures may be low because some of the induced abortions might otherwise have aborted spontaneously.

At birth and in the neonatal period there were also more complications in the gluing operatives than in controls. Pathology associated with incorrect implantation and detachment of the placenta was found in 8·8% of gluers compared with 4·2% of controls. Fetal asphyxia occurred in 6·8% of gluers and 2·6% of controls. The complications of pregnancy and labour may also have contributed to the higher perinatal mortality (predominantly stillbirths) in the gluers of 6·3%, compared with 1·8% in controls.

Whilst the differences in the events and outcomes of pregnancy listed above between gluing operatives and controls were not always statistically significant, they add up to a fairly convincing picture of an increased incidence of pregnancy and childbirth complications in the group exposed to petroleum and chlorinated hydrocarbons. However it should be noted that the percentages given in some instances are based on only 65 births in the exposed group and 79 births in controls, the majority of pregnancies in the original groups (510 in total) being terminated by induced abortion. It is also not known how closely the 2 groups were matched for factors other than age and being in work. There may have been nutritional and socio-economic differences between the 2 groups which could contribute to the pregnancy problems. Thus it is not known what relative contribution, if any, exposure to benzene and chlorinated hydrocarbons may have had to the outcomes observed, but this study clearly indicates there may be problems with exposure to such agents and further studies are urgently required.

In the study of Mikhailova *et al.* (1971), also discussed in detail in section B, the incidence of spontaneous abortions and premature births for women exposed to benzene and its homologues was given as 4·6%, compared with rates in other groups of 2·1% (noise), 2·8% (shop workers), 2·9% (lead), 4·6% (superphosphate), 6·5% (mercury), 9·8% (physical labour), 11·8% (vibrations) and 14·1% (shocks). The numbers of pregnancies these percentages are calculated from are not given.

A few case reports of benzene poisoning in pregnancy have appeared in the literature subsequent to the early reports up to 1930 (reviewed by Hunt, 1979). Ragucci (1969) mentioned 15 cases of benzene poisoning in pregnancy collected by Tara in 1938 (original reference not given); there were 4 normal births, 3 cases of uterine inertia, one stillbirth and 7 spontaneous abortions. No further details were given.

Riera-Bartra and Señor (1957) have recorded one case of a 29-year-old para 4 woman with no previous history of pregnancy complications, who was exposed to benzene through her work in toy manufacture and developed aplastic anaemia. She presented in the seventh month of pregnancy with severe haemorrhage and delivered a premature fetus which survived and had no visible morphological abnormalities nor any haematological abnormalities. However, after delivery, severe uterine bleeding continued and the woman died 36 h later. The child survived without problems to one year of age at the last ascertainment.

Messerschmitt (1972) has reviewed 5 cases of exposure to benzene inducing the onset of aplastic anaemia in pregnancy taken from the literature of 1934–1957. Three were exposed to "benzenic solvents" and 2 to "arsenobenzenes". The women were aged 22–32, 3 in their first pregnancy, one in the third and one in the fourth. Diagnosis of aplastic anaemia was in the fourth to ninth months of pregnancy. In 2 cases there was abortion at 5 months; the fetus died in both cases, one mother died, the other survived. In one case there was delivery at 7 months and the child survived but the mother died (this is the case of Reira-Bartra and Señor (1957) already mentioned). In the last 2 cases delivery was at 9 months, one child died and one survived but both the mothers died. Thus the fetal prognosis may be slightly better than the maternal prognosis with delivery after the 7th month.

Holmberg (1979) has published a study of 14 mothers of children with congenital central-nervous system defects with their matched pair controls (see Styrene section D for details). Case mothers had been exposed to organic solvents during the first trimester of pregnancy significantly more often than controls ($p < 0{\cdot}01$); of 120 cases of CNS defects collected from the Finnish Register of Congenital Malformations in 1976–1978, 16 had been exposed to organic solvents compared with 3 controls. Two of the 16 cases were excluded (one because of rubella infection, the other with diagnosis of Beckwith-Wiedemann syndrome). Of the remaining 14 cases, one had been exposed to benzene, dichloromethane, methanol and ether in a laboratory and the child was a stillborn anencephalic. The mother was aged 32 and had had no previous abortions or defective children and was not given any drugs during pregnancy. However, no conclusions can be drawn on the basis of this one case.

E. MUTAGENICITY

In vitro testing of human lymphocytes with benzene added to the culture medium has produced conflicting results. Koizumi *et al.* (1974) reported increased chromosome aberrations (breaks, gaps) at dose levels of benzene of $1{\cdot}1 \times 10^{-3}$ and $2{\cdot}2 \times 10^{-3}$ M. In a subsequent study Koizumi *et al.* (1979) could find no increase in the frequency of sister-chromatid exchange (SCE) using similar concentrations *in vitro*. Similarly, Gerner-Smidt and Friedrich (1978) failed to show any increase in SCE or chromosomal aberrations in human lymphocytes cultured *in vitro* with 15·2–1520 μg benzene/ml of culture medium.

There have been a number of studies of chromosomal changes in workers exposed to benzene following the first observation by Pollini and Columbi in 1964 of lymphocyte chromosome damage in patients with benzene-induced aplastic anaemia. These studies have been reviewed elsewhere (Committee on Toxicology, 1976; Frohberg, 1974) and will not be discussed in detail here. General conclusions emerging from these studies are that, excluding concurrent absorption from the skin, chromosomal changes have been found only after many years of exposure to high benzene concentrations in the air and no chromosomal changes have been detected so far where exposure levels in the air were below 15 ppm. In the studies published up to 1973, increased rates of chromosomal aberrations in the lymphocytes have been found in all patients with clinical signs of chronic benzene toxicity and in about 50% of those exposed to benzene but with no clinical signs of poisoning. None of the studies have shown a correlation between persistence of chromosomal changes and the degree of benzene poisoning or duration of benzene exposure, but quantitative data on total exposure is sparse and the accuracy of the levels that are quoted is not known. Age is also known to be an important factor (Tough *et al.*, 1970) and must be controlled for in studies attempting to relate cytogenetic damage to duration of exposure. In some cases in these studies, workers were also exposed to other chemicals besides benzene.

Three of the published studies are of particular interest for this review and will be discussed in more detail. Pollini *et al.* (1976) have shown persistent changes in DNA in 4 female subjects 10 years after the diagnosis of benzene-induced poisoning (haemopathy), despite substantial progress towards normalization of the karyotype; fine structural changes persisted in the DNA of the interphase nucleus, manifested as a quantitative increase in Feulgen-reactive nuclear material. In other subjects, of advanced age these same authors have noted close correlation between aneuploidy and increased Feulgen-reactive DNA.

Another study showing the persistence of benzene-induced changes has been carried out by Forni *et al.* (1971). They have shown persistence of chromosome aberrations which in most cases were still present several years after exposure to benzene had ceased. Many of these exposures were heavy, resulting in clinical signs of benzene poisoning. Abnormal clone formation in peripheral lymphocytes was noted in a few cases but it is not yet known if these are related to later development of leukaemia (see section F). Two of the 34 cases in this study were pregnant at the time of investigation and chromosome studies on the offspring were carried out in one case. This case presented with pancytopenia at 8 months of pregnancy from occupational exposure to benzene during the last year. Whilst still severely pancytopenic, the patient delivered an apparently normal boy, but herself had severe haemorrhagic problems. One year later, the patient delivered a normal girl. Chromosome studies of the mother showed an increased rate of aberrations at the time of both pregnancies, but cytogenetic analysis of the newborn baby boy revealed no abnormalities. The baby girl was not studied. No conclusions may be drawn from this single report and further studies in this area are needed.

One study of the children of exposed workers has been carried out by Funes-Cravioto *et al.* (1977). They studied the incidence of chromosome aberrations in cultured lymphocytes from 73 workers in chemical laboratories and the printing industry. They found a significantly increased incidence, approximately two-fold, of chromatid and iso-chromatid breaks when compared with 49 controls. A similar increased incidence was also observed in 14 children aged 4–11 years of 11 women laboratory workers who had worked during pregnancy. There was also an increased incidence of sister-chromatid exchange in 12 technicians and in the 4 children of 2 of the female technicians who had worked during pregnancy. The technicians came from 8 different laboratories but all were exposed to one or more of chloroform, toluene, benzene, cyclohexane, diethyl ether, isooctane, methanol, toluene or xylene, with chloroform, benzene and toluene being most common, though the atmospheric concentrations of these solvents was not measured in most instances. In a group of 34 of the subjects there was a correlation between the frequency of chromosome breaks and duration of exposure. There was no correlation between exposed mothers and their children, with sex or smoking habits. The subjects and controls in this study were not carefully matched and it is impossible to state that the chromosome aberrations were a direct result of exposure to organic solvents, but this was a common factor in all the working environments studied. The biological significance of the changes observed is unknown as far as the health of workers is concerned.

F. CARCINOGENICITY

IARC Monograph Vol. 7 (1974) reported that it is established that benzene or benzene-containing mixtures result in damage to the haematopoietic system and that a relationship between such exposure and the development of leukaemia is suggested by many case reports and a case-control study. A more recent evaluation (IARC Monograph Vol. 29, 1982 in press) concluded that there is now sufficient evidence that benzene is carcinogenic to man causing leukaemia.

SUMMARY AND EVALUATION

EXPERIMENTAL STUDIES

One study has reported damage to the testis of rats, guinea pigs and rabbits exposed to around 80 ppm for 8–10 months but no studies of effects on male fertility have been found. Limited studies have shown no adverse effects in females at non-toxic doses. The effects of benzene during pregnancy have been studied in mice, rats and rabbits, and the adequately controlled studies have consistently shown no embryolethal or teratogenic effects even at maternally toxic doses. Reduced fetal weight and retardation have been observed.

It is not mutagenic in bacterial systems but several reports show mutagenic activity *in vivo*. There is limited evidence that it is carcinogenic in animals.

HUMAN STUDIES

Women are more susceptible to benzene toxicity than men possibly because of greater uptake and fat storage. Benzene crosses the placenta and is present in fetal blood in amounts equal to or greater than in maternal blood. Anaemia and menstrual disorders have been reported in women exposed to benzene. No studies on male or female fertility from benzene exposure alone were found. Several reports have suggested an increased abortion rate in women exposed to benzene and in rare cases of aplastic anaemia due to benzene exposure, parturition has had a fatal outcome for the mother. Chromosomal damage has been reported in people exposed to toxic amounts of benzene or to high levels for many years. No chromosomal changes were seen below 15 ppm exposure. It is thought to cause leukaemia secondarily to its toxic effect on the haematopoietic system.

EVALUATION

Data on fertility is inadequate for assessment. There is sufficient evidence that it is not embryotoxic or teratogenic in animals though toxic doses may retard fetal development. There is limited evidence that it may cause menstrual disorders in exposed women, and with high or prolonged exposure may be mutagenic. Attention is drawn to the lack of data on effects in males and to the need for adequate data on effects in pregnancy. It is a human carcinogen and attention is drawn to the lack of data on transplacental carcinogenesis.

References

Avilova, G. G. and Ulanova, I. P. (1975). Comparative characteristics of the effect of benzene on the reproductive function of adult and young animals. *Gigiena Truda i Professional 'nye Zabolevaniya* **(2)**, 55–57.

Batra, B. K. (1959). The effect of methylcholanthrene painting of the ovaries on the progeny of mice. *Acta Unionis internationalis contra cancrum* **15**, 128–133.

Batra, B. K. (1966). A study of reproduction and ovarian histology in mice treated with a chemical carcinogen. *Indian Journal of Experimental Biology* **4**, (3), 139–143.

Committee on Toxicology, Assembly of Life Sciences, National Research Council (1976). Health effects of benzene: A review. National Academy of Sciences, Washington D.C., U.S.A.

Dean, B. J. (1969). Chemical-induced chromosome damage. *Laboratory Animals* **3**, (2), 157–174.

Dean, B. J. (1978). Genetic toxicology of benzene, toluene, xylenes and phenols. *Mutation Research* **47**, (2), 75–97.

Desoille, H., Philbert, M. and Albahary, C. (1962). Incidences hormonales sur le benzénisme chronique du lapin. III. Influence du sexe, de la castration et de l'hormonothérapie sexuelle homologue ou hétérologue sur les globules rouge du lapin soumis a une intoxication benzénique de courte durée (42 jours). IV. Influence des oestrogènes naturels et des androgènes administrés au long cours (105 jours) sur le taux des globules blancs et rouges du lapin mâle et femelle normaux. V. Influence du sexe, de la castration et de l'hormonothérapie sexuelle homologue ou hétérologue sur les globules blancs et rouges du lapin soumis a une intoxication benzénique au long cours (98 jours). *Archives des Maladies Professionelles de Médecine du Travail et de Sécurité Sociale* **23**, (12), 757–785.

Desoille, H., Albahary, C. and Philbert, M. (1963). Incidences hormonales sur le benzénisme chronique du lapin. IV. Influence de la gestation sur le taux des globules blancs et des globules rouges de la lapine soumise ou non à une intoxication benzénique modérée pendant toute la durée de la gravidité. *Archives des Maladies Professionelles de Médecine du Travail et de Sécurité Sociale* **24**, (12), 867–879.

Desoille, H., Albahary, C. and Philbert, M. (1965). Incidences hormonales sur le benzénisme chronique de la rate. Influence de la gestation sur le taux des globules blancs et des globules rouges de la rate soumise ou non à une intoxication benzénique modérée pendant toute la durée de la gravidité. *Archives des Maladies Professionelles de Médecine du Travail et de Sécurité Sociale* **26**, (4–5), 205–220.

Desoille, H., Philbert, M. and Albahary, C. (1967). Hormonal incidences of chronic benzene poisoning in guinea pigs. Influence of gestation on white and red corpuscle levels in guinea pigs submitted or not to moderate benzene poisoning during the entire gestation period. *Archives des Maladies Professionelles, de Médecine du Travail et de Sécurité Sociale* **28**, (3), 329–339.

Dobrokhotov, B. (1972). Mutagenic effect of benzene and toluene under experimental conditions. *Gigiena I Sanitariya* **37**, (10), 36–39.

Dobrokhotov, B. and Enikeev, M. I. (1977). Mutagenic action of benzene, toluene and a mixture of these hydrocarbons in a chronic experiment. *Gigiena I Sanitariya* **42**, (1), 32–34.

Dowty, B. J., Laseter, J. L. and Storer, J. L. (1976). The transplacental migration and accumulation in blood of volatile organic constituents. *Pediatric Research* **10**, 696–701.

Forni, A. M., Cappellini, A., Pacifico, E. and Vigliani, E. C. (1971). Chromosome changes and their evolution in subjects with past exposure to benzene. *Archives of Environmental Health* **23**, (5), 385–391.

Frohberg, H. (1974). Problems encountered in the toxicological testing of environmental chemicals. *Environmental Quality and Safety* **3**, 57–84.

Funes-Cravioto, F., Kolmodin-Hedman, B., Lindsten, J., Nordenskjold, M., Zapata-Gayon, C., Lambert, B., Norberg, E., Olin, R. and Swenson, A. (1977). Chromosome aberrations and sister-chromatid exchange in workers in chemical laboratories and a rotoprinting factory and in children of women laboratory workers. *Lancet* **ii**, 322–325.

Gerner-Smidt, P. and Friedrich, U. (1978). The mutagenic effect of benzene, toluene and xylene studied by the SCE technique. *Mutation Research* **58**, (2/3), 313–316.

Gofmekler, V. A., Pushkina, N. N. and Kletsova, G. N. (1968). Various biochemical shifts during a study of the embryotropic effect of benzene and formaldehyde. *Gigiena I Sanitariya* **33**, (7), 96–98.

Gofmekler, V. A. (1968). The embryotropic action of benzene and formaldehyde in experimental administration by inhalation. *Gigiena I Sanitariya* **33**, (3), 12–16.

Green, J. D., Leong, B. K. J. and Laskin, S. (1978). Inhaled benzene fetotoxicity in rats. *Toxicology and Applied Pharmacology* **46**, 9–18.

Holmberg, P. C. (1979). Central-nervous-system defects in children born to mothers exposed to organic solvents during pregnancy. *Lancet* **ii**, 177–179.

Hudák, A. and Ungváry, G. (1978). Embryotoxic effects of benzene, and its methyl derivatives: toluene, xylene. *Toxicology* **11**, 55–63.

Hunt, V. R. (1979). Work and the Health of Women. CRC Press, Inc., Florida, U.S.A.

IARC Monographs on the Evaluation of the Carcinogenic Risk of Chemicals to Humans: Some anti-thyroid and related substances, nitrofurans and industrial chemicals (1974). Vol. 7, Lyon, France.

Iwanaga, R., Suzuki, T. and Koizumi, A. (1970). Changes in growth and hematopoietic functions in mice, mothers of which had been injected with benzene during gestation period. *Japanese Journal of Hygiene* **25**, (5), 438–445.

Kissling, M. and Speck, B. (1971). Chromosome aberrations in experimental benzene intoxication. *Helvetica Medica Acta* **36**, (1), 59–66.

Koizumi, A., Dobashi, Y., Tachibana, Y., Tsuda, K. and Katsunuma, H. (1974). Cytokinetic and cytogenic changes in cultures of human lymphocytes HeLa cells induced by benzene. *Industrial Health (Japan)* **12**, 23–29.

Koizumi, A., Dobashi, Y. and Tachibana, Y. (1979). Chromosome changes induced by industrial chemicals. *Japanese Journal of Industrial Health* **21**, (1), 3–10.

Leong, B. K. J. (1977). Experimental benzene intoxication. *Journal of Toxicology and Environmental Health*, Supplement 2, 45–61.

Lyapkalo, A. A. (1973). Genetic activity of benzene and toluene. *Gigiena Truda I Professional 'nye Zabolevaniya* **17**, (3), 24–28.

Matsumoto, N., Ijima, S. and Katsunuma, H. (1975). Effect of benzene on fetal growth with special reference to the different stages of development in mice. *Congenital Anomalies* **15** (2), 47–58.

Messerschmitt, J. (1972). Bone marrow aplasias during pregnancy. *Nouvelle Revue Francaise d'Hematologie* **12**, (1), 15–28.

Michon, S. (1965). Disturbances of menstruation in women working in an atmosphere polluted with aromatic hydrocarbons. *Polski Tygodnik Lekarski* **20**, 1648–1649.

Mikhailova, L. M., Kobyets, G. P., Lyubomudrov, V. E. and Braga, G. F. (1971). The influence of occupational factors on diseases of the female reproductive organs. *Pediatriya Akusherstvo Ginekologiya* **33**, (6), 56–58.

Mukhametova, I. M. and Vozovaya, M. A. (1972). Reproductive power and the incidence of gynecological affections in female workers exposed to the combined effect of benzine and chlorinated hydrocarbons. *Gigiena Truda i Professional 'nye Zabolevaniya* **16**, (11), 6–9.

Murray, F. J., John, J. A., Rampy, L. W., Kuna, R. A. and Schwetz, B. A. (1979). Embryotoxicity of inhaled benzene in mice and rabbits. *American Industrial Hygiene Association Journal* **40**, (11), 993–998.

Nawrot, P. S. and Staples, R. E. (1979). Embryofetal toxicity and teratogenicity of benzene and toluene in the mouse. *Teratology* **19**, (2), 41A.

Philip, P. and Jensen, M. K. (1970). Benzene induced chromosome abnormalities in rat bone marrow cells. *Acta Pathologica et Microbiologica Scandinavica Section A* **78**, 489–490.

Pollini, G., Biscaldi, G. P. and de Stefano, G. F. (1976). Increase in Feulgen-reactive material in peripheral blood lymphocytes of subjects ten years after benzene poisoning. *Medicina del Lavoro* **67**, Suppl. No. 5, 506–510.

Ragucci, N. (1969). Exogenous poisonings and pregnancy. *Minerva Ginecologica* **21**, (18), 1163–1171.

Rickert, D. E., Baker, T. S., Bus, J. S., Carrow, C. S. and Irons, R. D. (1979). Benzene disposition in the rat after exposure by inhalation. *Toxicology and Applied Pharmacology* **49**, 417–423.

Riera-Bartra, L. and Señor, J.-C. (1957). Anemia aplastica y gestacion. *Medicina Clinica* **29**, 388–390.

Rusch, G. M., Leong, B. K. J. and Laskin, S. (1977). Benzene metabolism. *Journal of Toxicology and Environmental Health* Supplement **2**, 23–36.

Sato, A., Nakajima, T., Fujiwara, Y. and Hirosawa, K. (1974). Pharmacokinetics of benzene and toluene. *Internationale Archiv fur Arbeitsmedizin* **33**, (3), 169–182.

Sato, A., Nakajima, T., Fujiwara, Y. and Murayama, N. (1975). Kinetic studies on sex difference in susceptibility to chronic benzene intoxication—with special reference to body fat content. *British Journal of Industrial Medicine* **32**, 321–328.

Solomon, N. S. and Batra, B. K. (1964). Changes in the cleaving ova of mice following carcinogen treatment of the preovulatory eggs. *Nucleus* **7**, (2), 71–76.

Sridharan, B. N., Batra, B. K. and Savkur, L. D. (1963). The effect of a carcinogen on the progeny of treated mice. *Indian Journal of Pathology and Bacteriology* **6**, (1), 26–33.

Tough, I. M., Smith, P. G., Brown, W. M. C. and Harnden, D. G. (1970). Chromosome studies on workers exposed to atmospheric benzene. The possible influence of age. *European Journal of Cancer* **6**, (1), 49–55.

Watanabe, G. and Yoshida, S. (1970). The teratogenic effect of benzene in pregnant mice. *Acta Medica et Biologica Niigata* **17**, 285–291.
Wolf, M. A., Rowe, V. K., McCollister, D. D., Hollingsworth, R. L. and Oyen, F. (1956). Toxicological studies of certain alkylated benzenes and benzene. *A.M.A. Archives of Industrial Health* **14**, 387–398.

5. Benzo(a)pyrene

TECHNICAL DATA

Formula	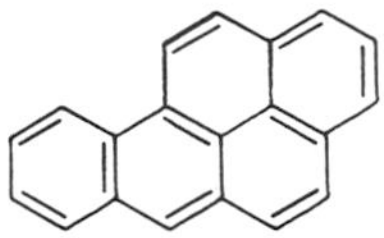 [structural formula]
CAS registry number	50–32–8
Chemical abstracts name	Benzo(a)pyrene
Synonyms	3,4-Benzopyrene; 1,2-Benzopyrene; 3,4-Benzpyrene; 1,2-Benzpyrene; B(a)P.
Uses	As a reagent for the determination of cadmium which is precipitated as $(C_{13}H_9N)_2\ H_2(CdI_4)$ from dilute nitric or sulfuric acid solution in the presence of potassium iodide.
TLV	None

ANIMAL STUDIES

A. RELEVANT PHARMACOLOGY AND TOXICOLOGY

Metabolism of benzo(a)pyrene (BP) by the liver is important since BP itself is not carcinogenic but its metabolites, which bind to protein and DNA, are. In rat liver homogenates, benzpyrene hydroxylase converts BP to 3-hydroxy-BP, 1,2-dihydro-1,2-dihydroxy BP, and 9,10-dihydro-9,10-dihydroxy BP (Sims, 1970). The capacity of maternal and fetal tissues to metabolize BP and the placental transfer of metabolites will influence the transplacental carcinogenicity of BP (see section F).

Placental transfer of BP has been shown in the mouse and the rat. Shendrikova *et al.* (1974) injected pregnant mice i.v. with 15 mg/kg BP on days 17–19 of pregnancy. Measurable levels of BP were found in the fetus within 5 min of administration to the dam and levels peaked at 1·3–3·2 ppm by 15 min. By 4–6 h only traces remained in the fetus. Levels in maternal liver also peaked around 15 min at 48–86 ppm and fell to very low levels by 6 h after injection. Placental levels were not measured.

Shendrikova and Aleksandrov (1974) have shown placental transfer of BP in the rat. On day 21 of pregnancy, rats were given 200 mg/kg BP orally by gavage and killed 3 h later. BP was found at mean concentrations of 2·8, 3·9 and 23·5 ppm in fetal, placental and maternal liver tissue respectively. Study of the pharmacokinetics of placental transfer in the mouse and rat shows that transfer of BP is by simple diffusion only (Baranova *et al.*, 1976).

Raimondi and Pagani (1967) have shown that passage of BP and/or its metabolites into the rat fetus may depend on the vehicle used for administration of the compound to the dam. When radiolabelled BP was given in oil from day 3 of pregnancy onwards, radioactivity levels in the fetuses increased gradually throughout gestation, but if BP was given in water-soluble 40% vitamin PP complexes, radioactivity levels in the fetus declined during gestation. These results mirrored placental levels of radioactivity which increased with administration of BP in oil and decreased with administration in water-soluble complexes. However if administration was continued after delivery of the litters, the reverse was seen; pup radioactivity levels increased in those suckled by dams given BP in water-soluble complexes, suggesting transfer into the milk, but decreased below levels found at birth in those suckled by dams given BP in oil. The major proportion of BP in the milk is known to be in the fat portion (West and Horton, 1976), and one explanation for the above findings may be that BP administered in water is readily partitioned into the milk fat from maternal blood, but BP administered in oil only disperses from the vehicle slowly.

It is not known whether the radioactivity measured in the fetuses and pups in Raimondi and Pagani's experiments (1967) was BP itself or its hydroxymetabolites. There have been no systematic studies of placental transfer of BP metabolites, which may be more important than BP transfer in transplacental carcinogenicity (see section F).

West and Horton (1976) have shown that transfer of BP given in the diet to maternal milk during lactation is low in the rabbit and sheep. In rabbits, only 0·003% of dietary BP was found in the milk and in sheep 0·01% was found in the milk. In the rat, as much as 3% of the dose of a similar polycyclic aromatic hydrocarbon, 3-methylcholanthrene, may be transferred into the milk. It is likely that BP behaves similarly, but no definitive studies have been done on transfer into the milk in rodents.

B. ENDOCRINE AND GONADAL EFFECTS

Males

Payne (1958) has noted marked changes in the testes of rats given a single i.p.

injection of 4 mg of BP at 6 months of age. They were killed 12 months after injection. In 3/30 males interstitial cell tumours were found compared with none in controls (number not specified). In the remaining BP-treated males there was complete absence of interstitial tissue and in many there was atrophy of the seminiferous tubules with absent spermatids and spermatozoa. In some tubules, only Sertoli cells and a few spermatocytes remained. Abdominal tumours and lesions of the liver, kidney and adrenal were also seen in these rats. Payne (1958) also refers to earlier reports of atrophy of the seminiferous tubules and reduced spermatogenesis following i.p. or s.c. injection of BP in the rat, in experiments carried out in the 1930s and 1940s (original papers not seen by us).

Wyrobek and Bruce (1975) have looked at the effect of BP on sperm morphology. Mice were given 5 consecutive, daily i.p. injections of 20 or 100 mg/kg and sperm morphology was examined at 0, 4 and 10 weeks after the end of dosing, covering exposure of spermatids, spermatocytes and spermatogonia respectively to BP. At 100 mg/kg, 15–20% of sperm were abnormal at 4 and 10 weeks after exposure. At other times and at all times after 20 mg/kg no increase was seen over the background control abnormality rate of 1–3%. Some animals died in the 100 mg/kg group.

Females

Rigdon and Rennels (1964) have studied the effect of BP in the diet on the rat oestrous cycle. Eight female rats were given 1 mg BP/g of food for 28 days. Cycles continued to be regular in all but one animal which had a 12-day dioestrous period, attributed to induction of pseudopregnancy by the vaginal smear technique used. Subsequent pregnancies in the BP fed group were abnormal (see section D).

Payne (1958) has looked at the effect of BP on ovarian and uterine histology. Ten female rats were injected with a single dose of 10 mg of BP i.p. and killed 12 months later. The ovaries were found to contain few normal follicles and mainly large cysts and the uteri were very hyperplastic. Abdominal tumours, and lesions of the liver, kidney and adrenal gland were also seen at autopsy. Payne (1958) also referred to earlier reports of cystic ovaries and suppression of ovulation in experiments carried out in the 1930s and 1940s where rats were given BP s.c. or i.p.

C. FERTILITY

Males

In a series of poorly controlled experiments, Rigdon and Neal (1965) have looked at fertility in male mice fed BP in the diet. In one experiment, 5 males were given 0·25 mg BP/g of food during the daytime. At night (no food allowed) they were mated with untreated females. After 6, 13 and 28 days on the diet they mated, but only 1/5, 0/5 and 2/5 females delivered young after each of these matings. In another experiment, however, equivocal effects on fertility were seen with 2/5 pregnancies resulting from mating after 21 days on the BP diet, 6/10 pregnancies after 31 days on the diet, and 4/10 pregnancies from the same males after being on BP diet for 34 days and returning to normal diet for 21 days. In another experiment, male mice were fed 0·5 mg BP/g of food. Before treatment 5/5 mated with untreated females who all delivered young. After 23 days on the diet each male was mated twice and 9/10 females delivered young. When killed after 30 days on the diet, spermatozoa were seen in the tubules of the testes, but no further information on testicular histology was given. No control data on fertility was given in these experiments.

In a dominant lethal study in the mouse, Epstein *et al.* (1972) have shown a decrease in pregnancy rate (13–29% pregnant) and a significant increase in early embryonic deaths or decreased implants/dam following a single i.p. injection of 500, 750 or 1000 mg/kg, doses which were lethal to some males. But in the six different experiments carried out at these doses using 3- or 8-week mating periods there was a lack of consistency in the parameter affected and in the magnitude of effect between experiments.

Females

Rigdon and Neal (1965) have also looked at female fertility during feeding of BP in the diet. Female mice were fed 0·25, 0·5 or 1·0 mg BP/g of food for varying periods before, during and after mating. Dietary levels of 0·25 and 0·5 mg/g were without effect in terms of number of litters produced and litter size, but no other details are given of these results. At a dietary level of 1 mg/g, equivocal results were obtained; 14 females were fed BP for 19–29 days then switched to normal diet during mating and pregnancy, and 7/14 delivered young compared with 3/6 controls. The 3 females on the BP diet for the longest period, 29 days, each had litters.

Males and females

Rigdon and Neal (1965) also mated BP-treated male mice with BP-treated females. Males were fed 0·25 mg/g of diet for 9 days then placed with females, both being fed 0·25 mg/g during the mating period. All 5 females became pregnant, 4 delivered live young and 1 female was thought to have delivered and eaten her young. In another experiment, where the duration of pre-mating treatment was not stated, Rigdon and Rennels (1964) mated BP-treated male rats with BP-treated female rats, using a dietary level of 1 mg/g of food, and continuing the diet throughout pregnancy. It resulted in 2 pregnancies from 7 mated females with complete fetal death and resorption in both cases.

Marked effects on fertility have been seen in male and female mice exposed prenatally to BP (see section D).

Conclusion
The studies of Rigdon and colleagues on effects of dietary BP on male and female fertility do not permit any conclusions to be drawn; only small numbers of animals were used, controls were not always included, and where they were, their fertility was often as poor as 50%. In BP-treated groups, results from different experiments using the same dose were inconsistent and effects seen at one dose were not seen at a higher dose. Inconsistent effects were also noted in a dominant lethal study, suggesting that BP may only affect a certain sub-group of exposed animals. Much larger experiments using adequate numbers of animals of proven fertility are needed to clarify the effects of BP. When BP is added to the diet, food consumption is known to vary widely, some animals showing a marked reduction in intake. Administration of BP should be such as to avoid this major confounding factor.

D. PREGNANCY

Mouse
Mackenzie *et al.* (1979) gave mice 10, 40 or 160 mg/kg/day BP orally on days 7–16 of pregnancy. At 160 mg/kg/day "pregnancy maintenance" was reduced by 25% and there was slight fetotoxicity with delayed ossification in the fetuses. The most dramatic effect, however, was on the fertility of offspring born to dams given 40 or 160 mg/kg. Ninety-seven percent of these offspring were completely infertile. Fertility was also decreased in those exposed prenatally to 10 mg/kg, female offspring giving birth to significantly fewer and smaller litters during several months of breeding and male offspring showing a 50% reduction in fertility. In female offspring many of the BP-exposed animals had no ovaries at all or hypoplastic remnants of ovarian tissue only, with delayed or absent follicular development. In male BP-exposed offspring the testes and seminiferous tubules were small and there was an increase in the quantity of interstitial tissue. There was also germ cell aplasia and altered spermatogenesis. This study is reported in abstract only and no further details are given.

Rigdon and Neal (1965) fed BP in the diet to 9 mice at a concentration of 1 mg/g of food from the fifth or the tenth day of pregnancy onwards through lactation. In these 2 groups 5/9 and 7/9 carried normal-sized litters. Of those that were allowed to deliver, the dams cannibalized part or the whole of their litters, the surviving young showed slow development and a number died before weaning. Maternal food consumption was decreased in the BP-fed groups. No further information and no control data are given. Subsequent experiments using very small numbers of mice fed 0·25 mg BP/g of food during pregnancy and/or lactation suggested that the effects on postnatal weight gain of the offspring were due not to prenatal exposure nor postnatal exposure to BP itself, but due to lower food consumption by the dams in the BP groups during lactation. However the methodology and reporting of these experiments is very inadequate, and the suggestion of no direct toxicity of BP on the offspring would require confirmation.

Rat

Rigdon and Rennels (1964) fed 8 female rats diet containing 1 mg BP/g of food for 28 days before mating and throughout pregnancy. Only 5/8 became pregnant compared with 3/3 controls. The 3 controls delivered normal litters of 3, 6 and 11 pups, but only 1/5 of the BP group delivered a litter, comprising 2 dead and 2 live pups, all of which were small and 1 grossly malformed. Three of the remaining 4 dams showed vaginal bleeding only at the expected delivery date, suggesting fetal resorption had occurred and the remaining dam was hysterectomized on day 20 of pregnancy and found to contain 6 grossly abnormal fetuses. The small numbers used in this experiment do not permit any firm conclusions to be drawn about the effects of BP in the rat.

Wolfe and Bryan (1939) injected 17 rats s.c. with 5 mg BP/day from the first day of pregnancy until killed between day 10 and day 18 of pregnancy. There was no effect on implantation, but profuse continuous vaginal bleeding was seen beginning around day 10–12 of pregnancy and there was extensive haemorrhaging around the lateral margins of the placentae with resorption of fetuses in all the dams.

Sheveleva (1978) has given a total of 100 rats 0, 0·05, 0·5 or 5 mg BP/kg/day orally by gavage on days 1–15, 3–4 or 9–10 of pregnancy. The dams showed signs of maternal toxicity including decreased weight gain and haematological changes with doses of 0·5 and 5 mg/kg on days 1–15. At these doses she noted dose-related increases in pre- and post-implantation losses, decreased live fetuses/dam and decreased fetal weights on day 20. Quantitative details were not given. Examination of the fetuses showed an increased incidence of liver haemorrhage, hydronephrosis and bladder dilatation in BP-exposed groups with no such effects in controls. Again, quantitative information was not given. At 0·05 mg/kg, fetuses showed generalized oedema (51%), hydronephrosis (6%), and bladder dilatation (1%) with 1 fetus showing multiple abnormalities. When BP was given on days 3–4 only, there were increased pre- and post-implantation losses, decreased fetal weight, and liver haemorrhages in the fetuses. When BP was given on days 9–10, post-implantation losses increased, fetal weights decreased, and fetal haemorrhages increased. No quantitative data were given and it is not clear if these results applied to all three dose levels.

Raimondi and Pagani (1967) have noted premature delivery in dams given

BP in water-soluble 40% vitamin PP complexes, but not in dams given BP in oil, using the intramuscular route, from day 15 of pregnancy onwards. No further details are given and the dose is not stated.

Conclusion

BP has a variety of unusual effects on the offspring after prenatal exposure. It does not appear to show conventional embryotoxic or teratogenic effects, but in the mouse, at doses causing slight fetotoxicity (160 mg/kg/day orally) or lower (down to at least 10 mg/kg/day orally), marked adverse effects on subsequent fertility of the offspring are seen in the absence of any other effects. Doses of 5 mg/kg/day s.c. in the rat totally disrupt pregnancy causing extensive placental haemorrhage. When given late in pregnancy BP is a transplacental carcinogen causing tumours at doses which are less tumourigenic in adults than offspring (see section F for details). One poorly reported study has shown embryolethality, teratogenicity and fetotoxicity in the rat at doses as low as 0·05 mg/kg/day orally. Replication of this study is needed before any conclusions can be drawn about a no-effect level for BP in pregnancy.

E. MUTAGENICITY

Sugiyama (1973) has shown increased chromosomal aberrations in dividing bone marrow cells from rats injected i.v. with 50 mg/kg BP. Twelve and 24 h after injection 14% and 9% of cells respectively had aberrations compared with 2% in controls.

Basler and Rohrborn (1976) have shown a similar increase in chromosome aberrations (mainly gaps) in dividing bone marrow cells of Chinese hamsters given BP orally at doses of 450 mg/kg × 2 (3% aberrations), 180 mg/kg × 5 (7% aberrations), or 450 mg/kg × 5 (13% aberrations) compared with controls (1% aberrations). They also showed mutagenic effects in mouse oocytes. After synchronizing ovulation, 450 mg/kg BP was given orally by gavage 24 h later. Nine percent of oocytes showed aberrations compared with 1% for controls.

F. CARCINOGENICITY

IARC Monograph Vol. 3 (1973) reported on studies showing BP was carcinogenic in all nine species tested following different routes of administration including oral, skin and intratracheal routes.

Transplacental carcinogenicity

As mentioned in section A, BP itself is not carcinogenic but its hydroxymetabolites are. Thus the time of appearance of significant benzpyrene hydroxylase activity in the placenta has a bearing on the potential of BP to act as a transplacental carcinogen. The benzpyrene hydroxylase activity of the fetal liver may also be relevant, but it should be noted that its activity is generally low, and that placental transfer of BP is thought to be small (see section A). However benzpyrene hydroxylase activity can be induced by exposure to BP.

In the mouse and rat the amounts of BP metabolites in the maternal blood and liver, following a single oral administration of 40 mg/kg BP on one of days 6, 8, 12 or 15 of pregnancy, were highest following treatment on day 15, suggesting an increasing capacity for metabolism as pregnancy advances (Lin *et al.*, 1976). This may be due to increasing placental enzyme activity.

In the rat, Juchau (1971) has shown a peak in placental benzpyrene hydroxylase activity on days 17–19 of pregnancy in animals pretreated on day 15 with another polycyclic aromatic hydrocarbon, 3-methylcholanthrene (MC). Without pretreatment, enzyme activity is fairly low in maternal liver, placenta and fetal liver. Gillette *et al.* (1973) have shown that fetal liver benzpyrene hydroxylase activity in the rabbit is also low without pretreatment. After pretreatment with MC in the rat, Bogdan and Juchau (1970) have shown benzpyrene hydroxylase activity is increased 30-fold, 11-fold, and 12-fold in maternal liver, placenta and fetal liver respectively. Welch *et al.* (1972) have shown that for enzyme induction in the rat, 40-fold higher doses of BP are needed to stimulate fetal liver activity than for stimulation of maternal liver activity.

Juchau (1971) has also shown a number of biochemical similarities between human and rat placental benzpyrene hydroxylase, including inhibition by oestrogens, which, as pregnancy advances, may offset the developmental increases in benzpyrene hydroxylase activity. This suggests that studies in the rat may serve as a suitable model for the human in this respect.

Clearly, prior treatment with BP or another polycyclic aromatic hydrocarbon in pregnancy increases the metabolic capacity for any subsequent BP exposure and increases the likelihood of transplacental carcinogenesis. Formation of tumours in mouse offspring exposed prenatally to BP was first shown by Bulay and Wattenberg (1970, 1971). The dams were injected with 4 mg BP i.p. on days 11, 13 and 15 of pregnancy and allowed to litter out. The pups were then reared by control dams to eliminate the possibility of postnatal exposure to BP in the milk. Lung adenomas developed in 67% of BP-exposed offspring compared with 11% and 14% in vehicle and untreated controls. Tumours of the peripheral nerves and kidneys have been seen in offspring of rabbits injected i.v. with 30 mg/kg on day 25/26 of pregnancy (Dimant and Beniashvili, 1978).

Since then, there have been several demonstrations of induction of hyperplasia and tumours in cultured fetal mouse kidney and lung cells taken just before term from dams injected with 4 mg BP in the last week of pregnancy (Sorokina, 1971; Shabad *et al.*, 1972, 1975).

Nikonova (1977) has shown increased susceptibility of offspring compared with their mothers following s.c. injections of 4–12 mg BP into mice on day 18–19 of pregnancy. Tumours of the lung, liver and mammary gland were seen in both offspring and dams, but the numbers of tumours and multiplicity of sites were always higher in the offspring compared with their mothers.

Andrianova (1971) has shown increased susceptibility of adult mice to BP-induced tumours from skin painting when also exposed prenatally to BP. For four generations, pregnant females were skin painted with one drop of 0·5% BP solution, twice a week throughout pregnancy. From 8 weeks of age onwards the male offspring were exposed once a week to the same dose of BP and the development of papillomas and carcinomas monitored. In prenatally exposed males the tumours appeared earlier than in non-prenatally exposed males also painted with BP. The effect was maximal in the second generation.

Conclusion

There is clear evidence that BP is a transplacental carcinogen causing tumours at doses which are less tumourigenic in adults than in offspring. Since no threshold level has been shown for this carcinogen in adults, it may be that there is not any no effect-level for BP transplacental carcinogenicity.

HUMAN STUDIES

A. RELEVANT PHARMACOLOGY AND TOXICOLOGY

There have been a number of studies to investigate whether human placental tissue and human fetal tissue is capable of metabolizing benzo(a)pyrene (BP) to its reactive intermediate epoxides, and if so, at what stage of gestation the capacity develops.

Studies on BP hydroxylase activity in the human placenta have been numerous since it was first shown in 1969 that maternal smoking induces BP hydroxylase activity (reviewed by Juchau, 1973) and only a few studies will be referred to here. BP hydroxylase, otherwise known as aryl hydrocarbon hydroxylase, may be induced by a variety of polycyclic aromatic hydrocarbons including BP, such as are present in car exhausts, some factory emissions and cigarette smoke. The latter is probably the most important source of exposure in pregnant women. BP hydroxylase activity in human placenta is higher at term than in the first two trimesters and is far higher on average in placentae of smokers as compared to non-smokers, but even in smokers, detectable levels do not appear until 11–13 weeks gestation (Juchau, 1971). The enzyme system is localized in the endoplasmic reticulum. Jones and Juchau (1977) have shown that placental microsome preparations from smokers, but not from non-smokers, can catalyse the activation of BP to metabolites which are mutagenic in bacteria. However, whilst there is little doubt that placentae from smokers have the capacity to metabolize BP to reactive intermediates, little is known about how quickly these products may be inactivated by further metabolism or conjugation *in vivo*, nor to what extent the high oestrogen and progesterone levels near term, which are known to inhibit BP hydroxylase (Juchau, 1971) may actually protect the fetus from exposure to mutagens.

BP hydroxylase activity is also found in a variety of fetal tissues, particularly the liver, adrenal gland and kidney (Pelkonen *et al.*, 1971; Juchau *et al.*, 1972). In fetal and placental tissue of 8–26 weeks gestation, enzyme activity levels in fetal liver are higher than in placenta and do not appear to increase markedly with gestational age (Pelkonen *et al.*, 1971). The enzyme activity in fetal liver preparations is generally lower than that in adult human liver microsomes, when based on microsomal protein (Rane *et al.*, 1973). Pelkonen *et al.* (1973) using fetal tissue from 9–22 weeks gestational age found fetal liver BP hydroxylase activity averaged only 2·4% of adult liver activity, but in adults there was wide variability (9-fold) between individuals. Pelkonen and Kärki (1973) have shown BP hydroxylase activity in human fetal liver as early as 6–7 weeks gestation in abortuses from both smokers and non-smokers and in those with no history of drug exposure during pregnancy. They could not detect activity in the placenta at 5–8 weeks gestation. They noted that the appearance of fetal liver activity coincides with the time of appearance of smooth endoplasmic reticulum in the fetal liver. Belitsky *et al.* (1977) have shown BP hydroxylase activity in human fetal liver at 10–12 weeks gestation with much lower activity in fibroblasts taken from the same embryos.

These *in vitro* studies show that fetal liver has a measurable but limited capacity to metabolize BP from 6–7 weeks gestation onwards, independent of maternal smoking habits, and that placental capacity does not develop until 11–13 weeks gestation in smokers and remains very low in non-smokers. There is clearly in smokers a fairly considerable capacity to metabolize BP in maternal liver, placenta, fetal liver and perhaps other fetal tissues such as the adrenal, though Jones and Juchau (1977) have shown minimal or no capacity *in vitro* for human fetal liver, adrenal, ovary, pancreas or spleen to generate BP metabolites mutagenic to bacteria. Whether sufficient reactive intermediates pass across the placenta and/or are generated in the fetus *in vivo* to induce mutagenic or carcinogenic changes is not known.

B. ENDOCRINE AND GONADAL EFFECTS

No relevant data found.

C. FERTILITY

No relevant data found.

D. PREGNANCY

No relevant data found. (Review of the numerous studies on the adverse effects of smoking on outcome of pregnancy, in which BP may possibly play a role, is beyond the scope of this review.)

E. MUTAGENICITY

Rüdiger *et al.* (1976) have shown a doubling of the background rate of sister-chromatid exchange (SCE) in cultured human lymphocytes exposed to 10^{-6} M BP for 70 h. Addition of alpha-naphthylflavone, which inhibits the formation of water-soluble products of BP metabolism by more than 95%, prevented the increase in SCE.

F. CARCINOGENICITY

There are no studies which have looked into the question of whether BP is a human transplacental carcinogen. The prediction has been made that if this were the case then the offspring of women smokers should have an increased risk of developing cancer compared with offspring of non-smokers (Everson, 1980; Hinds and Kolonel, 1980). No adequate studies to test this hypothesis have yet been carried out.

In an *in vitro* experiment by Lasnitzki (1956) explants of human fetal lung tissue taken from therapeutic abortion material of 12–20 weeks gestation and cultured in the presence of one or 4 μg BP/ml of medium for 4 weeks, showed hyperplasia of the bronchiolar epithelium. The newly formed cells showed irregular enlargement and abnormal mitosis. If cultured in the presence of 6 μg/ml, there were not only individual hyperplastic foci but also increased general proliferation resembling adenomatous change. Whilst this study may indicate the potential of human fetal tissue to undergo neoplastic change with exposure to BP and its metabolites, cells in culture for long periods of time may change their characteristics from the *in vivo* situation.

IARC Monograph Vol. 3 (1973) reported that at that time no epidemiological studies on the significance of BP exposure in humans were available, and other studies were insufficient to prove that BP is carcinogenic in humans.

SUMMARY AND EVALUATION

EXPERIMENTAL STUDIES

Placental transfer of BP has been shown in the mouse and the rat and limited transfer into the breast milk in the rabbit and sheep. In male rats a single injection i.p. of 4 mg BP causes loss of interstitial tissue and atrophy of the seminiferous tubules of the testis. At doses of 100 mg/kg/day i.p. for 5 days, lethal to some rats, abnormal sperm morphology has been seen 1 and 10 weeks after exposure. There is limited evidence that BP may cause suppression of ovulation and cystic ovaries in female rats. Poorly designed studies on fertility in male and female mice have produced equivocal results, and a single dominant lethal study has also produced equivocal results.

When given during pregnancy, BP at 40 or 160 mg/kg/day in the mouse is slightly fetotoxic and causes infertility in male and female offspring exposed prenatally. One poorly reported study in the rat claimed to show embryolethality, teratogenicity and fetotoxicity at doses as low as 0·05 mg/kg/day orally. An early study showed complete resorption of embryos in the rat following 5 mg/kg/day s.c.

BP is mutagenic to bone marrow cells and mouse oocytes in *in vivo* tests. It is carcinogenic in 9 species tested and has been shown to be a transplacental carcinogen in the mouse, causing tumours at doses which are less tumourigenic in adult mice than in offspring.

HUMAN STUDIES

No studies were found on endocrine or gonadal effects, or of effects on fertility or pregnancy. An increased frequency of sister-chromatid exchange has been shown in lymphocytes cultured *in vitro* in the presence of BP. There is insufficient evidence to show it is a carcinogen in humans and no evidence on its transplacental carcinogenicity, though the placenta and fetal tissues can metabolize BP to its reactive intermediates.

EVALUATION

There is limited evidence to suggest that BP may damage the testis in animals and may cause infertility in male and female offspring exposed prenatally. There is adequate evidence that it is a transplacental carcinogen in the mouse. Data on the effects of BP on the ovaries and on fertility are inadequate for assessment.

Attention is drawn to the lack of evidence on the effects of BP on reproduction in humans.

References

Andrianova, M. (1971). Transplacental action of 3-methylcholanthrene and benz(a)pyrene on four generations of mice. *Bulletin of Experimental Biology and Medicine (USSR)* **71**, (6), 677–680.

Baranova, L. N., Shendrikova, I. A., Aleksandrov, V. A., Likhachev, A., Ivanov-Galitsin, M. N., Dikun, P. P. and Napalkov, N. P. (1976). Problem of the mechanism of penetration of carcinogenic polycyclic hydrocarbons through the placenta of rats and mice. *Doklady-Akademii Nauk SSSR* **228**, 733–736.

Basler, A. and Rohrborn, G. (1976). Chromosome aberrations in oocytes of NMRI mice and bone marrow cells of Chinese hamsters induced with 3,4-benzpyrene. *Mutation Research* **38**, (5), 327–332.

Belitsky, G. A., Erizer, T. L., Grinberg, K. N. and Khesina, A. Y. (1977). Benz(a)pyrene metabolism in cultured liver cells of human embryo. *Voprosy Onkologii* **23**, (6), 69–73.

Bogdan, D. P. and Juchau, M. R. (1970). Characteristics of induced benzpyrene hydroxylase activity in the rat foeto-placental unit. *European Journal of Pharmacology* **10**, 119–126.

Bulay, O. M. and Wattenberg, L. W. (1970). Effects of administration of polycyclic hydrocarbon carcinogens during pregnancy on the progeny. *Federation Proceedings* **29**, (2), 818.

Bulay, O. M. and Wattenberg, L. W. (1971). Carcinogenic effects of polycyclic hydrocarbon carcinogen administration to mice during pregnancy on the progeny. *Journal of the National Cancer Institute* **46**, (2), 397–402.

Dimant, I. N. and Beniashvili, O. S. (1978). Some aspects of transplacental carcinogenesis in rabbits. *Bulletin of Experimental Biology and Medicine (USSR)* **85**, (3), 369–372.

Epstein, S. S., Arnold, E., Andrea, J., Bass, W. and Bishop, Y. (1972). Detection of chemical mutagens by the dominant lethal assay in the mouse. *Toxicology and Applied Pharmacology* **23**, 288–325.

Everson, R. B. (1980). Individuals transplacentally exposed to maternal smoking may be at increased cancer risk in adult life. *Lancet* **ii**, 123–126.

Gillette, J. R., Menard, R. H. and Strip, B. (1973). Active products of fetal drug metabolism. *Clinical Pharmacology and Therapeutics* **14**, 680–692.

Hinds, M. W. and Kolonel, L. N. (1980). Maternal smoking and cancer risk to offspring. *Lancet* **ii**, 703.

IARC Monographs on the Evaluation of the Carcinogenic Risk of Chemicals to Man: Certain polycyclic aromatic hydrocarbons and heterocyclic compounds (1973). Volume 3, Lyon, France.

Jones, A. H. and Juchau, M. R. (1977). Conversion of procarcinogens to mutagens by enzymes in human fetal and placental tissues. *Pharmacologist* **19**, (2), 201.

Juchau, M. R. (1971). Human placental hydroxylation of 3,4-benzpyrene during early gestation and at term. *Toxicology and Applied Pharmacology* **18**, 665–675.

Juchau, M. R., Pedersen, M. G. and Symms, K. G. (1972). Hydroxylation of 3,4-benzpyrene in human fetal tissue homogenates. *Biochemical Pharmacology* **21**, 2269–2272.

Juchau, M. R. (1973). Placental metabolism in relation to toxicology. *CRC Critical Reviews in Toxicology* **2**, (2), 125–158.

Lasnitzki, I. (1956). The effect of 3-4-benzpyrene on human foetal lung grown in vitro. *British Journal of Cancer* **10**, 510–516.

Lin, T. H., Sperling, F. and Ottley, M. S. (1976). Benzpyrene metabolism in induced rat pseudopregnant decidua and in placentas of pregnant rat and mice: developmental variations and comparisons. *Toxicology and Applied Pharmacology* **37**, 126–127.

Mackenzie, K. M., Lucier, G. W. and McLachlan, J. A. (1979). Infertility in mice exposed prenatally to benzo (a) pyrene (BP). *Teratology* **19**, (2), 37A.

Nikonova, T. V. (1977). Transplacental action of benzo(a)pyrene and pyrene. *Byulleten Eksperimental Noi Biologii I Meditziny* **84**, (7), 88–91.

Payne, S. (1958). The pathological effects of the intraperitoneal injection of 3:4-benzpyrene into rats and mice. *British Journal of Cancer* **12**, 65–74.

Pelkonen, O. and Kärki, N. T. (1973). 3,4-Benzpyrene and aniline are hydroxylated by human fetal liver but not by placenta at 6–7 weeks of fetal age. *Biochemical Pharmacology* **22**, 1538–1540.

Pelkonen, O., Arvela, P. and Kärki, N. T. (1971). 3,4-Benzpyrene and n-methylaniline metabolizing enzymes in the immature human foetus and placenta. *Acta Pharmacologica et Toxicologica* **30**, (5–6), 385–395.

Pelkonen, O., Kaltiala, E. H., Larmi, T. K. I. and Kärki, N. T. (1973). Comparison of activities of drug-metabolizing enzymes in human fetal and adult livers. *Clinical Pharmacology and Therapeutics* **14**, (5), 840–846.

Raimondi, L. and Pagani, G. (1967). Research on the placenta of pregnant rats after injection of tritiated benzpyrene. *Bollettino Societa Italiana di Biologia Sperimentale* **43**, (21), 1465–1466.

Rane, A., Sjoqvist, F. and Orrenius, S. (1973). Drugs and fetal metabolism. *Clinical Pharmacology and Therapy* **14**, (4), 666–672.

Rigdon, R. H. and Rennels, E. G. (1964). Effect of feeding benzpyrene on reproduction in the rat. *Experientia* **20**, (4), 224–226.

Rigdon, R. H. and Neal, J. (1965). Effects of feeding benz(a)pyrene on fertility, embryos, and young mice. *Journal of the National Cancer Institute* **34**, 297–305.

Rüdiger, H. W., Kohl, F., Mangels, W., von Wichert, P., Bartram, C. R., Wöhler, W. Y. and Passarge, E. (1976). Benzpyrene induces sister chromatid exchanges in cultured human lymphocytes. *Nature* **262**, 290–292.

Shabad, L. M., Sorokina, J. D., Golub, N. I. and Bogovski, S. P. (1972). Transplacental effect of some chemical compounds on organ cultures of embryonic kidney tissue. *Cancer Research* **32**, 617–627.

Shabad, L. M., Kolesnichenko, T. S. and Nikonova, T. V. (1975). Transplacental and direct action of benzo(a)pyrene studied in organ cultures of embryonic lung tissue. *Neoplasma* **22**, (2), 113–122.

Shendrikova, A. and Aleksandrov, V. A. (1974). Comparative penetration of polycyclic hydrocarbons through the rat placenta into the fetus. *Bulletin on Experimental Biology and Medicine (USSR)* **77**, 169–171.

Shendrikova, I. A., Ivanov-Golitsyn, M. N. and Likchachev, A. Y. (1974). The transplacental penetration of benz(a)pyrene in mice. *Voprosy Onkologii* **20**, (7), 53–56.

Sheveleva, G. A. (1978). On the effect of 3,4-benzpyrene on the development of the foetus applied at different stages of gestation. *Gigiena Truda I Professional'nye Zabolevaniya* **7**, (54).

Sims, P. (1970). The metabolism of some aromatic hydrocarbons by mouse embryo cell cultures. *Biochemical Pharmacology* **19**, 285–297.

Sorokina, Y. D. (1971). Transplacental action of benz(a)pyrene in organ cultures of mouse embryonic kidneys. *Bulletin of Experimental Biology and Medicine (USSR)* **71**, 294–297.

Sugiyama, T. (1973). Chromosomal aberrations and carcinogenesis by various benz(a)anthracene derivatives. *Gann* **64**, 637–639.

Welch, R. M., Gommi, B., Alvares, A. P. and Conney, A. H. (1972). Effect of enzyme induction on the metabolism of benzo(a)pyrene and 3′-methyl-4-monomethylaminoazobenzene in the pregnant and fetal rat. *Cancer Research* **32**, 973–978.

West, C. E. and Horton, B. J. (1976). Transfer of polycyclic hydrocarbons from diet to milk in rats, rabbits and sheep. *Life Sciences* **19**, 1543–1552.

Wolfe, J. M. and Bryan, W. R. (1939). Effects induced in pregnant rats by injection of chemically pure carcinogenic agents. *American Journal of Cancer* **36**, 359–368.

Wyrobek, A. J. and Bruce, W. R. (1975). Chemical induction of sperm abnormalities in mice. *Proceedings of the National Academy of Sciences of the U.S.A.* **72**, (11), 4425–4429.

6. Beryllium

TECHNICAL DATA

Formula	Be
CAS registry number	7440–41–7
Chemical abstracts name	Beryllium
Synonyms	Glucinium
Uses	Source of neutrons when bombarded with alpha particles. In beryllium copper and beryllium aluminium alloys. In aerospace structures.
TLV	$0{\cdot}002\ mg/m^3$

ANIMAL STUDIES

A. RELEVANT PHARMACOLOGY AND TOXICOLOGY

Sex differences in beryllium distribution in the principal sites of retention, after transthoracic injection of beryllium sulphate into the lung, have been shown in the mouse by Clary *et al.* (1972). Two months after injection, females had significantly higher liver and lung contents and significantly lower skeletal contents than males. This finding may be relevant to the onset of disease, since translocation from the bone to the liver triggers systemic disease, characterized by weight loss and liver necrosis (Clary *et al.*, 1972).

The influence of pregnancy on beryllium-induced disease has been investigated since it has been postulated that situations of adrenal imbalance, such as the "stress" of pregnancy, might trigger the onset of chronic disease (Clary and Stokinger, 1973). However, in the rat, repeated pregnancies after a single intratracheal dose of beryllium oxide had no effect on the number, severity, or time of onset of lung lesions, whilst renal tubular necrosis was increased in one experiment at 12 and 15 months after injection but not in a replicate experiment (Clary *et al.*, 1975). Adrenal function is altered during pregnancy in many species including humans. However, free, biologically active corticosteroid levels are generally increased in pregnancy, whereas studies on non-pregnant animals show it is primarily reduced adrenal function which increases susceptibility to beryllium-induced disease (Clary and Stokinger, 1973; Clary *et al.*, 1972) and ACTH and adrenal steroids are used in treatment of disease (Clary *et al.*, 1975). Clearly, there is no adequate delineation of the factors involved in the onset of formerly latent disease, nor confirmation in animals of pregnancy altering the course of disease.

Placental transfer of beryllium in the rat has been shown by Clary *et al.* (1975). Low but detectable levels of radiolabelled beryllium were found in fetuses from dams in the last third of pregnancy following a single intratracheal dose of beryllium oxide. Schulert *et al.* (1969) have also shown very low transfer of radiolabelled beryllium to the fetus after maternal i.v. injection in the rat; on day 14 of pregnancy, placental and fetal levels were 0·14% and 0·006% of the dose respectively, and on day 20, 0·16% and 0·017% of the dose respectively.

B. ENDOCRINE AND GONADAL EFFECTS

No relevant data found.

C. & D. FERTILITY AND PREGNANCY

Low fertility, increased stillbirths and retarded postnatal growth has been recorded in cattle herds in Missouri, U.S.A. by Case *et al.* (1972) where geochemical studies revealed high levels of a number of elements including beryllium, but the role of beryllium, if any, in these disturbances is impossible to assess and the metabolic disturbances observed resembled molybdenosis.

Clary *et al.* (1975) gave a single intratracheal administration of 0·2 mg beryllium as beryllium oxide to male and female rats which were bred repeatedly over the subsequent 15 months. There were no effects on fertility, number of live and dead pups at birth, postnatal survival or weaning weight. If anything, the breeding performance of beryllium treated males and females was better than controls.

E. MUTAGENICITY

IARC Monograph Vol. 23 (1980) reviews mutagenicity tests showing beryllium sulphate is inactive in the Ames test and host-mediated assay, but beryllium chloride has caused chromosome aberrations and mitotic delay in cultured peripheral lymphocytes and primary kidney cells of the domestic pig.

F. CARCINOGENICITY

IARC Monograph Vol. 23 (1980) reports that beryllium compounds are carcinogenic in the rabbit, rat and monkey. There have been no studies on the transplacental carcinogenicity of beryllium.

HUMAN STUDIES

A. RELEVANT PHARMACOLOGY AND TOXICOLOGY

An important general paper has been published by Creason *et al.* (1976) on the levels of 16 trace elements in normal term "fetal" blood, in placenta and in maternal blood and hair samples. Analysis was carried out on 25 maternal-fetal sets from each of 8 areas co-operating in a Community Health surveillance programme in the U.S.A. and were analysed for As, B, Ba, Be, Cd, Cr, Co, Cu, Fe, Pb, Li, Mn, Hg, Ni, Se, Ag, Sn, V and Zn. The samples were obtained from patients in obstetric hospitals and were from normal pregnancies and deliveries. Values are given for the levels of trace elements in maternal scalp and pubic hair, maternal venous blood, cord blood and placenta. Significant geographic differences were found in the levels of many of the elements but overall the values provide base-line data which would be useful for comparison with other studies. Levels of arsenic, beryllium and cobalt were not reported because very many of the values were below the level of detection (limit not stated).

B. ENDOCRINE AND GONADAL EFFECTS

No relevant data found.

C. FERTILITY

No relevant data found.

D. PREGNANCY

Hardy and Stoeckle (1959), in a review of beryllium disease, distinguish a number of causes of disease either from industrial exposure or neighbourhood exposure. Of over 40 cases from neighbourhood exposure, more than half were in persons exposed to fine dust brought home on the work clothes. The majority of the remainder lived close to the factories where it was used. The disease may be manifest as two separate syndromes—acute or chronic. The chronic disease usually develops some time after exposure ceases, less than 1 year in half of the cases but up to 15 years later in some. In some cases the acute form may resolve and later reappear as the chronic disease.

The majority (92%) of 247 cases on the beryllium register in 1959 with acute disease were men, but of the 382 cases with chronic disease, half were women. It was not known if this reflected exposure patterns or whether women were more susceptible than men to the chronic disease. The mortality was about one third of those who developed the disease within 5 years of exposure but fell to one fifth or less with longer intervals. The advent of steroid therapy, however, brought some improvement in these figures. Furthermore, the decision to omit beryllium from fluorescent lamps in 1949 markedly decreased the incidence of this disease. A maximum average exposure level of 2 $\mu g/m^3$/8 h day was proposed in 1949 and this was followed by a dramatic drop in the incidence of the disease. The peak concentration should not exceed 25 $\mu g/m^3$ and the neighbourhood concentration should not exceed an average of 0·01 $\mu g/m^3$.

In a subsequent most interesting review of beryllium poisoning, Hardy (1965) presented an analysis of the cases on the beryllium register up to 1965. There was then a total of 725 records since its inception in 1952. In general there was a correlation between intensity of exposure and severity of disease, though precise details of exposure amount and type were often lacking. However, she pointed out that certain physiological or pathological events could trigger the onset of symptoms. Analysis of 161 fatal cases is shown in Table 5 (a modified version of Table 11 in the original paper).

The precipitating role of pregnancy in 66% of the women who died is, as Hardy states, impressive. It is clear that in women with chronic berylliosis the risks of pregnancy are very high.

In the U.K. the incidence of beryllium poisoning is very low and in a recent review, Constantinidis (1978) estimated from the published literature that probably not more than 30 cases had ever been reported.

Kline *et al.* (1951) published the first report of the use of ACTH and cortisone in the treatment of a pregnant woman with chronic beryllium poisoning. From 17 to 19 years of age she had worked in a fluorescent tube factory and she was in good health when she had her first pregnancy at 23

TABLE 5
Possible precipitating factors in fatal cases (Beryllium Registry Data 1965)

Group	Factor	Number of cases
161 dead persons (includes 95 females)	Pregnancy related in time*	63
	Other toxic exposures	27
	Infections	31
	Surgery	11
	Others/excessive dieting, combat duty, etc.	49

* 18 of 28 dead in neighbourhood cases.

years of age. At 25 years she became pregnant for a second time and immediately began to lose weight with increasing dyspnoea, cough and weakness. She was admitted to hospital at 7 months of gestation with marked lung involvement, cyanosis and dyspnoea on the slightest exertion. She was treated with ACTH and later cortisone acetate. She improved steadily and 7 weeks later delivered a 2·75 kg boy. The mother continued to improve and was discharged on cortisone acetate. The boy was normal at birth but became severely hypoglycaemic after 48 h, probably from adrenal insufficiency. After cortisone and ACTH he improved and was discharged in good health. Twenty-four-hour urine specimens from the child taken on the second and third day of life contained a total of 0·4 and 0·015 mg of beryllium. Among the interesting features of this case are the delay between the exposure to beryllium and the onset of clinical disease which coincided with conception of the second pregnancy, although the pregnancy 2 years previously was uneventful. This is the only case we have found where the outcome of pregnancy was described.

E. MUTAGENICITY

IARC Monograph Vol. 23 (1980) reports on a single mutagenicity study where no chromosome aberrations were noted with 0·01 and 1 μM beryllium sulphate in human fibroblasts and human leukocytes *in vitro*.

F. CARCINOGENICITY

IARC Monograph Vol. 23 (1980) noted that the epidemiological evidence that occupational exposure to beryllium may lead to an increased risk of lung cancer is small. They concluded that beryllium should be considered suspect of being carcinogenic to humans.

SUMMARY AND EVALUATION

EXPERIMENTAL STUDIES

Low but detectable amounts of beryllium cross the placenta in the rat. One study in rats failed to demonstrate any effect of a single, intratracheal dose of beryllium on fertility of males or females or on pregnancy. No studies on endocrine or gonadal function or teratogenicity were found.

Mutagenicity tests on bacterial systems were negative, but positive results were obtained with mammalian somatic cells. It is carcinogenic in several species but no studies on transplacental carcinogenicity were found.

HUMAN STUDIES

No studies were found on endocrine or gonadal effects, or of effects on fertility. Records in a beryllium registry show that pregnancy may precipitate onset of disease symptoms, often with a fatal outcome. There is inadequate evidence on the effects of beryllium on the fetus.

Mutagenicity was not detected in one study on human fibroblasts and leucocytes *in vitro*. It is a suspected carcinogen in humans.

EVALUATION

There is inadequate data to assess the effects of beryllium on reproduction in animals. There is evidence of increased susceptibility to the toxicity of beryllium in pregnant women. There is inadequate data to assess the effects on the fetus.

References

Case, A. A., Selby, L. A., Hutcheson, D. P., Ebens, R. J., Erdman, J. A. and Feder, G. L. (1972). Infertility and growth suppression in beef cattle associated with abnormalities in their geochemical environment. *In* "Sixth Annual Conference on Trace Substances in Environmental Health" (Ed. Hemphill, D. A.), pp. 15–21. Memorial Union, University of Missouri, Columbia, MO, U.S.A.

Clary, J. J., Bland, L. S. and Stokinger, H. E. (1975). The effect of reproduction and lactation on the onset of latent chronic beryllium disease. *Toxicology and Applied Pharmacology* **33**, 214–221.

Clary, J. J., Hopper, C. R. and Stokinger, H. E. (1972). Altered adrenal function as an inducer of latent chronic beryllium disease. *Toxicology and Applied Pharmacology* **23**, 365–375.

Clary, J. J. and Stokinger, H. E. (1973). The mechanism of delayed biologic response following beryllium exposure. *Journal of Occupational Medicine* **15**, (3), 255–259.

Constantinidis, K. (1978). Acute and chronic beryllium disease. *British Journal of Clinical Practice* **32**, (5), 127–136, and 153.

Creason, J. P., Svendsgaard, D., Bumgarner, J., Pinkerton, C. and Hinners, T. (1976). Maternal-fetal tissue levels of 16 trace elements in 8 selected continental United States communities. *Trace Substances in Environmental Health* **10**, 53–62.

Hardy, H. L. (1965). Beryllium poisoning—Lessons in control of man-made disease. *New England Journal of Medicine* **273**, 1188–1199.

Hardy, H. L. and Stoeckle, J. D. (1959). Beryllium disease. *Journal of Chronic Diseases* **9**, 152–160.

IARC Monographs on the Evaluation of the Carcinogenic Risk of Chemicals to Humans: Some metals and metallic compounds (1980). Volume 23, Lyon, France.

Kline, E. M., Inkley, S. R. and Pritchard, W. H. (1951). Five cases from the fluorescent lamp industry. (Treatment of chronic beryllium poisoning with ACTH and cortisone.) *Archives of Industrial Health and Occupational Medicine* **3**, 549–564.

Schulert, A. R., Glasser, S. R., Stant, E. G., Brill, A. B., Koshakji, R. P. and Mansour, M. M. (1969). Development of placental discrimination among homologous elements. *Atomic Energy Commission Symposium Series* **17**, 145–152.

7. Boric Acid (Boron)

TECHNICAL DATA

Formula	H_3BO_3
CAS registry number	10043–35–3
Chemical abstracts name	Boric acid
Synonyms	Boracic Acid, orthoboric acid.
Uses	For weatherproofing wood and fireproofing fabrics; as a preservative; manufacturing cements, crockery, porcelain, enamels, glass, borates, leather, carpets, hats, soaps, artificial gems; in nickeling baths, cosmetics; printing and dyeing; painting, photography; for impregnating wicks; electric condensers; hardening steel.
TLV	None (other boron-containing compounds 1–10 mg/m^3).

ANIMAL STUDIES

A. RELEVANT PHARMACOLOGY AND TOXICOLOGY

The acute oral toxicity of boric acid in male and female rats has been investigated by Weir and Fisher (1972). The 14-day LD50 was marginally higher in females (4·08 g/kg) than in males (3·45 g/kg).

Truhaut *et al.* (1964) have stated, without giving any quantitative data, that boron compounds cross the placenta and "accumulate in the fetus".

B. ENDOCRINE AND GONADAL EFFECTS

Males

The adverse effects of boric acid on the testes have been studied using acute, sub-chronic and chronic dosing regimes by a variety of routes of administration. The majority of studies have been in the rat but a limited study in the dog confirms similar findings.

Boussou and Castagnol (1965) have studied the effect of single, large, oral doses of boric acid 1–5 g/kg given by gavage in rats over 7 weeks of age. Dose-related testicular lesions (not specified) were seen at all doses used, commencing 20–30 days after administration, reaching maximum intensity at 45–60 days and decreasing thereafter. By 130 days after dosing, all the rats bred normally. At single doses of 3 and 4 g/kg which were fatal to some rats (LD50 for boric acid in rats is 3–4 g/kg, Weir and Fisher (1972)), many tubules were normal, but slight atrophy of the seminiferous tubules was frequently seen and occasionally considerable atrophy accompanied by the absence of germ cells with a few intact Sertoli cells. The interstitial tissue was fibrous with Leydig cell hyperplasia. In a sub-chronic experiment by the same workers, similar changes were seen after oral dosing with 0·8 g/kg for 30 days, except that lesions were more extensive than after single doses. Dosing rats with the same schedule, 0·8 g/kg for 30 days, before puberty or around the time of puberty showed that damage similar to that in adults only occurred when boric acid was given at the onset of spermatogenesis. Administration before this time was without effect.

Ultrastructural changes in the testes have been described by Silaev *et al.* (1977) after oral administration of boric acid, 1 g/kg by gavage, to 12 rats for 2 weeks. Multinucleate cells, characteristic of testicular damage, were seen both in the spermatogenic epithelium and free in the seminiferous tubules. Germ cells were absent or reduced in number in some tubules. Dystrophic changes in the cellular organelles, cytoplasm and nucleus were evident in large numbers of spermatogenic cells.

Weir and Fisher (1972) investigated the effects of the sub-chronic feeding of boric acid in the diet of rats, including lower dose groups than those in the previously described studies. Addition of boric acid at 0, 52·5, 175, 525, 1750 or 5250 ppm as boron to the diet for 90 days, followed by autopsy (10 males per group), resulted in significantly decreased absolute and relative testicular weights at 1750 ppm, the lowest dose which reduced growth and food consumption. At 5250 ppm all rats died within 3–6 weeks. Histological examination of the testes showed complete atrophy in all males at 1750 ppm and partial atrophy in 1/10 males at 525 ppm. No adverse effects were seen at 175 or 52·5 ppm.

In a chronic experiment, Weir and Fisher (1972) added 117, 350 or

1170 ppm boron as boric acid to the diet of rats for 2 years with 35 males per group. By the 5th week of the study, signs of toxicity, including shrunken appearance of the scrotum, were evident in the 1170 ppm group, a dose which initially reduced food consumption and affected growth rate throughout the study. Autopsies at 6, 12 and 24 months showed significantly decreased absolute and relative testicular weights in all 1170 ppm males, with atrophy of the seminiferous epithelium and decreased tubular size. No testicular effects were seen at 117 or 350 ppm.

The studies of Truhaut *et al.* (1964) also show that chronic administration of high doses of boric acid to the rat adversely affect the testes. Groups of 10 males were given boric acid by one of 3 routes; 0·4 g/kg in aqueous solution by gavage for 24 months; 2·5 g/l in the drinking water (equivalent to 25–50 mg/rat/day or 125–250 mg/kg body weight for a 200 g rat) for 12 months; or 0·5 and 1·0 g boric acid/kg of diet (i.e. 87·5 and 175 ppm boron) for 8 months followed by 2 and 3 g/kg (350 and 525 ppm) respectively for the next 12 months. The results of the study were reported in qualitative terms only. Those given boric acid by gavage or in the drinking water became totally sterile, but there was no effect in the dietary groups until the doses were increased to 350 or 525 ppm. These males then became sterile by the eleventh month of the study. Their method of ascertaining sterility was not described, neither was histology carried out after the first 8 months of dietary feeding at 87·5 and 175 ppm to ascertain whether there really was no effect at these levels. At autopsy at the end of the study, all sterile males showed marked testicular atrophy with necrotic lesions in the seminiferous tubules. Some males were aspermatogenic with hyperplasia of the Sertoli cells. Spermatids were not destroyed but showed changes (unspecified) accompanied by formation of multinucleate cells. They also reported that only small amounts of boron could be detected in the testes.

In a chronic study on the rat, Krasovskii *et al.* (1976) added boric acid to drinking water in concentrations as low as 0·3, 1·0 and 6·0 mg/l boron, equivalent to 0·08, 0·3 and 1·7 mg/kg body weight of boric acid, for 6 months. At autopsy, a number of parameters of testicular function were impaired in a dose-related manner. Small, but statistically significant decreases in relative testicular weight, and number, motility, acid and osmotic resistance of spermatozoa were seen at 1·7 mg/kg, with smaller but still significant decreases in number and motility of spermatozoa at 0·3 mg/kg. Smaller, but non-significant reductions were seen in these parameters at 0·08 mg/kg.

Weir and Fisher (1972) also studied the effect of boric acid administration in the diet (17·5, 175 and 1750 ppm boron) to the dog, with 5 dogs per group. At levels of 175 and 1750 ppm for 90 days there were significant reductions in relative testicular weights. At 175 ppm, histological appearance of the testes was normal, but at 1750 ppm severe atrophy and almost complete degeneration of the spermatogenic epithelium was seen in all dogs. The effect on the testes was relatively selective since general appearance, body weight, food consumption and histological appearance of other organs was relatively normal in both dose groups. No adverse effects were seen at 17·5 ppm. In dogs fed 58, 117 or 350 ppm boron as boric acid in the diet for 2 years (4 dogs per group), no changes were seen in histology, relative or absolute organ weights. In view of the absence of effects at 350 ppm in the 2-year study (see below), it seems likely that the reduction in relative testicular weight at 175 ppm is of no biological significance. Additional dogs given 1170 ppm in the diet for 38 weeks confirmed the selective adverse effects of high doses on the testis; testicular degeneration with spermatogenic arrest and atrophy of the seminiferous epithelium occurred in all 4 treated dogs, but no other organ changes were seen. Two of the treated dogs were then put onto control diet for 25 days at the end of which period relative and absolute testicular weights were similar to controls and moderately active spermatogenesis was seen in one dog, indicating possible reversibility of the effects of boric acid.

Tarasenko *et al.* (1972) have exposed male rats to 3·8 or 19·2 ppm (9·6 or 48·6 mg/m^3) by inhalation 4 times a day for 4 months (English abstract only seen by us). Generally toxicity was "insignificant", but morphological changes and profound functional disturbances were seen in the testes, which led to sterility by the end of the experiment.

Females

Weir and Fisher (1972) also investigated the effect of boric acid on the rat ovary. In a sub-chronic study where 52·5, 175, 525, 1750 and 5250 ppm boron as boric acid were fed in the diet for 90 days (10 females per group), a significant decrease in absolute, but not relative, ovarian weight was seen at 1750 ppm, which was the lowest dose affecting food consumption and body weight. Histological changes in the ovary were not reported. At 5250 ppm the changes were described only as "small gonads". In the chronic, 2-year study (117, 350 and 1170 ppm boron equivalent in the diet, 35 females per group) no adverse effects on the ovaries were reported, though in a multigeneration experiment the same authors found evidence of reduced ovulation at 1170 ppm (see section C/D). It therefore seems possible that the reduction in absolute ovarian weight noted at 1750 ppm was simply secondary to the reduced body weight, the ovarian/body weight ratio remaining unchanged.

In the study by Truhaut *et al.* (1964) where boric acid was given by gavage (0·4 g/kg for 24 months), or in the drinking water (2·5 g/l for 12 months), or in the diet (0·5 and 1·0 g/kg of diet for 8 months followed by 2 and 3 g/kg for 12 months), with 10 females per group, no lesions of the reproductive tract were seen.

Conclusion

The effects of boric acid on the histological appearance of the gonads seem confined to the male, where a selective toxic effect on the testes has been seen in both the rat and the dog. In the rat, although doses which resulted in microscopical pathological changes in the testes also reduced body weight, caused inflammation of the eyes and paws, and desquamated skin on the paws and tail, they did not cause histological changes in any other internal organs.

Testicular effects were observed in the dog in the absence of any other changes at 1 dose level. Limited information from the rat and dog suggests that these changes may be reversible. The similarity of the general toxic effects and reproductive toxicity of various boron compounds suggests that it is the boron itself which is the damaging agent, not just boric acid which has been considered in detail here. The specific toxicity to the testis is further underlined by the observation that only small amounts of boron reach the testis.

Although details of food and water intake were not given in all cases, estimates of the intake of boric acid can be made. These show that in rats a daily intake equivalent to 150 mg/kg boric acid or above, produces histological evidence of damage to the seminiferous tubules and sterility. There was either focal damage to segments of tubule or generalized effects on spermatozoa at low doses, or more extensive damage involving the stem cells at high doses. One study in rats showed small but significant reductions in sperm count and motility with doses as low as 0·3 mg/kg. The fertility of these animals was not tested.

In dogs similar results were found at doses approximately equivalent to 480 mg/kg, but no effect was found at about 150 mg/kg fed for 2 years.

C. & D. FERTILITY AND PREGNANCY

Weir and Fisher (1972) studied the effects of boric acid in a multigeneration test in the rat. Groups of 8 males and 16 females received 117, 350 or 1170 ppm boron as boric acid in the diet, commencing 14 weeks before the first breeding. Three generations were bred in a conventionally designed study with derivation of subsequent generations from second litters. Treated males were mated with treated females. At 117 and 350 ppm there were no adverse effects on reproduction; fertility and lactation indexes were generally higher in the boric-acid treated groups than in controls. No gross abnormalities were seen in either parents or weanlings.

As expected from their observations of severe testicular damage at 1170 ppm in the 2-year study (described in section B), Weir and Fisher found that in the 1170 ppm group the Fo males were completely sterile and at autopsy no viable spermatozoa were found in the atrophied testes. More surprisingly, 1170 ppm treated females mated with control males failed to produce litters and at autopsy evidence of decreased ovulation (presumably reduced numbers of corpora lutea) was found. No histological changes in the ovary were seen however in their 2-year study at 1170 ppm (Weir and Fisher, 1972).

Truhaut *et al.* (1964) in a descriptive study giving no quantitative data also noted absence of ovarian lesions and normal fertility in female rats given similar doses of boric acid by gavage (0·4 g/kg for 24 months) or in the drinking water (2·5 g/l for 12 months), when mated to control males. However, the offspring were stillborn or died within 3–4 days of birth. When boric acid was fed in the diet at 0·5 g/kg of diet (87·5 ppm boron equivalent) for 8 months, there was no effect on reproduction, but at 1·0 g/kg (175 ppm) for 8 months, litter size at birth was decreased by about 25%, and when dietary levels were increased in these 2 groups to 2 and 3 g/kg of diet (350 and 525 ppm) for the next 12 months, high perinatal mortality was again seen. These results are at variance with those of Weir and Fisher (1972) who found 350 ppm was without effect.

Conclusion

In multigeneration studies with boric acid given in the diet one study reports a no-effect level between 350 and 1170 ppm, and another study reports a no-effect level between 87·5 and 175 ppm. Due to inadequate reporting of details the latter study cannot be assessed. Further studies are needed to establish a clear no-effect level for fertility and no studies have been carried out where boric acid is given during embryogenesis and fetogenesis only, to ascertain whether it has any teratogenic effects.

E. MUTAGENICITY

No relevant data found.

F. CARCINOGENICITY

No relevant data found.

HUMAN STUDIES

A. RELEVANT PHARMACOLOGY AND TOXICOLOGY

Ploquin (1967), in a review of boron in food, stated that boron, especially in the form of boric acid and borates, is widespread in our environment. The average daily intake in man is 25 mg boron/day with a range (in France) of 4–40 mg/day. Blood levels of boron in man averaged 9·85 μg/100 g with a range from 3·9–36·5 μg/100 g, with blood boric acid values in children of 0·4–0·6 mg/100 ml (equivalent to 70–100 μg boron/100 ml). Levels of 8 mg/100 ml have been found in children after accidental ingestion of boric acid solution without symptoms and in true poisoning cases levels are of the order of 350 mg/100 ml (equivalent to 62 mg/100 ml of boron). Although boron is usually considered as a chronic poison, it has been estimated that effects are unlikely to be seen at an intake of less than 100 mg boron/day. Although boron is known to be an essential element for plants, it is not known whether it is essential for man.

B. & C. ENDOCRINE AND GONADAL EFFECTS AND FERTILITY

Following experiments in rats given boric acid in the drinking water (see Animal studies), Krasovskii *et al.* (1976) stated that three local drinking water sources contained 0·015, 0·05 and 0·3 mg (boron)/kg (this seems from another part of the paper to relate to the total dose taken in per day and should probably be 0·3, 1·0 and 6·0 mg/l) and they were able to study a small number (not stated) of people using those sources. They used a questionnaire of the Scientific Research Institute of Psychiatry of U.S.S.R. Ministry of Public Health to study sexual function of some of the men. They observed reduced function in the men consuming the highest amount of boron, 0·3 mg/kg, compared with a control group. Values of $32{\cdot}24 \pm 0{\cdot}37$ for control versus $27{\cdot}97 \pm 0{\cdot}49$ for exposed ($P < 0{\cdot}001$) are given. Unfortunately, the authors do not state how many men were studied in each group, what was actually studied, what the numbers quoted above refer to or where the control group was obtained. It is thus impossible to assess the value of this study. However the authors recommend that further work on boron should be carried out and that a concentration of 0·3 mg/l should be recommended as the state standard for boron in drinking water.

Tarasenko *et al.* (1972) have reported "weakened sexual activity" and generally low level of "genital functions" in 28 male workers engaged in the production of boric acid (English abstract only seen by us). Analysis of seminal fluid in 6 workers showed pathological changes; there was reduced volume, low sperm count, low sperm motility and elevated fructose content.

Boric acid 2% in a PEG ointment base had no effect on the motility of human sperm in *in vitro* tests but did slightly potentiate the action of quinine bisulphate (Kassem *et al.*, 1977). It is not possible from the paper to estimate the actual concentration of boric acid in the aqueous suspension of sperm.

D. PREGNANCY AND NEONATAL PERIOD

In the past, boric acid powders were commonly used to treat nappy rash in babies, often with disastrous consequences; vomiting, diarrhoea, erythema, convulsions and death occurred in up to 70% of infants under 1 year of age (Goldbloom and Goldbloom, 1953; Anonymous, 1970). Since 1966, following action by the British Paediatric Association and the Pharmaceutical Society, boric acid and its related compounds were dropped from the majority of baby preparations. The problem seemed especially to relate to the use of undiluted boric acid powder for dusting rather than the use of borated talcum powder (Samuel, 1970), and 5% boric acid in talc seems satisfactory for use on intact skin since the calcium hydroxide in the talc reacts with the boric acid to produce the highly insoluble calcium borate (Anonymous, 1966). However, poisonings have occurred even with the use of medicated talcum powders (Skipworth *et al.*, 1967), and considering the serious nature of the toxicity, all such use of boric acid should be avoided.

E. MUTAGENICITY

No relevant data found.

F. CARCINOGENICITY

No relevant data found.

SUMMARY AND EVALUATION

EXPERIMENTAL STUDIES

No studies were found on endocrine effects. Boron has been shown to have a toxic action in the testis to damage the seminiferous tubules as judged mainly by histology. This has been shown in several studies in rats to occur with oral doses of 150 mg/kg boric acid and above, with a no effect level possibly around 100 mg/kg. With the lower doses, the effect may be localized or confined to the later stages of spermatogenesis, but with higher doses, damage of the germ cells occurs. One study on rats showed that reduced sperm counts and motility could occur at doses as low as 0·3 mg/kg in drinking water.

Studies in dogs showed similar effects of testicular tubular damage at 1170 ppm of boron and above in the diet within 38 weeks, but not at 350 ppm in the diet over 2 years. This is equivalent to about 480 mg/kg and 150 mg/kg boric acid respectively. Limited studies in female rats suggest that the ovaries are not affected at doses up to 400 mg/kg given for 2 years. One well conducted multigeneration study showed no effects at about 100 mg/kg boric acid in the diet, but infertility in both males and females at 300 mg/kg.

No data on teratogenicity, mutagenicity or carcinogenicity were found.

HUMAN STUDIES

Two reports of reduced sexual function in men exposed occupationally or through the drinking water are available. Due to lack of details neither of these could be assessed. Boric acid powder used to treat nappy rash in babies has resulted in fatalities.

EVALUATION

There is adequate data to show that boron in the form of boric acid can damage the testis and cause infertility in rats and dogs. The data are insufficient to define a no effect level. There is also limited evidence that infertility may be produced in females. There are no teratogenicity data in animals.

Attention is drawn to the lack of adequate evidence about the reproductive toxic effects in humans.

References

Anonymous (1966). Boric Acid and Babies (editorial). *British Medical Journal* **2**, 188–189.

Anonymous (1970). Deadly Diapers (editorial). *British Medical Journal* **2**, 314.

Bouissou, H. and Castagnol, R. (1965). Action of boric acid on the testicle of the rat. *Archives de Maladies Professionnelles, de Medecine du Travail et de Securite Sociale* **26**, (6), 293–306.

Goldbloom, R. B. and Goldbloom, A. (1953). Boric acid poisoning. Report of four cases from the world literature. *Journal of Paediatrics* **43**, (6), 631–643.

Kassem, A. A., Elbary, A. A. and Nour, S. A. (1977). Spermicidal activity of quinine bisulphate with and without other spermicides in ointments using human sperms. *Bulletin of the Faculty of Pharmacy of Cairo University* **14**, (2), 199–206.

Krasovskii, G. N., Varshavskaya, S. P. and Borisov, A. I. (1976). Toxic and gonadotropic effects of cadmium and boron relative to standards for these substances in drinking water. *Environmental Health Perspectives* **13**, 69–75.

Ploquin, J. (1967). Boron in food. *Bulletin de la Societé scientifique d'Hygiène alimentaire* **55**, 70–113.

Samuel, D. L. (1970). Deadly Diapers. *British Medical Journal* **2**, 603.

Silaev, A. A., Kasparov, A. A., Korolev, V. N. and Nevstrueva, V. V. (1977). Electron microscopic study of the seminiferous tubules of albino rats with the action of boric acid. *Byulleten Eksperimentalnoi Biologii I Meditsiny* **83**, (4), 496–499.

Skipworth, G. B., Goldstein, M. and McBridge, W. P. (1967). Boric acid intoxication from "Medicated Talcum Powder". *Archives of Dermatology* **95**, (1), 83–86.

Tarasenko, N. Y., Kasparov, A. A. and Strongina, O. M. (1972). The effect of boric acid on the generative function in males. *Gigiena Truda I Professional 'Nye Zabolevaniya* **(16)**, 13–16.

Truhaut, R., Phu-Lich, N. and Loisillier, F. (1964). On the effects of repeated ingestion of small doses of boron compounds on the reproductive functions of the rat. *Comptes Rendus Academie des Sciences, Paris* **258**, (20), 5099–5102.

Weir, R. J. and Fisher, R. S. (1972). Toxicologic studies on borax and boric acid. *Toxicology and Applied Pharmacology* **23**, 351–364.

8. Cadmium and its compounds

TECHNICAL DATA

(a) *Cadmium*

Formula	Cd
CAS registry number	7440–43–9
Chemical abstracts name	Cadmium
Synonyms	None

(b) *Cadmium compounds* (Reviewed by IARC, 1976)

Formula	CAS registry number	Chemical abstracts name
$Cd(CH_3COO)_2$	543–90–8	Cadmium acetate
$CdCO_3$	513–78–0	Cadmium carbonate
$CdCl_2$	10108–64–2	Cadmium chloride
$Cd(BF_4)_2$	14486–19–2	Cadmium fluoroborate
CdF_2	7790–79–6	Cadmium fluoride
$CdMoO_4$	13972–68–4	Cadmium molybdate
$Cd(NO_3)_2$	10325–94–7	Cadmium nitrate
CdO	1306–19–0	Cadmium oxide
$CdSO_4$	10124–36–4	Cadmium sulphate
CdS	1306–23–6	Cadmium sulphide

Uses Constituent of easily fusible alloys; soft solder and solder for aluminium; electroplating (major use), deoxidiser in nickel plating; process engraving; electrodes for cadmium vapour lamps, photoelectric cells; photometry of ultraviolet sunrays; in nickel-cadmium storage batteries. Powder used (with mercury) as

	amalgam in dentistry. To charge Jones reductors.
TLV	0·05 mg/m^3 (as cadmium).

ANIMAL STUDIES

A. RELEVANT PHARMACOLOGY AND TOXICOLOGY

The absorption, distribution and excretion of cadmium (Cd) in adult animals have been reviewed by Probst (1979). Absorption of inhaled Cd from the air is efficient, with evidence from mice, rats, rabbits and dogs of absorption of 10–40% of the inhaled dose. Absorption from the gastro-intestinal tract, on the other hand, is poor; retention of around 1–5% of the administered dose has been shown in mice, rats, sheep and monkeys. With injection, approximately 80% of the administered dose is retained, irrespective of the injection route used. Absorbed Cd is found in nearly all tissues, but is highest in liver, kidney and testes and is retained over extended periods of time.

There are, however, important differences between adult and neonatal animals in oral absorption of Cd. Kostial *et al.* (1978) have shown absorption of 25% of an orally administered dose in 1-week old suckling rats compared with only 7% in 6-week old animals on a cows' milk diet or 0·5% in 6-week old animals on a standard diet. The acute oral LD50 reflects this difference in absorption, e.g. for cadmium chloride in the rat it is around 47 mg/kg at 2 weeks of age but 240 mg/kg at 3 weeks of age, falling gradually to 109 mg/kg by 54 weeks of age (Kostial *et al.*, 1978). This difference is important for consideration of the neonatal toxicity of Cd.

Kello *et al.* (1979) have shown a sex difference in the rat in retention of orally administered Cd; female rats retained approximately twice as much Cd as males, probably due to differences in absorption rather than excretion. Experiments with gonadectomised male and female rats showed that this sex difference was dependent on the presence or absence of male sex hormones.

Pregnant animals appear to be more susceptible than non-pregnant females to Cd toxicity. Pařízek (1965) showed a high mortality rate of 76% within 1–4 days of i.v. or s.c. injection of cadmium acetate or cadmium lactate during the last 4 days of pregnancy in the rat, with generalized venous congestion, pulmonary congestion and severe kidney pathology. In non-pregnant females or females which had given birth 3 days before the injection of Cd, no such effects were seen. It seems likely that this increased toxicity may be dependent on the presence of the placenta which begins to break down within hours of Cd injection and by 24 h is transformed into an extensive blood clot with just a little remaining necrotic tissue (Pařízek, 1964). Breakdown products from the placenta may thus contribute in part or wholly to the observed maternal toxicity. Prigge (1978) has also noted increased toxicity of inhaled Cd in pregnant compared with non-pregnant rats in terms of haematological changes, but could not find any increase in proteinuria to support Pařízek's suggestion (1965) that Cd may cause toxaemia of pregnancy as its primary effect.

Webb (1972) has shown in the rat that Cd retained in the tissue from injection prior to mating is not mobilized during a subsequent pregnancy; histological changes in the liver and kidney were similar in gravid or non-gravid rats injected in this way, and fetal and placental damage slight. However, if the same dose was injected in the second half of pregnancy, liver and kidney Cd content was lower than in gravid rats injected before mating, yet tissue damage to these organs was more severe and placental and fetal damage was extensive. The explanation for these findings may well be related to the binding of Cd by protein. Much of the Cd in the body is bound to the protein metallothionein and the synthesis of this protein is stimulated by the presence of Cd in the body (see review by Probst, (1979)). The extent to which binding may protect tissue from Cd toxicity is not known, but clearly there may not necessarily be any connection between tissue levels of Cd and toxicity.

Placental transfer

Placental transfer of Cd has been studied in the mouse, rat and hamster. Berlin and Ullberg (1963) could find no Cd in the mouse fetus after maternal i.v. injection of radiolabelled cadmium chloride at intervals of 20 min–16 days before sacrifice on day 18 of pregnancy. This may have been due to the relative insensitivity of the whole body radioautography technique used. Wolkowski (1974) has shown passage of radiolabelled Cd into the mouse embryo within 1 h of maternal s.c. injection on day 10. He also found Cd in the embryo, fetus and placenta at 4 h and 24 h after injection on day 13 or 17 of pregnancy. However, Cd may not be retained for long in fetal tissues; Ishizu *et al.* (1973) have failed to find Cd in fetal tissue of mice on day 18 of pregnancy after a single s.c. injection of 5 mg/kg of cadmium chloride into the dam on day 7 of pregnancy, despite high maternal liver, kidney and placental Cd concentrations. Matsumoto *et al.* (1975) have also noted very low levels of transfer to the mouse fetus after maternal s.c. injection of 0·25 or 0·5 mg/kg/day of cadmium chloride on days 7–18 of pregnancy. Dencker (1976) has shown embryonic uptake of radiolabelled Cd in the mouse by radioautography techniques, 4–24 h after maternal i.v. injection on day 8 or 9 of pregnancy. Traces of radioactivity were present in the embryonic gut up to 3 days after injection but not thereafter. With injection on day 11 or 16 of pregnancy, however, no radioactivity could be detected in the embryo or fetus 4–8 h afterwards, though there were high Cd levels in the chorioallantoic placenta. Dencker has suggested that in early pregnancy, Cd can pass from the visceral yolk sac into the primitive gut via the so-called "vitelline duct", but by day 8–9 of pregnancy this closes and passage of Cd into the embryo and fetus is then negligible.

There have been several studies of placental transfer of Cd in the rat, using different routes of administration. Lucis *et al.* (1972) first noted high Cd levels in the placenta and low Cd levels in the gastro-intestinal tract, liver and brain of newborns after s.c. injection into the dam in late pregnancy. Ariyoshi *et al.* (1977) found much higher levels of up to 1·7 ppm Cd in the placenta compared with levels of 0·02 ppm in the fetus, 3 days after a single s.c. injection of 3 mg/kg cadmium chloride on day 15 of pregnancy.

Sonawane *et al.* (1975) made a systematic study of Cd transfer in the rat in relation to dose and gestational age. The dams were injected i.v. with 0·1, 0·4 or 1·6 mg Cd/kg as cadmium chloride on day 12, 15 or 20 of pregnancy. Transfer to the fetus was dose-related, and increased with advancing gestation, but at no time exceeded a mean of 0·016% of the total dose 24 h after the injection. Maternal blood levels were similarly low (0·01–0·02% of the dose) but placenta levels were high (up to 8% of the dose on day 20). Similar results were obtained by Ahokas *et al.* (1976) following oral administration of 10 μg–10 mg Cd/rat on day 17 of pregnancy; 24 h after administration fetal levels were very low (0·00006–0·0002% of the dose) with similarly low maternal blood levels but placental levels were 400-fold higher than fetal levels (0·025–0·092% of the dose). In a subsequent experiment on the rat, Ahokas and Dilts (1977) showed that, as in the mouse, passage of Cd into the embryo was higher than in the fetus, with embryonic levels of 0·008% and 0·004% of the dose 24 h after oral administration on day 6 or 10 of pregnancy and fetal levels of 0·0003% and 0·0002% of the dose 24 h after administration on day 14 or 17. By 96 h embryonic and fetal levels were negligible.

Pietrzak-Flis *et al.* (1978) have also confirmed very low transfer of Cd to the fetus with high placental retention in rats given Cd in the drinking water throughout gestation. Cd was only detectable at a range of <0·4–1·2 ppm in the liver, kidney, brain and blood of newborns from dams given 5 ppm Cd in the drinking water with placental levels of around 20 ppm. It was not detectable in newborns from dams on 0·1, 0·2 or 1·1 ppm Cd in the drinking water, where placental levels ranged from <0·4–1·4 ppm.

Prigge (1978) has shown low transfer of Cd to the rat fetus following maternal inhalation of 0·1 ppm (0·4 mg/m^3) Cd throughout pregnancy. On day 21 fetal liver levels averaged 0·04 ppm compared with maternal liver levels of 3·3 ppm.

Placental transfer in the hamster has also been shown to occur. Ferm *et al.*

(1969) injected i.v. radiolabelled Cd on day 8 of pregnancy and found embryonic levels generally similar to or slightly higher than maternal blood levels 24 h after injection, but 25–50-fold lower than maternal blood levels 96 h after injection.

In a study using radioautography, Dencker (1976) has shown the presence of Cd in the embryonic gut 4–24 h after maternal i.v. administration of radiolabelled cadmium chloride on day 7–8 of pregnancy, but no transfer to the embryo with injection on day 9 of pregnancy. Placental levels were high. The possible relationship of this to closure of the vitelline duct has already been mentioned in relation to studies on the mouse.

The effect of other ions on the transfer of Cd into the embryo and fetus has also been investigated. Zinc protects against Cd-induced teratogenesis in the hamster, but does not block the placental transfer of Cd in this species (Ferm *et al.*, 1969). Neither does dietary zinc deficiency, which potentiated Cd-induced fetotoxicity in the rat, affect placental transfer of Cd, though maternal liver, kidney and placental levels were higher in zinc-deficient rats, suggesting that the fetotoxicity may be secondary to increased maternal toxicity (Rohrer *et al.*, 1978a). Samarawickrama and Webb (1979) have looked at the interaction between Cd and zinc in another way; injection of Cd i.v. at teratogenic doses in the rat markedly reduces placental transfer of zinc, and in the embryo, zinc-dependent thymidine kinase is inhibited and DNA concentration reduced. This may be pertinent to the mechanism of action of Cd as a teratogen, and would explain the protective and potentiating effects of high and low zinc levels in the absence of any effect on placental transfer of Cd.

Pond and Walker (1975) have shown that placental transfer of Cd from the maternal diet is influenced by dietary calcium levels. Maternal liver, kidney and newborn pup levels of Cd are lower on a high calcium diet than on a low calcium diet, and pup weight at birth in Cd-exposed litters is marginally higher in dams on a high calcium diet.

Transfer of Cd in the milk has been less extensively studied than placental transfer but is generally low. Lucis *et al.* (1972) showed injection of radiolabelled Cd into dams on the day of parturition resulted in only very low levels of Cd in the milk, with some uptake of Cd by the suckling pup in the intestine but low pup liver levels. Mammary tissue levels were high, however, as has also been noted by Berlin and Ullberg (1963) but most of the Cd remained bound to macromolecules in the tissue and did not pass into the milk. Pietrzak-Flis *et al.* (1978) also found only low Cd levels in milk of rats following dosing throughout pregnancy with 5·1 ppm Cd in the drinking water. Cd was not detectable in the milk of dams given 0·1–1·1 ppm Cd in the drinking water.

Conclusion

A fairly consistent picture of very limited Cd transfer across the placenta and into milk has been seen in all 3 species studied, viz. the mouse, rat and hamster. Studies showing no placental transfer of Cd have employed the relatively insensitive technique of autoradiography, and should therefore be discounted. However, transfer is generally very low and embryonic and fetal levels drop rapidly after single administration. In those studies where quantitative measurements have been made, embryonic and fetal levels rarely exceed 0·02% of the total maternal dose, regardless of route of administration. Transfer across the yolk-sac placenta may be slightly greater than across the chorioallantoic placenta, but the fetus may retain Cd longer than the embryo, due to binding of Cd by macromolecules in the fetal liver. Binding of Cd to macromolecules in the placenta and mammary tissue has also been proposed to account for the very high levels found in these tissues, which seemingly protects the embryo, fetus and neonate from exposure to high levels of Cd. However, clearly, in the case of the placenta, such binding does not protect the tissue from damage (see section D). The relevance of these observations to the mechanisms by which Cd may damage embryos and fetuses will be discussed in section D.

B. ENDOCRINE AND GONADAL EFFECTS

Males

The necrotizing effect of parenteral Cd on the testes in animals is perhaps one of the best documented examples of reproductive toxicity in the male and so the literature will be surveyed briefly.

The effects are confined to animals with scrotal testes, are seen at doses well below the lethal dose, and can occur in the absence of any other signs of Cd toxicity to other organs with much higher Cd contents than the testes. Damage is seen with testicular Cd levels as low as 0·15 ppm in the mouse (Gunn *et al.*, 1968) and 0·3 ppm in the rat (Kotsonis and Klaassen, 1977). The Cd is primarily associated with the interstitial tissues of the testes, epididymides, seminal vesicles and prostate. It does not appear to penetrate the seminiferous tubules or become associated with sperm cells (see review by Probst, 1979). There are marked species and strain differences in the testicular toxicity of parenteral Cd, but there is conflicting evidence on whether this is a function of difference in testicular Cd levels or differing sensitivity to the same Cd level in the testis (see review by Probst, 1979). Genotype certainly has some influence on testicular toxicity of Cd given s.c. or i.p. (Taylor *et al.*, 1973). Intratesticular injection of Cd has caused necrosis in all species so far investigated (Chiquoine and Suntzeff, 1965; Donelly and Monty, 1977).

The first report of Cd toxicity to the testis was by Pařízek and Zahor (1956). A single s.c. injection of 0·02 or 0·04 m mol/kg (3·7 or 7·4 mg/kg) of cadmium chloride into adult male rats caused rapid changes. Within a few hours, testicular size increased as they become oedematous, and they changed colour from pink to red to blue-purple. Over the next few days they decreased in size, becoming small, firm, yellow scars. Histologically, cells in the tubules began desquamating and showed nuclear changes within hours of injection. In the interstitial tissue there was oedema, hyperaemia, haemorrhage and thrombosis. Eventually there was complete testicular necrosis. Similar effects could be produced by other Cd salts given s.c. or i.p. (Pařízek, 1960). With necrosis of the testis there is a loss of androgen production and the secondary sex organs lose weight. With time, there is a variable recovery of androgen production but no regeneration of the tubules in the testis (Pařízek, 1960). Testicular sensitivity of Cd toxicity develops very early, between the 7th and 15th day of life (Pařízek, 1960).

Since that first report, Pařízek and a number of other workers have confirmed these findings in the rat and other species, following injection of Cd salts (see review by Lohiya, 1976); species sensitive to i.p. or s.c. injection of Cd include the mouse, hamster, rabbit, guinea pig, dog and squirrel, though some species such as the opossum and ferret are insensitive, possibly due to insufficient Cd levels being attained in the testis (Chiquoine and Suntzeff, 1965). Testicular damage has been seen in the opossum, goat and monkey following intratesticular injection of Cd. In the recovery phase, revascularization and proliferation of Leydig cells with restoration of androgen production is seen in all species, while limited regeneration of seminiferous tubules and renewed spermatogenesis may occur in a few instances.

Pařízek (1960) has reported he is unable to produce testicular necrosis in the rat after chronic oral administration of Cd (dose unspecified), but Kotsonis and Klaassen (1977) have found reduced fertility and focal testicular necrosis in the rat following a single oral dose of 100 or 150 mg Cd/kg but not after lower doses of 25 or 50 mg Cd/kg.

With chronic dosing, adverse effects on spermatogenesis have been seen at lower doses than with acute dosing. Krasovskii *et al.*, (1976) have found significant reductions in sperm number and motility and a significant increase in desquamation of spermatogenic epithelium in rats given 0·005 or 0·0005 mg/kg orally for 6 months. There were no adverse effects at 0·00005 mg/kg. Details of the oral dosing were not given, but other information given in the paper suggests the Cd may have been given in the drinking water. Dwivedi *et al.* (1977) have found depression of spermatogenesis, increased production of abnormal sperm and atrophy of the seminal vesicles with daily doses of 0·001 m mol/kg (0·2 mg/kg) i.p., given for 1 month which was similar to that produced by a single i.p. dose of 0·01 m mol/kg

(2 mg/kg). They also noted marked inhibition of choline acetyl transferase activity in the spermatozoa, a change known to be associated with impaired sperm function and sterility. Senczuk and Zielinska-Psuja (1977) have noted damage to the spermatogenic tubules and interstitial tissue hypertrophy following administration of cadmium chloride at 8 or 88 mg/kg in the diet for 12–15 months. These changes were not seen after 3 or 6 months on the diet.

Changes in blood androgen and gonadotrophin levels have been shown to parallel the extent of histological damage to the interstitial tissue of the testes (Favino *et al.*, 1966; Saksena *et al.*, 1977; Lau *et al.*, 1978; Dutt *et al.*, 1978). Changes in secondary sex organs following Cd injection are thought to be due to these hormone changes, but Timms *et al.* (1977) have evidence in the rat suggesting Cd may itself have a direct effect on the prostate gland, which is of interest in view of an increased incidence of prostatic disease amongst Cd-exposed workers which has been observed.

Over the years, a number of hypotheses have been put forward to explain Cd-induced testicular damage, including haemorrhagic necrosis, hypoxia, increased vascular permeability, impairment of the vascular cooling mechanism, and a direct action of Cd on the seminiferous tubules. However, there now seems to be general agreement (see reviews by Probst (1979) and Aoki and Hoffer (1978)) that the chronology of Cd damage involves localization of Cd in the capillary endothelium, causing damage which increases capillary permeability, resulting in massive oedema. This is followed by increased blood flow, then by failure of vessels to fill adequately as the microvasculature becomes obstructed by the increased concentration of erythrocytes following leakage of plasma fluids through the capillary walls and by thrombus formation initiated around the platelet plugs in the leaky capillary walls. The resulting ischaemia is thought to be responsible for all subsequent damage to the interstitial tissue and seminiferous tubules, rather than any direct effect of the Cd itself.

The damaging effects of Cd on the testis may be prevented by simultaneous administration of zinc (Pařízek, 1957), selenium (Gunn *et al.*, 1968), cysteine, BAL (Gunn *et al.*, 1966) or oestrogen (Gunn *et al.*, 1965). The possible mechanisms underlying these protective effects have been discussed elsewhere (White and Holland, 1977; Singhal and Merali, 1979), but none are proven. Pretreatment with small non-toxic doses of Cd also protects the testis against larger doses of Cd, and this is thought to be due to stimulation of metallothionein formation which binds the Cd (Nordberg, 1971).

Der *et al.* (1978) have shown that a combination of 25 μg of Cd i.m. and 25 μg of lead i.p., which do not by themselves cause testicular damage, results in enlargement of seminiferous tubules and absence of spermatogenesis in some tubules in the rat. Histological damage to the testes was not seen with doses of up to 250 μg of either Cd or lead alone, suggesting that the threshold for testicular damage by Cd may vary depending on the presence of other environmental metals.

Females

Dencker (1976) has shown heavy accumulation of radioactive Cd in the ovaries of mice and hamsters, concentrated in the corpora lutea and follicular walls, after i.v. injection. Watanabe *et al.* (1977) have found ovarian levels of 2·5 and 5 ppm Cd 12 h after the s.c. injection of 3 and 6 mg/kg cadmium chloride respectively in the mouse.

Changes in the oestrous cycle of rats have been noted. Tsvetkova (1970) exposed female rats to cadmium sulphate by inhalation. They inhaled 3 g/day for 4 months. It is not known how the inhalation exposure was carried out. Two months after the start of exposure, 50% of the animals had prolonged cycles, and after 4 months, 75% had prolonged cycles; dioestrus lasted an average of 6·2 days compared with 1·2 days in controls. Exposed females had a 35% lower weight gain than controls.

Der *et al.* (1977) have also shown altered oestrous cycles in rats given 250 μg/day of cadmium chloride by i.m. injection for 54 days. After 25 days, regular cycles ceased and the animals went into persistent dioestrus. The dose of 250 μg/day caused other signs of toxicity, viz. lower weight gain, coarse hair coat, sluggish movements and significant reductions in uterine, ovarian and pituitary weights, but no histological changes in the uterus or ovary. Injection of 50 μg/day produced few toxic signs and had no effect on oestrous cycles or reproductive organ weights.

Pařízek and Zahor (1956) and Gunn *et al.* (1965) have also reported absence of any effect on ovarian histology of a single s.c. injection of 0·02–0·04 m mol/kg (3·7–7·4 mg/kg) cadmium chloride in the rat, but Pařízek *et al.* (1968b) have reported massive ovarian haemorrhages after injection of the same dose into rats in persistent oestrus. Watanabe *et al.* (1977), using s.c. doses of 3 and 6 mg/kg cadmium chloride in the normal mouse, found severe, diffuse ovarian haemorrhages. In those given 3 mg/kg, 10/30 had ovarian haemorrhages, and in those given 6 mg/kg, 14/44 died and 22/30 survivors had ovarian haemorrhages. Oocytes recovered from induced ovulations in these mice were reduced from a mean of 22·6 in controls, to 18·1 after 3 mg/kg and 15·6 after 6 mg/kg. The mutagenic effects induced in these oocytes by Cd are discussed in section E.

The most comprehensive report on ovarian changes following Cd treatment has been published by Kar *et al.* (1959), but only prepubertal rats were studied. Females 6–8 weeks old were given a single s.c. injection of 10 mg/kg cadmium chloride and killed at intervals up to 360 h later. Beginning 6 h after injection the follicles underwent mass atresia and there was vascular engorgement and haemorrhage in the theca. The primordial oocytes, however, survived and the germinal epithelium was not damaged. The stroma showed deposition of yellow pigment and chromatin extruded from the nuclei of dead cells. By 96 h recovery had begun with disappearance of haemorrhagic changes and aberrant luteinisation, and new follicles differentiated from primordial oocytes. By 168 h recovery was complete and the ovary appeared histologically normal.

It may be that the capacity of the ovary for recovery may be the reason why some workers have failed to find any ovarian changes after Cd treatment. The time at which the ovaries were examined in the negative studies described above is not known, but is clearly important for interpretation of the results.

Conclusion

Acute parenteral administration of Cd has been shown to cause severe damage to the testis in a variety of species at doses below those causing other signs of toxicity, though the precise dose needed may vary between species and even between strains. There is some recovery of the interstitial tissue and restoration of androgen production, but recovery of the seminiferous epithelium is rare. Absorption of Cd when given orally is poor (see section A) but testicular damage has been seen following chronic oral dosing with doses as low as 0·0005 mg/kg (probably given in the drinking water) and 8 mg/kg given in the food. Further studies are needed to confirm the effects of such chronic low dosing and no studies of the testis have been carried out using the inhalational route. Testicular damage is thought to be caused by Cd-induced vascular changes leading to ischaemia, but the reason for the peculiar susceptibility of the testis to such changes is not known. The consistent precipitate fall in androgen levels following initial acute Cd damage to the testis and clear effects on sperm count and motility could provide the means for non-invasive investigation of Cd-exposed workers.

Ovarian haemorrhage, follicular damage and oestrous cycle changes have been seen by some workers following Cd treatment, but the effects appear to be transitory and, unlike the testis, complete recovery can occur.

C. FERTILITY

Males

From studies summarized in section B it will be clear that single, acute, parenteral dosing with Cd causes complete sterility which rarely recovers. Impairment of sexual behaviour, however, due to falling androgen levels, does recover with the gradual recovery of androgen production by the Leydig cells of the testis.

Madlafousek *et al.* (1971) noted complete loss of copulatory ability in male rats during the first 3 weeks after Cd injection, but by 2 months there was only slight impairment of sexual behaviour in comparison with pretreatment performance. In the early phase normal sexual behaviour could be restored by injection of testosterone.

Saksena *et al.* (1977) have investigated the effects of different doses on fertility. A single s.c. injection of 1 mg cadmium chloride to adult male rats significantly reduced sperm count in the caput and cauda epididymis and vas deferens at 15 days after the injection but 5/5 mated and produced litters of normal size at 7 and 15 days after the injection, despite the reduction of 87% in sperm count. A single s.c. injection of 5 mg further reduced total sperm population by 93% compared with controls 15 days after the injection. From pairings on the 7th day after injection only 2/5 females mated and became pregnant, one with only 2 implantation sites. From the pairings on the 15th day after injection, 0/6 mated. Serum testosterone levels were significantly decreased in the 5 mg group at 7 and 15 days after injection.

Kotsonis and Klaassen (1977) gave groups of 6 rats a single oral dose of 0, 25, 50, 100 or 150 mg Cd/kg as cadmium chloride and placed each male with one untreated female between 14 and 21 days after dosing. At 0, 25 and 50 mg/kg, 5/6 females became pregnant, but at 100 and 150 mg/kg only 1/6 became pregnant. Litter size in those pregnant was normal. The 2 highest dose group males showed slight loss of body weight in the first 4 days after dosing. Histopathological examination of males treated 2 or 14 days before sacrifice, showed focal testicular necrosis and reduced spermatogenesis at 100 and 150 mg/kg but no changes in any other tissues in any of the dose groups.

Lee and Dixon (1973) have investigated the effects of Cd on fertility in the mouse. Although this experiment was carried out using methods appropriate for dominant lethal testing, numbers of pre- and post-implantation deaths were not reported. Ten male mice were injected with a single i.p. dose of 1 mg/kg cadmium chloride and each paired with one untreated female/week for 9 weeks. Ten uninjected males served as controls. Fertility was defined as the presence of a litter of more than 4 implantation sites. Fertility decreased from 90% in the first week to 80% in the second week, declining steadily to 40% by the seventh week and recovering to 70% in the eighth and ninth weeks. This indicated an adverse effect on spermatids, spermatocytes and spermatogonia, but not on mature spermatozoa present in the epididymis and vas deferens. Pretreatment with zinc reversed the effect of Cd on spermatids and spermatocytes, but not those on spermatogonia. Gross appearance of the testes was normal, and histological appearance was normal except for a few spermatocytes with pyknotic chromosomes. However, injection of a slightly higher dose of 3 mg/kg caused gross haemorrhagic and oedematous changes in the testes.

Epstein *et al.* (1972) carried out a dominant lethal test in the mouse. Groups of 7–9 males were given single i.p. doses of 1·35, 2·7, 5·4 or 7·0 mg/kg cadmium chloride. A total of 5/32 males died, with deaths occurring in all dose groups except 5·4 mg/kg. Each male was mated with 3 untreated females/week for 8 weeks. There was no effect on pre- or post-implantation losses, but the number of females becoming pregnant was reduced (details not given). It is not known at what times this reduction in fertility was seen, nor whether it occurred in all dose groups.

Gilliavod and Léonard (1975) have also carried out a dominant lethal test in the mouse, after injection of a single i.p. dose of 1·75 mg/kg cadmium chloride. However, each male was mated with 3 untreated females/week for only 3 weeks after dosing. The number of males treated is not stated. There were no significant effects on pre- or post-implantation losses, but the pregnancy rate dropped to 45% in the third week of mating, compared with rates of 68–70% in the first 2 weeks in the Cd group and 57–68% in controls.

Sutou *et al.* (1980) have found no effect on fertility and no dominant lethal effects in male rats given 0·1, 1, or 10 mg Cd/kg/day (salt unspecified) orally for 6 weeks and mated with one control female/week during the 6 dosing weeks.

Paufler and Foote (1969) have injected 5 male rabbits with a single s.c. dose of 0·05 m mol cadmium chloride/kg (10 mg/kg). Two of the rabbits died. Semen was collected from the remaining 3 and used in artificial inseminations of 6 does at intervals of 1–2, 6–8, and 9–11 weeks after treatment. Only 1/6 or 2/6 does became pregnant on each occasion. Histologically, the males showed marked testicular atrophy and oligospermia, bordering on aspermia, by 4 weeks with poor motility and increased morphological abnormalities in surviving sperm. There was little evidence of recovery during the 17 weeks of the study.

Females

There have been fewer studies on the effects of Cd on female fertility. Pařízek (1960) has found no effect on fertility in female rats given single s.c. injections of 0·04 m mol/kg (7·5 mg/kg), a dose causing complete and irreversible sterility in male rats.

Sutou *et al.* (1980), however, have found adverse effects on fertility when male and female rats both treated with 10 mg/kg Cd orally for 3 weeks were mated during the dosing period. Only 5/13 pairs mated and in these 5 pregnancies there was a significant increase in resorptions/dam. Surprisingly, treatment of males only with this dose had no effect on fertility, so the effects seen in their initial experiment are assumed to be due to Cd in the females. Treatment of males and females with 0·1 or 1 mg/kg orally for 3 weeks was without effect on fertility.

Schroeder and Mitchener (1971) have carried out a multigeneration study on the effect of Cd in the drinking water at 10 ppm, in the mouse. Five pairs of mice were given Cd in the drinking water from weaning and allowed to breed freely up to 6 months of age. In the F_1 litters, average litter size at birth was normal but there was a 14% incidence of runts and a 21% incidence of postnatal deaths of the young compared with none in controls. By the F_2 generation, 2/5 litters were born dead and postnatal deaths had increased to 47% of the young. Kinked tail was seen in both F_1 and F_2 offspring. Breeding of an F_3 generation was not attempted.

Conclusion

Complete and generally irreversible infertility following parenteral administration of Cd in doses which have severe necrotic effects on the testes is not surprising. However, resumption of normal sexual behaviour with infertile matings may be seen as recovery of the androgen-producing Leydig cells proceeds after single acute doses. One study in the mouse has shown that adverse effects on fertility are seen even after doses which do not cause any histological damage to the testis (1 mg/kg i.p.). Dominant lethal studies have been negative, but reduction in fertility is again seen in the mouse at parenteral doses of 1–2 mg/kg. In the rat, histological damage to the testis and effects on fertility occur at parenteral doses of 3·7 mg/kg but are not seen at one tenth of this dose. Intermediate doses have not been studied. Oral dosing is less effective, presumably because of poor absorption of Cd from the oral route. Single oral doses of up to 50 mg/kg and subchronic doses of 10 mg/kg/day are without effect. Single oral doses of 100 mg/kg diminish fertility and affect testicular histology. In males showing subfertility, however, embryos fertilized are normal, confirming the dominant lethal studies.

In females, single parenteral doses affecting the males have no effect, though there is evidence suggesting impaired fertility during subchronic dosing with 10 mg/kg/day, but this result requires confirmation. Further studies are needed on the effects of different doses and routes of administration of Cd on female fertility. Inhalational studies on fertility are required for both males and females.

D. PREGNANCY

Numerous teratology studies on Cd exposure during pregnancy have been carried out in rodents. Those studies with adequate methodology will be briefly reviewed, but with particular emphasis on oral and inhalational studies.

Mouse

Webster (1978) has exposed mice to Cd in the drinking water throughout pregnancy. Cd at levels of 10, 20 or 40 ppm was given as cadmium chloride to groups of 26–65 pregnant mice. Maternal food consumption was not affected but water intake was reduced by 15–20% in the 40 ppm group. Litter size was not affected but there was a dose-related reduction in fetal weight, the mean fetal weight in the 40 ppm group being 14% below that of controls. Haematological investigation of mothers and newborns in another group given 40 ppm throughout pregnancy showed moderate anaemia in the mothers and severe anaemia in the newborns. Both the fetal growth retardation and the anaemia could be prevented in the mice given 40 ppm Cd by administration of iron dextran on days 1 and 14 of pregnancy, though the dams still showed reduced water consumption, showing that this factor did not contribute to the fetotoxicity of maternal Cd consumption. Matsumoto *et al.* (1975) have also found a reduction in fetal body weight after s.c. injection of 0·5 mg Cd/kg on days 7–18 of pregnancy in the mouse.

Chiquoine (1965) gave a total of 25 mice a single s.c. injection of 0·02 m mol/kg (3·7 mg/kg) cadmium chloride on one of days 1–17 of pregnancy. Injection up to day 5 had no effect, but with injection on day 5, only 1/5 carried litters to term. Injections on any of days 6–17 caused necrosis of the decidual tissue or placenta and intrauterine death of all the embryos and fetuses.

Ishizu *et al.* (1973) have looked at the effect of s.c. injection of 0·33, 0·63, 2·5 or 5·0 mg/kg cadmium chloride given to groups of 20 mice once on day 7 of pregnancy. At 5 mg/kg, 40% of mice "aborted" and 10–15% "aborted" in the lowest dose groups. It is not known if this was true abortion, or lack of implantation of fertilized ova. There was a dose-related incidence of resorptions ranging from 9·9–17·5% in Cd-exposed groups compared with 9·7% in controls. A dose-related increase in malformations was seen in all Cd-exposed groups except the 0·33 mg/kg group; 0·97%, 19·5% and 59·0% of fetuses were malformed in the 0·63, 2·5 and 5·0 mg/kg groups respectively, the principal malformations being exencephaly and open eye.

Similar findings of increases in resorptions and malformations, with exencephaly predominating, were reported by Semba *et al.* (1977) following i.p. injection of 5 mg/kg cadmium sulphate on day 7 of pregnancy, except that the proportions of affected implants were not so high as in the experiments of Ishizu *et al.* (1973) using cadmium chloride. These effects could be partly prevented by prior injection of 1 mg/kg Cd on day 6 of pregnancy, perhaps due to the induction of the Cd-binding protein, metallothionein. In a further study, Keino and Yamamura (1974) allowed mice given 5 mg/kg cadmium sulphate i.p. on day 7 to litter out. In addition to the skeletal abnormalities induced by Cd which are recognizable at the late fetal stage, those surviving also developed leg fractures and extreme sinuosity of the spine and limb bones.

Injection of Cd i.p. on day 9 of pregnancy as cadmium sulphate by Layton and Layton (1979) caused 17% and 34% resorptions and 30% and 71%

malformations in survivors in groups given 0·012 or 0·024 m mol Cd/kg (2·2 or 4·4 mg/kg) respectively. At this stage of pregnancy Cd caused predominantly limb malformations.

Rat

In the rat, as in the mouse, exposure to Cd during pregnancy causes anaemia in the offspring and to a lesser extent in the dams. Choudhury *et al.* (1979) fed 8·6 or 17·2 ppm Cd in the diet throughout pregnancy and neonates had significantly lower total body iron levels and lower haematocrits than controls. However, the haematocrits returned to normal by 2 weeks of age. Kelman *et al.* (1978) have also observed significant reductions in maternal and fetal haemotocrits when 10 or 25 ppm Cd was given in the drinking water throughout pregnancy. The induction of anaemia by Cd may account for the increased prenatal and postnatal mortality of offspring from dams on iron deficient diets compared with those on iron-replete diets, given a single oral dose of 0·1 m mol Cd on day 18 of pregnancy, noted by Martin *et al.* (1978). However, they found that low birth weights in the Cd groups were independent of dietary iron level, and it is possible that higher supplements must be given to reverse this effect, as has been shown in the mouse.

Prigge (1978) has looked at the effect of inhaled Cd. Groups of 12–13 rats were exposed to 0·04, 0·08 or 0·12 ppm Cd (0·2, 0·4 or 0·6 mg Cd/m^3) for 24 h/day throughout pregnancy. There was a dose-related reduction in maternal weight gain which was significant at all doses. Weight gain in the highest dose group was only one third of that in controls. Resorption and malformation rates were not ascertained. Fetal body weight on day 21 of gestation was also reduced in a dose-related manner but the reduction was only significant in the highest dose group, which showed a 19% reduction in comparison with controls. However, in contrast to other experiments already described, maternal haemoglobin and haematocrit were increased in a dose-related way, significantly so at the highest dose, whilst fetal haemoglobin and haematocrit, as in other studies, were decreased in a dose-related manner. Serum alkaline phosphatase activity in the dams decreased with increasing Cd exposure, but in the fetuses it increased with increasing Cd exposure, possibly reflecting the known skeletal damage caused by Cd in the fetus.

Effects of inhaled Cd have also been studied by Tsvetkova (1970). A group of 40 rats were exposed to 0·6 ppm (2·8 mg/m^3) for 24 h/day throughout pregnancy. Nineteen rats served as controls. Maternal weight gain was not mentioned but newborn weight was significantly reduced by 20% and lower weight persisted up to 8 months of age. By 3 months of age, 26% of Cd-exposed offspring had died compared with 7% in controls. This difference was largely due to death of 17% of the Cd-exposed offspring between 10 and 14 days of age. Exposure to the same level of Cd (0·6 ppm) for 4 or 7 months before pregnancy, but not during pregnancy, also reduced offspring body weight, but effects on viability were not mentioned.

Pond and Walker (1975) have investigated the effects of low (0 ppm) and high (200 ppm) Cd in the diet combined with low (0·07%) and high (0·96%) calcium, throughout pregnancy. The dams were allowed to litter out, then they and their pups were killed for tissue ion analysis. High Cd depressed daily food consumption and markedly reduced weight gain in the dams. These effects were only slightly worsened by low calcium in the diet. Average litter size at birth was slightly, but not significantly decreased in high Cd groups, and average pup weight at birth was significantly decreased by high Cd, being lowest in the high Cd, low calcium group. Mean Cd level in the pups in the high Cd, low calcium group was double that in the high Cd, high calcium group.

Sutou *et al.* (1980) have given Cd orally in doses of 0, 0·1, 1·0 or 10 mg Cd/kg/day throughout pregnancy. Numbers of animals used and teratology methods were not described, though it is clear from the results given that external, internal and skeletal abnormalities were evaluated. Fetal body weight was reduced in a dose-related way but was only significantly reduced in the highest dose group, which had a 33% reduction in comparison with controls. Placental weight was increased in a dose-related way which may reflect compensation for Cd-induced anaemia. Resorption rates were not given. There were no effects on malformation rates, though, not surprisingly, retarded ossification was increased in the highest dose group.

Kelman *et al.* (1978) have investigated the effect of Cd in the drinking water, at 0, 10 or 25 ppm, throughout pregnancy. When killed on day 20, there were no effects on implants/dam, live litter size or gross malformation rates, but increases in fetal bone-stable calcium and decreases in fetal liver and kidney-stable calcium were seen, indicating a disturbance of calcium metabolism.

Nolen *et al.* (1972b) have given groups of 15–20 rats Cd in the drinking water as cadmium chloride, in notional doses of 0·01, 1 and 4 mg Cd/kg on days 6–14 of pregnancy. Acceptable teratological methods were used. Maternal weight gain during the dosing period was reduced only in the high dose group (85% reduction). Food consumption was slightly reduced and water consumption considerably reduced during dosing. At the end of dosing, however, the high dose group gained weight quickly and by day 21 of pregnancy were not significantly different from controls. Because of the effect on body weight the ingestion of Cd was actually higher than the notional dose of 4 mg/kg in the highest dose group. There were no significant effects on implants/dam, live fetuses/dam, resorptions/dam or fetal weight, though Cd-exposed fetuses weighed less than controls. There was an increase in abnormalities in all Cd-exposed groups, the difference between treated and controls being significant at 4 mg/kg, with 46% abnormal fetuses/litter compared with 13% in controls. Genitourinary defects were most common, including hydronephrosis, hydroureter, bladder defects and undescended testes. There were no significant effects on overall skeletal anomalies, but extra ribs were significantly decreased and retarded ossification significantly increased in the 4 mg/kg group. However, in a subsequent study, Nolen *et al.* (1972a) could not confirm the teratogenicity of 4 mg/kg given in the drinking water on days 6–15 of pregnancy, and maternal weight gain was not so severely affected. They did confirm absence of embryolethal or fetotoxic effects at this dose.

Rohrer *et al.* (1979) investigated the effects of single i.p. injections of 1 or 2 mg Cd/kg as cadmium acetate on one of days 12, 14, 18 or 20 of pregnancy. Rats treated on day 12 or 14 were killed 2 days after dosing; resorptions were not affected and fetal weight was only reduced in those injected on day 14. Rats injected on day 18 or 20 were killed on day 21 and fetal deaths were significantly increased in both groups given 2 mg/kg. A small number of rats from these groups were allowed to litter out; stillbirths and neonatal mortality were very high in those given 2 mg/kg on day 20, but not in other groups.

Vare and Monie (1976) injected cadmium sulphate i.p. at very high doses of 8–32 mg/kg on one of days 9, 10, 11, 15 or 16 of pregnancy. There was a high incidence of maternal mortality and fetal deaths but no malformations were found. Malformations were seen, however, with intra-amniotic injection of 8–32 μg of cadmium sulphate on day 13 or 17 of pregnancy, primarily hydrocephalus, jaw defects and cleft palate. These results suggest that, under some circumstances, Cd may cause fetal death by damaging the placenta before sufficient may cross the placenta to cause malformations.

Barr (1972) has shown that Cd in a dose of 0·016 m mol/kg (3 mg/kg) given on day 9, 10 or 11 of pregnancy by the s.c. route is not teratogenic, but is teratogenic if given by the i.p. route. Following treatment, maternal weight loss was seen in those given Cd i.p. but not in those given Cd s.c. Fetal weight was significantly reduced by up to 23% and resorption and abnormality rates significantly increased after single i.p. injections on day 9, 10 or 11. The pattern of malformations differed depending on the day of injection, but anophthalmia, microphthalmia, hydrocephaly, undescended testes and dysplastic tail predominated.

Ariyoshi *et al.* (1977) have also found no effect on fetal weight of single s.c. injections of 3 mg/kg cadmium chloride on days 7, 9 or 15 of pregnancy. There is evidence that blood levels of Cd are higher following i.p. than s.c. injections, which may explain the differing teratogenicity of these 2 routes of administration. However, s.c. injections of higher doses for longer periods are teratogenic. Chernoff (1973) injected 4–12 mg/kg cadmium chloride on days 13–16 of pregnancy and noted a dose-related decrease in fetal weight and increases in resorption and malformation rates. At 12 mg/kg, 52% of implants were resorbed and 100% of survivors malformed. Jaw defects, cleft palate and hypoplastic lungs predominated. Jaw defects were still seen with injections commencing as late as day 16.

Samarawickrama and Webb (1979) have shown that single i.v. injections of 1·25 mg Cd/kg on one of days 9–15 of pregnancy are highly teratogenic, causing hydrocephalus. The dose was critical; 1·1 mg/kg was not teratogenic, whilst 1·35 mg/kg killed all the embryos. Sonawane *et al.* (1975) have shown 1·6 mg Cd/kg i.v. on day 12 was teratogenic, but lower doses of 0·4 or 0·1 mg Cd/kg were not.

A high incidence of hydrocephalus has been seen with Cd treatment during embryogenesis and other work with injection of non-lethal doses of Cd in late pregnancy and the early neonatal period suggest that the developing brain may be particularly susceptible to Cd injury. Rohrer *et al.* (1978b) have shown formation of vacuoles in the endothelial cells of capillaries of the fetal brain, following i.p. injection of 2 mg Cd/kg as cadmium acetate on day 20 of pregnancy, but no such effect with lower doses of 0·5 or 1·0 mg/kg. The possible consequences of such changes are not yet known. Gabbiani *et al.* (1967) have shown widespread haemorrhage in the cerebrum and cerebellum of young rats and rabbits, given a single s.c. injection of 10 mg/kg cadium chloride at 1, 5, 10 or 20 days of age. This is in contrast to the specific action of Cd on sensory ganglia in adult animals.

Possible later manifesting effects of Cd exposure in the developing brain have been investigated by Howell and Cooper (1979). Rats were given 0, 8·6 or 17·2 ppm Cd as cadmium chloride in the drinking water throughout pregnancy. Birth weight was not affected but postnatal weight gain was reduced in Cd-exposed groups. Wheel running activity in the offspring at 12–21 weeks of age was significantly increased in the 17·2 ppm group and this group also took significantly longer in reversal learning of a spatial discrimination task (described incorrectly by the authors as a visual discrimination task). These effects could not be accounted for by the reduced body weights in this group and were attributed directly to the Cd exposure. However, in a different publication by the same group of workers (Hastings *et al.*, 1978), conflicting results were obtained. Male and female rats were exposed to 17·2 ppm in the drinking water for 90 days, then mated and continued on exposure to 17·2 ppm throughout pregnancy. In this experiment, pup weight at birth was significantly reduced, but postnatal weight gain was normal, activity in the running wheel was significantly decreased, and performance on the same spatial discrimination task with reversal, as used before, did not differ in Cd and control offspring. The authors do not comment on these totally conflicting findings, the only difference between the 2 groups being that in the second experiment the rats were exposed before pregnancy as well as during pregnancy. However, this could have built up metallothionein levels, thus protecting the offspring from Cd exposure during gestation and lessening its effects.

Hamster

Ferm and co-workers have carried out several experiments in the hamster. Ferm and Carpenter (1967) showed that i.v. injection of 2 mg/kg cadmium sulphate on day 8 of pregnancy caused a high incidence of resorptions and malformations. It caused a specific type of malformation of the face and jaw, ranging from a simple mid-line cleft to almost complete obliteration of the normal facial features. Anophthalmia, digital and limb defects, rib fusions and exencephaly were also occasionally seen. The relative proportions of resorptions and malformations differed depending on the precise timing of dosing on day 8. Resorptions and facial abnormalities were not seen after injection on day 9 of pregnancy, though malformations were seen (Ferm, 1971). Detailed examination of skeletal defects after i.v. injection of 2 mg/kg cadmium sulphate on day 8 showed a wide ranging variety of defects of the skull, vertebrae, ribs and limbs, depending on the precise timing of dosing (Gale and Ferm, 1971). As in the mouse, pretreatment with a lower s.c. or i.p. dose of cadmium (1 mg/kg) on day 6 or 7 considerably reduced the embryolethality and teratogenicity of Cd injected i.v. on day 8, though prior oral dosing with Cd did not. The mechanism is presumably by induction of methallothionein binding, if adequate amounts of Cd enter the blood on day 6 or 7.

Rabbit

Datnow (1928) has injected colloidal Cd i.v. into pregnant rabbits on one of days 7–14 of pregnancy. A dose of 10 ml of a 0·1% suspension was lethal to 6/12 rabbits and one aborted. Three of the rabbits littered normally at term and one littered 5 days prematurely. In the rabbits which died or were killed when moribund, all showed signs of vasocongestion and haemorrhage in the litters and placentae.

Interaction with other metals

Simultaneous zinc administration reduces Cd-induced embryolethality and teratogenicity in the hamster (Ferm and Carpenter, 1967) and in the mouse (Chiquoine, 1965), whilst a zinc-deficient diet enhances the embryolethality of Cd in the rat (Parzyck *et al.*, 1978).

Simultaneous administration of selenium has been shown to protect against Cd-induced embryolethality and teratogenesis in the hamster (Holmberg and Ferm, 1969), and against Cd-induced placental necrosis and fetal death in later pregnancy in the rat (Pařícek *et al.*, 1968a). There is some evidence to suggest that selenium may increase the amount of Cd bound to macromolecules in the blood, thus protecting the tissues.

Lead has also been shown to interact with Cd in the hamster (Ferm, 1972). Cd-induced malformation of the head was decreased by simultaneous administration of lead with Cd, but malformation of the tail and lower extremities were exacerbated. Lead itself caused tail defects.

Mechanism of action of Cd in pregnancy

The mechanism by which high doses of Cd cause rapid embryonic or fetal death has been speculated about ever since Pařízek (1964) first observed drastic placental changes following s.c. injection of Cd salts in the rat. By 24 h after injection on one of days 17–21 of pregnancy, the whole of the placenta was transformed into an extensive blood clot with little remaining necrotic tissue. Pařízek (1964) described the fetal part of the placenta as the most affected, but Samarawickrama and Webb (1979) have disputed this, finding more extensive damage in the maternal part of the placenta at the earlier time of 8 h after Cd injection. Levin and co-workers have investigated the chronology of placental changes in relation to fetal death. The earliest changes observed were increased mitochondrial calcium levels in the placenta, indicative of cell injury, by 8 h after Cd injection (Levin *et al.*, 1980). At 8–10 h after injection, placental blood flow was normal, but by 12–14 h it decreased significantly and by 18 h there was a 50% reduction in placental blood flow, accompanied by 40% fetal mortality (Levin and Miller, 1979). Histological necrosis of the placenta was concurrent with the decreased blood flow, but early cell injury seen at 8 h suggests that early placental injury precedes the vascular changes which ultimately cause fetal death. The sequence of these changes resembles the Cd-induced ischaemia seen in the testis (see section B).

Conclusion

Cd is clearly embryolethal, teratogenic and fetotoxic in all species tested so far when given during pregnancy, but the effects are crucially dependent on route of administration and dose. Because of poor oral absorption of Cd, dosing by this route generally only causes a reduction in fetal weight, but with high oral doses (4 mg/kg in the rat) malformations are also seen. Parenteral administration causes successively fetotoxicity, teratogenicity and intrauterine death over a very narrow dose range; with high doses, placental damage precedes fetal death, whilst with lower doses, small amounts of Cd cross the placenta and are likely to be the primary cause of malformations since intra-amniotic injections cause similar abnormalities to parenterally administered Cd. Inhaled Cd has been shown to cause fetal weight retardation (0·04–0·12 ppm) and low birth weight with high postnatal mortality (0·6 ppm) in the rat.

Exposure to higher doses of Cd by inhalation, which might cause prenatal death and malformation, has not been investigated.

A number of unusual teratogenic effects of Cd are worth noting. Anaemia in the dam, fetus and neonate has been observed in the mouse and the rat, but the effects on the offspring are greater than those on the dam. Fetal anaemia may be partly or wholly responsible for the growth retardation caused by Cd. There are also unusually severe effects on the bones. Calcium metabolism in the fetus is known to be disturbed by Cd exposure, and as well as the occurrence of multiple skeletal defects, later-developing limb fractures and extreme sinuosity of the bones have been observed in prenatally exposed offspring. These effects somewhat resemble the adult bone disease of itai-itai which has been observed in humans exposed to Cd in Japan.

Finally, the specific effects of Cd on developing brain observed in some studies warrant further evaluation of postnatal development and behaviour in prenatally exposed offspring.

E. MUTAGENICITY

Since Cd has a particular toxic effect on the gonads, the potential for mutagenic effects in the germ cells has been examined. Gilliavod and Léonard (1975) gave male mice single i.p. injections of 0·5, 1·75 or 3·0 mg/kg cadmium chloride. Three months later they were killed and spermatocytes examined for translocations. None were found, suggesting that there had been no mutagenic effect on the spermatogonia at the time of treatment. They also examined spermatocytes from F_1 male offspring sired by males injected with 1·75 mg/kg i.p. and mated to control females for 3 weeks after dosing. Again, no translocations were found. Negative dominant lethal studies have already been reported above.

Shimada *et al.* (1976) have looked at the effect of Cd on mouse oocytes. In mice with stimulated ovulation, injection of 3 or 6 mg/kg of cadmium chloride 12 h before sacrifice decreased the numbers of oocytes ovulated in a dose-related way and caused ovarian haemorrhage (see section B for details). More chromosome anomalies were seen in the Cd-treated groups, the increase in the 6 mg/kg group being statistically significant in comparison with controls. The anomalies were hypoploidy, hyperploidy and diploidy found in 4/155 oocytes at 3 mg/kg and in 6/126 oocytes at 6 mg/kg, compared with 1/199 in controls. Chromosome gaps, breaks and rearrangements were not seen, probably due to the relatively short exposure period. In a similar experiment in the hamster, Watanabe *et al.* (1976) showed an increase in hyperploidy and diploidy in oocytes from females given 1·5 or 3·0 mg/kg of cadmium chloride. In the 3 mg/kg group more than one third of treated animals had oocytes with anomalies, suggesting this species is more susceptible than the mouse to Cd-induced chromosome anomalies.

F. CARCINOGENICITY

IARC Monograph Vol. 11 (1976) reports on studies showing local tumours in rats following s.c. or i.m. injection of several cadmium compounds. Oral and inhalational studies were not adequate for evaluation. No studies on the possible transplacental carcinogenicity of cadmium and its compounds have been carried out.

HUMAN STUDIES

A. RELEVANT PHARMACOLOGY AND TOXICOLOGY

The absorption, distribution and excretion of cadmium has been reviewed by Probst (1979). In humans the 2 major routes for cadmium absorption are through the respiratory tract and the gastrointestinal tract. For non-occupationally exposed persons consumption of contaminated food and water are the most likely sources of exposure, but absorption from the gastrointestinal tract is limited, reducing the severity of poisoning by this route. When there are high levels of atmospheric cadmium from industrial pollution the risk of poisoning is greater since absorption of cadmium through the respiratory mucosa is very efficient. Absorbed cadmium is deposited in nearly all body tissues, with liver, kidney, pancreas and testes showing the highest levels.

Sex differences

The occurrence of widespread environmental contamination from a metal mine in the Fuchu area within the Toyama prefecture of Japan, resulting in the development of itai-itai (ouch-ouch) disease, largely confined to postmenopausal women living in that area, provides some information on possible sex differences in cadmium toxicity. Tsuchiya (1969) has reviewed the epidemiology and hypotheses of causation of the disease and Murata *et al.* (1970) have described the clinical course of the disease. The disease is characterized by sharp pain and pain on pressure of the bones and waddling gait due to bone deformation; X-rays usually revealed bone atrophy and multiple fractures similar to those seen in osteomalacia. Clinical findings include hypochromic anaemia, low serum iron and phosphorus, very high serum alkaline phosphatase, atrophic gastritis and enteropathy, albuminuria in all cases and glycosuria in most cases. Serum cadmium levels are raised and serum zinc levels reduced. By 1970 there were a total of 300 registered patients with the disease, 56 deaths attributed to the disease and further suspected cases, the majority being registered from the mid-1950s onwards, though it is likely that many cases went unrecognized for some time before this.

The age and sex distribution of the disease was remarkably unusual. Onset of the disease is assumed to occur between 35 and 65 years of age and clinically apparent disease, up to 1970 was confined to women over 47 years of age, nearly all of whom were multiparous. In the 60 cases seen by Murata *et al.* (1970), the average age of the patients when first examined was 53·4 years, with reproductive histories averaging 6·2 deliveries/woman.

The source of pollution was a mine upstream along the Jintsu river; waste cadmium, lead and zinc from the mine contaminated the river water, drinking water and locally grown food consumed by the inhabitants living downstream where itai-itai disease became endemic. It has been estimated that the daily cadmium intake in the area averaged about 600 μg compared with 60 μg in non-endemic areas (studies reviewed by Chaube *et al.*, 1973). Metal production began in the mine in 1874 and only lead was produced until 1943 when production of cadmium and zinc began. It is agreed that cadmium is a major factor in the causation of the disease, but the participation of lead and zinc and the possible interactions between the 3 metals cannot be discounted. The clinical course of the disease, with such severe effects on bone certainly differs somewhat from other cases of industrial cadmium poisoning where renal involvement is more prominent.

There has been speculation as to the reason for the clinical disease being confined to older women and nutritional and hormonal deficiencies have been postulated. It was suggested that due to the nature of the society in that area (80% were farming families) the housewives may have eaten less and poorer quality food than others. A nutritional survey in 1965 found no evidence of malnutrition and a similar nutritional intake in the areas where itai-itai disease was endemic compared with neighbouring areas of similar socio-economic status where it was not. However, this may not have reflected the nutritional situation in the 1940s and 1950s when onset of the disease may have occurred. Others have postulated specific calcium and vitamin D deficiency or hormonal changes due to a high number of pregnancies, though there is no good human evidence to support these hypotheses. Kello *et al.* (1979) quote a study showing that women accumulate more cadmium than men (Sumino, K. *et al.*, *Arch. Environ. Hlth* **30**, 487, 1975, original not seen by us). It is possible that in women, sub-clinical poisoning from a higher retention of cadmium, ingested over a long period of time, becomes unmasked around the time of the menopause when hormonal changes accelerate the natural rate of bone loss. These natural changes may synergise with the effects of cadmium on bone, resulting in a clinical picture where skeletal rather than renal symptoms predominate. Whether multiparity may also affect bone density in women with adequate nutrition but exposure to cadmium is not known.

In other studies where there have been apparent sex differences suggesting an increased resistance of women to cadmium toxicity, it is likely that the true explanation lies in lower exposure levels of women compared with men in the industries studied (see U.S. Department of Health, Education and Welfare, 1976, for review).

Placental transfer

A number of studies have confirmed placental transfer of cadmium in the human. Fox first reported in 1969 in a personal communication to Flick *et al.* (1971) finding levels around 50 μg/kg in the human fetus, though earlier workers using less sensitive methods had been unable to detect cadmium in the human fetus at term.

Chaube *et al.* (1973) reported on cadmium levels in abortuses of 31–261 days' gestation from Japanese women. None of the women came from areas where cadmium poisoning was known to exist but it is recognized that the Japanese diet generally contains more cadmium than the average Western diet due to its high fish, shellfish and rice content. The daily intake has been estimated as around 60 μg in Japan compared with around 50 μg in the United States (studies reviewed by Chaube *et al.*, 1973). In embryos aged 31–78 days cadmium was below detectable levels in 4/8 pooled samples and ranged from 0·032–0·101 μg/g of wet tissue in the remaining samples. In second trimester fetuses, cadmium was detectable in only 4/14 fetal kidney samples (mean 0·05 μg/g) and in 2/12 fetal brain samples (mean 0·114 μg/g), but was found in 10/12 fetal liver samples (mean 0·114 μg/g). A single third trimester fetus contained traces of cadmium in the liver. There was no relationship between cadmium concentrations in the fetal tissues and age or sex of the fetuses.

Schulte-Löbbert *et al.* (1978) have reported cadmium concentrations of 14–33 μg/kg in the liver and 22–33 μg/kg in the kidneys of fetuses and stillborns. Postnatally, liver and kidney concentrations in infants up to 2 months of age were similar to fetal levels and kidney levels began to increase from 3–6 months of age, reaching concentrations around 3–5 times higher than those in the liver by 5 years of age. No details about the mothers, age of fetuses, or source of the samples were given. Bryce-Smith *et al.* (1977) have reported bone cadmium levels about 10 times above what might be expected in stillbirths, averaging 5·2 μg/g in 26 rib samples and 2·2 μg/g in 42 vertebral samples. However, they did not analyse cadmium levels in normal infants for comparison but, expected values were taken from studies on people aged 6–82 years in which cadmium levels were reported to be independent of age.

Baglan *et al.* (1974) measured cadmium levels in placenta, maternal and fetal blood of normal term deliveries in Nashville, Tennessee, U.S.A.

Placental levels averaged 1·7 μg/100 g wet weight in 135 samples, maternal blood 1·7 μg/100 g wet weight in 83 samples and fetal blood 1·6 μg/100 g wet weight in 123 samples, with a significant correlation between placental and fetal blood levels.

Thürauf *et al.* (1975) measured placental cadmium levels in a total of 179 normal term deliveries, premature deliveries and abortions in 3 different areas of West Germany with differing levels of industrialization. Average cadmium content in the industrial Ruhr area was 17·6 μg/100 g wet weight compared with 12·9 and 15·2 μg/100 g in the less industrialized Frankonian and Bavarian Forest areas respectively. Thieme *et al.* (1977) have also shown higher cadmium levels in placentae from women living in the industrial area of Essen (12 μg/100 g) compared with those living in Munich or the rural areas of Bavaria (2–3 μg/100 g).

Lauwerys, Buchet, Roels and Hubermont have published a series of papers on cadmium levels in placenta, maternal and cord blood of 500 Belgian women living in different areas surveyed in 1975 to 1976. Samples were taken at delivery. In their first paper (Lauwerys *et al.*, 1978) they reported maternal blood cadmium levels of 0·01–1·01 μg/100 ml and newborn blood levels of 0·01–1·03 μg/100 ml, but the median value for newborn blood was 50% lower than for maternal blood, suggesting a partial placental barrier to cadmium transfer. There was a small but statistically significant correlation between maternal and newborn blood levels ($r = +0{\cdot}38$, $p < 0{\cdot}001$). Smoking was associated with a significant increase in average maternal blood cadmium levels (0·12 μg/100 ml in non-smokers, 0·20 μg/100 ml in smokers) but not with any similar increase in newborns (Buchet *et al.*, 1978). In fact the average newborn blood level in the smoking group was marginally lower (0·07 μg/100 ml) than in the non-smokers (0·10 μg/100 ml). Mean placental cadmium level in the total sample was 1·08 μg/100 g wet weight compared with a mean maternal blood level of 0·10 μg/100 ml (Roels *et al.*, 1978), suggesting the placenta concentrates cadmium about 10-fold, and this may explain the lower levels in newborn compared with maternal blood. Placental concentrations in smokers were about 25% higher than in non-smokers and the authors have speculated that cadmium from smoking may induce metallothionein synthesis in the placenta which can then bind more cadmium, thus "protecting" the fetus from the higher maternal blood cadmium levels. However, it should be pointed out that high placental cadmium levels may be damaging to placental function (see below and Animal Studies) and thereby have a secondary effect on the fetus, despite low fetal blood levels. Unlike other authors, Roels *et al.* (1978) could not find any effect of place of residence related to industrialization and placental cadmium levels, after controlling for smoking habits.

Roels *et al.* (1978) have also reviewed 3 other studies of placental cadmium levels not reviewed here in which reported levels ranged from means of $<1{\cdot}0$–$15{\cdot}2\ \mu g/100$ g wet weight. Taken together with their own study and those of Thürauf *et al.* (1975) and Baglan *et al.* (1974) already reviewed, 4/6 studies have reported mean levels of 1–2 $\mu g/100$ g, and the 2 remaining studies levels of 12–18 $\mu g/100$ g. Methodology differences in cadmium estimation may account for this disparity.

Goodman *et al.* (1978, 1979) have shown adverse effects of cadmium on facilitated diffusion and active transport of γ-aminoisobutyric acid (AIB) across human placental membranes. Using membrane vesicle preparations taken from the maternal, microvillous surface of the human placental syncytiotrophoblast, they added 100 μM cadmium chloride and observed a depression of AIB uptake. At a concentration of 200 μM there was a 21% inhibition of the initial rate of AIB facilitated diffusion and at 800 μM a 19% inhibition of active transport of AIB. The authors suggest that cadmium therefore may affect amino-acid transport across the placenta to the fetus thus contributing to fetotoxicity. Dawson *et al.* (1969) have looked at the effect of cadmium *in vitro* on succinic dehydrogenase and cytochrome oxidase activities of mitochondria from human term placentae. Cadmium in concentrations up to 43 mμM caused no significant inhibition of these mitochondrial enzymes, suggesting there are no major effects on placental metabolism.

Transfer in the milk

There is sufficient evidence that cadmium may be passed to the infant in the breast milk. Murthy and Rhea (1971) found a mean level of $0{\cdot}019 \pm 0{\cdot}027$ ppm in samples of breast milk from 13 mothers living in the Cincinnati area of Ohio, U.S.A. Generally higher levels were found in evaporated and formula milk products (0·021–0·042 ppm). In a later study from the same group (Pinkerton *et al.*, 1972) they reported a mean level of 0·0111 ppm (range 0·0088–0·13335 ppm) in samples from 14 Cincinnati mothers aged 21–37 years (median 25·5 years), who had been breast feeding for 2–46 weeks (median 12 weeks). Levels in bovine milk were approximately double those in human milk. It is not known whether the subjects in these 2 studies overlapped.

Schulte-Löbbert *et al.* (1978) took samples of human breast milk from 42 women aged 19–37 years between the third and eleventh day after the beginning of lactation. Cadmium levels in the milk ranged from 0·005–0·05 ppm and were dependent on maternal age and duration of lactation. Higher levels were found in older women. The relationship to duration of lactation was further investigated by daily collection of "mid-stream" milk from 6 women aged 24–36 years. For the 4 subjects aged 24–27 years, cadmium content in the colostrum of the first 3 days of lactation was 0·022–0·025 ppm and in the 2 subjects aged 30 and 36 years it was 0·030 and

0·035 ppm. After the first 3 days, levels fell to a mean of 0·010 ppm in all subjects. From these values and known contents in various foodstuffs, the authors calculate that the weekly intake of cadmium in babies in the first month of life would average 0·04 mg, rising to 0·12 mg by 8–12 months of age.

B. ENDOCRINE AND GONADAL FUNCTION

There are only 2 reports in the literature relating to testicular function in men occupationally exposed to cadmium. Smith *et al.* (1960) have reported on 5 autopsy cases where there had been intermittent exposure to high levels of cadmium fume in the manufacture of copper-cadmium alloy, due to inadequate ventilation of the working area. In one case, results of the testis examination, if carried out, were not mentioned. In the second case of a 46-year-old male, exposed to cadmium from 32–41 years of age before being transferred to light work because of respiratory problems, the testes were found to contain no spermatids or spermatozoa, though the tubular epithelium was normal and there were abundant mitoses. There was no fibrosis or tubular atrophy and interstitial cells were normal. The third case was a male aged 55, exposed to cadmium fume from 42–49 years of age, and then transferred to other work within the factory because of emphysema. The picture was very similar to the previous case with normal appearance of the testicular tissues except for absence of spermatids and spermatozoa. The fourth case aged 57 was exposed to cadmium fume from 30–38 years of age before being transferred to lighter work due to dyspnoea. Emphysema was later diagnosed. The testes showed some areas of tubular atrophy with peritubular fibrosis. Many mitoses were present but spermatids and spermatozoa were infrequent. In the fifth case, aged 67, exposure had occurred at 49–57 years of age. He was then transferred to office work due to dyspnoea. The testes showed no fibrosis or hyaline thickening of the tubules, but only occasional spermatozoa were seen and the interstitial cells were inconspicuous. In all 4 cases the testes were macroscopically normal. Tissue cadmium levels were measured in the last 4 cases. Levels were highest in kidney and liver (65–39 μg/g wet weight). In one case levels of 54, 37, 24, 38 and 94 μg/g were found in the epididymis and vas, prostate, seminal vesicles, body and tunica of the testis. In another case levels of 18, 9 and 18 μg/g were found in the prostate, body and tunica of the testis. In a third case levels of 3·5 mg/g were found in the testis. No levels in the testis and accessory organs are recorded for the fourth case. These levels were compared with levels of 0·10–0·18 μg/g in the prostate, 0·16–0·20 μg/g in the body of the testis, and 0·30–0·34 μg/g in the tunica of the testis in 3 men of comparable age at autopsy with no known exposure to cadmium fume. Smith *et al.* (1960) in discussing these results noted the concentration of cadmium in the testes but felt that the plentiful mitotic activity of the spermatocytes suggested that effects on later stages of spermatogenesis were an effect of the terminal illness rather than cadmium intoxication. In view of the long time lag (5–19 years) between last exposure to cadmium fume and autopsy and the lack of any gross histological lesions in the testes which could give rise to persistent effects, these authors' interpretation may well be correct. However, the specificity of the effect on spermatids and spermatocytes also suggests the possibility of a specific causal agent, and cadmium, which persists in the body for a long time with an estimated half-life in humans of 9–30 years (Probst, 1979), cannot be ruled out.

Favino *et al.* (1968) have studied androgenic function in 10 males working in manufacture of nickel-cadmium storage batteries. Some had worked for 2–5 years or more and were still working in the cadmium area at the time of the study, whilst others had been exposed to cadmium for some years but then employed in other areas of the factory when signs of cadmium toxicity such as nose ulcers and anosmia developed. Some had left the plant some years before. The numbers in each category were not given. Results were compared with 10 controls working in other areas of the factory not exposed to cadmium, the majority working in lead storage battery manufacture. There were no significant differences in mean urinary 17-ketosteroid, androsterone, aetiocholanolone, testosterone or epitestosterone levels between exposed and control groups. However, in the cadmium exposed group, one man aged 38 years complained of impotence and inability to have more children, though he had 2 before starting work with cadmium, and his urinary testosterone level was below normal (50 μg/24 h compared with the group mean of 110 μg/24 h). His urinary cadmium level was also above the normal range (details not given). A second man in the cadmium group aged 47 years with nasal septal ulcers from cadmium poisoning also complained of impotence, but hormone levels were within the normal range. He had no children but it was not stated whether he had been trying to have children. The number of children for the other 8 cadmium exposed subjects, aged 32–75 years, ranged from 1–3 (mean for whole group 1·5). Information on numbers of children is not given for the control group. There are a number of problems with this study. Firstly, the exposure history of those in the cadmium group was highly variable and only some of the subjects in the cadmium exposed group had elevated urinary cadmium levels and these are not identified in the text or tables. Secondly, hormone levels show considerable variability in both control and exposed groups. Thirdly, subjects chosen as controls were exposed to lead which may affect testicular function, though so far there is no evidence that hormone levels are affected (Lancranjan *et al.*, 1975). From such a small, poorly controlled study it is not possible to draw any conclusions about the effects of cadmium on testicular and sexual function.

Cadmium exposure has been associated with cancer of the prostate in 2 epidemiological studies and one case report (reviewed by Owen, 1976) and there has been some speculation that cadmium may interact with zinc, which appears to have a special metabolic role in the prostate, and that the alteration in enzyme activity brought about by zinc deficiency may predispose to neoplasia.

There have been no studies on the effect of cadmium on endocrine and gonadal functions in women, except for the study of Tsvetkova (1970), showing no effect on the menstrual cycle in 106 women working with cadmium except for isolated endocrine and gynaecological disorders which had developed before the subjects had begun working with cadmium (see section D for details of this study).

C. FERTILITY

The study of Favino *et al.* (1968) discussed in detail in section B, indicated a small family size (average 1·5 children) in 10 men exposed to cadmium, but insufficient details are given of numbers conceived before exposure to cadmium, desired family size, etc., to evaluate fertility. One of the 2 workers complaining of impotence also complained of inability to have more children. Kazantzis *et al.* (1963) interviewed cadmium workers and took fertility histories but found no definitive evidence of sterility (no further details given).

In the cases of itai-itai disease, discussed in detail in section A, the high fecundity of those women succumbing to clinical symptoms suggests there is not any major effect on female fertility.

D. PREGNANCY

Tsvetkova (1970) has reported on the menstrual and reproductive histories of 106 women, aged 18–48 years, working with cadmium compounds for 2–16 years. They came from 3 different factories, one where alkaline batteries were produced where concentrations of cadmium oxide ranged from 0·1–25 mg/m^3, a chemical reagent kit factory with air concentrations of soluble cadmium salts from 0·16–35 mg/m^3, and a zinc moulding factory where sulphoxide, sulphurous and metallic cadmium levels were 0·02–25 mg/m^3. Controls were women not exposed to cadmium (no further details given). There were a total of 67 births in the cadmium-exposed group and 20 births in controls. It is not known if some women had more than one child in this study. The course and duration of pregnancy was normal in both groups but mean birth-weight of children born to those working the alkaline storage battery and zinc moulding factories (3·084 and 3·351 kg respectively) were significantly lower than controls (3·630 kg). Mean birth-weight in those working in the chemical reagents factory was also lower than controls (3·202 kg), but was not significantly so because of small sample size and large variability in this group.

In 4 of the 27 children born to the women working in zinc moulding there were clear signs of rickets, 1 child had retarded tooth eruption and 2 had dental disorders (not specified). No such effects were observed in controls. Whilst the sample size is small and further details would be required to permit proper evaluation of these findings, the similarity between these effects on bone and teeth and those involving the skeletal system in animals exposed prenatally to cadmium (see Animal Studies), cannot be ignored.

Bryce-Smith *et al.* (1977) have shown elevated levels of lead and cadmium in bones of stillbirths (see section A for details) but the aetiological significance of these observations cannot be assessed until there is data available on liveborns succumbing to accidental death shortly after birth, for comparison.

Brill *et al.* (1974) have published data on various trace elements, including cadmium, in placenta and newborn blood from cases of respiratory disease of the newborn compared with normal newborns. The ratios of cadmium for respiratory disease:normal newborn were 1·11 for placenta, and 1·36 for fetal blood. Ratios for other elements (Hg, Se, Rb, Zn, Fe, Co and Pb) ranged from 0·72–1·03 for placenta and 0·97–1·52 for newborn blood. These results suggested that levels of lead and cadmium in the blood of newborns with respiratory disease is slightly higher than that in controls, but no definite conclusions can be drawn.

E. MUTAGENICITY

A number of workers have shown chromosome damage to human lymphocyte cultures exposed to cadmium *in vitro*. Shiraishi *et al.* (1972) added cadmium sulphide to lymphocytes in culture at a final concentration of $6{\cdot}2 \times 10^{-2}$ μg/ml and found significant increases in cells with chromatid or isochromatid breaks, translocations and dicentric chromosomes after 4 and 8 h incubation. Zasukhina *et al.* (1977) have cultured human lymphocytes in the presence of cadmium chloride at $2{\cdot}5 \times 10^{-5}$–$3{\cdot}5 \times 10^{-6}$ M and shown increased DNA degradation, as assessed from profiles of DNA sedimentation. Combined treatment with cadmium and gamma-irradiation (the latter induces repair) suggested that cadmium probably acts by inducing non-repairable DNA damage. Koizumi *et al.* (1979) have also shown significant increases in chromosome breaks in human lymphocytes cultured in the presence of 1×10^{-6} M cadmium chloride, and Voroshilin *et al.* (1978) have shown increases in chromosome aberrations in the presence of cadmium acetate. However, besides these 4 positive studies, Paton and Allison (1972) have found no cytogenetic effects in human lymphocytes cultured in the presence of $5{\cdot}0 \times 10^{-8}$ M cadmium chloride. This is a lower concentration than that used by Koizumi *et al.* (1979) who did find effects with cadmium chloride.

There have been a number of *in vivo* studies on people exposed environmentally or occupationally to cadmium. Shiraishi and Yosida (1972) published a preliminary study on chromosome aberrations in itai-itai patients (see section A for description) and these patients were also included in a larger study published later by Shiraishi (1975). Twelve patients, all female aged 52–72 years, exposed to cadmium pollution for up to 30 years were examined in 1972 and some of them again in 1973. Results were compared with 6 female and 3 male controls aged 58–78 (no further details given). Eight of the 12 patients showed a very high frequency of chromatid aberrations and some chromosomal aberrations of both the unstable and stable type, and aneuploidy. The remaining 4 patients showed a much lower frequency of aberrations but a significant number of stable aberrations were still observed in this latter group. At the 1972 examination in the itai-itai group a total of 31·2% of the cells examined were cytogenetically abnormal compared with 2·6% in controls. At the 1973 examination structural aberrations were seen in 23·5% of itai-itai patients' cells compared with 2·5% in controls, and numerical aberrations in 13·3% of patients' cells compared with 2·5% in controls. In the itai-itai disease group aberrations were found in both 50 h and 72 h cultures, suggesting that aberrations were in the blood stem cells. It is not known whether the itai-itai patients had received therapeutic drugs or diagnostic radiation which might have induced chromosome damage, though in their preliminary publication on 7 of the 12 patients Shiraishi and Yosida (1972) stated that drugs had not been given. However, given the nature of the disease, it is likely that the patients had been X-rayed for signs of bone damage.

Bui *et al.* (1975) have compared Japanese itai-itai patients and Japanese controls with Swedish workers exposed to cadmium from work in the electrode department of an alkaline storage battery manufacturer and Swedish controls. The Swedish workers had been exposed to cadmium for 5–24 years (mean 12 years) and exposure levels taken in 1969–1972, thought to be representative of conditions since 1961, indicated average air levels of 35 $\mu g/m^3$ in the electrode department whilst personal air samples indicated twice this value. Blood and urinary cadmium levels were measured in all 4 groups. Blood cadmium was highest in the Swedish workers indicating higher recent exposure (26–61 ng/g) followed by the itai-itai patients (15–29 ng/g). Japanese controls (4–6 ng/g) and Swedish controls (1–3 ng/g). Urinary cadmium was highest in itai-itai patients, probably reflecting more pronounced renal tubular damage and higher body burden (12–31 μg/g creatinine), followed by the Swedish workers (2–31 μg/g), Japanese controls (5–11 μg/g) and Swedish controls (1–4 μg/g). Cytogenetic analysis of the itai-itai patients and the 4 Japanese controls (of similar age and from the same prefecture as the patients but living in uncontaminated areas) showed no significant differences between the 2 groups; structural aberrations were found in 6·6% of patients' cells compared with 6·0% in controls, chromatid breaks, chromosome breaks and aneuploidy being found in both groups. In the Swedish groups the mean frequency of structural aberrations in 72 h and 48 h cultures was 2·0% and 2·4% respectively in the 5 workers and 4·7% and 3·3% respectively in the 3 controls of the same sex and similar age to the workers. The results of this study do not agree with those of Shiraishi (1975). The itai-itai patients did not have a chromosome aberration rate higher than Japanese controls, though the blood and urinary cadmium levels of the controls and their geographical proximity to the area where itai-itai disease is endemic suggest the controls may have had some cadmium exposure from the environment too. Nevertheless the rate of aberrations in the itai-itai group (6·6%) is still substantially lower than the rates in Shiraishi's (1975) study of 9–12% in "low frequency" patients and well below the "high frequency" patients' rates of 11–50%. The results from the 2 Swedish groups also suggest no cytogenetic effect of cadmium. The aberration frequency in these groups was slightly lower than that in the 2 Japanese groups as might be expected from the age difference. Unfortunately the small sample sizes in this study do not permit firm conclusions to be drawn. It is possible that some, but not all, itai-itai patients have increased chromosome aberrations and that these were missed in the present study where only 4 patients were examined. It is further possible that cadmium alone is insufficient to induce chromosome aberrations, but exposure to cadmium, lead and zinc as is known to be the case for itai-itai patients, is necessary.

Léonard *et al.* (1975) have published in abstract only observations of chromatid and chromosome aberrations in peripheral blood lymphocytes from workers in the cadmium industry, but no rates and no control data were given. In another abstract (Deknudt and Léonard, 1976) they reported finding a higher rate of severe chromosome anomalies (chromatid exchange, disturbance of spiralisation, translocation, ring and dicentric chromosomes) but a lower total number of structural aberrations in workers exposed to high levels of lead and cadmium (dust and fume) compared with workers exposed mostly to zinc but also to lower levels of lead and cadmium. No further details were given.

Bauchinger *et al.* (1976) have observed increased chromosome damage in 24 workers in a zinc smelting plant (1·35% of cells with structural aberrations) compared with 15 controls (0·47% of cells with aberrations). Damage was mainly of the chromatid type (breaks and exchanges) accompanied by acentric fragments. The workers, however, were exposed to zinc and lead as well as cadmium and blood levels of lead and cadmium were elevated to 19 μg/100 ml for cadmium, compared with expected values (not given) for adults not occupationally exposed to heavy metals. Bauchinger *et al.* (1976) suggest from their other negative studies on lead workers that cadmium alone or in synergism with the other metals may well be responsible for the increase in aberrations observed in the present study. However, other workers claim lead does have cytogenetic effects and so it is not possible definitely to identify the causal agent(s).

O'Riordan *et al.* (1978) have studied 40 men actively employed in the manufacture of cadmium pigments and compared the results with 13 controls employed as laboratory and administrative staff in the same plant, and 285 controls from the general population examined in a previous study. In the exposed group, aged 17–61 years, occupational exposure varied from 6 weeks to 34 years (mean not given). Atmospheric cadmium levels were 0·6–1·0 mg/m^3 between 1964 and 1968 and 0·2 mg/m^3 from 1968 onwards. Blood cadmium levels in the exposed group averaged 1·9 μg/100 ml (range 0·2–14·0 μg/100 ml) and in controls from the same plant 0·6–2·9 μg/100 ml in 5 cases and <0·2 μg/100 ml in 8 cases. Two of the exposed group had proteinuria, suggesting cadmium toxicity had occurred. In the exposed group 6·6% of cells were cytogenetically abnormal. In the control workers in the same plant 7·6% were abnormal and in the general population 3·4% were abnormal. The authors state there were no significant differences between the groups, which is surprising in view of the lower frequency of aberrations in the general population group. Within the occupationally exposed group, no significant correlations could be found between the extent of chromosome damage and past occupational history nor blood cadmium level. However, some doubt remains about the authors' claim of negative findings since the exposed and control groups working in the plant showed a higher overall frequency of aberrations than general population controls and there was some evidence from blood cadmium levels that workers in the plant "control" group may have had some cadmium exposure.

In summary, there is evidence from 4/5 *in vitro* studies that cadmium is mutagenic. The *in vivo* studies suggest that cadmium in combination with other heavy metals such as lead may have mutagenic effects but evidence that cadmium alone has cytogenetic effects is as yet unconvincing.

F. CARCINOGENICITY

IARC Monograph Vol. 11 (1976) reported that available studies indicate that occupational exposure to cadmium increases the risk of prostate cancer and one of these studies also suggests an increased risk of respiratory cancer.

SUMMARY AND EVALUATION

EXPERIMENTAL STUDIES

Cadmium is well absorbed by inhalation and to a lesser extent orally, except in neonatal animals which absorb cadmium well by the oral route. Toxicity is higher in pregnant than non-pregnant or post-partum animals due to a specific toxic action on the placenta. Studies in mice, rats and hamsters have shown that very little cadmium, usually less than 0·02% of a maternal dose, crosses the placenta into the fetus. Fetal levels soon decrease after a single dose to the dam, though some binding to fetal liver occurs. Little cadmium is excreted via the milk. Studies in mice, rats, hamsters, rabbits, guinea pigs, dogs and squirrels have shown that injections of cadmium salts can produce severe testicular damage both in the tubules and in the interstitial cells. Several studies have also shown that this damage can be produced following oral dosing, if given chronically. Changes in secondary sex organs are probably a result of reduced interstitial cell production of testosterone though there is some evidence of a direct toxic effect on the prostate. The testicular damage is thought to be due to damage to the microvasculature resulting in ischaemia and tissue necrosis. Interaction with other substances also occurs so that the effects may be potentiated by simultaneous exposure to lead, or inhibited by exposure to zinc, selenium, cysteine, BAL or oestrogen. The ovary has also been shown to accumulate cadmium but ovarian damage with disturbed cycles is only seen with doses producing other signs of toxicity. Unlike the changes in the seminiferous tubules, the ovarian effects are reversible.

Reduced fertility is seen in male rodents following parenteral doses around 1 mg/kg or oral doses around 100 mg/kg.

If administered during pregnancy cadmium is embryolethal, fetotoxic and teratogenic in all species studied. The margin between the teratogenic and the embryolethal dose is small, and because of the poor oral absorption higher doses are needed orally ($\sim$4 mg/kg) to produce malformations. At high doses, some of the effects observed may be secondary to damage to the placenta but at lower doses a direct effect of cadmium on the embryo seems likely. Inhalation of 0·04–0·6 ppm affect fetal and postnatal development in rats. Among the adverse effects of cadmium exposure is anaemia in both the dam and fetus with the latter being more severely affected. Abnormal calcium metabolism in the fetus may result in skeletal abnormalities as well as very brittle bones causing postnatal fractures. Brain development also appears to be affected.

Conflicting results have been obtained in mutagenicity studies. Local tumours have been produced in rats following s.c. or i.m. injections. Studies of other routes are inadequate for evaluation. No transplacental carcinogenicity studies have been found.

HUMAN STUDIES

The evidence from Japanese studies suggests that post-menopausal women are most susceptible to the toxic effects of environmental cadmium contamination. Intakes of around 600 μg per day caused a variety of defects in bone resulting in pain and increased brittleness. Cadmium crosses the placenta and levels in the fetus are generally slightly less than in the maternal blood. Placental levels are usually higher than those in blood and may provide some barrier to transfer to the fetus. The levels in the placenta but not in the fetus are higher in smokers than in non-smokers. There is some evidence that women living in industrial areas have higher blood and placental levels than those in rural areas. Small amounts around 0·01 ppm are present in breast milk giving a weekly intake of about 0·04–0·1 mg cadmium to the baby. There is limited evidence that exposure to very high levels of cadmium repeatedly may induce testicular damage in men as well as respiratory problems. Cadmium does not seem to affect fertility in women. There are inadequate data to define any effects on pregnancy. The majority of *in vitro* studies have suggested that cadmium has mutagenic activity but despite several studies on occupationally exposed workers equivocal results have been obtained. There is evidence that cadmium exposure increases the risk of prostatic and possibly also respiratory cancer.

EVALUATION

There is sufficient evidence that cadmium can exert a specific toxic effect on the testis in chronically exposed animals. It is embryolethal, fetotoxic and teratogenic and affects postnatal development. In humans there is evidence that exposure to high levels may be especially toxic to post-menopausal women. There is inadequate data to assess its toxicity to the testis in men or its effects on pregnancy. It may have a low degree of mutagenic activity in occupationally exposed persons and may pose a carcinogenic hazard.

Attention is drawn to the need for studies on fertility in men, and on pregnancy and postnatal development in children of occupationally exposed women.

References

Ahokas, R. A., Herman, W. K. and Dilts, P. V. (1976). Placental accumulation of cadmium. *Gynecologic and Obstetric Investigation* **7**, 66–67.

Ahokas, R. A. and Dilts, P. V. (1977). Cadmium uptake in the rat embryo as a function of gestational age. *Gynecologic and Obstetric Investigation* **8**, 46–47.

Aoki, R. A. and Hoffer, A. P. (1978). Reexamination of the lesions in rat testis caused by cadmium. *Biology of Reproduction* **18**, (4), 579–591.

Ariyoshi, T., Tenda, N., Yoshitake, S. and Yamada, H. (1977). Placenta distribution and accumulation of cadmium in pregnant rats. *Shokuhin Eisegaku Zasshi* **18**, (6), 516–523.

Baglan, R. J., Brill, A. B., Schulert, A., Wilson, D., Larsen, K., Dyer, N., Mansour, M., Schaffner, W., Hoffman, L. and Davies, J. (1974). Utility of placental tissue as an indicator of trace element exposure to adult and fetus. *Environmental Research* **8**, (1), 64–70.

Barr, M. Jr. (1972). The teratogenicity of cadmium chloride in two stocks of Wistar rats. *Teratology* **7**, 237–242.

Bauchinger, M., Schmid, E., Einbrodt, H. J. and Dresp, J. (1976). Chromosome aberrations in lymphocytes after occupational exposure to lead and cadmium *Mutation Research* **40**, 57–62.

Berlin, M. and Ullberg, S. (1963). The fate of Cd109 in the mouse. *Archives of Environmental Health* **7**, 686–693.

Brill, A. B., Baglan, R. J., Fleet, W., Schaffner, W. and Schulert, A. (1974). A network to determine causality between abnormal trace element levels in congenital defects. *Proceedings—First Annual NSF Trace Contamination Conference (1973)*, pp. 522–527.

Bryce-Smith, D., Deshpande, R. R., Hughes, J. and Waldron, H. A. (1977). Lead and cadmium levels in stillbirths. (Letter). *Lancet* **i**, 1159.

Buchet, J. P., Roels, H., Hubermont, G. and Lauwerys, R. (1978). Placental transfer of lead, mercury, cadmium, and carbon monoxide in women. *Environmental Research* **15**, (3), 494–503.

Bui, T.-H., Lindsten, J. and Nordberg, G. F. (1975). Chromosome analysis of lymphocytes from cadmium workers and itai-itai patients. *Environmental Research* **9**, 187–195.

Chaube, S., Nishimura, H. and Swinyard, C. A. (1973). Zinc and cadmium in normal human embryos and fetuses. *Archives of Environmental Health* **26**, 237–240.

Chernoff, W. (1973). Teratogenic effects of cadmium in rats. *Teratology* **8**, 29–32.

Chiquoine, A. D. (1965). Effect of cadmium chloride on pregnant albino mouse. *Journal of Reproduction and Fertility* **10**, 263–265.

Chiquoine, A. D. and Suntzeff, V. (1965). Sensitivity of mammals to cadmium necrosis of the testis. *Journal of Reproduction and Fertility* **10**, 455–457.

Choudhury, H., Hastings, L., Cooper, G. P. and Petering, H. G. (1979). Gestational cadmium exposure: effects on maternal and neonatal hematopoiesis. Annual Report of Program 1978–1979—Center for the Study of the Human Environment, Department of Environmental Health, Kettering Laboratory, University of Cincinnati, pp. 23–28.

Datnow, M. M. (1928). An experimental investigation concerning toxic abortion produced by chemical agents. *Journal of Obstetrics and Gynaecology of the British Commonwealth* **35**, 693–724.

Dawson, E. B., Cravy, W. D., Clark, R. R and McGanity, W. J. (1969). Effect of trace metals on placental metabolism. *American Journal of Obstetrics and Gynecology* **103**, 253–256.

Deknudt, G. and Léonard, A. (1976). Cytogenic investigations on leucocytes of workers from a cadmium plant. *Mutation Research* **38**, (2), 112–113.

Dencker, L. (1976). Cadmium: accumulation in the embryos, placentas and ovaries related to effects on reproduction. *Acta Pharmacologica et Toxicologica* **39**, (Suppl. 1, Chapter 1), 9–25.

Der, R., Fahim, Z., Youset, M. and Fahim, M. (1977). Effects of cadmium on growth, sexual development and metabolism in female rats. *Research Communications in Chemical Pathology and Pharmacology* **16**, (3), 485–505.

Der, R., Fahim, Z., Youset, M. and Fahim, M. (1978). Environmental interaction of lead and cadmium on reproduction and metabolism of male rats. *Trace Substances in Environmental Health* **10**, 505–507.

Donnelly, P. A. and Monty, D. E. (1977). Toxicological effects of cadmium chloride on the canine testis following various routes of administration. *Toxicology Letters (Amsterdam)* **1**, (1), 55–58.

Dutt, N. H. G., Wakabayashik, K. and Inouye, S. (1978). Effect of cadmium chloride on the serum levels of follicle stimulating hormone (FSH), luteinizing hormone (LH) and androgens in the adult male rat. *Proceedings—Indian Academy of Sciences Section B* **87**, (7), 161–167.

Dwivedi, C., Singh, D. N., Crump, E. P. and Harbison, R. D. (1977). Reproductive toxicity of cadmium. *Toxicology and Applied Pharmacology* **41**, 194.

Epstein, S. S., Arnold, E., Andrea, J., Bass, W. and Bishop, Y. (1972). Detection of chemical mutagens by the dominant lethal assay in the mouse. *Toxicology and Applied Pharmacology* **23**, 288–325.

Favino, A., Baillie, A. H. and Griffiths, K. (1966). Androgen synthesis by the testes and adrenal glands of rats poisoned with cadmium chloride. *Journal of Endocrinology* **35**, 185–192.

Favino, A., Candura, F., Chiappino, G. and Cavalleri, A. (1968). Study on the androgen function of men exposed to cadmium. *Medicina del Lavoro* **59**, 105–110.

Ferm, V. H. (1971). Developmental malformations induced by cadmium. A study of timed injections during embryogenesis. *Biology of the Neonate* **19**, 101–107.

Ferm, V. H. (1972). The teratogenic effects of metals on mammalian embryos. *Advances in Teratology* **5**, 51–75.

Ferm, V. H. and Carpenter, S. J. (1967). Teratogenic effect of cadmium and its inhibition by zinc. *Nature* **216**, 1123.

Ferm, V. H., Hanlon, D. P. and Urban, J. (1969). The permeability of the hamster placenta to radioactive cadmium. *Journal of Embryology and Experimental Morphology* **22**, (1), 107–113.

Flick, D. F., Kraybill, H. F. and Dimitroff, J. M. (1971). Toxic effects of cadmium. A review. *Environmental Research* **4**, (2), 71–85.

Gale, T. F. and Ferm, V. H. (1971). Skeletal malformations resulting from cadmium treatment in the hamster. *Biology of the Neonate* **19**, 101–107.

Gabbiani, G., Baic, D. and Deziel, C. (1967). Toxicity of cadmium for the central nervous system. *Experimental Neurology* **18**, 154–160.

Gilliavod, N. and Léonard, A. (1975). Mutagenicity tests with cadmium in the mouse. *Toxicology* **5**, 43–47.

Goodman, D. L., Fant, M. and Harbison, R. D. (1978). Placental toxicity of mercury and cadmium; evidence for direct effects on placental plasma membranes. *Pharmacologist* **20**, 262.

Goodman, D. R., Fant, M. E. and Harbison, R. D. (1979). Direct effects of the heavy metals mercury and cadmium on α-aminoisobutyric acid transport across human placental membranes. *Federation Proceedings* **38**, 535.

Gunn, S. A., Gould, T. C. and Anderson, W. A. D. (1965). Protective effect of estrogen against vascular damage to the testis caused by cadmium. *Proceedings of the Society for Experimental Biology and Medicine* **119**, 901–905.

Gunn, S. A., Gould, T. C. and Anderson, W. A. (1966). Protective effect of thiol compounds against cadmium-induced vascular damage to testis. *Proceedings of the Society for Experimental Biology and Medicine* **122**, 1036–1039.

Gunn, S. A., Gould, T. C. and Anderson, W. A. D. (1968). Selectivity of organ response to cadmium injury and various protective measures. *Journal of Pathology and Bacteriology* **96**, 89–96.

Hastings, L., Choudhury, H., Petering, H. G. and Cooper, G. P. (1978). Behavioral and biochemical effects of low-level prenatal cadmium exposure in rats. *Bulletin of Environmental Contamination and Toxicology* **20**, 96–101.

Holmberg, R. E. and Ferm, V. H. (1969). Interrelationships of selenium, cadmium and arsenic in mammalian teratogenesis. *Archives of Environmental Health* **18**, 873–877.

Howell, W. and Cooper, G. P. (1979). Biochemical and behavioral evaluation of gestational cadmium exposure. Annual Report of Program—Center for the Study of the Human Environment, Department of Environmental Health, Kettering Laboratory, University of Cincinnati, pp. 170–177.

IARC Monographs on the Evaluation of the Carcinogenic Risk of Chemicals to Humans: Cadmium, nickel, some epoxides, miscellaneous industrial chemicals and general considerations on volatile anaesthetics (1976). Vol. 11, Lyon, France.

Ishizu, S., Minami, I., Suzuki, A., Yamada, M., Sato, M. and Yamamura, K. (1973). An experimental study on teratogenic effects of cadmium. *Industrial Health* **11**, 127–139.

Kar, A. B., Das, R. P. and Karkun, J. N. (1959). Ovarian changes in prepuberal rats after treatment with cadmium chloride. *Acta Biologica et Medica Germanica* **3**, 372–379.

Kazantzis, G., Flynn, F. V., Spowage, J. S. and Trott, D. G. (1963). Renal tubular malfunction and pulmonary emphysema in cadmium pigment workers. *Quarterly Journal of Medicine, New Series* **32**, 165–192.

Keino, H. and Yamamura, H. (1974). Effects of a cadmium salt administered to pregnant mice on postnatal development of the offspring. *Teratology* **10**, (1), 87.

Kello, D., Dekanic, D. and Kostial, K. (1979). Influence of sex and dietary calcium on intestinal cadmium absorption in rats. *Archives of Environmental Health* **34**, 30–33.

Kelman, B. J., Walter, B. K., Jarboe, G. E. and Sasser, L. B. (1978). Effect of dietary cadmium on calcium metabolism in the rat during late gestation. *Proceedings of the Society for Experimental Biology and Medicine* **158**, 614–617.

Koizumi, A., Dobashi, Y. and Tachibana, Y. (1979). Chromosome changes induced by industrial chemicals. *Japanese Journal of Industrial Health* **21**, (1), 3–10.

Kostial, K., Kello, D., Jugo, S., Rabar, I. and Maljkovic, T. (1978). Influence of age on metal metabolism and toxicity. *Environmental Health Perspectives* **25**, 81–86.

Kotsonis, F. N. and Klaassen, C. D. (1977). Toxicity and distribution of cadmium administered to rats at sublethal doses. *Toxicology and Applied Pharmacology* **41**, 667–680.

Krasovskii, G. N., Varshavskaya, S. P. and Borisov, A. I. (1976). Toxic and gonadotropic effects of cadmium and boron relative to standards for these substances in drinking water. *Environmental Health Perspectives* **13**, 69–75.

Lancranjan, I., Popescu, H. I., Gavanescu, O., Klepsch, I. and Serbanescu, M. (1975). Reproductive ability of workmen exposed to lead. *Archives of Environmental Health* **30**, 396–401.

Lau, I. F., Saksena, S. K., Dahlgren, L. and Chang, M. C. (1978). Steroids in the blood serum and testes of cadmium chloride treated hamsters. *Biology of Reproduction* **19**, (4), 886–889.

Lauwerys, R., Buchet, J. P., Roels, H. and Hubermont, G. (1978). Placental transfer of lead, mercury, cadmium and carbon monoxide in women. 1. Comparison of the frequency distributions of the biological indices in maternal and umbilical cord blood. *Environmental Research* **15**, (2), 278–289.

Layton, W. M. Jr. and Layton, M. W. (1979). Cadmium induced limb defects in mice: strain associated differences in sensitivity. *Teratology* **19**, 229–236.

Lee, I. P. and Dixon, R. L. (1973). Effects of cadmium on spermatogenesis studied by velocity sedimentation cell separation and serial mating. *Journal of Pharmacology and Experimental Therapeutics* **187**, (3), 641–652.

Léonard, A., Deknudt, G. and Gilliavod, N. (1975). Genetic and cytogenetic hazards of heavy metals in mammals. *Mutation Research* **29**, (2), 280–281.

Levin, A. A., Cary, D. I. and Miller, R. K. (1980). Fetal toxicity of cadmium in Wistar rats: maternal endocrine status and placental viability. *Teratology* **21**, (3), 53A.

Levin, A. A. and Miller, R. K. (1979). Fetal toxicity of cadmium: decreased placental blood flow in the Wistar rat. *Teratology* **19**, (2), 36–37A.

Lohiya, N. K. (1976). Effects of cadmium chloride on the testis and sex accessory glands of the Indian palm squirrel, funambulus pennanti (Wroughton). *Acta Europaea Fertilitatis* **7**, (3), 257–265.

Lucis, O. J., Lucis, R. and Shaikh, Z. A. (1972). Cadmium and zinc in pregnancy and lactation. *Archives of Environmental Health* **25**, 14–22.

Madlafousek, J., Hlinak, Z. and Pařízek, J. (1971). Sexual behaviour of male rats sterilized by cadmium. *Journal of Reproduction and Fertility* **26**, 189–196.

Martin, P. G., Hitchcock, B. B. and King, J. F. (1978). Postnatal changes in the anemic rat after exposure to Cd during gestation. *Trace Substances in Environmental Health* **12**, 191–197.

Matsumoto, N., Iijama, S. and Katsunuma, H. (1975). Fetal body burden of chemicals and its effect on fetal growth. *Congenital Anomalies* **15**, (4), 245–246.

Murata, I., Hirono, T., Saeki, Y. and Kakagawa, S. (1970). Cadmium enteropathy, renal osteomalacia ("Itai Itai" disease in Japan). *Bulletin de la Société International de Chirurgie* **29**, (11), 34–42.

Murthy, G. K. and Rhea, U. S. (1971). Cadmium, copper, iron, lead, manganese and zinc in evaporated milk, infant products, and human milk. *Journal of Dairy Science* **54**, (7), 1001–1005.

Nolen, G. A., Bohne, R. L. and Buehler, E. V. (1972a). Effects of trisodium nitrilotriacetate, trisodium citrate and a trisodium nitrilotriacetate-ferric chloride mixture on cadmium and methylmercury toxicity and teratogenesis in rats. *Toxicology and Applied Pharmacolgy* **23**, 238–250.

Nolen, G. A., Buehler, E. V., Geil, R. G. and Goldenthal, E. H. (1972b). Effects of trisodium nitrilotriacetate on cadmium and methylmercury toxicity and teratogenicity in rats. *Toxicology and Applied Pharmacology* **23**, 222–237.

Nordberg, G. F. (1971). Effects of acute and chronic cadmium exposure on the testicles of mice. *Environmental Physiology* **1**, (4), 171–187.

O'Riordan, M. L., Hughes, E. G. and Evans, H. J. (1978). Chromosome studies on blood lymphocytes of men occupationally exposed to cadmium. *Mutation Research* **58**, 305–311.

Owen, W. L. (1976). Cancer of the prostate: a literature review. *Journal of Chronic Diseases* **29**, (2), 89–114.

Pařízek, J. (1957). The destructive effect of cadmium ion on testicular tissue and its prevention by zinc. *Journal of Endocrinology* **15**, 56–63.

Pařízek, J. (1960). Sterilization of the male by cadmium salts. *Journal of Reproduction and Fertility* **1**, 294–309.

Pařízek, J. (1964). Vascular changes at sites of oestrogen biosynthesis produced by parenteral injection of cadmium salts: the destruction of placenta by cadmium salts. *Journal of Reproduction and Fertility* **7**, 263–265.

Pařízek, J. (1965). The peculiar toxicity of cadmium during pregnancy—an experimental 'toxaemia of pregnancy' induced by cadmium salts. *Journal of Reproduction and Fertility* **9**, 111–112.

Pařízek, J., Oštádalová, I., Benes, I. and Babický, A. (1968a). Pregnancy and trace elements: the protective effect of compounds of an essential trace element—selenium—against the peculiar toxic effects of cadmium during pregnancy. *Journal of Reproduction and Fertility* **16**, 507–509.

Pařízek, J., Oštádalová, I., Benes, I. and Pitha, J. (1968b). The effect of a subcutaneous injection of cadmium salts on the ovaries of adult rats in persistent oestrus. *Journal of Reproduction and Fertility* **17**, 559–562.

Pařízek, J. and Záhoř, Z. (1956). Effect of cadmium salts on testicular tissue. *Nature* **177**, 1036.

Parzyck, D. C., Shaw, S. M., Kessler, W. V., Vetter, R. J., Sickle, D. C. and Mayes, R. A. (1978). Fetal effects of cadmium in pregnant rats on normal and zinc deficient diets. *Bulletin of Environmental Contamination and Toxicology* **19**, 206–214.

Paton, G. R. and Allison, A. C. (1972). Chromosome damage in human cell cultures induced by metal salts. *Mutation Research* **16**, (3), 332–336.

Paufler, S. K. and Foote, R. H. (1969). Effect of triethylenemelamine (TEM) and cadmium chloride on spermatogenesis in rabbits. *Journal of Reproduction and Fertility* **19**, 309–319.

Pietrzak-Flis, Z., Rehnberg, G. L., Favor, M. J., Cahili, D. F. and Laskey, J. W. (1978). Chronic ingestion of cadmium and/or tritium in rats. *Environmental Research* **16**, 9–17.

Pinkerton, C., Hammerton, D. I., Bridbord, K., Craeson, J. P., Kent, J. L. and Murthy, G. K. (1972). Human milk as a dietary source of cadmium and lead. *In* "Sixth Annual Conference on Trace Substances in Environmental Health" (Ed. Hemphill, D. D.), pp. 37–43. Memorial Union, University of Missouri, Columbia, on June 13–15, 1972.

Pond, W. G. and Walker, E. F. (1975). Effect of dietary Ca and Cd level of pregnant rats on reproduction and on dam and progeny tissue mineral concentrations. *Proceedings of the Society for Experimental Biology and Medicine* **148**, 665–668.

Prigge, E. (1978). Inhalative cadmium effects in pregnant and fetal rats. *Toxicology* **10**, 297–309.

Probst, G. S. (1979). Cadmium: absorption, distribution, and excretion in mammals. *In* "Cadmium Toxicity" (Ed. Mennear, J. H.), Chapter 2, pp. 30–59. Marcel Dekker, Inc., New York and Basel.

Roels, H., Humbermont, G., Buchet, J. P. and Lauwerys, R. (1978). Placental transfer of lead, mercury, cadmium and carbon monoxide in women. *Environmental Research* **16**, 236–247.

Rohrer, S. R., Shaw, S. M., Born, G. S. and Vetter, R. J. (1978a). The maternal distribution and placental transfer of cadmium in zinc deficient rats. *Bulletin of Environmental Contamination and Toxicology* **19**, 556–563.

Rohrer, S. R., Shaw, S. M. and Lamar, C. H. (1978b). Cadmium induced endothelial cell alterations in the fetal brain from prenatal exposure. *Acta Neuropathologica* **44**, (2), 147–149.

Rohrer, S. R., Shaw, S. M. and Lamar, C. H. (1979). Cadmium fetotoxicity in rats following prenatal exposure. *Bulletin of Environmental Contamination and Toxicology* **23**, 25–29.

Saksena, S. K., Dahlgren, L., Lau, I. F. and Chang, M. C. (1977). Reproductive and endocrinological features of male rats after treatment with cadmium chloride. *Biology of Reproduction* **16**, (5), 609–613.

Samarawickrama, G. P. and Webb, M. (1979). Acute effects of cadmium on the pregnant rat and embryo-fetal development. *Environmental Health Perspectives* **28**, 245–249.

Schroeder, H. A. and Mitchener, M. (1971). Toxic effects of trace elements on the reproduction of mice and rats. *Archives of Environmental Health* **23**, 102–106.

Schulte-Löbbert, F. J., Bohn, G. and Ackov, L. (1978). Studies on exogenous cadmium uptake in newborns and small children. *Beitraege zur Gerichtlichen Medizin* **36**, 491–495.

Semba, R., Yamamura, H. and Murakami, U. (1977). Effect of cadmium pretreatment on teratogenicity and fetolethality of cadmium. *Okajimas Folia Anatomica Japonica* **54**, 283–287.

Senczuk, W. and Zielinska-Psuja, B. (1977). Morphological and histoenzymatic changes in rat testicles after prolonged administration of cadmium. *Folia Histochemica et Cytochemica* **15**, (2), 162.

Shimada, T., Watanabe, T. and Endo, A. (1976). Potential mutagenicity of cadmium in mammalian oocytes. *Mutation Research* **40**, 389–396.

Shiraishi, Y. (1975). Cytogenetic studies in 12 patients with itai-itai disease. *Humangenetik* **27**, 31–44.

Shiraishi, Y., Kurahashi, K. and Yosida, T. H. (1972). Chromosomal aberrations in cultured human leucocytes induced by cadmium sulphide. *Proceedings of the Japan Academy* **48**, (2), 133–137.

Shiraishi, Y. and Yosida, T. H. (1972). Chromosomal abnormalities in cultured leucocyte cells from Itai Itai disease patients. *Proceedings of the Japan Academy* **48**, (4), 248–251.

Singhal, R. L. and Merali, Z. (1979). Biochemical toxicity of cadmium (Parts III and IV). *In* "Cadmium Toxicity", (Ed. Mennear, J. H.), Chapter 3, pp. 80–112. Marcel Dekker, Inc., New York and Basel.

Smith, J. P., Smith, J. C. and McCall, A. J. (1960). Chronic poisoning from cadmium fume. *Journal of Pathology and Bacteriology* **80**, 287–296.

Sonawane, B. R., Nordberg, M., Nordberg, G. F. and Lucier, G. W. (1975). Placental transfer of cadmium in rats: influence of dose and gestational age. *Environmental Health Perspectives* **12**, 97–102.

Sutou, S., Yamamoto, K., Sendota, H. and Sugiyama, M. (1980). Toxicity, fertility, teratogenicity, and dominant lethal tests in rats administered cadmium subchronically. *Ecotoxicology and Environmental Safety* **4**, 51–56.

Taylor, B. A., Heiniger, H. J. and Meier, H. (1973). Genetic analysis of resistance to cadmium-induced testicular damage. *Proceedings of the Society for Experimental Biology and Medicine* **143**, 629–633.

Thieme, R., Schramel, P. and Kurz, E. (1977). Die Spurenelementkonzentration der menschlichen Plazenta in stark kontaminiertter Umwelt. *Geburtshilfe und Frauenheilkunde* **37**, (9), 756–761.

Thurauf, J., Schaller, K.-H., Engelhardt, E. and Gossler, K. (1975). Cadmium-content in the human placenta. *International Archives of Occupational and Environmental Health* **36**, 19–27.

Timms, B. G., Chandler, J. A., Morton, M. S. and Groom, G. V. (1977). The effect of cadmium administration in vivo on plasma testosterone and the ultrastructure of rat lateral prostate. *Virchows Archiv B (Cell Pathology)* **25**, (1), 33–52.

Tsuchiya, K. (1969). Causation of ouch ouch disease (Itai-Itai Byo)—An introductory review. Part II. Epidemiology and evaluation. *Keio Journal of Medicine* **18**, (4), 195–211.

Tsvetkova, R. P. (1970). Materials on the study of the influence of cadmium compounds on the generative function. *Gigiena Truda i Professional'Nye Zabolevaniya* **14**, (3), 31–33.

U.S. Department of Health, Education and Welfare (1976). Occupational exposure to cadmium: criteria for a recommended standard. HEW publication No. (NIOSH) 76–192.

Vare, A. M. and Monie, I. W. (1976). Effect of cadmium sulphate on Long-Evans rat fetuses. *Journal of the Anatomical Society of India* **25**, (3), 118–123.

Voroshilin, S. I., Plotko, E. G., Fink, T. V. and Nikiforova, V. Jr. (1978). Cytogenetic effect of inorganic compounds of tungsten, zinc, cadmium, and cobalt on animal and human somatic cells. *Tsitologiya i Genetika* **12**, (3), 241–243.

Watanabe, T., Shimada, T. and Endo, A. (1976). Mutagenic effects of cadmium in hamster oocyte chromosomes. *Teratology* **14**, (2), 259.

Watanabe, T., Shimada, T. and Endo, A. (1977). Mutagenic effects of cadmium on the oocyte chromosomes of mice. *Nippon Eisegaku Zasshi* **32**, (3), 472–481.

Webb, M. (1972). Persistence of stored Cd2+ in the livers and kidneys of female rats during pregnancy. *Journal of Reproduction and Fertility* **30**, 99–103.

Webster, W. S. (1978). Cadmium-induced fetal growth retardation in the mouse. *Archives of Environmental Health* **33**, 36–42.

White, I. G. and Holland, M. K. (1977). Aspects of the involvement of heavy metals in reproduction and fertility control. *Inorganic Perspectives in Biology and Medicine* **1**, (2), 137–172.

Wolkowski, R. M. (1974). Differential cadmium-induced embryotoxicity in two inbred mouse strains. 1. Analysis of inheritance of the response to cadmium and of the presence of cadmium in fetal and placental tissues. *Teratology* **10**, (3), 243–261.

Zasukhina, G. D., Sinelschikova, T. A., Lvova, G. N. and Kirkova, Z. S. (1977). Molecular-genetic effects of cadmium chloride. *Mutation Research* **45**, 169–174.

9. Carbon Monoxide

TECHNICAL DATA

Formula	CO
CAS registry number	630–08–0
Chemical abstracts name	Carbon monoxide
Synonyms	Carbonic oxide; exhaust gas; flue gas.
Uses	As reducing agent in metallurgical operations especially in the Mond process for the recovery of nickel; in organic synthesis especially in the Fischer-Tropsch processes, petroleum-type products and in the oxo reaction; in the manufacture of metal carbonyls.
TLV	50 ppm

ANIMAL STUDIES

A. RELEVANT PHARMACOLOGY AND TOXICOLOGY

Sex differences in the toxicity of inhaled carbon monoxide (CO) have been investigated in the mouse and the rat by Stupfel and co-workers (1971a, 1971b, 1972). In one experiment male and female intact and gonadectomized mice were exposed to 2000 ppm (0·2%) CO for 3 h 7 min at 70 days of age. Mortality was 80% in intact males, 31% in castrated males, 13% in ovariectomized females and 10% in intact females, suggesting that the presence of male sex hormones may render the animal more susceptible to CO poisoning. In another experiment intact male and female mice were exposed to 3300 ppm (0·33%) CO for 25–35 min. At 60 days of age mortality was 32% and 0%, and at 81 days of age it was 89% and 13% in males and females respectively. They also compared mortalities in male, "pregnant" and virgin female mice exposed to 4500 ppm (0·45%) CO for 2 h 15 min. The "pregnant" group were females housed with males of which 50–60% were actually pregnant. Mortality was 100%, 79% and 56% in males, "pregnant" females and virgin females. In the "pregnant" group there was no difference in mortality between those carrying fetuses and those not. A similar sex difference is seen in the rat; males and females exposed to 2100 ppm (0·21%) CO for 93 min at 122 days of age had mortalities of 78% and 32% respectively. Williams and Smith (1934) have also noted higher mortality amongst male rats than female rats exposed to 3400 ppm (0·34%) CO for up to 1 h/day.

Thus mortality amongst males would seem to be consistently greater than amongst females, with no difference between pregnant and non-pregnant females. However, in none of these experiments were animals matched for body weight, and in all of them, mortality increased with increasing body weight. Since the amount of CO absorbed into the body during inhalation will be greater in larger animals, it is not clear to what extent the above findings represent a true sex difference in the toxicity of CO or simply reflect differences in body weight and vital capacity.

Placental transfer of CO has been demonstrated in a number of species including the rat, rabbit, guinea pig, dog and sheep (see Medico-Legal Bulletin, 1978; Bissonnette and Wickham, 1977; Longo and Ching, 1977; Bissonnette *et al.*, 1977) and CO is in fact used as a test gas in the measurement of placental diffusion capacity. In general, the diffusion of CO across the placenta into fetal blood is proportional to the length of exposure of the mother to CO in the atmosphere and the concentration of CO in that atmosphere. However, there are considerable species differences in CO diffusion capacity of the placenta (see, for example, discussion by Longo and Ching, 1977) and it is clear that, in some cases, early on during maternal exposure to CO little passes across to the fetus, yet considerable fetal damage may occur because of the secondary hypoxic effect caused by the decreased diffusion of oxygen across to the fetus when maternal carboxyhaemoglobin (HbCO) levels are high. There is evidence in the guinea pig (Bissonnette *et al.*, 1977), rabbit and sheep (Longo and Ching, 1977) that placental diffusion capacity for CO increases with gestational age and is correlated with increases in fetal weight but not placental weight. There is some debate as to whether there exists a placental carrier for CO based on cytochrome P450, or whether passage into the fetus is by simple diffusion only (see for example Longo and Ching, 1977; Bissonnette *et al.*, 1977).

As transfer of CO across the placenta proceeds, fetal HbCO levels will exceed those of the mother, for most species by a factor of around 2·2, due to the higher affinity of fetal haemoglobin for CO. In the human however CO-affinities of maternal and fetal haemoglobin are similar and fetal:maternal HbCO ratio is only 1·1 (Garvey and Longo, 1978).

A further factor which may contribute to fetal vulnerability to CO exposure is that in fetal blood the partial pressure of oxygen (pO_2) is much lower than in maternal blood, and is normally close to the critical values for maintenance of adequate tissue oxygenation. So with maternal CO exposure, the decreases in fetal arterial pO_2, resulting from increased maternal and fetal HbCO levels, are likely to result in tissue hypoxia or anoxia at a much earlier stage than in the mother (Longo, 1976).

B. ENDOCRINE AND GONADAL EFFECTS

Males

In an early study, Williams and Smith (1934) investigated the effects of exposure to sublethal levels of illuminating gas in a mixture with air, such that the final CO content was 3400 ppm (0·34%). Male rats were exposed to the gas for 1 h/day for 2 weeks to 120 days. Weight gain, food intake and muscle tone were reduced and alopecia developed over time. After exposure they were mated with control females, but few pregnancies resulted and no young survived (see section C for details). At autopsy, the testes and spermatozoa were examined. After short treatment periods, sperm motility was sluggish, but after 60 days treatment non-motile sperm predominated, and with longer treatments no sperm were seen. Litter mate controls showed active sperm at all times. After 120 days exposure, the testes weighed $\frac{1}{2}$–$\frac{1}{3}$ of control weights but sperm were found on histological examination. Numbers killed at each time period were not given.

Stupfel and Bouley (1970) exposed male rats to 50 ppm CO for 95 h/week during 5 days of the week for up to 3 months and examined organ weights. There were no significant effects on mean testis weight or water content in 18 males killed at unspecified intervals during the 3-month exposure period nor in 10 males killed at the end of the exposure period. In another group of males exposed to 50 ppm for 2 weeks reproduction was normal (see section C for details).

Females

Effects of CO exposure on the oestrous cycle of rats have been studied. Williams and Smith (1934) exposed 12 female rats to 3400 ppm CO for 1 h/day for 68 days. As in the males, weight gain, food intake and muscle tone were reduced during exposure. The mean length of the cycle in these rats over 73 days before exposure was 4·74 days, and during exposure it increased significantly to 5·56 days. It was not further prolonged in females exposed for 250 days. Ovarian histology showed normal follicle development and corpora lutea but they noted the ovaries were "somewhat reduced" in size and there was a "great excess" of red blood cells in all sections. Reproduction in female rats similarly exposed was abnormal (see section C for details).

Mamatsashvili (1970) has also studied the oestrous cycle in rats exposed to CO. Groups of 10 females were exposed to 0, 0·9 or 1·7 ppm CO (0, 1 or 2 mg/m^3) for 72 days. The daily duration of exposure was not given. In the first month of exposure there was a significant decrease in the length of dioestrus and metoestrus and an increase in pro-oestrus and oestrus in comparison with controls at both 0·9 and 1·7 ppm. The average duration of the cycle increased during the second and third months of exposure. At 1·7 ppm oestrous cycles did not return to normal until 190 days after exposure stopped. No numerical data are given. The ovaries of those exposed to 0·9 ppm were histologically normal but the appearance of the pituitary glands suggested increased activity. No information is given on those exposed to 1·7 ppm. Reproduction in both these groups was abnormal (see section C for details).

Conclusion

Adverse effects on spermatogenesis in the rat have only been seen at very high, toxic doses (3400 ppm) and not with prolonged exposure to a low dose of 50 ppm. In female rats there is an overall lengthening of the oestrous cycle at 3400 ppm and it has been claimed that similar effects are seen with doses as low as 0·9 and 1·7 ppm.

C. FERTILITY

Males

Effects on fertility have been investigated in the mouse and the rat. Stupfel and Bouley (1970) exposed separately male and female mice to 50 ppm CO for 24 h/day, 5 days a week for 2 weeks, and then mated them, one exposed male to 10 control females, over the next 3 weeks. Females were killed 15 days after placing with the male. There were no significant effects on pregnancy rate, live fetuses/dam or dead fetuses/dam in comparison with controls exposed to filtered air only.

Williams and Smith (1934) studied the effect of male exposure only or female exposure only in the rat. Of 6 males exposed to 3400 ppm (0·34%) CO for 1 h/day for 14 days, then caged with 2 control females/male for the next 3 weeks (unexposed), only 2 pregnancies occurred and none of the delivered young survived. With 6 male rats similarly exposed for 50 days, only one pregnancy occurred and no young survived, and in 3 males exposed for 75 days no pregnancies occurred as was the case with even longer exposures. Pregnancies were ascertained from weight records only and delivery of young. During the same experimental period 9 control males fathered 14 healthy litters which survived to maturity. The results in the CO-exposed males accord with the observations on spermatozoa in these same males at autopsy (see section B for details).

Females

Stupfel and Bouley (1970) exposed separately male and female mice to 50 ppm CO for 24 h/day, 5 days a week for 2 weeks and then mated them, one control male to 10 exposed females, over the next 3 weeks. Females were killed 15 days after placing with the male. There were no significant effects on pregnancy rate, live fetuses/dam or dead fetuses/dam in comparison with controls exposed to filtered air only. Exposure of female rats (Williams and Smith, 1934) to 3400 ppm CO for 1 h/day for 3 months halved litter production. Seven exposed females were mated with control males and 13 litters were born compared with 26 from 7 control females over the same time period. Average litter size at birth was reduced and most pups destroyed by the CO-exposed dams, only 2 pups surviving to weaning. Five females exposed to 3400 ppm CO for 1 h/day for 150 or 250 days had no pregnancies. It is not clear from the description of methods given whether females in these experiments were mated during or after the exposure period. Females similarly exposed showed some disturbance of the oestrous cycle but no gross ovarian changes (see section B for details).

Mamatsashvili (1970) also showed reduced fertility in females with disturbed oestrous cycles exposed to 0·9 or 1·7 ppm CO (10/group) for 72 days (daily duration of exposure not given). After exposure they were mated with control males and fertility, average duration of pregnancy and postnatal weight gain between 7 and 14 days of age were all affected by maternal CO exposure. Fertility was increased in terms of live litter size, as might be predicted from the increased duration of oestrus and increased pituitary activity. The female offspring also showed alterations in their oestrous cycle similar to those described in the dams (see section B). The study is reported descriptively with no numerical data given on the pregnancies.

Conclusion

In both the male and the female exposed to CO, effects on the gonads correlate with changes in fertility. At low exposures of 50 ppm there is no effect in males or females though one study suggests that very low exposures of 2 ppm may enhance fertility in the female but adversely affect the offspring. At higher exposures of 3400 ppm exposure of either males or females results in reduced fertility and very high postnatal mortality of the offspring.

D. PREGNANCY

The effects of exposure to CO during pregnancy have been investigated in a number of species including the mouse, rat, rabbit, sheep, pig and monkey.

Mouse

Kato (1958) exposed groups of 30 mice to 5%, 7·5% and over 8% fuel-gas by inhalation for 1 h on day 8 of pregnancy. The CO content of the air-fuel-gas mixture was not given. The females were killed on day 13 of pregnancy. In those exposed to over 8% gas 11/30 dams died. There were no other deaths. Significance levels for changes were not given, but dead implants increased from 4·7% in controls to 12·9% in the 5% gas group, 22·4% in the 7·5% gas group and 14·5% in the over 8% group. There was no effect on the mean weight of embryo plus placenta, membranes or amniotic fluid, but embryonic length was decreased in a dose-related manner. The stage of embryonic development was also retarded in a dose-related way. Malformations increased from 4·1% in controls to 8·8%, 9·7% and 30·4% in 5%, 7·5% and >8% fuel-gas groups respectively. Both the severity and variety of malformations increased with increasing dose, from mild hydrocephalus only in controls, to exencephaly, encephalocoele, marked hydrocephalus, spina bifida, jaw abnormalities, twisting of the body axis and haemorrhage in treated groups. Details of how the embryos were examined were not given.

Schwetz *et al.* (1979) exposed groups of 17–28 mice to 0 or 250 ppm CO by inhalation for 7 or 24 h/day on days 6–15 of pregnancy. Acceptable teratological methods were used. Maternal HbCO levels immediately after exposure ranged from 7–11%, compared with 0·5% or less in controls. HbCO levels fell to control values within 24 h after the last exposure. There was no dose-related effect on maternal weight gain. There was no effect on dams carrying to term, implants/dam or live fetuses/dam. Resorptions/dam were significantly increased in the 7 h exposure group but not in the 24 h group. Fetal weight was significantly increased in the 7 h group and decreased in the 24 h group. Two fetuses with exencephaly and ablepharia were seen in the 24 h CO group and one fetus with cleft palate in each of the 7 h CO and 24 h 0 ppm control groups. These differences are not significant. However, there was a significant increase in the incidence of extra lumbar ribs and lumbar spurs in the 24 h CO group and a significant increase in lumbar spurs in the 7 h CO group. Ossification was unaffected.

Abbatiello and Mohrmann (1979) have examined the effect of maternal CO exposure on offspring maze-learning ability. Mice were exposed to an unspecified concentration of CO for 90 sec/day throughout pregnancy. Maternal HbCO levels were determined periodically (presumably immediately after exposure, though this is not stated) and litters from dams with HbCO levels in the range of 6–11% were designated test animals. Control litters were from unexposed dams. At 40 days of age onwards 2 males and 2 females/litter were tested in a Y-maze. There was no significant effect on days taken to learn the maze, but the number of errors made during learning was significantly increased in male and female offspring exposed prenatally to CO compared with controls, indicating some deficit in learning ability.

Rat

In rat studies, there has been no comprehensive screen with exposure throughout organogenesis. Yun (1978) exposed groups of 20 females to 500 ppm CO by inhalation for 1 h/day for 20 days before mating and throughout pregnancy or throughout pregnancy only. The dams were killed on day 20 of pregnancy. There was no significant effect on the proportion of dams carrying to term. Live litter size was unaffected but mean fetal weight was significantly decreased from 5·1 g in controls to 3·8 g in litters from dams exposed before mating and throughout pregnancy and to 3·5 g in litters from dams exposed during pregnancy only. No further information on the litters was given.

Yun (1978) also exposed groups of 21–24 rats acutely to higher levels of 4500–5000 ppm (0·45–0·50%) CO for 15 minutes on day 6 or 7 or on day 13 or 14 of pregnancy. Maternal HbCO levels after exposure were 42–58%. Live fetuses/dam were unaffected but fetal weight was significantly reduced from 5·1 g in controls to 4·4 g in those exposed during late gestation on day 13/14. Choi and Oh (1975) exposed rats to 0 or 750 ppm by inhalation for 3 h/day on days 7–9 of pregnancy. Implants/dam were unaffected but the resorption rate in 15 exposed rats was 32% compared with 0% in controls, and mean fetal weight was significantly reduced from 4·1 g in controls to 2·6 g in the treated group. Malformations increased from 2·6% in controls to 4·1% in exposed fetuses.

Petter *et al.* (1971) exposed 4 rats to domestic lighting gas for 3 h on day 16 of pregnancy. The CO content was not stated. The dams were killed 24 h later. Of a total of 36 fetuses, 18 were dead and 9 of the survivors had haemorrhages on the extremities. The importance of this small study is that the authors also showed similar disturbances of the fetal circulation following other hypoxia-inducing treatments.

Several workers have examined the detailed effects of CO exposure on brain and heart development. Garvey and Longo (1978) exposed groups of 12–16 rats to 0, 30 or 90 ppm CO for 24 h/day from days 3–20 of pregnancy and examined its effects on the fetal brain. On day 20, maternal and fetal HbCO concentrations were 4·8% and 11·3% respectively in the 30 ppm group and 8·8% and 17·0% respectively in the 90 ppm group, but other maternal haematological parameters were unchanged, suggesting that the CO exposure was insufficient to induce physiological adaptation in the mother. Of those mated, the numbers carrying to term were reduced in the CO groups in a dose-related manner, from 100% in controls, to 69% at 30 ppm and 38% at 90 ppm. Resorption sites were not visible suggesting that fertilized eggs were lost before implantation. Of those carrying to term, there were no effects on implants/dam, live fetuses/dam, resorptions/dam, full-term dead fetuses/dam or external gross malformation rate. Fetal body and organ weights were unaffected, except in the 90 ppm group where brain wet weight was significantly increased by 17% and lung weight significantly decreased by 25% in comparison with controls. Total brain protein, DNA, 5-HT and noradrenaline levels were similar to controls in the 90 ppm group but the concentration/g of wet tissue was decreased at 90 ppm. These findings, together with a decreased dry weight expressed as a percentage of the wet weight, suggest that brain oedema had occurred in fetuses exposed to 90 ppm. No other abnormalities were reported but it should be remembered that only visible external malformations were ascertained.

Dydyk *et al.* (1975) have examined the effects of maternal CO exposure on respiratory activity and ultrastructure of cells in the brain stem of mother and fetus. Rats on day 18 of pregnancy were exposed to CO by inhalation for 1 h, such that at the end of exposure, maternal HbCO was 73% and fetal HbCO was 10·3%. Directly after exposure the oxygen consumption of fetal giant cells in the brain stem reticular formation was increased 4-fold whereas the equivalent maternal cells showed a 77% decrease in oxygen consumption. However no histological changes occurred as a result of these changes in fetuses and newborns up to 72 h old exposed on day 18 of gestation.

Prigge and Hochrainer (1977) have exposed rats to 60, 125, 250 or 500 ppm CO for 24 h/day on days 1–21 of pregnancy and examined fetal haematological and cardiac parameters. Details of maternal weight gain were not given but fetal weight was significantly reduced in a dose-related manner in 125–500 ppm groups, and at 500 ppm was only 63% of the control weight. A significant decrease in fetal haemoglobin and haematocrit was seen at 250 and 500 ppm, no change at 125 ppm, and an increase in these parameters at 60 ppm. There was a significant, dose-related increase in heart weight at all doses. The reason for the cardiac hypertrophy is unknown. Since adaptational changes are not seen in adult rats exposed to 60 ppm, these findings suggest a greater vulnerability of the fetus to CO exposure.

Penney *et al.* (1980) have confirmed the above findings using continuous exposure to 200 ppm CO from days 4–21 of pregnancy and extended observations into the postnatal period. At birth maternal and newborn HbCO levels were similar at 27–28%. Newborn but not maternal body weight was significantly reduced by 13% and mean litter size was decreased from 13·0 in controls to 10·2 in CO-exposed litters. However in rats exposed prenatally only to CO there was complete reversibility of the effects on body weight, heart weight and haematological parameters by 105 days of age, whereas rats exposed prenatally and for 4 weeks postnatally to 200 ppm CO continuously, still showed persistent changes in the above parameters.

Hoffman and Campbell (1977) could not confirm a decrease in litter size at birth in rats exposed continuously to 230 ppm CO by inhalation from day 2 of pregnancy through to delivery, but weights 24 h after birth were significantly reduced by 15%. The dams and their litters continued to be exposed to 230 ppm CO for the 21 days of lactation. Survival to 21 days was markedly reduced from 94% in controls to only 34% in the CO group and daily weight gain was reduced by one-third. Increase of haematocrit, haemoglobin and cardiac weight changes at 5 days of age were similar to those seen by others described above. Comparison of this study with the results of a previous unpublished study from the same laboratory, where litters were exposed postnatally only to 550 ppm CO, suggest that prenatal exposure may enhance the toxicity of postnatal exposure in terms of survival and weight gain, though prenatal exposure alone has only a small effect on these parameters (see later).

Grabowski (1976) has studied the postnatal effects of prenatal exposure to 1000 ppm for 6–9 h or 300 ppm for 3–6 days during different times of pregnancy in the rat. In general, prolonged exposure to low concentrations had more adverse effects than acute exposure to high concentrations. The same is true of adult CO poisoning (Sokal, 1975), Later stages of gestation were more sensitive than early ones. There was little or no effect on postnatal weight gain, but retarded development of standing and startle reflexes, later onset of grooming and escape activity, and higher open field activity were seen in pups from CO-exposed dams. There was evidence of fatty degeneration in the livers of treated pups that died. The study is reported in abstract only and no further details are given.

Fechter and Annau (1971, 1976) have also examined postnatal development in rats exposed prenatally to CO. Groups of 26–27 rats were exposed to 0 or 150 ppm CO from day 1 of pregnancy to delivery, such that maternal HbCO levels during exposure were 15%. Mean birth weight was reduced, though not significantly, but postnatal growth rates were adversely affected and pup body weight in the CO group was significantly lower than controls from 4 days of age onwards at least up to day 21. Cross fostering to control mothers did not alter the effect on growth rates. There was no effect on litter size or mortality of pups on the day of birth. Subsequent postnatal mortality is not mentioned. At one day of age the ratio of wet weight of the brain to body weight was increased significantly and brain protein concentration/g wet tissue was decreased significantly in the prenatal CO group, similar to the findings of Garvey and Longo (1978) after prenatal exposure to 90 ppm CO, suggesting oedema of the brain. At one and 4 days of age, brain dopamine and noradrenaline levels in response to saline injection were not affected but after s.c. injection of L-dopa, which normally increases central dopamine levels and induces vigorous activity, dopamine levels were significantly decreased in pups exposed prenatally to CO compared with controls. Activity levels after the injection were correspondingly reduced as was spontaneous open field activity at 14 and 21 days of age. These observations on activity are contrary to those of Grabowski (1976), who found increased open field activity after prenatal exposure for a shorter period to 300 or 1000 ppm CO.

Rabbit

Schwetz *et al.* (1979) exposed groups of 9–12 rabbits to 0 or 250 ppm CO for 7 or 24 h/day on days 6–18 of pregnancy and looked for prenatal effects. Acceptable teratological methods were used. Maternal HbCO levels immediately after the 7 h exposure periods were 13–15% compared with <1% in controls. By 24 h after the last exposure they had returned to normal. No determinations were made on the group exposed for 24 h/day. There was no effect on maternal weight gain, implants/dam, live fetuses/dam or resorptions/dam. Fetal body weight was significantly increased in the 7 h/day exposure group but was unaffected in the 24 h/day group. A similar increase in fetal weight was seen in mice exposed to 250 ppm for 7 h/day in the same study (see earlier for details). Major malformations were seen only in the 24 h/day 250 ppm group, which had 2 fetuses with umbilical hernia. There were no significant differences between treated and control groups in the incidence of skeletal anomalies. Schwetz *et al.* (1979) also discuss unpublished observations on postnatal survival following prenatal exposure to 250 ppm on days 6–28 in the rabbit. Survival to weaning was comparable in treated and control groups.

Astrup *et al.* (1972) have exposed groups of 14–17 rabbits to 0, 90 or 180 ppm CO by inhalation from days 1–30 of pregnancy. Maternal HbCO levels were 9–10% in the 90 ppm group and 16–18% in the 180 ppm group. There was no effect on mean litter size at birth, but birth weights were reduced in a dose-related manner by 12% at 90 ppm and 17% at 180 ppm. Stillbirths and neonatal deaths within 24 h of birth were increased from 0·9% and 4·5% in the 2 control groups to 10% and 35% in the 90 and 180 ppm groups respectively. Three offspring in the 190 ppm groups were noted to have leg deformities (unspecified). In another publication, Astrup (1972) described the deformities as absent leg, and also noted that mortality from 2–21 days of age was unaffected in litters from these same exposed dams.

Sheep

In the sheep, fetal death occurs with maternal exposure to 100 ppm or above. Longo and Hill (1977) exposed ewes during the last quarter of gestation to 30, 50, 100 or 300 ppm CO by inhalation. At 30–100 ppm equilibration between maternal and fetal HbCO was not reached until 36–48 h of exposure, and at steady-state, fetal HbCO levels were around 60% higher than maternal levels. When fetal HbCO levels exceeded 15% for more than 30 minutes the fetuses began to die. At 100 ppm, 5/11 died, and at 300 ppm, where exposure only lasted 2–3 h, 3/3 fetuses died. At fetal HbCO concentrations of 15–20% fetal pO_2 falls by 6–10 torr, the fetus is unable to increase its cardiac output to compensate, and tissue hypoxia results.

Pig

Keller (1976) has noted a high incidence of stillbirths in pigs inhaling CO. Sows placed in rooms containing up to 150 ppm CO emitted from uncleaned gas radiators, a few days before farrowing, gave birth to 369 litters containing 4369 piglets, of which 760 (17·4%) were stillborn. The normal stillbirth rate was around 5%. Sows and surviving piglets appeared to be unaffected.

Monkey

Ginsberg and Myers (1974, 1976) have exposed 9 near-term rhesus monkeys to 1000–3000 ppm (0·1–0·3%) CO for 1–3 h. The mothers tolerated HbCO levels of up to 60% during exposure without any clinical sequelae. In the fetuses, hypoxia developed very rapidly, fetal arterial pO_2 falling rapidly during the first 15–30 minutes of exposure. Fetal HbCO levels rose only gradually over the 1–3 h of maternal exposure, indicating that the fetal hypoxia is largely due to falling maternal arterial pO_2 and is not much further affected by the later-onset increase in HbCO levels, though the accumulation of CO in fetal blood would shift the oxygen dissociation curve so that release of oxygen to the fetal tissues is further decreased. The fetal hypoxia was associated with bradycardia, hypotension, metabolic and later respiratory acidosis. At the end of the CO exposure the fetuses were delivered surgically. Four of the 9 newborns were normal and remained so until killed 3 months later. The brains of these monkeys appeared grossly and microscopically normal at sacrifice. A fifth newborn with hypotonia, lethargy, poor suckling response and apnoeic periods was killed at 5 days of age due to development of gangrene in one leg (following the fetal surgery) and inadequate feeding. The brain showed bilateral haemorrhagic necrosis of the globus pallidus and putamen and bilateral cerebral cortical necrosis. The remaining 4 newborns required mechanical ventilation and displayed nystagmus, opisthotonus and extensor spasms with signs of increased intracranial pressure. They were killed within 12–72 h of delivery when near to death. At autopsy, their brains were swollen and showed widespread haemorrhagic necrosis of the cerebral cortex, basal ganglia and thalamus. The degree of damage in the newborns correlated with the fall in fetal arterial pO_2 during maternal CO exposure and the results suggest that severe brain injury only occurs if fetal arterial oxygen content falls below 2 ml/100 ml for periods somewhere between 10 and 45 minutes or longer.

Conclusion

In summary, maternal exposure to CO has an adverse effect on fetal and postnatal weight gain and survival in a variety of species from around 90 ppm upwards, especially with exposure in later pregnancy. However, it does not produce a wide variety of malformations, though the frequency of malformations is increased to a small extent in some studies. It does however have a marked effect on brain development; adverse effects on learning ability and evidence of brain oedema have been seen in the rat, for example, with exposures that raise maternal HbCO levels to 6–11% (equivalent to exposures around 100 ppm); higher exposures in the primate cause extensive oedema and damage to the brain incompatible with life, even at exposure levels that have no lasting consequences for the dam. There is clear evidence in other species too of fetal or neonatal death in the absence of effects on the dam. The majority of effects on the fetus appear to be secondary to fetal hypoxia which occurs early in maternal CO exposure, well before fetal HbCO levels rise substantially. It is presumably for this reason that it is the fetus rather than the embryo which is most at risk, since the embryo is less dependent than the fetus on oxygen from circulating blood. The reasons for the particular vulnerability of the fetus to maternal CO exposure have been discussed in section A. Cardiovascular changes in the fetus brought about by prenatal CO exposure would appear to be reversible, but the effects on the brain are not.

E. MUTAGENICITY

No relevant data found.

F. CARCINOGENICITY

No relevant data found.

HUMAN STUDIES

A. RELEVANT PHARMACOLOGY AND TOXICOLOGY

Longo (1970, 1977) has published very extensive reviews of the effects of carbon monoxide (CO) on the pregnant woman, fetus and newborn infant, and most of the data discussed in this section will be drawn from these reviews, unless otherwise stated.

Sex differences in susceptibility to CO poisoning have been claimed. Stupfel *et al.* (1971b), reviewing the literature, mention a paper suggesting that accidental or provoked lethality by CO was higher in men than in women, which may be related to a sex difference in the haemoglobin-oxygen dissociation curve (F. Gremy *et al.*, *Presse Med.* **76**, 1099, 1968, original paper not seen by us).

Endogenous CO production varies considerably between individuals, but on average, men produce about 0·42 ml of CO per hour. Women produce a similar amount during the oestrogenic phase of the menstrual cycle, but during the progestational phase, CO production is almost doubled, and during pregnancy is increased even further, rapidly decreasing in the *postpartum* period. Only about 15% of this increase in endogenous CO production in pregnancy is attributable to fetal production, about 30–40% is due to the increased red cell mass, and the remainder may be due to progesterone induction of hepatic microsomal enzymes. It is perhaps partly because of this increased endogenous CO production that Longo (1977) has suggested that (fetal considerations aside) the pregnant woman is probably more sensitive to CO than the non-pregnant woman. Certainly, oxygen consumption increases by 15–20% in pregnancy and blood oxygen capacity decreases during pregnancy, from which one would predict an increased susceptibility to CO poisoning in pregnancy. There is suggestive evidence that this is the case in animals (see section A, Animal studies), but none as yet in humans. Exposure to the TLV of 50 ppm for 6–8 h produces a carboxy-haemoglobin level of about 8–10%.

Placental transfer

There is no doubt that CO is exchanged across the human placenta. Blood carboxyhaemoglobin concentrations in normal non-smoking pregnant women are around 0·5–1·0%, though values ranging from 0·4–2·6% have been reported. Fetal carboxyhaemoglobin levels have been reported to vary from 0·7–2·5% and the ratio of fetal:maternal carboxyhaemoglobin from 0·6–1·6. Fetal carboxyhaemoglobin concentration varies not only as a function of maternal carboxyhaemoglobin concentration, but also as a function of the rate of fetal CO production, the placental diffusion capacity for CO, the relative affinity of haemoglobin for CO as compared with oxygen, and the affinity of blood as a whole for CO and oxygen.

The theoretical relationship between fetal and maternal carboxyhaemoglobin levels in humans has been worked out using a mathematical model (Hill *et al.*, 1977). As the mother breathes in CO, fetal carboxyhaemoglobin concentrations would lag behind maternal concentrations for the first few hours. By 14–24 h they would equal maternal concentrations and then eventually equilibrate at concentrations 10–15% higher than the maternal concentrations. During subsequent maternal elimination of CO, fetal CO elimination would lag behind, with maternal carboxyhaemoglobin levels falling by half in about 2 h, while that in the fetus would take about 7 h to fall by half.

Reviewing studies published up to 1972, Longo (1977) summarized that in pregnant women who smoke, maternal carboxyhaemoglobin levels of 2–14% have been reported, with fetal levels obtained at the time of delivery of 2–10%. In these different studies, fetal carboxyhaemoglobin levels were higher, equal to or lower than maternal levels. In a later study of maternal and fetal carboxyhaemoglobin levels in 103 normal deliveries to Belgian women who smoked, Buchet *et al.* (1978) have reported higher levels of carboxyhaemoglobin (1·84%) in the fetus than in the maternal blood (1·37%). In non-smokers maternal and fetal carboxyhaemoglobin levels were 0·67% and 0·66% respectively. Longo and Hill (1977) have estimated that in a pregnant woman exposed to 30 ppm CO in air for prolonged periods, as in industrial exposure or excessive air pollution, the increases in carboxyhaemoglobin concentration and decreases in fetal oxygen tension should be equivalent to smoking one packet of cigarettes a day.

In 6 cases of CO poisoning reviewed by Longo (1970), where both maternal and fetal carboxyhaemoglobin levels were measured, maternal levels ranged from 48–95% and fetal levels from 0–23%. In all cases the mother died and in all but one case the fetus died. Longo has pointed out that several authors have assumed that the cases in which no CO was detected in fetal blood indicate that CO does not cross the placenta, but if maternal death is rapid there will be insufficient time for CO to cross the placenta, fetal levels lagging behind maternal levels, as mentioned earlier. Fetal carboxyhaemoglobin levels higher than 23% have been recorded in 2 cases of maternal CO poisoning. In one case reported by Muller and Graham (1955), the fetal carboxyhaemoglobin level was 49% (maternal level not measured) after accidental maternal inhalation of CO for some hours. In a case of twins reported by Piette *et al.* (1978), the maternal level was 85%, umbilical cord levels in the fetuses 47% and 41%, and fetal heart blood levels 28% and 32%. Thus there is no doubt that large quantities of CO can cross the human placenta, given time.

B. ENDOCRINE AND GONADAL FUNCTION

No relevant data found.

C. FERTILITY

No relevant data found.

D. PREGNANCY

After the introduction of coal gas for illumination in the mid-nineteenth century, reports of CO poisoning in pregnancy began to appear in the literature. Longo (1970) has reviewed over 20 cases, the first ones being reported in 1859. Bankl and Jellinger (1967) have reviewed an additional 7 cases not mentioned by Longo and other cases have also appeared (Kamraj-Mazurkiewicz, 1967; Beaudoing *et al.*, 1969; Matsuyama, 1969; Stokowski and Kesiak, 1969; Raimondi and Gardoni, 1975). In some cases both mother and fetus died, in some the mother survived and the fetus or infant died, and in some both mother and fetus survived. The sources of CO in these cases were illuminating gas, store gas, coal gas or smoke from fires. Duration of exposure varied from $\frac{1}{2}$–12 h and cases have been recorded at all stages of pregnancy.

In 6 cases where the mothers and fetuses died and carboxyhaemoglobin levels were measured, reviewed by Longo (1970) maternal levels were 48–88% and fetal levels 0–24%. In one case of maternal death, the maternal carboxyhaemoglobin level was 95% and that in the 8 month fetus which survived, 10%. In 3 cases where the mother survived but the fetus was stillborn 11–72 h after CO poisoning, fetal carboxyhaemoglobin levels were 20%, 23% and 49%, but maternal levels were not measured. In no other cases (except 2, see below) where mother or mother and fetus survived have carboxyhaemoglobin levels been measured, so it is not known what levels and durations of poisoning may be endured without any fatal or neurological consequences for the infant. Stokowski and Kesiak (1969) have reported a single case where a woman 7 months pregnant inhaled town gas for 6 h in a suicide attempt. She was unconscious when found and had a carboxyhaemoglobin level of 8%, though it is not clear how soon after discovery the maternal blood sample was taken. She remained unconscious for 22 h but recovered. However, the fetal heart beat was not audible and the mother reported absence of fetal movements. Two weeks later, labour was induced and a macerated fetus was delivered. Beaudoing *et al.* (1969) reported a case where the mother was poisoned, causing a 4 h coma and with unspecified maternal carboxyhaemoglobin levels. The baby survived but with severe neurological impairment (see later for details).

In cases recorded in the literature where the baby was liveborn following maternal CO poisoning at various stages of pregnancy from the first to the eighth month, psychomotor disturbances have been observed in the infant and severe brain damage at autopsy where postnatal death occurred. In 8/23 cases mentioned by Longo (1970) where death did not occur *in utero* (these cases originally reviewed by Muller and Graham 1955) all exhibited psychomotor disturbances and mental retardation, with some cases of hypotonia of the neck, hypertonia of the extremities, anatomical abnormalities and hydrocephalus. Four of these 8 cases died in infancy and 3 of these were autopsied; all showed evidence of brain damage, in one case involving softening of the basal ganglia, similar to that seen in adults with delayed death from CO poisoning (Muller and Graham, 1955).

In 7 cases not mentioned by Longo (1970) where the baby was liveborn, reviewed by Bankl and Jellinger (1967), with poisoning occurring in the first to eighth month of pregnancy, 5 died within one year of birth. The 2 remaining cases lived until 68 years and 81 years of age. All exhibited trembling, athetosis or convulsions and at autopsy various types of brain pathology were detected with damage to the basal ganglia seen in all but one case. In the case reported by Beaudoing *et al.* (1969), after CO poisoning in the seventh month of gestation, a child of normal weight and height was delivered at term, but there was diffuse hypertonicity with lively reflexes and the head was thrown back. The EEG was abnormal. At 7 months of age general growth was normal but hypertonicity persisted and there was microcephaly. Convulsions appeared and the EEG worsened. At $2\frac{1}{2}$ years the child was still surviving and hypotonia had superseded the hypertonicity. A gas pneumo-encephalographic examination showed dilation of the ventricle and cortical atrophy. In the case reported by Matsuyama (1969), where poisoning occurred near the end of the eighth month of pregnancy, a low birth weight baby was born 6 days later. The day after birth fever and spasms developed and the infant died. At autopsy extensive lesions were found in the midbrain and cerebral cortex, including the basal ganglia. Raimondi and Gardoni (1975) reported on a birth occurring 12 days after an episode of CO poisoning at $8\frac{1}{2}$ months gestation. The mother was unconscious for 1 h but was not treated or admitted to hospital at that time. Delivery was normal but the infant was sluggish, hypotonic and with minor tremors in the arms. There were brief episodes of apnoea and bronchial pneumonia with convulsions developed at 15 days of age. Hypotonia and convulsions continued with further attacks of bronchial pneumonia and the child finally succumbed to one of these attacks at 6 months of age. Extensive lesions were found in the cerebral and cerebellar cortices at autopsy.

One case has been reported of absence of neurological impairment following substantial maternal CO poisoning (Larcan *et al.*, 1970). A woman near the end of the second month of gestation awoke with severe headache and muscle pain, lost consciousness for a brief period and had clonic movements. Two hours later maternal carboxyhaemoglobin was 35% and therapy was begun. By 6 h after waking her carboxyhaemoglobin level was 5%. Delivery occurred at $8\frac{1}{2}$ months and no neurological impairments could be detected in the infant on examination up to 2 months of age. Subsequent development is not reported, but the usual signs of prenatal CO poisoning, if they had occurred, would probably be evident by 2 months of age. However, the possibility of more subtle effects on intellectual development cannot be discounted.

Conclusion

It is clear from the foregoing review that CO poisoning in pregnancy can result in fetal and infant death or severe neurological impairment in the offspring whilst the mother fully recovers, as far as can be ascertained. In the majority of cases where the fetus was liveborn but neurologically impaired, the episode of CO poisoning had been sufficient to render the mother unconscious. Unfortunately, there are insufficient measurements of maternal carboxyhaemoglobin levels in those cases where the mother or mother and fetus survived to indicate the exposure levels which may affect fetal development. It is clear, however, that because of the kinetics of placental transfer of CO (see section A), both level and duration of exposure are important factors. The human case reports do not answer the question of whether it is fetal hypoxia consequent to increased carboxyhaemoglobin levels or the CO itself which is damaging to brain development. It is likely that the lack of oxygen is the most important factor and experiments on monkeys support this (see Animal studies).

A more difficult question is whether the raised carboxyhaemoglobin levels in smokers may contribute to the increased risk of adverse outcome of pregnancy in that group. The relationship between low birth weight and maternal smoking is now firmly established and other problems such as pregnancy complications, increased perinatal death and congenital heart disease have been reported by some workers (see Longo, 1977, for review). However, the numerous other components of tobacco smoke may contribute to the effects and reported negative correlations between birth weight and maternal carboxyhaemoglobin concentrations in smokers (e.g. see Astrup *et al.*, 1972) are insufficient to establish cause and effect.

E. MUTAGENICITY

No relevant data found.

F. CARCINOGENICITY

No relevant data found.

SUMMARY AND EVALUATION

EXPERIMENTAL STUDIES

Carbon monoxide readily crosses the placenta, and although fetal haemoglobin in rodents has a higher affinity for CO than in the dam, the carboxyhaemoglobin ratio in humans between mother and fetus is near unity. The fetus is more sensitive to the anoxia produced however, so that fetal toxicity is observed at lower levels than in the mother.

Rats exposed for prolonged periods to high toxic doses (around 3000 ppm) show reduced testicular activity with absence of sperm, but no effects have been demonstrated following repeated exposure to 50 ppm. In female rats lengthening of the oestrous cycle has been demonstrated at doses as low as 0·9 ppm but this requires confirmation in further studies. Fertility of male rats is reduced following exposure to high toxic doses, but not at 50 ppm. In females, fertility is reduced at high exposure levels (around 3000 ppm) but data is inadequate to assess effects at lower levels.

Exposure to CO during pregnancy adversely affects both fetal and postnatal weight gain and survival, from about 90 ppm upwards. The effects are primarily due to reduced oxygenation of the fetus and in general the longer the period of anoxia, the more severe the effect. Since equilibration across the placenta takes some hours, brief exposure to high concentrations is less damaging than chronic exposure to lower concentrations. In general, only a low incidence of teratogenic effects is observed. At HbCO levels around 10% or greater, brain oedema, haemorrhages and permanent damage may result. The effects are more marked in late pregnancy, and in general it can be concluded that the fetus is much more susceptible to the toxic effects of CO than the dam.

No studies were found on mutagenicity or carcinogenicity.

HUMAN STUDIES

CO crosses the placenta in humans but since equilibration between maternal and fetal blood may take 12–24 hours, and the half-lives in the mother and fetus are 2 hours and 7 hours respectively, the ratio of maternal to fetal levels varies depending on duration of exposure and time since last exposure. In women who smoke, HbCO levels may be 2–14% with similar levels in the fetus. Exposure to 30 ppm CO throughout the day is about equivalent to smoking 20 cigarettes a day.

No studies on endocrine or gonadal function, or on fertility were found. It is difficult to predict the outcome of pregnancy in women exposed to CO. The effect on the fetus depends on both the degree and the duration of exposure. Where exposure is sufficient to cause unconsciousness in the mother, then there seems a high risk that the fetus will die, or that if a live-born baby is delivered it will have brain damage. Lower levels of CO exposure may still adversely affect the fetus producing neurological damage or reduced fetal growth. Whether the well established relationship between maternal smoking and reduced birth weight and higher neonatal mortality is due to CO is unknown. It would however be expected that any reduction in fetal oxygen availability would be disadvantageous. There is no evidence that CO is teratogenic in humans although it is clearly fetotoxic. No studies on mutagenicity or carcinogenicity were found.

EVALUATION

In animals, CO does not appear to exert any specific reproductive toxic effects in exposed males. Exposure of females, however, produces alterations in cycles and in fertility and data are inadequate to define the lowest level producing effects. There is sufficient evidence that CO exerts toxic effects on the embryo and fetus in animals. At low levels there is risk of fetal brain damage, though it is not teratogenic. In humans, exposure to high levels, sufficient to cause unconsciousness, can cause fetal death or severe neurological damage in survivors. There is no evidence whether it is teratogenic in humans. Exposure to the current TLV of 50 ppm CO produces about 8–10% carboxyhaemoglobin levels. Since this is at the high end of the range observed in smokers it should be regarded as unsatisfactorily high for pregnant women, and especially so for women who smoke in whom even higher HbCO levels might be produced. Attention is drawn to the lack of evidence of the effects of low levels of CO alone during pregnancy.

References

Abbatiello, E. R. and Mohrmann, K. (1979). Effects on the offspring of chronic low exposure carbon monoxide during mice pregnancy. *Clinical Toxicology* **14**, (4), 401–406.

Astrup, P. (1972). Some physiological and pathological effects of moderate carbon monoxide exposure. *British Medical Journal* **4**, 447–452.

Astrup, P., Trolle, D., Olsen, H. M. and Kjeldsen, K. (1972). Effect of moderate carbon monoxide exposure on fetal development. *Lancet* **ii**, 1220–1222.

Bankl, H. and Jellinger, K. (1967). Central nervous system injuries following fetal carbon monoxide poisoning. *Beitrage zur Pathologie und Anatomie* **135**, (3), 350–376.

Beaudoing, A., Gachon, J., Butin, L. and Bost, M. (1969). Foetal consequences of carbon monoxide poisoning of the mother. *Pediatrie* **24**, (5), 539–553.

Bissonnette, J. M. and Wickham, W. K. (1977). Placental diffusing capacity for carbon monoxide in unaesthetized guinea pigs. *Respiration Physiology* **31**, 161–168.

Bissonnette, J. M., Wickham, W. K. and Drummond, W. H. (1977). Placental diffusing capacities at carbon monoxide tensions. *Journal of Clinical Investigation* **59**, 1038–1044.

Buchet, J. P., Roels, H., Hubermont, G. and Lauwerys, R. (1978). Placental transfer of lead, mercury, cadmium, and carbon monoxide in women. *Environmental Research* **15**, (3), 494–503.

Choi, K. D. and Oh, Y. K. (1975). A teratological study on the effects of carbon monoxide exposure upon the fetal development of albino rats. *Korean Central Medical Journal* **29**, (2), 209–212.

Dydyk, L., Smialek, M. and Dambska, M. (1975). Respiration activity of isolated giant cells of reticular formation and ultrastructure of neurons from rat brain stem in carbon monoxide intoxication during pregnancy. *Neuropatologiya Polska* **13**, (3–4), 389–396.

Fechter, L. D. and Annau, Z. (1971). Toxicity of mild prenatal carbon monoxide exposure. *Science* **197**, 680–682.

Fechter, L. D. and Annau, Z. (1976). Effects of prenatal carbon monoxide exposure on neonatal rats. *Adverse Effects of Environmental Chemicals and Psychotropic Drugs* **2**, 219–227.

Garvey, D. J. and Longo, L. D. (1978). Chronic low level maternal carbon monoxide exposure and fetal growth and development. *Biology of Reproduction* **19**, (1), 8–14.

Ginsberg, M. D. and Myers, R. E. (1974). Fetal brain damage following maternal carbon monoxide intoxication: an experimental study. *Acta Obstetrica et Gynecologica Scandinavica* **53**, (4), 309–317.

Ginsberg, M. D. and Myers, R. E. (1976). Fetal brain injury after maternal carbon monoxide intoxication. Clinical and neuropathologic aspects. *Neurology* **26**, 15–23.

Grabowski, C. T. (1976). Postnatal effects on rats of prenatal exposure to carbon monoxide. *Teratology* **13**, 23A.

Hill, E. P., Hill, J. R., Power, G. G. and Longo, L. D. (1977). Carbon monoxide exchanges between the human fetus and mother: a mathematical model. *American Journal of Physiology* **232**, (3), H311–H323.

Hoffman, D. J. and Campbell, K. I. (1977). Postnatal toxicity of carbon monoxide after pre- and postnatal exposure. *Toxicology Letters* **1**, 147–150.

Kamraj-Mazurkiewicz, K. (1967). Effect of carbon monoxide poisoning in the course of pregnancy on the fetal central nervous system, according to our case. *Ginekologia Polska* **38**, (3), 291–294.

Kato, T. (1958). Embryonic abnormalities of the central nervous system caused by the fuel-gas inhalation of the mother animal. *Folia Psychiatrica et Neurologica Japonica* **11**, (4), 301–324.

Keller, H. (1976). Still births in a pig breeding unit due to high carbon monoxide content in the air. *Schweizer Archiv fur Tierheilkunde* **118**, (10), 425–428.

Larcan, A., Landes, P. and Vert, P. (1970). Carbon monoxide poisoning during the second month of pregnancy without neonatal abnormality. *Bulletin de la Fédération des Societés de Gynecologie de d'obstetrique de langue francaise* **22**, (3), 338–339.

Longo, L. D. (1970). Carbon monoxide in the pregnant mother and fetus and its exchange across the placenta. *Annals of the New York Academy of Sciences* **174**, (1), 313–341.

Longo, L. D. (1976). Carbon monoxide: effects on oxygenation of the fetus in utero. *Science* **194**, 523–525.

Longo, L. D. (1977). The biological effects of carbon monoxide on the pregnant woman, fetus and newborn infant. *American Journal of Obstetrics and Gynecology* **129**, 69–103.

Longo, L. D. and Ching, K. S. (1977). Placental diffusing capacity for carbon monoxide and oxygen in unaesthetized sheep. *Journal of Applied Physiology* **43**, (5), 885–893.

Longo, L. D. and Hill, E. P. (1977). Carbon monoxide uptake and elimination in fetal and maternal sheep. *American Journal of Physiology* **232**, (3), H324–H330.

Mamatsashvili, M. J. (1970). Toxic effect of carbon monoxide, sulphur dioxide and their combinations on the fertility of female rats. *Gigiena I Sanitariya* **35**, (5), 100–101.

Matsuyama, H. (1969). Effect of maternal fuel-gas poisoning on the fetal brain. *Advances in Neurological Sciences (Tokyo)* **13**, (1), 34–38.

Medico-Legal Bulletin (1978). Carbon monoxide poisoning during pregnancy. *Medico-Legal Bulletin* **17**, (1). Commonwealth of Virginia Department of Health, Office of the Chief Medical Examiner.

Muller, G. L. and Graham, S. (1955). Intrauterine death of the fetus due to accidental carbon monoxide poisoning. *New England Journal of Medicine* **252**, 1075–1078.

Penney, D. G., Baylerian, M. S. and Fanning, K. E. (1980). Temporary and lasting effects of pre- and postnatal exposure to carbon monoxide. *Toxicology and Applied Pharmacology* **53**, 271–278.

Petter, C., Bourbon, J., Maltier, J. and Jost, A. (1971). Production of hemorrhages of the extremities in the rat fetus subjected to hypoxia in utero. *Comptes Rendus des Academies des Sciences Serie D* **272**, (19), 2488–2489.

Piette, M., Timperman, J., Majelyne, W. and Heyndrickx, A. (1978). Carboxhemoglobine bij Moeder en Foetussen bij een Fatale Accidentele Koolstofmonoxidevergiftiging. *Archives Belges de Medecine Sociale, Hygiene, Medecine du Travail et Medecine Legale (Bruxelles)* **36**, (8), 504–511.

Prigge, E. and Hochrainer, D. (1977). Effects of carbon monoxide inhalation on erythropoiesis and cardiac hypertrophy in fetal rats. *Toxicology and Applied Pharmacology* **42**, 225–228.

Raimondi, C. and Gardoni, L. (1975). Neonatal encephalopathy due to maternal carbon monoxide poisoning. *Minerva Pediatrica* **27**, (40), 2239–2245.

Schwetz, B. A., Smith, F. A., Leong, B. K. J. and Staples, R. E. (1979). Teratogenic potential of inhaled carbon monoxide in mice and rabbits. *Teratology* **19**, 385–392.

Sokal, J. A. (1975). Lack of the correlation between biochemical effects on rats and blood carboxyhemoglobin concentrations in various conditions of single acute exposure to carbon monoxide. *Archives of Toxicology* **34**, (4), 331–336.

Stokowski, C. and Kesiak, J. (1969). Carbon monoxide intoxication in pregnancy. *Ginekologia Polska* **40**, (7), 801–804.

Stupfel, M. and Bouley, G. (1970). Physiological and biochemical effects on rats and mice exposed to small concentrations of carbon monoxide for long periods. *Annals of the New York Academy of Sciences* **174**, (1), 342–368.

Stupfel, M., Bouley, G. and Polianski, J. (1971a). Castration and mortality of mice due to carbon monoxide. *Journal of Physiology-Paris* **63**, (2), 99A–110A.

Stupfel, M., Bouley, G. and Roussel, A. (1971b). Difference of experimental toxicity of several air pollutants related to sex. *Proceedings of the Second International Clean Air Congress*, pp. 180–186.

Stupfel, M., Magnier, M., Polianski, J. and Romary, F. (1972). Pregnancy and mortality in mice induced by hypoxia and carbon monoxide. *Journal de Physiologie* **65**, (Supplement 1), 166A.

Williams, I. R. and Smith, E. (1934). Blood picture, reproduction and general condition during daily exposure to illuminating gas. *American Journal of Physiology* **110**, (3), 611–615.

Yun, D. R. (1978). An experimental study of the effects of acute and chronic carbon monoxide poisoning on the gestation patterns of rat. *The Seoul Journal of Medicine* **19**, (4), 187–192.

10. Carbon Tetrachloride

TECHNICAL DATA

Formula	CCl_4
CAS registry number	56–23–5
Chemical abstract name	Tetrachloromethane
Synonyms	Carbona; carbon chloride; carbon tet; methane tetrachloride; perchloromethane; tetrachlorocarbon.
Uses	As fire extinguisher; for cleaning clothing; rendering benzin nonflammable; as azeotropic drying agent for wet spark plugs in automobiles; as solvent for oils, fats, lacquers, varnishes, rubber waxes, resins; extracting oil from flowers, seeds; exterminating destructive insects; solvent; starting material in manufacture of many organic compounds.
TLV	10 ppm (skin) (1980 Intended change to 5 ppm).

ANIMAL STUDIES

A. RELEVANT PHARMACOLOGY AND TOXICOLOGY

Sex differences in the toxicity of carbon tetrachloride have been found in the rat. In acute studies, adult males are more susceptible than females to the hepatotoxic effects of s.c. injection of 1·5 ml/kg carbon tetrachloride (Chaturvedi, 1969). A comparison of the two sexes and with respect to different stages of the oestrous cycle by Yakobson *et al.* (1978) showed that the hepatotoxicity seen in females during prooestrus, when oestrogen levels are rising, was equivalent to that seen in males, but was less marked at other stages of the cycle. Ovariectomy reduced hepatic damage, but was less marked at other stages of the cycle, whilst exogenous oestradiol increased it. After chronic s.c. injection of 1·5 ml/kg/day for 13 days, however, there were no adult sex differences in mortality or degree of hepatic injury (Chaturvedi, 1969).

Pre-pubertal, one month old rats were reported by Chaturvedi (1969) to be less susceptible than adults and show no sex differences in mortality following acute injection. With chronic injection, young males are more susceptible than young females, though both are still less susceptible than adults. One study however has reported changes in the liver of the 5–7 day old neonates "identical" with those seen in adult rats after s.c. injection of 1 ml/kg, but it is not clear whether the changes were qualitatively or quantitatively "identical" (Bhattacharyya, 1965).

In mice, an experimental study failed to show any sex difference in LD50 or hepatotoxicity as measured by serum glutamic pyruvic transaminase levels after i.p. administration of carbon tetrachloride, in contrast to an earlier report where increased susceptibility of male mice was reported following accidental exposure (Klaassen and Plaa, 1967).

From a comparative study of lipoperoxidation in the pregnant and non-pregnant rat following acute oral administrations, it has been suggested that there is slower absorption and metabolism of carbon tetrachloride during pregnancy (Gualandi and Faccioli, 1969). Two studies have shown that the extent of hepatic injury decreases the later in pregnancy carbon tetrachloride is given (Dobrovolskaya *et al.*, 1973; Douglas and Clower, 1968) and mortality was lower amongst pregnant than non-pregnant animals given the same dosage (Wilson, 1954). This is not simply due to slower absorption since in some of these experiments the carbon tetrachloride was given by non-oral routes. In view of the rising oestrogen levels in late pregnancy, these findings of reduced toxicity are unexpected in the light of the study described earlier showing enhanced hepatotoxicity when oestrogen levels were high (Yakobson *et al.*, 1978).

Indirect evidence for the transfer of carbon tetrachloride in the milk comes from observation of histological changes in the livers of neonatal rats suckled by dams given 1–2 ml/kg s.c. on the tenth day of lactation (Bhattacharyya, 1965). Placental transfer has not been investigated, though, being a small lipophilic molecule, transfer is unlikely to be impeded.

B. ENDOCRINE AND GONADAL EFFECTS

Males

A number of studies in the rat have shown that a single i.p. injection of

1·5 ml/kg carbon tetrachloride caused a decrease in the weight of the testes and seminal vesicles accompanied by significant increases in pituitary weight and histological evidence of testicular atrophy and abnormal spermatogenesis, though the nature of the abnormality was not described (Chatterjee, 1966, 1967a, 1967b). There were no changes in body weight, but adrenal hypertrophy and hepatic damage were also evident at this dose level.

In a chronic study on the rat 1·5 ml/kg/day was given i.p. for 10, 15 or 20 days and the males killed at the end of the treatment period (Kalla and Bansal, 1975). Body weight and relative weights of the testes, seminal vesicles, epididymis and prostate were decreased in all groups, whilst relative adrenal weight was increased. Histological examination of the testes showed no damage in the males dosed for 10 days. In the 15-day group there was slight damage to spermatids with a reduction in the number of spermatogenic cells and an increase in size of the lumen of the seminiferous tubules. After 20 days of treatment, a further increase in lumen size with shrinkage of the tubules was seen. There was a disruption of the germ cells with early gonadal cells appearing in the lumen and complete absence of spermatids. Interstitial cells were also damaged. Hepatoxicity was not reported but would be expected at the dose level used, even after single injection.

In the rat liver, reduction of microsomal cytochrome P-450 is one of the earliest observable effects of carbon tetrachloride. The same effect is seen in the testes within 3 h of an i.p. injection of 1 ml/kg (De Toranzo *et al.*, 1978). However, the toxicological significance of this observation is unknown.

A chronic toxicity study by Adams *et al.* (1952) on inhaled carbon tetrachloride in the rat included information on testicular weights and histology. Exposure to 400 ppm for 1 h/day, 5 days/week for 6 weeks had no effect on the testes but caused a slight decrease in body growth and some liver toxicity. Exposure to 200 or 400 ppm for 7 h/day, 5 days/week for 25 weeks caused moderate to marked degeneration of the germinal elements of the testes but also severe general toxicity; 9/15 rats died during treatment at 200 ppm and 13/15 died at 400 ppm. Unfortunately, at lower exposure levels of 10, 25 and 100 ppm, no data on the testes are reported. In the same study, exposure of guinea pigs to 400 ppm for 7 h/day, 5 days/week, caused death of most animals within 4 weeks and at autopsy "minor non-specific" pathological changes were seen in the testes. Data on lower concentrations were not reported.

In an acute study on the mouse, males were given a single dose of 2000 mg/kg carbon tetrachloride orally and subsequent uptake of (^{3}H)-thymidine into testicular DNA was measured. Carbon tetrachloride caused a significant reduction in uptake to 50% of the concurrent control level (Seiler, 1977). Considering the testicular toxicity of the substance this might be expected and is not necessarily indicative of a specific genetic effect as was suggested by the author.

Females

The effects of carbon tetrachloride on oestrogen activity are unclear. In immature rats given doses of 0·17–1·7 ml/kg p.o. it inhibited the metabolism of oestrogen by the liver both *in vitro* and *in vivo*, and potentiated the uterotropic effect of endogenous or exogenous oestrogens as measured by an increase in uterine wet weight (Levin *et al.*, 1970; Talbot, 1939). However, a similar experiment in the immature mouse, where carbon tetrachloride was given in a dose of approximately 2 ml/kg i.p., the uteroptropic effect of exogenous oestrogen was not potentiated, and the increase in uterine weight normally seen in response to low doses of HCG and PMS was inhibited (Hipkin, 1969). Despite this contradictory finding, it would seem logical that an agent such as carbon tetrachloride, causing extensive liver damage, would reduce the capacity of the liver to metabolize oestrogen and thereby enhance its biological activity. However, the possibility of an effect on oestrogen secretion as well as metabolism cannot be ruled out; there have been no measurements of FSH, LH or oestrogen secretion rates and data on ovarian weight changes are conflicting (see below).

Three studies by Chatterjee and Mukherji (1966) and Chatterjee (1967a, 1967b) have shown that carbon tetrachloride arrests the oestrous cycle and alters ovarian and uterine weights in rats, but in an inconsistent way. Doses of 1·5–2 ml/kg, which did not affect body weight but were hepatotoxic, were given i.p. Injection during pro-oestrus induced persistent vaginal oestrus for the subsequent 15 days and autopsy at the end of this period showed a significant increase in uterine weight. After injection on the first day of dioestrus, the rats remained in dioestrus for the next 12 days and showed, in one experiment, increased ovarian weight and decreased uterine weight, and in another experiment, decreased ovarian and uterine weights. All weight changes described were significant. A direct effect of carbon tetrachloride on the organs after i.p. injection cannot be ruled out.

In a study by Khominska (1974), normally cycling female rats were injected s.c. with 3 ml/kg of carbon tetrachloride, 4 times on one day, and the oestrous cycles followed for one month after the injections. There was a significant increase in the mean length of the cycle from 4·56 to 5·21 days and the oestrous phase was prolonged by over a day.

The significance of the above observations is difficult to assess since the hepatotoxicity would potentiate oestrogenic effects by inhibiting oestrogen metabolism, whilst the direct toxic effect of i.p. injection on the ovary would tend to reduce oestrogen production.

It has been suggested that the gonadal inhibition in both males and females injected with carbon tetrachloride may be stress-related, since in both sexes it is accompanied by adrenal hypertrophy and is prevented by ascorbic acid, which blocks the release of ACTH (Chatterjee, 1967a) or by phentolamine, which blocks the action of catecholamines (Chatterjee, 1967b). However, both these agents also protect not only against carbon tetrachloride-induced adrenal hypertrophy but also against hepatotoxicity, and hepatic damage is regarded as a specific primary toxic effect of carbon tetrachloride, not stress-induced, so the mechanism of gonadal inhibition is unclear. No work has been done to show whether lower doses which are not hepatotoxic still affect male or reproductive functions.

C. FERTILITY

In a chronic study on the effects of feeding carbon tetrachloride in the diet to rats at 80 or 200 ppm Alumot *et al.* (1976) detected no adverse effects on reproduction in either males or females. There were 18 females and 9 males per treatment group. The diet was commenced 2 weeks after weaning and the females were mated for 5 successive pregnancies beginning at 3 months of age. For the first pregnancy they were mated with control males and subsequently with males from the corresponding treatment group. No adverse effects attributable to either treated males or treated females were seen in terms of pregnancy rate, delivery rate, live litter size, offspring weight or mortality. At the highest dose (200 ppm) the rats consumed 10–18 mg carbon tetrachloride/kg/day, a dose causing no observable liver damage or alteration to body weight.

D. PREGNANCY

In an early teratology study in the rat by Wilson (1954) carbon tetrachloride was given orally (0·3 ml/rat) or s.c. (0·8 ml/rat) on 2 or 3 days beginning between days 7 and 11 of pregnancy, and the dams killed on day 20. The reported results did not distinguish between the 2 routes of administration. Of the 29 rats treated, 6 died and 11 lost entire litters due to early resorption. The remaining 12 pregnant animals had a resorption rate within "normal limits" (no control data given). There were no malformed fetuses, and only 1 litter was growth retarded.

In a preliminary experiment in the rat, reported only briefly, carbon tetrachloride at a dose of 1 ml/kg s.c., given at various unstated times during pregnancy and for varying, unstated numbers of days, had no effect on resorption or abnormality rates (Roussel, 1967). However, the details were not presented and numbers of animals used and precise timing of treatments cannot be ascertained.

Khominska (1974) has investigated the course of pregnancy in rats with carbon tetrachloride-induced hepatotoxicity. Rats were given 3 ml/kg in 4 s.c.

injections on one day and mated not earlier than 7 days after the injections. Pre-implantation losses were increased from 5% in controls to 21% in treated dams, and post-implantation losses from 7% in controls to 18% in treated rats. The author suggested that the high pre-implantation losses were due to high oestrogen levels, though these were not measured. In the same study, this treatment was also reported to cause prolongation of the oestrous stage of the cycle in rats (see section B). Khominska also noted a disturbance of maternal corticosterone levels (decreased adrenal venous blood levels and increased peripheral blood levels), which was attributed to increased oestrogen levels and/or liver damage affecting levels of the corticosterone carrier protein, transcortin. In the fetuses, corticosterone levels in the treated group were double control levels, which was attributed to possible hepatic damage in the fetuses.

Inadequately reported studies in the rabbit by Heine *et al.* (1964) and Neumann (1977) stated that no malformations were found following oral administration of 50 or 60 mg/kg on day 6 of pregnancy. Adams *et al.* (1961) have shown that i.p. injection of 1 ml/kg on days 4 and 5 of pregnancy in the rabbit caused some cellular degeneration in the embryonic discs and trophoblasts contained very large nuclei with prominent nucleoli. Injection of 0·6 ml/kg i.p. on day 5 of pregnancy had no effect on blastocysts recovered at 6·5 days' gestation.

Oral administration of 0·15 ml/kg carbon tetrachloride, on one of days 12, 14, 16 and 18 of pregnancy in the rat, reduced glycogen levels and increased the number of dividing cells in the chorionic epithelium of the placenta (Tsirelnikov and Tsirelnikova, 1976). After administration on days 12 or 14 of pregnancy, destruction of the chorionic epithelium of the labyrinthine portion of the placenta was observed. However, in these experiments the rats were killed 48 h after administration of carbon tetrachloride and no data on fetal viability was reported. It is thus not possible to tell whether the placental changes were secondary to fetal death or a primary pathological change induced by carbon tetrachloride. One study by Roschlau and Rodenkirchen (1969) in the mouse reported extensive fetal deaths on day 19 of pregnancy following s.c. or i.p. injection of 0·04 ml carbon tetrachloride on day 16 or 18, accompanied by placental necrosis, but again it is not clear whether necrosis preceded or followed fetal death.

Inhalation exposure to 300 or 1000 ppm for 7 h/day on days 6–15 of pregnancy in the rat has been investigated by Schwetz *et al.* (1974) in a well designed study using large numbers of animals. During the dosing period, food consumption by the dams was reduced by as much as 40% (300 ppm) and 55% (1000 ppm) on some days, resulting in a mean decrease in body weight of 7% (300 ppm) and 15% (1000 ppm) by day 21 in comparison with controls. Evidence of maternal hepatotoxicity was seen in both groups; serum glutamic-pyruvic transaminase (SGPT) was significantly elevated during exposure but had returned to normal by day 21 when relative liver weights were significantly increased but absolute weights unchanged. No other signs of toxicity were observed. There was no statistically significant effect on resorptions, although 1/23 of the litters in the 1000 ppm group was completely resorbed compared with 0/43 in controls. No gross external abnormalities were seen in any group. The data on internal and skeletal anomalies is difficult to evaluate since only information on the number and percentage of litters affected is given, with no data on the numbers of fetuses affected. However, the authors report no significant increases in anomalies, except for subcutaneous oedema in the 300 ppm group and sternebral anomalies in the 1000 ppm group. These increases are unlikely to be of any biological significance since oedema was not significantly elevated in the 1000 ppm group and the incidence of sternebral anomalies varied considerably in the two control groups. It was low in the control group run concurrently with the 1000 ppm group but in the control group exposed to air concurrently with the 300 ppm group the incidence was as high as in the group exposed to 1000 ppm. Fetal body weight and crown-rump length were significantly decreased in a dose-related manner but this is not unexpected in view of the severe effect on food consumption in the dams.

In a study by Gilman (1971), reported in abstract only, exposure of rats to 250 ppm for 8 h/day for 5 days between days 10 and 15 of pregnancy had no significant effect on skeletal abnormalities, live versus stillbirths, litter size or resorptions, but postnatally there was a significant increase in pup deaths between 1 and 4 days and between 4 and 21 days of age. However, a proper assessment of this work is not possible in the absence of any information on methods or more detail of results other than that given above.

The effect of carbon tetrachloride on the liver of offspring from treated rats has been specifically studied. Tsirelnikov and Dobrovolskaya (1973) gave 3 ml/kg carbon tetrachloride (route not specified) on one of days 12–20 of pregnancy, and killed the dams two days after dosing for examination of the fetal liver. Administration on days 12–15 caused fetal death in the majority of cases. From day 16, fetal body weight in the treated groups was significantly lower than controls, and at 15–16 days relative liver weight was lower, but subsequently higher in treated fetuses compared with controls. In the fetal liver, morphological changes were not seen until day 19, but biochemical changes appeared earlier. Altered lipid metabolism was evident by day 16 and the appearance of glycogen was delayed by one day until day 19 and its quantity at term much reduced. However, the authors noted that damage to the fetal liver was considerably less than damage to the maternal liver.

Kyutukchiev and Matrova (1971) have also demonstrated relative resistance of the fetal liver to carbon tetrachloride. Rats were injected with 0·3 ml/kg i.p. on day 13 or 17 of pregnancy and killed on day 16 or 20 respectively. Changes in liver enzyme levels were more marked in the mother than the fetus, though this is not perhaps surprising in view of the relative immaturity of the fetal liver enzyme system before term.

Doses of 0·5–2·0 ml/kg s.c. on days 19–20 of pregnancy in the rat, which could cause extensive liver damage in adults, caused very few histological changes and only occasional necrosis in the offspring (Bhattacharyya, 1965). Even fetal s.c. or intra-amniotic injections of 0·04 ml carbon tetrachloride on one of the last 3 days of gestation failed to cause significant fetal liver damage.

In the mouse, dilation and hyperaemia of liver sinusoids was seen in many fetuses and liver necrosis in some fetuses, following s.c. or i.p. injection of 0·04 ml carbon tetrachloride on day 16 or 18 of pregnancy with autopsy on day 19 (Roschlau and Rodenkirchen, 1969). However, the effect on maternal liver was more pronounced and many fetuses died as a result of treatment, possibly because of placental necrosis.

Doses of 1–2 ml/kg but not 0·5 ml/kg given s.c. to suckling rat dams on the tenth day of lactation resulted in histological changes in the liver of the pups but no extensive damage (Bhattacharyya, 1965).

Exposure of rats before pregnancy to hepatotoxic doses of carbon tetrachloride has been shown to render their offspring more susceptible to liver damage induced by oral carbon tetrachloride given at 4 weeks of age (Khominska, 1974). However, the interval between injection of the adult female and pregnancy commencing was not stated and the mechanism of such specific transgenerational effects remains obscure.

Conclusion

In summary it would seem that in the one species tested, the rat, carbon tetrachloride is not teratogenic but may be embryo- and fetotoxic at doses which are also toxic to the dam. Severe embryotoxicity has only been shown at doses which are also lethal to some adults. The mechanism may be by induction of placental damage. The fetal, neonatal and young rat appears to be more resistant than adults to the hepatotoxic effects of carbon tetrachloride, but the suggestion of higher postnatal mortality following exposure *in utero* requires further investigation.

E. MUTAGENICITY

IARC Monograph Vol. 20 (1979) reports that carbon tetrachloride is not mutagenic in the Ames test either with or without metabolic activation.

F. CARCINOGENICITY

IARC Monograph Vol. 20 (1979) summarizes studies showing carbon tetrachloride is carcinogenic in the mouse, rat and hamster. There are no studies on the transplacental carcinogenicity of carbon tetrachloride.

HUMAN STUDIES

A. RELEVANT PHARMACOLOGY AND TOXICOLOGY

Dowty *et al.* (1976) collected 11 paired samples of maternal and cord blood at delivery in 11 normal, uneventful pregnancies. All infants were normal except for one with lumbosacral meningomyelocoele and were all of normal weight. Many volatile low molecular weight compounds were detected in maternal and cord blood including halogenated hydrocarbons, plastic components and food preservatives. Benzene, carbon tetrachloride and chloroform were present in cord blood in amounts equal to or greater than in maternal blood. No quantitative details were given. This indicates that carbon tetrachloride crosses the placenta.

B. ENDOCRINE AND GONADAL EFFECTS

No relevant data found.

C. FERTILITY

No relevant data found.

D. PREGNANCY

No relevant data found.

E. MUTAGENICITY

No relevant data found.

F. CARCINOGENICITY

IARC Monograph Vol. 20 (1979) notes the carcinogenicity of carbon tetrachloride in animals, and suggestive case reports of liver cancer in humans, and concludes that in the absence of adequate data, it is reasonable, for practical purposes, to regard carbon tetrachloride as if it presented a carcinogenic risk to humans.

SUMMARY AND EVALUATION

EXPERIMENTAL STUDIES

Sex differences in the toxicity of carbon tetrachloride to rodents has been demonstrated with males more susceptible than females. As well as hepatotoxicity, large doses cause testicular damage both to the seminiferous tubules and to the interstitial cells. The effects of sub-hepatotoxic doses on the testes have not been investigated. Effects of toxic doses on the oestrous cycle have also been described in females but the significance of these is impossible to assess. The effects of low doses have not been studied.

Chronic administration of 80 and 200 ppm in the diet (10–18 mg/kg/day at the top dose) to male and female rats had no effect on fertility, offspring weight or survival.

One satisfactory teratology study has been reported in which pregnant rats were exposed by inhalation to 300 or 1000 ppm daily. No embryolethal or teratogenic effects were observed. There was reduced fetal body weight but this may well have been secondary to reduced food intake in the dams. A number of studies have suggested that very large doses may result in fetal death, but in general the fetal liver seems slightly more resistant than the maternal liver to the toxicity of carbon tetrachloride. It is not mutagenic in bacterial systems. It is carcinogenic in rodents but no reports of transplacental carcinogenicity were found.

HUMAN STUDIES

Carbon tetrachloride crosses the placenta producing levels in cord blood similar to that in maternal blood. No studies were found on endocrine or gonadal effects or of effects on fertility, pregnancy, or mutagenicity. It is regarded as a potential human carcinogen.

EVALUATION

There is evidence that testicular and ovarian damage may be induced at toxic doses. There is limited evidence that it is not teratogenic or embryolethal in rats but fetotoxicity may occur at maternally toxic doses. There is lack of evidence about effects at non-toxic doses.

Attention is drawn to the lack of human reproductive toxicity data, so no evaluation can be made.

References

Adams, E. M., Spencer, H. C., Rowe, V. K., McCollister, D. D. and Irish, D. D. (1952). Vapor toxicity of carbon tetrachloride determined by experiments on laboratory animals. *Archives of Industrial Hygiene and Occupational Health* **6**, 50–66.

Adams, C. E., Hay, M. F. and Lutwak-Mann, C. (1961). The action of various agents upon the rabbit embryo. *Journal of Embryology and experimental Morphology* **9**, (3), 468–491.

Alumot, E., Nachtomi, E., Mandel, E. and Holsten, P. (1976). Tolerance and acceptable daily intake of chlorinated fumigants in the rat diet. *Food and Cosmetics Toxicology* **14**, 105–110.

Bhattacharyya, K. (1965). Foetal and neonatal responses to hepatotoxic agents. *Journal of Pathology and Bacteriology* **90**, (1), 151–161.

Chatterjee, A. (1966). Testicular degeneration in rats by carbon tetrachloride intoxication. *Experientia* **22**, 395–396.

Chatterjee, A. (1967a). Role of ascorbic acid in the prevention of gonadal inhibition by carbon tetrachloride. *Endokrinologie* **51**, (5–6), 319–322.

Chatterjee, A. (1967b). Effect of phentolamine (Regitine) in the prevention of carbon tetrachloride-induced gonadal inhibition of rats. *Endocrinology* **80**, (5), 983–985.

Chatterjee, A. and Mukherji, M. (1966). Effect of carbon tetrachloride in the gonadal activity of female rats. *Endokrinologie* **50**, (1–2), 1–3.

Chaturvedi, V. C. (1969). Influence of sex on hepatic injury in albino rats. *Indian Journal of Medical Science* **23**, 374–379.

De Toranzo, E. G. D., Villarruel, M. C. and Castro, J. A. (1978). Early destruction of cytochrome P-450 in testis of carbon tetrachloride poisoned rats. *Toxicology* **10**, (1), 39–44.

Dobrovolskaya, S. G., Tsirelnikov, N. I. and Yakobson, G. S. (1973). Morphohistochemical characteristics of the liver of pregnant rats under conditions of carbon tetrachloride administration. *Byulleten Eksperimental Noi Biologii I Meditsiny* **75**, (2), 114–117.

Douglas, B. H. and Clower, B. R. (1968). Hepatotoxic effect of carbon tetrachloride during pregnancy. *American Journal of Obstetrics and Gynecology* **102**, (2), 236–239.

Dowty, B. J., Laseter, J. L. and Storer, J. L. (1976). The transplacental migration and accumulation in blood of volatile organic constituents. *Pediatric Research* **10**, 696–701.

Gilman, M. R. (1971). A preliminary study of the teratogenic effects of inhaled carbon tetrachloride and ethyl alcohol consumption in the rat. *Dissertation Abstracts International B* **32**, (4), 2021.

Gualandi, L. and Faccioli, G. (1969). A study of lipoperoxidation of the tissue in pregnant and non pregnant female rats intoxicated with CC14. *Rivista Italiana di Ginecologia* **53**, (8), 560–567.

Heine, W., Kirchmair, H., Fiedler, M. and Stuwe, W. (1964). Thalidomide embryopathy in rabbits following transient liver damage in the mother by carbon tetrachloride. *Klinische Wochenschrift* **42**, 592.

Hipkin, L. J. (1969). Nonspecific inhibition of gonadotropin in the uterine weight assay. *Endocrinology* **84**, (3), 482–487.

IARC Monographs on the Evaluation of the Carcinogenic Risk of Chemicals to Humans: Some halogenated hydrocarbons (1979). Volume 20, Lyon, France.

Kalla, N. R. and Bansal, M. P. (1975). Effect of carbon tetrachloride on gonadal physiology in male rats. *Acta Anatomica (Basel)* **91**, (3), 380–385.

Khominska, Z. B. (1974). Change in function of ovaries and adrenal glands in rats under experimental toxic hepatitis. *Fiziologicheskii Zhurnal* **20**, (6), 747–751.

Klaassen, C. C. and Plaa, G. L. (1967). Susceptibility of male and female mice to the nephrotoxic and hepatotoxic properties of chlorinated hydrocarbons. *Proceedings—Society for Experimental Biology and Medicine* **124**, (4), 1163–1166.

Kyutukchiev, B. and Matrova, T. (1971). A comparative study on the enzymic changes in liver, kidney and placenta of rats and fetuses after administration of estrogen and carbon tetrachloride. *Eksperimentalnaya Meditsina* **10**, (3), 164–171.

Levin, W., Welch, R. M. and Conney, A. H. (1970). Effect of carbon tetrachloride and other inhibitors of drug metabolism on the metabolism of estradiol-17β and estrone in the rat. *Journal of Pharmacology and Experimental Therapeutics* **173**, 247–255.

Neumann, H. J. (1977). Contribution to the embryotoxic effect of chloramphenicol in animal experiment. *Zahn Mund und Kieferheilkunde* **65**, 25–32.

Roschlau, G. and Rodenkirchen, H. (1969). Histological examination of the diaplacental action of carbon tetrachloride and allyl alcohol in mice embryos. *Experimentelle Pathologie* **3**, (4–5), 255–263.

Roussel, C. (1967). Effect of liver damage on the responses of pregnant rats to a teratogen, Triton W. R. 1339. *Comptes Rendus des Seances Societe de Biologie* **161**, (4), 758–762.

Schwetz, B. A., Leong, B. K. J. and Gehring, P. J. (1974). Embryo- and fetotoxicity of inhaled carbon tetrachloride, 1,1-dichloroethane and methyl ethyl ketone in rats. *Toxicology and Applied Pharmacology* **28**, 452–464.

Seiler, J. P. (1977). Inhibitions of testicular DNA synthesis by chemical mutagens and carcinogens. Preliminary results in the validations of a novel short term test. *Mutation Research* **46**, 305–310.

Talbot, N. B. (1939). The inactivation of endogenous estrogen by the liver. *Endocrinology* **25**, 601–604.

Tsirelnikov, N. I. and Dobrovolskaya, S. G. (1973). Morphohistochemical study of the liver in embryos in case of administration of carbon tetrachloride at various stages of ontogenesis. *Byulleten Eksperimentalnoi Biologii I Meditsiny* **76**, (12), 95–97.

Tsirelnikov, N. I. and Tsirelnikova, T. G. (1976). Morphohistochemical study of the placenta of rats after administration of hepatotrophic poison at various periods during pregnancy. *Byulleten Eksperimentalnoi Biologii I Meditsiny* **82**, (8), 1007–1009.

Wilson, J. G. (1954). Influence on the offspring of altered physiologic states during pregnancy in the rat. *Annals of the New York Academy of Sciences* **57**, 517–525.

Yakobson, G. S., Dobrovolskaya, S. G. and Vakulin, G. M. (1978). Dependence of the intensity of the process of damage and recovery in the rat liver following acute carbon tetrachloride poisoning in the sex and estrous cycle phase. *Byulleten Eksperimentalnoi Biologii I Meditsiny* **85**, (4), 460–464.

11. Chlordecone

TECHNICAL DATA

Formula

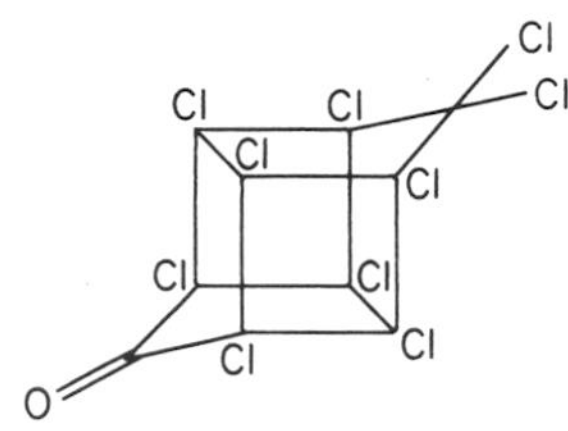

CAS registry number 143–50–0

Chemical abstracts name Decachlorooctahydro-1,3,4-metheno-2H-cyclobuta(c,d)pentalen-2-one

Synonym Kepone; Decachloroketone; decachlorooctahydro-1,3,4-metheno-2H-cyclobuta(c,d) pentalen-2-one; decachloropentacyclo $(5.2.1.0^{2,6}.0\text{-}^{3,9}0^{5,8})$ decan-4-one; decachlorotetracyclodecanone.

Uses Insecticide, fungicide.

TLV None

ANIMAL STUDIES

A. RELEVANT PHARMACOLOGY AND TOXICOLOGY

Sex differences in toxicity in juvenile and adult mice have been investigated by Huber (1965). Chlordecone (Kepone) was fed in the diet at 0–100 ppm with an interval of 10 ppm between each treatment group, and a minimum of 12 mice/group. There were no sex differences in mortality, which occurred at 50 ppm and above.

Huber (1965) also demonstrated placental transfer of Kepone and transfer to suckling neonates through the milk in the mouse, though in a very limited number of animals. Seven embryos, averaging 0·3 g in weight each and placentae were removed from a pregnant female that had been fed 40 ppm Kepone in the diet for 6 days. The embryos contained 5 ppm and the placentae 12 ppm Kepone. Offspring of dams fed 40 ppm in the diet during lactation only, from the day of parturition, were found to contain Kepone; at 6 days of age one pup had a whole body level of 3 ppm, and another pup had stomach, liver and brain contents of 16·8, 33·6, 16·8 ppm respectively, while at 15 days of age one pup had liver and brain levels of 47 and 36 ppm respectively.

B. ENDOCRINE AND GONADAL EFFECTS

Epstein (1978) has published a comprehensive review of Kepone toxicity using literature and documentation available up to June 1976. The data on avian toxicity are drawn largely from this review and the original papers are not separately referenced. Some of the work referred to by Epstein appears only in documents deposited with U.S. agencies such as the F.D.A. and E.P.A.

Avian toxicity

Whilst the scope of this review does not generally include avian species, in the case of Kepone, effects on birds and mammals are not dissimilar and are therefore reviewed here. In avian species, feeding Kepone in the diet has been shown to generally inhibit their reproduction and been described as having "oestrogen-like effects".

De Witt and co-workers reported that male pheasants fed 50 ppm developed female plumage, histologically abnormal testes and malformed spermatozoa. Feeding pheasants (sex unspecified) 1 ppm during winter and spring markedly inhibited reproduction, whilst at other times, 25 ppm almost completely inhibited reproduction. A later study from this same group of workers confirmed the reproductive toxicity of Kepone in quail, pheasant and duck.

McFarland and co-workers investigated the effects of Kepone on immature and mature quail. After feeding 300 ppm to immature males for 3 weeks, there was a significant increase in liver weight and a significant decrease in testicular weight. Adult males fed 400 ppm died within 7–15 days and showed decreased width of the cloacal gland, indicative of LH and testosterone deficiency. The effects on the testes were variable; weights were within control limits but some were atrophic, containing degenerating seminiferous tubules, whilst others were enlarged with increased tubular diameters and partially degenerated seminiferous epithelium. Immature females fed 300 ppm for 2 weeks had increased body and liver weights with a greatly increased oviduct weight. These effects were still seen in ovariectomized or hypophysectomized immature females, though the effects were much reduced in the latter group. Mature females fed 200 ppm for 30 days showed increased liver and ovarian weights, the latter due to increased numbers of follicles. There was no effect on oviduct weight or egg production. The effects in female quail are consistent with increased FSH secretion.

Eroschenko and co-workers feeding quail 200 ppm for 3 weeks have found significant increases in liver, oviduct and testicular weights in immature birds, and significant increases in testicular weight but not oviduct or ovarian weights in mature birds. Some of these results are at variance with those of McFarland *et al.* but histological studies of the testes from mature quail confirmed previous findings of extensive oedema, disrupted seminiferous epithelium and morphologically abnormal spermatozoa. In a later study Eroschenko (1978) also confirmed the findings of McFarland *et al.* of variable effect on the testes: after feeding 200 ppm in the diet to quail for 6 weeks, both enlarged and atrophic testes were seen, the difference being due to the presence or absence of oedema which greatly distended the seminiferous tubules. Disruption of germinal epithelium, reduced sperm production and abnormal spermatozoa were all found in both oedematous and non-oedematous testes. In hens, Naber and Ware have shown that feeding 75 or 150 ppm for 16 weeks reduced egg production, hatchability and survival of the hatched chicks.

Reversibility of the reproductive effects of Kepone in avians has been shown by De Witt, within 60–90 days of return to a control diet. Eroschenko (1978) has found improvements in testicular morphology of the quail beginning 20 days after return to a control diet. However, in many birds, foci of necrosis and degeneration and lymphocytic infiltration were evident in the testes, epididymides and vasa deferentia. Samples taken 60 days after return to a control diet indicated irreversible damage to the testes and ducts in a number of cases.

Mammalian toxicity

Males

In studies carried out on behalf of Allied Chemical Company in 1958–1961 and published in 1979, Larson *et al.* fed young male rats 0, 1, 5, 10, 25, 50, or 80 ppm Kepone in the diet for 2 years. There were initially 40 rats/group. All those fed 50 or 80 ppm died within the first 6 months and 2-year survival was reduced in a dose-related manner in all other treated groups. Five rats/group were killed at 3 months and 1 year after the start of the study. At 3 months, dose-related testicular atrophy was seen in 1/5 rats at 10 ppm, 4/5 at 25 ppm, 4/5 rats at 50 ppm and 5/5 rats at 80 ppm. At 50 and 80 ppm degenerative changes were also seen in the liver but their severity was unrelated to the severity of the testicular atrophy. Testicular pathology at 1 and 2 years is not mentioned in the published paper. However, Epstein (1978), reviewing the data from this study submitted to the F.D.A. noted that at 2 years testicular atrophy was seen in 44% of males at 10 ppm compared with only 12% of controls. Other signs of toxicity noted at 10 ppm were proteinuria and liver hyperplasia.

In a further study on behalf of Allied Chemical reviewed by Epstein (1978), Kepone was applied percutaneously to male rabbits for 8 h/day, 5 days/week for 3 weeks. Bran bait containing 2% Kepone was applied to shaved skin in quantitites equivalent to 5 and 10 mg/kg. Testicular atrophy was seen in 2/6 rabbits at 5 mg/kg and 1/6 rabbits at 10 mg/kg. No other toxic effects were noted. These doses are well below the acute percutaneous LD50 for the rabbit, determined in another Allied Chemical study as 410–435 mg/kg (quoted by Epstein, 1978).

Huber (1965) fed male mice 40 ppm Kepone in the diet for 6 months. After withdrawal of the diet, examination of the testis (time of autopsy in relation to feeding Kepone not stated) revealed normal spermatogenesis and interstitial cell content, despite a reduction in average litter size from matings with untreated females (see section C for details). All treated males produced litters. Kepone levels in the testis were also measured (Huber, 1965) after 100 and 300 days on a 40 ppm diet. Testicular levels were 26 and 17 ppm compared with liver levels of 65 and 113 ppm at 100 and 300 days respectively.

Hammond *et al.* (1978) have recorded a similar reduction in litter size to that seen by Huber (1965) in the litters of male rats fed 30 ppm Kepone in the diet for 8 weeks, when mated with females at 7 weeks after starting treatment. Testosterone levels were higher (level of significance not stated) at 4 weeks than at 1, 2 or 8 weeks and LH levels fluctuated irregularly in the Kepone-fed males. Testicular weight was not affected but seminal vesicle weight was decreased at 8 weeks. The study is reported in abstract only and no further details are given.

Females

The effects of Kepone in the diet on female rats and mice have also been studied. Huber (1965) fed groups of 14–20 female mice 0, 10, 30, 37·5 or 40 ppm. Constant oestrus appeared in the majority of females in groups fed 30 ppm or above and occurred as early as 3 weeks after starting the Kepone diet in the 40 ppm group. It was not seen in the 10 ppm group, even after 240 days on the diet. Histological examination of the ovaries of the mice showed normal follicle development but few corpora lutea at 30 ppm or above. Kepone levels in the ovaries from mice fed 40ppm ranged from 13–26ppm and in the liver 64–168ppm, in measurements made 30–500 days after starting on the Kepone diet. Bioassay of pituitary FSH and LH activities in females fed

40 ppm for 3 months showed no change in FSH levels but a 25% reduction in LH levels. These results are consistent with the histological findings in the ovary.

Hammond *et al.* (1978) also reported constant oestrus in female rats fed 30 ppm after 8–10 weeks on the Kepone diet. At 10 weeks the rats were killed and at this time oestradiol and LH levels were decreased, while FSH levels were unchanged. The uterine horns were fluid-filled and the uterine weight increased while ovarian weights were decreased in comparison with controls.

Gellert (1978) has administered 1, 10 or 100 mg/kg to female rats as a single s.c. injection at 22 days of age and measured their uterotrophic response 24 h later. Uterine weight was increased in a dose-related manner and the differences between treated and control rats were significant at 10 and 100 mg/kg. The response at 10 mg/kg was similar to that elicited by 1 μg/kg oestradiol-17β.

The effects of neonatal exposure to Kepone on subsequent reproductive function in rats and mice have also been studied. Since the effects are similar to those seen after prenatal exposure they will be considered in section D.

Conclusion

The mammalian experiments indicate that adverse effects on the testes may be seen at doses as low as 10 ppm Kepone in the diet when fed for a prolonged period, a dose well below that causing overt toxicity. In avian species, the nature of the atrophic effect on the testes is such that some changes produced by Kepone may be irreversible. It is not known if this is also the case in mammalian species. In females, effects on rats and mice are very similar (persistent oestrus and anovulation) but do not appear at doses as low as 10 ppm. At 30 ppm the effects are marked even after only a few weeks on the diet. The mechanism by which Kepone affects reproductive function in males and females is not known. Results from avian and mammalian experiments indicate FSH secretion may be increased, LH secretion may be decreased, or Kepone may have direct oestrogenic effects itself. Any one or combination of these effects may be taking place.

C. FERTILITY

The general inhibition of reproduction caused by Kepone in avian species has already been mentioned in section B. In mammalian species Kepone affects fertility in both males and females, but the effects in females are generally more marked.

Males

Huber (1965) fed 40 ppm Kepone in the diet of male mice for 2 months before mating and during a 100-day mating period. Males mated to control females produced litters but no further information on fertility, litter size, litter viability, etc., was given. Following withdrawal of Kepone after feeding 40 ppm in the diet for 6 months, all treated males mated with control females produced litters, but average litter size was reduced; first litters averaged 5·5 pups/litter compared with 7·4 in controls and second litters averaged 5·7 pups/litter compared with 7·0 in controls. In the treated group, 10/10 produced first litters but only 6/10 produced second litters compared with 4/5 controls. There was no adverse effect on pup survival in litters from treated males.

Hammond *et al.* (1978) recorded a similar reduction in litter size to that seen by Huber (1965) in the litters of male rats fed 30 ppm in the diet for 8 weeks.

Epstein (1978) has summarized the results of an E.P.A. study. Adult male rats were given 10 mg/kg/day Kepone orally for 6 days and then mated with untreated females over several weeks. Severe neurological symptoms were observed during the dosing period and there was a significant loss in "fertility" lasting up to 3 weeks after dosing stopped. The study did not indicate whether this loss was due to failure to mate, infertile matings or dominant lethal effects.

Simon *et al.* (1978) have carried out a dominant lethal study in rats. Groups of 10 males were given 0, 3·6 or 11·4 mg/kg orally for 5 consecutive days (toxic effects are not specifically mentioned) and then mated with 2 untreated females/week for 14 weeks. The females were killed on day 14 of pregnancy and corpora lutea counted and the contents of the uterus examined. Kepone caused no "compound-related effects", whereas dominant lethal mutations were seen in positive controls given triethylenemelamine. The study is reported in abstract only and no further details were given.

Cannon and Kimbrough (1979) fed groups of 20 male rats 0 or 25 ppm Kepone in the diet for 3 months followed by a 4·5 month "recovery" period during which they were paired twice with control females. Kepone intake during treatment ranged from 1·17–1·58 mg/kg/day and was sufficient to cause tremors and a significant reduction in body weight both at the end of treatment and at the end of the recovery period. Males killed at the end of the treatment period had enlarged, histologically abnormal livers and abnormalities were still present at the end of the recovery period. None of the rats died and reproduction during the recovery period was normal; successful matings, litters produced, litter size at birth, litter size at weaning and average weaning weight were similar for control and treated groups.

Females

Huber (1965) fed groups of 8 female mice 0, 10, 30 or 37·5 ppm Kepone in the diet for one month before mating and during a 100-day test period, during which they were paired twice with control males. Dose-related reductions in numbers of litters produced, average young/litter and increased time to mating were seen in all treated groups. At 10 ppm, survival of pups to weaning was 87% compared with 89% in controls, but at 30 ppm it was only 26% and at 37·5 ppm it was 42%. No second litters were produced following pairings at 30 or 37·5 ppm. Fourteen females fed on 40 ppm for 2 months before mating and during a 100-day test period produced no litters at all. Following withdrawal of Kepone diet from 10 females in this group, reproduction resumed within 7 weeks and 8/10 females paired with control males produced litters. However, first litters were smaller than controls averaging 4·3 young/litter compared with 7·4 in controls and survival to weaning was only 65% compared with 89% in controls. Second litters were also small, averaging 4·6 pups/litter compared with 7·0 in controls, but survival to weaning was similar in treated and control groups.

Good *et al.* (1965) also investigated the effects of feeding up to 37·5 ppm Kepone in the diet to mice, but in their experiments treated females were paired with treated males after one month on the diet and treatment of both sexes continued during the 4–5 months of pairing. Groups of 7–36 pairs were fed 0, 5, 10, 17·5, 25, 30 or 37·5 ppm. In all treated groups there was a dose-related reduction in average number of litters produced and in litter size, and an increased time to mating. At the lowest dose of 5 ppm, first litter size was not affected but second litter size averaged only 5·7 pups compared with 7·3 in controls. At 5 ppm, 81% produced a first litter compared with 96% in controls and 50% a second litter compared with 78% in controls. A similar but more marked effect was seen at 10 ppm, 71% producing a first litter (controls 100%) and only 21% a second litter (controls 96%). These data suggest that at low doses duration of treatment is a significant variable. The most marked deterioration occurred between 25 and 30 ppm; at 25 ppm 11 pairs produced 12 litters of average size 6·1 but at 30 ppm 7 pairs produced only 2 litters of average size 3·0, and at 37·5 ppm, 10 pairs produced only 2 litters of average size 5·0.

Cannon and Kimbrough (1979) fed female rats 0 or 25 ppm for 3 months followed by a 4–5 month "recovery" period during which they were paired twice, first with control males, then later with treated males (given 25 ppm). Kepone did not affect male reproduction at 25 ppm (see earlier in this section for details). Kepone intake ranged from 1·62–1·71 mg/kg/day, which caused tremors and a reduction in body weight at the end of the treatment period. Females killed at this time showed enlarged, histologically abnormal livers and adrenal glands. At the end of the recovery period, body weight and adrenals were normal, but livers still showed abnormal histology. None of the rats died but 20/20 showed complete reproductive failure when paired with control males at the end of the treatment period. No litters were produced and it is not known if they mated. When paired again with treated males 9 weeks after the withdrawal of the Kepone diet, 9/20 mated and produced litters compared with 13/20 in control females mated to control males. Average litter size at birth and at weaning were slightly reduced by 12–17% in comparison with controls but average weight at weaning was normal.

Conclusion

In the previous section, it was noted that male rats fed 25 ppm (equivalent to 1·2–1·6 mg/kg) or doses as low as 10 ppm showed testicular atrophy after 3 months on a Kepone diet, but the potential for recovery was unknown. The experiments reviewed in this section indicate that after feeding 25 ppm for 3 months in the rat, complete recovery, in terms of normal reproductive capacity, occurs after withdrawal of treatment. However, with higher doses (40 ppm in the mouse or 30 ppm in the rat) partial impairment, in terms of reduced litter size, remains after withdrawal of treatment. Results from experiments in rats where much larger doses of 10 or 11 mg/kg are given by gavage over a short period of time are conflicting, with one group of workers finding a significant loss of fertility and another group not.

In female rodents, clear adverse effects on reproduction are seen during treatment with Kepone in the diet at 25 ppm and above, though partial recovery does occur after withdrawal of the Kepone diet. However, impaired reproduction is also seen in females fed doses as low as 10 ppm which do not seem to affect oestrous cycles or ovulation (see section B), and if both male and female in a mating pair are treated then impaired reproduction is seen at 5 ppm. The effects of levels between 0 and 5 ppm have not yet been investigated so no conclusion can be drawn about a no-effect level.

D. PREGNANCY

The teratogenic potential of Kepone in rats and mice has been studied by Chernoff and Rogers (1976). Acceptable teratological methods were used. Mice were given 0, 2, 4, 8 or 12 mg/kg/day orally by gavage on days 7–16 of pregnancy. Groups of 12–26 animals were used. There was a dose-related reduction in maternal weight gain between days 6–18 of pregnancy, reaching significant levels in the 8 and 12 mg/kg groups. At 12 mg/kg there was actually a loss in body weight averaging −2·8 g compared with a weight gain of +4·3 g in controls. Liver:body weight ratios were significantly increased at all doses except 12 mg/kg. There was one maternal death in the 12 mg/kg group. Only 5/12 mice carried to term at 12 mg/kg compared with 16/26 controls, a number of litters being completely resorbed at this dose level. Average fetal mortality (excluding complete resorptions) was significantly increased to 53% at 12 mg/kg compared with 16% in controls. There were no significant effects on fetal mortality in lower dose groups, and no significant effects on implants/dam, fetal weight or degree of ossification at any dose level. Sporadic malformations seen in fetuses were one with encephalocoele at 4 mg/kg, one with cleft palate at 8 mg/kg and three with club foot at 12 mg/kg. The latter differs significantly from controls. Thus significant effects were only seen at doses which caused considerable maternal toxicity.

Rats (Chernoff and Rogers, 1976) were given 2, 6 or 10 mg/kg/day orally by gavage on days 7–16 of pregnancy. Groups of 26–42 animals were used. As in the mice, there was a dose-related reduction in maternal weight gain, significant at all three dose levels. Controls gained twice as much weight as those given 6 or 10 mg/kg. Liver:body weight ratios were significantly increased at 6 and 10 mg/kg. At 10 mg/kg 8/42 rats died. Only one other animal died, in the 2 mg/kg group. There were no significant effects on implants/dam or average fetal mortality at any dose level. However, there was a dose-related reduction in fetal body weight and degree of ossification, reaching significant levels at 6 and 10 mg/kg. The number of abnormalities seen was increased in all treated groups; in controls there were two malformations, at 2 and 6 mg/kg six malformations/group, and at 10 mg/kg, 32 malformations were seen. The commonest were enlarged renal pelvis, oedema, undescended testis, and enlarged cerebral ventricles, all of which were significantly increased in the 10 mg/kg group in comparison with controls. Thus, as with the mice, severe effects were only seen at doses toxic to the dam. The reductions in fetal weight and degree of ossification seen at lower doses may have been secondary to the reductions in maternal weight gain.

Chernoff *et al.* (1979) also gave mice and rats Kepone during lactation only. Mice were given 6–24 mg/kg/day and rats 2·5–10 mg/kg/day orally by gavage from days 1–4 *post-partum*. In both cases the highest dose approached the maternal LD50. In the mouse 24 mg/kg killed 4/9 dams and by 16 days of age all pups in the remaining 5 litters were dead. At 18 mg/kg pup mortality was 64% at 16 days of age compared with 11% in controls. In rats 10 mg/kg significantly reduced offspring body weight at 37 days of age to 136 g compared with 145 g in controls. No further details were given. In view of the high doses used, and the likely interference with maternal care and lactation, these effects on the offspring may well be secondary to the maternal toxicity, rather than an effect on the offspring through exposure to Kepone in the milk.

Epstein (1978) has also reviewed an E.P.A. study on humans, in which reference is made to experiments showing a reduction in litter viability of mice given 12 and 24 mg/kg/day for 4 days and a reduction in litter weight of rats given 10 mg/kg/day. However no further details are given, and this may be a reference to the study of Chernoff *et al.* (1979) described above.

Rosenstein *et al.* (1977) have investigated the effects of Kepone administration throughout pregnancy and lactation. Rats were given 1, 2 or 4 mg/kg/day orally by gavage beginning on day 2 of pregnancy. Maternal weight gain was significantly reduced in the 2 and 4 mg/kg groups. Deliveries were normal in control and 1 mg/kg groups, but of those given 2 mg/kg, only one-third delivered healthy pups and the remainder had abortions and stillbirths. At 4 mg/kg no healthy pups were delivered. At 24 days of age, electroencephalograms (EEGs) and visual-evoked responses (VERs) were obtained from the pups. EEGs differed significantly from controls but the nature of the differences was not described. VERs were all normal. The study is reported in abstract only and no further information is given.

Because of the nature of Kepone's effects on the endocrine and gonadal systems of adults, the effects of Kepone on the reproductive function of animals exposed prenatally during gestation or in the neonatal period, have been specifically studied. Chernoff and Rogers (1976) found no effect on reproductive capacity of male offspring of rats exposed to 2, 6 or 10 mg/kg from days 7–16 of gestation given orally by gavage to the dam. At 90 days of age they were paired with untreated females for 7 days. Conception rate, average litter size and intrauterine mortality were similar to controls in all treated groups. Similarly, exposure of rats during late gestation had no effect on male offspring reproductive capacity. Gellert and Wilson (1979) gave rats 15 mg/kg/day orally by gavage on days 14–20 of gestation. At 6 months of age, 14/14 male offspring produced litters when paired with control females and there were no significant effects on testis or ventral prostate weights.

Good *et al.* (1965) have studied reproduction in offspring from dams exposed to 5 ppm Kepone in the diet for one month before pairing and during a 120-day pairing period during which two litters were produced. Offspring were segregated, paired and put onto control diet or continued on the 5 ppm Kepone diet. The age(s) at which these events took place was not specified. Three groups of 20–23 pairs of offspring were set up; treated males with treated females on treated diet, treated males with treated females on control diet, and control females with control males on control diet. Reproduction was markedly reduced in both treated groups. In control pairs 71% produced first litters and 29% second litters, whereas in treated groups on control diet 30% had first litters and 9% second litters, and in treated groups on treated diet 25% had first litters and 15% second litters. Litter sizes were smaller in both treated groups but not significantly so. There were no marked differences between treated pairs on control or treated diet indicating that the effects were induced entirely in the prenatal and/or preweaning periods.

Female offspring are markedly affected by prenatal exposure. Gellert and Wilson (1979) gave rats 15 mg/kg orally by gavage on days 14–20 of pregnancy. At 6 months of age female offspring were of normal body weight and normal uterine weight but had a significant reduction in mean ovarian weight which was 59 mg compared with 96 mg in vehicle-treated controls, and a significant increase in adrenal weight which was 85 mg compared with 68 mg in vehicle controls. Vaginal smears taken for two weeks showed 12/21 Kepone treated offspring had persistent vaginal oestrus. At autopsy, there were no corpora lutea in any of the 21 offspring. Only 1/21 controls showed these features. Serum oestradiol-17β levels in Kepone treated offspring with persistent vaginal oestrus were intermediate between the high pro-oestrus and low oestrus levels of controls.

Neonatal treatment of rats or mice produces similar effects. Gellert (1978) gave s.c. injections of 0·2 or 1·0 mg Kepone at 3 and 4 days of age in the rat. Vaginal opening occurred significantly earlier than in controls; the mean age of opening was 41 days in controls, <31 days at 0·2 mg and <23 days at 1·0 mg. Vaginal smears were taken from 2 months of age onwards. Cycles were abnormal in both treated groups at 2 months of age, and persistent vaginal oestrus appeared at 4 months in the 1·0 mg group (5/12 affected) and at 6 months in the 0·2 mg group (6/19 affected). No abnormalities were seen in controls. At autopsy at 8 months of age complete absence of corpora lutea was seen in 11/11 in the 1·0 mg group, in 11/19 in the 0·2 mg group, and in 1/20 of controls. This was reflected in ovarian weights which were significantly reduced in the 1·0 mg group and much lower in anovulatory than in ovulatory rats in the 0·2 mg group. Body weight was significantly increased in the 1·0 mg group and uterine weight significantly increased in the 0·2 mg group. Adrenal and anterior pituitary weights were not affected.

Eroschenko and Mousa (1979) have injected neonatal mice with Kepone. Starting on day of birth, they gave 10 daily injections i.p. of 0·015, 0·03, 0·06 or 0·125 mg Kepone. Higher doses of 0·18 and 0·25 mg were given daily for 4 days, then every other day for the remaining 6 injections. Mortality seen in groups given 0·06 mg or more ranged from 14–31%. A portion of the neonates (5–7) were killed after every 2 injections and the reproductive tract examined histologically. There was a dose-related acceleration in development and maturation of the vagina and uterus. For example, uniform keratinization of the vagina was seen in groups given 0·125 mg and above after the fourth injection. Daily injections of 10 μg of oestradiol-17β produced a similar acceleration. Vehicle-injected controls showed no keratinization even after 10 injections. In related experiments, Eroschenko and Mousa (1979) showed that the effects of Kepone on the reproductive tract were still present 30 days after the last neonatal injection.

Conclusion

The teratology studies employing prenatal exposure only, show that in rats and mice significant embryotoxicity and teratogenicity are only seen at doses which are severely toxic to the dam, killing a proportion of those treated (10–12 mg/kg). Reductions in fetal body weight, retarded ossification and slight increases in malformations seen at doses below 10 mg/kg in the rat may be secondary to the reduction in maternal weight gain, particularly since the majority of malformed fetuses at lower doses had enlarged renal pelvis, a common spontaneous malformation in the strain of rat used (Charles River CD), which can simply reflect immature kidney development. Other common malformations seen at 10 mg/kg (undescended testis, enlarged cerebral ventricles) are also often associated with immature fetuses and may disappear as development proceeds. Thus Kepone does not appear to be a gross, structural teratogen, though it must be emphasized that thorough studies have only been done by one group of workers (Chernoff and co-workers). However lower doses of Kepone of 2 mg/kg, a dose which has been reported to cause tremors and reduce weight gain, during the whole of pregnancy have been shown to cause high fetal and neonatal mortality.

There is no evidence of any effect on male reproductive capacity following prenatal exposure to Kepone. However, postnatal functional changes in the reproductive capacity of female offspring appear after even lower exposure during the prenatal and/or neonatal period. Females exposed to high levels of Kepone prenatally and/or neonatally develop persistent vaginal oestrus and anovulation, just as do mature females when treated with Kepone. After lower exposure (5 ppm in the diet) during gestation and lactation, offspring showed reduced fertility. Thus the greatest potential hazard of Kepone to the offspring surviving prenatal or neonatal treatment is an adverse effect on the subsequent reproductive capacity of females. The effect observed is similar to that seen following neonatal steroid-induced sterility and thus may reflect an oestrogenic action of Kepone on the developing brain.

E. MUTAGENICITY

No relevant data found. Dominant lethal tests have been reviewed in section C.

F. CARCINOGENICITY

IARC Monograph Vol. 20 (1979) reported that chlordecone was carcinogenic in rats and mice following oral administration.

HUMAN STUDIES

A. RELEVANT PHARMACOLOGY AND TOXICOLOGY

Like other organochlorine compounds with high fat solubility, Kepone has been reported to concentrate in breast milk (Giacoia and Catz, 1979). (No figures or references quoted.) Kepone was also reported in breast milk of women in a Mirex spray area (quoted by Huff and Gerstner, 1978). Kepone is a breakdown product of Mirex in the environment.

B. ENDOCRINE AND GONADAL EFFECTS

Cannon *et al.* (1978) published details of an epidemic of Kepone poisoning in workers producing it at Life Science Products Company (LSPC), Hopewell, U.S.A. The insecticide Kepone had been produced in small amounts by Allied Chemical Corporation since the early 1950s, and the amount gradually increased to about 200,000 kg by 1973. From March 1974 to July 1975 total world production was taken over by LSPC with an annual production of 400,000 kg of powdered Kepone. This was the only product for the Company. Following investigation of one patient with severe tremors who worked at LSPC and who had a blood Kepone level of 7·5 μg/ml, all workers, the factory and surrounding neighbourhood were investigated and found to be heavily contaminated. Work conditions were very poor and the workers became covered with white Kepone dust. No protective clothing was used, and in the 16 months of operation, the turnover was such that the workforce had been replaced 5 times due to the poor conditions and the frequent development of a symptom complex known as "Kepone shakes". The Virginia State Health Department obtained a list of the 148 persons employed in the plant during its operation (33 current employees and 115 former employees). All the current employees and 100 of the former employees were located and agreed to be investigated. In addition 270 family members, 39 employees of Allied Chemical Corporation and 214 people selected from the neighbourhood of the plant up to 1·6 km distance were investigated. Large volume air sample filters which happened to be 200 metres from the plant also provided evidence of air contamination levels.

The syndrome observed in the workers closely paralleled those previously observed in animal toxicological studies, and were primarily neurological. The three commonest symptoms were subjective sensation of nervousness, objective signs of tremor especially of the hands but which could affect the entire body, and visual difficulty in fixation and focussing with bursts of rapid, erratic eye movements. Numerous other symptoms were recorded, and sperm counts showed oligospermia with a predominance of abnormal and non-motile forms.

Using the criteria of the first two symptoms above, 76 cases of Kepone poisoning in the 133 past and present workers were identified (57%). Of these, 49 had objective neurologic abnormalities. Average time of onset of symptoms after starting employment was 6 weeks, and average length of employment was 17·8 weeks, with production workers being more commonly affected (64%) than non-production (16%). The Kepone blood levels in affected workers averaged 2·53 μg/ml (range 0·009–11·8) and in unaffected workers averaged 0·60 μg/ml (range 0·003–4·1). A high proportion of all other groups tested had detectable blood Kepone levels, although none of the general community survey participants had the clinical syndrome of Kepone poisoning. Two of the workers' wives however did have objective tremor and in 32 family members who had blood samples analysed, Kepone was detected in 30 (mean 0·10 μg/ml, range 0·003–0·39). Environmental air samples between March 1974–April 1975 averaged 7·0 $\mu g/m^3$ (maximum 54·8 $\mu g/m^3$). Significant contamination was also detected in river water and cumulation occurred in fish and shellfish along the James river and right into Chesapeake Bay, 64 km from the plant.

Some evidence of the effect of Kepone on testicular function is given in a paper by Cohn *et al.* (1978) on the treatment of Kepone poisoning with cholestyramine. They studied 32 former male employees of Life Science Products Corporation, some of whom had left the Company up to 13 months earlier and all of whom still had symptoms and with blood Kepone levels greater than 0·6 μg/ml. Because Kepone is highly fat soluble it is only slowly eliminated from the body, mainly in the bile and faeces. In untreated subjects the half-life in blood, which reflected total body levels, was found to be 165 $\pm$ 27 days (mean $\pm$ S.E.M.) and that treatment with cholestyramine could increase the rate of excretion, reducing the half-life to 80 $\pm$ 4 days ($P < 0{\cdot}005$). During the 18-month observation period, as the blood levels of Kepone fell the neurological signs also decreased in severity, and the number of subjects unable to work because of these fell from 11 to 3. Because of the difficulty of quantifying the neurological effects, the authors studied sperm counts in relation to blood Kepone. In 19 of 20 subjects with blood Kepone of greater than 1 μg/ml, the motile sperm count was less than 25×10^6 per ml, (details of collection procedures, number of samples studied, and individual results were not given in the paper). Of 21 subjects with blood Kepone less than 1 μg/ml, 7 showed abnormal sperm counts ("abnormal" is not defined in the paper) and it is stated that the motile sperm count increased as blood Kepone levels fell in 12 of 13 subjects. The period of treatment with cholestyramine was stated to be too brief to determine whether the rapid reduction of blood Kepone level was paralleled by a rapid rise in sperm count. No further details are given but it would appear that in the majority of cases recovery from oligospermia is to be expected following Kepone poisoning.

Huff and Gerstner (1978) in a review of the Kepone history, refer to an obscure publication by Guzelian in 1976 that semen analysis of 14 exposed workers had shown abnormal morphology, decreased motility and oligospermia, probably sufficient to cause sterility (no other details).

C. FERTILITY

No relevant data found.

D. PREGNANCY

No relevant data found.

E. MUTAGENICITY

No relevant data found.

F. CARCINOGENICITY

IARC Monograph Vol. 20 (1979) reported that no case reports or epidemiological studies on the carcinogenicity of chlordecone in humans were available but that there is sufficient evidence that it is carcinogenic in rodents, therefore it is reasonable, for practical purposes, to regard chlordecone as if it presented a carcinogenic risk to humans.

SUMMARY AND EVALUATION

EXPERIMENTAL STUDIES

Limited studies indicate that there are no sex differences in acute toxicity. It is transferred across the placenta and in the breast milk in mice.

Experiments in rats and mice have shown testicular atrophy in the absence of other overt toxic effects following prolonged administration of doses as low as 10 ppm in the diet. In rabbits similar effects have been observed following percutaneous administration of 5 mg/kg. A no-effect level has not been established by either route.

In female rats and mice there is evidence of reduced ovulation and reduced LH levels at oral doses of 30 ppm and above.

There is some evidence that levels of 30–40 ppm Kepone in the diet fed to mice and rats can reduce male fertility as evidenced by reduced litter size. An abstract of one study reported no dominant lethal effects at doses to male rats up to 11·4 mg/kg orally.

One study at 25 ppm in the diet to male rats (equivalent to 1·2–1·6 mg/kg/day) showed no adverse effects on fertility during a recovery period although the dose was sufficient to cause tremors. In female mice and rats Kepone exerts a clear adverse effect. Reduction of number of litters and of litter size were observed in mice at doses down to 5 ppm in the diet, and in rats at doses of 25 ppm. No no-effect level was established in either species. Complete infertility was observed in mice at 40 ppm and in rats at 25 ppm. In mice there was evidence of some recovery following cessation of treatment.

Studies in mice showed that maternally toxic doses of 12 mg/kg orally are embryolethal but probably not teratogenic. Doses of 8 mg/kg and below were without effect. In rats, doses of 6–10 mg/kg orally, lethal to some dams, were fetotoxic, and teratogenicity was reported at 2, 6 and 10 mg/kg. The abnormalities reported however were indicative of retarded development rather than specific malformations. When rats were treated throughout pregnancy, instead of just during embryogenesis, marked embryo- and fetal lethality was observed from doses as low as 2 mg/kg/day. No effect was observed from 1 mg/kg/day. All of the above doses cause some degree of maternal toxicity.

Following treatment during pregnancy and/or in the neonatal period, fertility of male offspring was unaffected, but female offspring showed persistent oestrus and infertility. This may be due to an oestrogenic effect of Kepone on the developing brain. Effects of this type were seen with doses down to 5 ppm in the diet, equivalent to 0·3 mg/kg.

Other than one negative dominant lethal test in rats, no mutagenicity data were found. It is carcinogenic in rats and mice but no reports on transplacental carcinogenicity were found.

HUMAN STUDIES

Kepone has been found in breast milk. Workers exposed to high levels of Kepone developed a variety of symptoms, particularly neurological, characterized by nervousness, tremor and visual problems. Among other effects reported were reduced sperm count and motility and abnormal sperm morphology. Nineteen of 20 workers with blood Kepone levels greater than 1 μg/ml had motile sperm counts of less than 25×10^6 per ml, compared with 7 of 21 workers with blood levels below 1 μg/ml. However, as the blood Kepone levels fell, sperm counts increased, so that the adverse effect on the testis would seem to be reversible. No studies were found of effects on fertility or on pregnancy. No reports on mutagenicity were found or epidemiological studies for carcinogenicity.

EVALUATION

There is sufficient evidence that Kepone causes testicular and ovarian damage in males and females in a variety of mammalian and avian species. There is limited evidence that it may have a low degree of teratogenicity at doses toxic to the dam and is also embryolethal. The significance of the neonatally induced sterility in female rodents for humans is uncertain. This phenomenon is well known in rodents following steroid exposure but has never been recorded in humans.

There is clear evidence for both neurotoxicity and testicular toxicity in men occupationally exposed to high levels of Kepone. Attention is drawn to the lack of data on pregnancy outcome in exposed humans.

References

Cannon, S. B. and Kimbrough, R. D. (1979). Short-term chlordecone toxicity in rats including effects on reproduction, pathological organ changes, and their reversibility. *Toxicology and Applied Pharmacolgy* **47**, 469–476.

Cannon, S. B., Veazey, J. M., Jackson, R. S., Burse, V. W., Hayes, C., Straub, W. E., Landrigan, P. J. and Liddle, J. A. (1978). Epidemic Kepone poisoning in chemical workers. *American Journal of Epidemiology* **107**, (6), 529–537.

Chernoff, N., Linder, R. E., Scotti, T. M., Rogers, E. H., Carver, B. D. and Kevlock, R. J. (1979). Fetotoxicity and cataractogenicity of Mirex in rats and mice with notes on Kepone. *Environmental Research* **18**, 257–269.

Chernoff, N. and Rogers, E. H. (1976). Fetal toxicity of Kepone in rats and mice. *Toxicology and Applied Pharmacology* **38**, 189–194.

Cohn, W. J., Boylan, J. J., Blanke, R. B., Fariss, M. W., Howell, J. R. and Guzelian, P. S. (1978). Treatment of chlordecone (Kepone) toxicity with cholestyramine. (Results of a controlled clinical trial.) *New England Journal of Medicine* **298**, (5), 243–248.

Epstein, S. S. (1978). Kepone-hazard evaluation. *Science of the Total Environment* **9**, (1), 1–62.

Eroschenko, V. P. (1978). Alterations in the testes of the Japanese quail during and after the ingestion of the insecticide Kepone. *Toxicology and Applied Pharmacology* **43**, 535–545.

Eroschenko, V. P. and Mousa, M. A. (1979). Neonatal administration of insecticide chlordecone and its effects on the development of the reproductive tract in the female mouse. *Toxicology and Applied Pharmacology* **49**, 151–159.

Gellert, R. J. (1978). Kepone, Mirex, Dieldrin, and Aldrin: Estrogenic activity and the induction of persistent vaginal estrus and anovulation in rats following neonatal treatment. *Environmental Research* **16**, 131–138.

Gellert, R. J. and Wilson, C. (1979). Reproductive function in rats exposed prenatally to pesticides and polychlorinated biphenyls (PCB). *Environmental Research* **18**, 437–443.

Giacoia, G. P. and Catz, C. S. (1979). Drugs and pollutants in breast milk. *Clinics in Perinatology* **6**, (1), 181–196.

Good, E. E., Ware, G. W. and Miller, D. F. (1965). Effects of insecticides in the Labsaton mouse. I. Kepone. *Journal of Economic Entomology* **58**, 754–757.

Hammond, B., Bahr, J., Dial, O., McConnel, J. and Metcalf, R. (1978). Reproductive toxicology of Mirex and Kepone. *Federation Proceedings* **37**, 501.

Huber, J. J. (1965). Some physiological effects of the insecticide Kepone in the laboratory mouse. *Toxicology and Applied Pharmacology* **7**, 516–524.

Huff, J. E. and Gerstner, H. B. (1978). Kepone: A literature summary. *Journal of Environmental Pathology and Toxicology* **1**, (4), 377–395.

IARC Monographs on the Evaluation of the Carcinogenic Risk of Chemicals to Humans: Some halogenated hydrocarbons (1979). Volume 20, Lyon, France.

Larson, P. S., Egle, J.L. Jr., Hennigar, G. R., Lane, R. W. and Borzelleca, J. F. (1979). Acute, subchronic, and chronic toxicity of chlordecone. *Toxicology and Applied Pharmacology* **48**, 29–41.

Rosenstein, L., Brice, A., Rogers, N. and Lawrence, S. (1977). Neurotoxicity of Kepone in perinatal rats following *in utero* exposure. *Toxicology and Applied Pharmacology* **41**, 142–143.

Simon, G. S., Kipps, B. R., Tardiff, R. G. and Borzelleca, J. F. (1978). Failure of Kepone and hexachlorobenzene to induce dominant lethal mutations in the rat. *Toxicology and Applied Pharmacology* **45**, 330–331.

12. Chloroform

TECHNICAL DATA

Formula	$CHCl_3$
CAS registry number	67–66–3
Chemical abstracts name	Trichloromethane
Synonyms	Trichloromethane
Uses	As a solvent for fats, oils, rubber alkaloids, waxes, gutta-percha, resins; as cleansing agent; in fire extinguishers to lower the freezing temperature of carbon tetrachloride; in the rubber industry.
TLV	10 ppm

ANIMAL STUDIES

A. RELEVANT PHARMACOLOGY AND TOXICOLOGY

A number of reports of accidental exposure of rodents to high concentrations of chloroform have noted the death of male animals but not females (Hill, 1977). Experimental studies of sex differences in the toxicity of chloroform have confirmed that males are more susceptible than females.

In acute studies of the LD50 for i.p. chloroform in mice by Klaassen and Plaa (1967), there was no sex difference in the 24 h-mortality resulting from narcosis but males showed nephrotoxicity at doses 15 times lower than the lethal dose (ED50 0·078 ml/kg) whereas in females there were no signs of kidney damage even at lethal doses. In another study, when mice were anaesthetized for 1 h with 1–2% chloroform in air, 47% of the males died within 48 h whereas no females died (Cascorbi *et al.*, 1976). In the same study, pretreatment of males with oestradiol or females with testosterone for 12 days before chloroform anaesthesia, reversed the susceptibility of the sexes with 27% of females dying compared with only 7% males. No sex differences in the hepatotoxicity of chloroform have been found (Hill, 1977).

Metabolism of chloroform and binding of the metabolites to tissue macromolecules are important determinants of toxicity. In intact male mice, necrosis of the renal proximal convoluted tubules was associated with binding of the label after (^{14}C)-chloroform administration, whereas castrated males or intact females failed to show binding or necrosis unless treated with exogenous testosterone (Hill, 1977). The mechanism by which testosterone increases renal damage is not known. Increased microsomal enzyme activity, enhancing the production of toxic metabolites (Cascorbi *et al.*, 1976) and sensitization of the kidney via a testosterone receptor mechanism (Hill, 1977) have both been suggested as possible mechanisms.

A series of studies have been carried out by Torkelson *et al.* (1976) where exposures were more closely related to conditions likely to be encountered in the workplace. Rats, rabbits, guinea pigs and dogs were exposed to 25, 50 or 85 ppm chloroform by inhalation for 7 h/day, 5 days/week for 6 months. At 50 and 85 ppm male rats showed more lung pathology than females, with an excess mortality of males at 85 ppm, largely due to pneumonia. Changes in liver and kidney weights and microscopical appearance were similar however in both sexes. At 25 ppm minor changes were seen in the liver and kidney of exposed males only, but they were reversible; within 6 weeks of their last exposure there was complete recovery. In the guinea pig studies, mortality in all groups including air-exposed controls was high, and dog and rabbit studies employed too few animals to permit any conclusions to be drawn on sex differences.

B. ENDOCRINE AND GONADAL EFFECTS

The effect of chloroform on the ovaries is not known. In the study of Torkelson *et al.* (1976), where rats, guinea pigs, rabbits and dogs were exposed to 25, 50 or 85 ppm chloroform for 7 h/day, 5 days/week, for 6 months, testicular weights were measured at the end of the exposure period. In rats exposed to 50 or 85 ppm, testicular weights relative to body weight were significantly elevated compared with air-exposed or untreated controls. However, the authors point out that the control testicular weights were unusually low and attach no biological significance to these results, especially since there were no detectable histopathological changes in the testes of chloroform-exposed rats. In guinea pigs exposed to 85 and 50 ppm chloroform, relative but not absolute testicular weights were increased, but not significantly, and no histopathological changes were seen. Too few rabbits and dogs were used for evaluation of effects on the testes.

C. FERTILITY

No relevant data found.

D. PREGNANCY

An early study by Whipple (1912) on chloroform anaesthesia in pregnant dogs near term indicated that 2 h anaesthesia, which was invariably hepatotoxic to the dam, also caused placental necrosis sometimes accompanied by placental separation, haemorrhage and premature delivery. Fetal tissues including the liver were reported as normal however.

Schwetz (1970) reported in abstract only a study on chloroform anaesthesia in pregnant mice and rats. Anaesthesia with 2·5 volumes % of chloroform (equivalent to 25,000–37,000 ppm) for 15 mins/day on days 8–10 or 12–14 of pregnancy in the mouse, or for 1 h/day on days 9–11 or 13–15 of pregnancy in the rat, was reported as embryotoxic but not highly teratogenic. However, the incidence of fetal resorptions, skeletal and soft tissue anomalies was high and fetal body weight and length were decreased in both species. The numbers of animals used and numbers of abnormal offspring are not stated, and some of the fetal malformations described as "anomalies", such as exencephaly and cleft palate, might be more appropriately classified as major malformations. Chloroform had a marked adverse effect compared with other anaesthetics such as ether, methoxyfluorane or halothane. Preventing hypoxia in the chloroform-exposed rats decreased the lethal and growth retarding effects, but chloroform-induced "anomalies" were not reduced. Furthermore, hypoxia controls and methoxyfluorane-exposed animals became more hypoxic than chloroform-exposed animals during treatment and did not show such effects.

Oral administration of chloroform has been studied in mice, rats and rabbits. In a study by Thompson *et al.* (1974), employing around 20 rats and 15 rabbits per treatment group, acceptable teratological methods were used. Doses which were just toxic to the dams, reducing food consumption and weight gain (126 mg/kg days 6–15 in the rat, 50 mg/kg days 6–18 in the rabbit), reduced fetal weight but were not embryolethal or teratogenic. Higher doses, causing nephrotoxicity, hepatotoxicity and occasionally death (316 and 501 mg/kg in the rat, 100 mg/kg in the rabbit) increased the incidence of resorptions as well as reducing fetal weight of surviving offspring, but no increase in abnormalities was seen.

Administration of chloroform in the drinking water has been reported in a preliminary study by McKinney *et al.* (1976). Mice were given 0, 152, 760 or 3800 ppb of chloroform in the drinking water, equivalent to approximately 0,

40, 200 and 1000 μg/kg for a 30 g mouse, before mating (time unspecified) and during pregnancy. There was a dose-related decrease in "embryonic development" and fewer females in the 152 ppb group mated, but no other details were given.

Inhalation studies of chloroform exposure during pregnancy have confirmed effects of intrauterine mortality and growth retardation, but not demonstrated any teratogenic effects. In a study reported in abstract only, Dilley *et al.* (1977) exposed rats to up to 4080 ppm (20 g/m^3) from days 7–14 of pregnancy. They noted increased fetal mortality and decreased fetal weight gain but no teratogenic effects.

Two further inhalation studies have investigated effects in the mouse and rat. Mice were exposed to 100 ppm or filtered room-air for 7 h/day on days 1–7, 6–15 or 8–15 of pregnancy (Murray *et al.*, 1979). They employed 34–40 mice per group and used acceptable teratological methods. All chloroform-exposed groups showed a decrease in maternal body weight gain and reduced food consumption during the treatment period. Absolute and relative maternal liver weights were significantly increased in those exposed during mid-pregnancy, and maternal serum glutamic pyruvic transaminase (SGPT) was also elevated in the one group where it was measured, indicating hepatotoxicity. There was a significant reduction in the percentage of mice found pregnant at term in those where exposure began before or around the time of implantation (days 1–7 or 6–15). The incidence of resorptions was significantly increased in those exposed on days 1–7 only, largely due to 2/11 litters which were completely resorbed. Fetal body weight and crown-rump length was reduced in all groups, significantly so in those exposed on days 1–7 or 8–15. The overall incidence of malformations was not increased by chloroform. Cleft palate was significantly elevated in the group exposed on days 8–15 but 6/10 affected fetuses were from one severely growth retarded litter and no clefts were seen in those exposed on days 6–15. Delayed ossification, paralleling the changes in fetal growth retardation, was seen in all chloroform-exposed groups. Thus embryo- and fetotoxic but not teratogenic effects have been observed at a dose which was also toxic to the dam. It is not possible to determine from this experiment whether the effects on the offspring were independent of, or secondary to, the maternal toxicity.

Rats were exposed to 30,100 or 300 ppm of chloroform (around 20 rats per group) or filtered room-air (77 rats) for 7 h/day on days 6–15 of pregnancy (Schwetz *et al.*, 1974). Maternal weight gain and food consumption was significantly decreased in all chloroform exposed groups. Absolute and relative maternal liver weights were not affected by 30 ppm, were increased by 100 ppm and decreased by 300 ppm. SGPT levels were unaffected. In the 300 ppm group, only 15% of the rats were pregnant at term, compared with 88% of controls. Significantly increased fetal resorptions and decreased fetal body weight and crown-rump length were also found. In lower dose groups these parameters were not affected in any dose-related way. No increase in gross abnormalities was seen in the 30 ppm group but there was a significant increase in acaudia or short tail accompanied by imperforate anus in the 100 ppm group. The effects at 100 ppm were quantitatively and qualitatively similar to those reported in Schwetz's (1970) earlier study on chloroform anaesthesia. There were significant increases in delayed ossification of the skull and wavy ribs at 30 ppm and in missing ribs and delayed ossification of the sternebrae at 100 ppm. Only 2 litters with viable fetuses were available for examination in the 300 ppm group. To control for the anorectic effects of the treatment, an additional air-exposed control group was fed only 3·7 g of food/day on day 6–15, well below the consumption in the 30 and 100 ppm groups. A significant reduction in fetal body weight but no significant increases in gross, skeletal or soft tissue abnormalities, including delayed ossification, were found. Retarded ossification in the absence of significant fetal body weight reductions and increased anomalies or malformations at 30 and 100 ppm therefore suggests a true teratogenic effect of chloroform at doses which do not cause any significant maternal toxicity other than anorexia which was controlled for. A no-effect level for chloroform inhalation has not been established. Clearly, it is below 30 ppm, a dose causing no hepatotoxicity and which is only 3 times the TLV of 10 ppm. However, at a given air concentration, the dose absorbed is likely to be higher in rats than humans because of the greater amount of air inhaled in proportion to body weight.

Direct depressant effects of chloroform on uterine contractions have been shown in the dog and rat by Whalley and Riley (1977) during anaesthesia, but the effects of lower concentrations are not known. *In vitro* studies have indicated that chloroform can inhibit the aggregation of embryonic brain cells which may indicate a potential *in vivo* for interference with recognition processes by which cells are assembled into tissues. These studies and the observed teratogenicity at comparatively low doses indicate a need for postnatal investigation of prenatal chloroform exposure.

E. MUTAGENICITY

Chloroform is not mutagenic in the Ames test with metabolic activation (IARC Monograph Vol. 20, 1979). Chloroform did not increase the frequency of sister-chromatid exchange in cultured Chinese hamster ovary cells after 24 h exposure (White *et al.*, 1979).

F. CARCINOGENICITY

IARC Monograph Vol. 20 (1979) reported that chloroform is carcinogenic in rats and mice.

HUMAN STUDIES

A. RELEVANT PHARMACOLOGY AND TOXICOLOGY

As mentioned in section A of carbon tetrachloride, a study of Dowty *et al.* (1976) of volatile organic constituents in maternal plasma and cord blood in 11 normal pregnancies showed that chloroform could be detected in fetal blood at levels equal to or greater than in maternal blood. Quantitative data were not given in the paper nor speculation as to the source of the chemical.

B. ENDOCRINE AND GONADAL EFFECTS

No relevant data found.

C. FERTILITY

No relevant data found.

D. PREGNANCY

Tylleskar-Jensen (1967) reported that 2 women who worked in the same chemical laboratory both developed eclampsia of pregnancy within 6 months of each other. The laboratory was poorly ventilated and various liquids, chloroform, ether-chloroform-butanol, carbon tetrachloride, acetic, phosphoric and sulphuric acids were often handled in open vessels. A further 6 laboratory employees were examined and all showed evidence of liver damage with raised transaminases in the blood. Measurement of the laboratory atmosphere showed concentrations of 300–1000 ppm chloroform at face level, which were well above the recommended limits at the time of 50 ppm. Whilst it cannot be proven that the chloroform vapour caused the eclamptic toxaemia, it is a remarkable coincidence to observe 2 cases from the one work place when the incidence of eclampsia in the hospital clinic was only 1 in 4000 pregnancies.

E. MUTAGENICITY

Funes-Cravioto *et al.* (1977) studied the incidence of chromosome aberrations in cultured lymphocytes from 73 workers in chemical laboratories and the printing industry. They found a significant increase of approximately 2-fold in the incidence of chromatid and isochromatid breaks when compared with 49 controls. A similar increased incidence was also observed in 14 children aged 4–11 years of 11 women laboratory workers who had worked during pregnancy. There was also an increased incidence of sister-chromatid exchange in 12 technicians and in the 4 children of 2 of the female technicians who had worked during pregnancy. The technicians came from 8 different laboratories but all were exposed to one or more of chloroform, toluene, benzene, cyclohexane, diethyl ether, isooctane, methanol, toluene or xylene, with chloroform, benzene and toluene being most common, though the atmospheric concentrations of these solvents were not measured in most instances. In a group of 34 of the subjects there was a correlation between the frequency of chromosome breaks and duration of exposure. The subjects and controls in this study were not carefully matched and it is impossible to state that the chromosome aberrations were a direct result of exposure to organic solvents, but this was a common factor in all the working environments studied. The biological significance of the changes observed is unknown as far as the health of the workers is concerned.

F. CARCINOGENICITY

IARC Monograph Vol. 20 (1979) states that, in the absence of adequate data in humans, but evidence of carcinogenicity in animals, it is reasonable for practical purposes to regard chloroform as if it presented a carcinogenic risk to humans.

SUMMARY AND EVALUATION

EXPERIMENTAL STUDIES

Many studies have shown that male rodents are more susceptible to the acute and chronic toxic effects of chloroform than females. There is limited evidence that inhalation of up to 85 ppm in rats and guinea pigs for 6 months caused no testicular pathology.

Several studies have shown that administration both orally and by inhalation during pregnancy results in embryolethal and fetotoxic effects but only at doses producing some evidence of toxicity in the dams. Studies in mice and rabbits showed no teratogenic effects even at maternally toxic doses. In rats however, an increase in congenital abnormalities has been observed in two studies, at doses down to 100 ppm in one of these. At 30 ppm there was also an increase in anomalies which could not be accounted for by maternal toxicity. It is not mutagenic in bacterial systems or in cultured mammalian germ cells. It is carcinogenic in rodents but no reports of transplacental carcinogenicity were found.

HUMAN STUDIES

Chloroform crosses the placenta and is found in similar concentrations in maternal and cord blood. No studies were found of effects on endocrine or gonadal function or fertility. There is one report of two women working in the same laboratory and exposed to a variety of organic chemicals, including chloroform at 300–1000 ppm, developing eclampsia of pregnancy. Another study has shown an increased incidence of chromosomal abnormalities in laboratory workers and their children. They were exposed to a variety of organic solvents, with chloroform, benzene and toluene, in unknown concentrations, being the most common.

Chloroform is regarded as potentially carcinogenic for humans.

EVALUATION

There is sufficient evidence that chloroform is embryolethal and fetotoxic at maternally toxic doses. There is limited evidence that it may be teratogenic, independent of maternal toxicity, in rats but not in mice and rabbits.

There is insufficient evidence in humans to evaluate the reproductive toxicity of chloroform. Attention is drawn to the lack of evidence of effects on fertility and pregnancy in humans.

References

Cascorbi, H. F., Gesinski, R. M. and Komar, M. K. (1976). Biotransformation, sex hormones, and toxicity of two volatile anesthetics in mice. *Journal of Toxicology and Environmental Health* **1**, (5), 839–842.

Dilley, J. V., Chernoff, N., Kay, D., Winslow, N. and Newell, W. G. (1977). Inhalation teratology studies of five chemicals in rats. *Toxicology and Applied Pharmacology* **41**, 196.

Dowty, B. J., Laseter, J. L. and Storer, J. L. (1976). The transplacental migration and accumulation in blood of volatile organic constituents. *Pediatric Research* **10**, 696–701.

Funes-Cravioto, F., Kolmodin-Hedman, B., Lindsten, J., Nordenskjold, M., Zapata-Gayon, C., Lambert, B., Norberg, E., Olin, R. and Swenson, A. (1977). Chromosome aberrations and sister-chromatid exchange in workers in chemical laboratories and a rotoprinting factory and in children of women laboratory workers. *Lancet* **ii**, 322–325.

Hill, R. N. (1977). Differential toxicity of chloroform in the mouse. *Annals of the New York Academy of Sciences* **298**, 170–175.

IARC Monograph on the Evaluation of the Carcinogenic Risk of Chemicals to humans: Some halogenated hydrocarbons (1979). Volume 20, Lyon, France.

Klaassen, C. O. and Plaa, G. B. (1967). Susceptibility of male and female mice to the nephrotoxic and hepatotoxic properties of chlorinated hydrocarbons. *Proceedings Society for Experimental Biology and Medicine* **124**, (4), 1163–1166.

McKinney, J. D., Maurer, R. R., Hass, J. R. and Thomas, R. O. (1976). Possible factors in the drinking water of laboratory animals causing reproductive failure. *In* "Identification and Analysis of Organic Pollutants in Water" (Ed. Keith, L. W.), pp. 417–432. Ann. Arbor Science.

Murray, F. J., Schwetz, B. A., McBride, J. G. and Staples, R. E. (1979). Toxicity of inhaled chloroform in pregnant mice and their offspring. *Toxicology and Applied Pharmacology* **50**, 515–522.

Schwetz, B. A. (1970). Teratogenicity of maternally administered volatile anesthetics in mice and rats. *Dissertation Abstracts International B*, **31**, 3599-B.

Schwetz, B. A., Leong, B. K. and Gehring, P. J. (1974). Embryo and fetotoxicity of inhaled chloroform in rats. *Toxicology and Applied Pharmacology* **28**, 442–451.

Thompson, D. J., Warner, S. D. and Robinson, V. B. (1974). Teratology studies on orally administered chloroform in the rat and rabbit. *Toxicology and Applied Pharmacology* **29**, 348–357.

Torkelson, T. R., Oyen, F. and Rowe, V. K. (1976). The toxicity of chloroform as determined by single and repeated exposure of laboratory animals. *American Industrial Hygiene Association Journal* **37**, (12), 697–705.

Tylleskar-Jensen, J. (1967). Chloroform—a cause of pregnancy toxaemia? *Nordisk Medicin* **77**, (26), 841–842.

Whalley, E. T. and Riley, A. J. (1977). The action of various volatile anaesthetics on the motility of the rat uterus *in vivo*. *Journal of Pharmacy and Pharmacology* **29**, 571–573.

Whipple, G. H. (1912). Pregnancy and chloroform anesthesia. A study of the maternal, placental, and fetal tissues. *Journal of Experimental Medicine* **15**, 246–258.

White, A. E., Takehisa, S., Eger, E. I., Wolff, S. and Stevens, W. C. (1979). Sister chromatic exchanges induced by inhaled anaesthetics. *Anesthesiology* **50**, 426–430.

13. Chloroprene

TECHNICAL DATA

Formula	$CH_2{=}CClCH{=}CH_2$
CAS registry number	None
Chemical abstracts name	None
Synonyms	Chlorobutadiene; 2-chlorobuta-1,3-diene.
Uses	In manufacture of synthetic rubber.
TLV	10 ppm (skin)

ANIMAL STUDIES

A. RELEVANT PHARMACOLOGY AND TOXICOLOGY

The possibility that there might be sex differences in toxicity of chloroprene was investigated in an early study by von Oettingen *et al.* (1936). Exposure of mice to 140 ppm (500 mg/m^3) chloroprene for 8 h killed 2/10 males and 3/10 females. Young mice of 6–32 days of age, sex unspecified, were similarly exposed and showed, if anything, increased resistance compared with adults with 22/22 surviving. It is not possible to draw specific conclusions from this one small experiment.

Sanotskii *et al.* (1976) have investigated the relative sensitivities of pregnant and non-pregnant rats to chloroprene. The animals were exposed to 1·1 or 0·17 ppm (4 or 0·6 mg/m^3) for 4 h/day for 20 days, i.e. through most of pregnancy. Of the 13 indices of toxicity used in the study, at 1·1 ppm, four were changed in the pregnant animals (body weight, oxygen consumption, spontaneous motor activity and liver function as measured by urinary hippuric acid excretion following sodium benzoate loading), compared with only one in non-pregnant rats (spontaneous motor activity). At 0·17 ppm hypoproteinaemia was seen in pregnant but not non-pregnant rats.

B. ENDOCRINE AND GONADAL EFFECTS

Males

Von Oettingen *et al.* (1936) investigated the effects of chloroprene on the male reproductive system, using a variety of routes of administration and several species. In the rat, single doses which were lethal within a few hours or days, given either orally (0·4–0·8 ml/rat) or s.c. (0·02 ml/rat), caused extensive hyperaemia and haemorrhage in a number of tissues and marked testicular changes. Macroscopically, the testes were soft and small. Microscopically, there was degeneration of spermatozoa and spermatogonia, with the formation of multinucleated giant cells and atypical mitoses. Within four days of administration, there was complete atrophy and calcification of the spermatogenic epithelium. In the cat, similar hyperaemia of the internal organs and degenerative changes in the testes were seen after lethal s.c. doses. The authors claimed that a dose as minute as 0·1 μl/cat was sufficient to cause death. With non-lethal doses of chloroprene (1·5 mg/day) applied cutaneously in the rat for 34 days, degeneration and calcification of the testes was again observed at autopsy 15 days after the last application, along with loss of body weight, and pathology of the liver, kidney and spleen. With inhalation as the route of exposure at doses of 110–12,000 ppm (400–43,800 mg/m^3) for 8 h, where 600 ppm upwards caused 100% lethality, no information on testicular changes was given, but the authors noted that "toxic and pathologic symptoms are the same as those observed in other forms of administration".

The work of Davtyan and co-workers has produced conflicting results on the effect of chloroprene on testicular function. In one study (Davtyan, 1972) a total of 100 male rats were exposed to 0·47, 0·042, 0·014, or 0 ppm (1·69, 0·15 or 0·051 mg/m^3) for 4 h/day for 5·5 months. At the two higher doses, significant reductions in sperm motility, viability and acid resistance were reported together with a reduction in the number of spermatogonia and testicular atrophy in some males. All changes were dose-related. No effects were reported at 0·014 ppm. However, in another experiment (Davtyan *et al.*, 1973) where male rats were exposed to higher concentrations of 1·1 or 11 ppm (3·8 or 39 mg/m^3) for 4 h/day for 48 days (12 rats per group), sperm motility was reported as unchanged. Sperm viability and acid resistance were not studied and testicular weights were measured but the results not reported. In this second paper, no mention was made of Davtyan's earlier findings with lower doses. The doses of 0·042, 1·1 and 11 ppm were also reported to increase embryonic mortality when these males were mated to untreated females, but the dose of 0·47 ppm apparently had no effect on embryonic deaths. Fertility was unaffected (see section C for details) at any dose level.

In a study commissioned by the Joint Industry Committee on Chloroprene, carried out by Immel and Willems (1979), groups of five male rats were exposed to 0, 10, 33 or 100 ppm chloroprene for 6 h/day, 5 days/week for 3 or 6 months. Whilst no dose-related changes in sperm concentration or morphological abnormalities were found, the study is difficult to evaluate since treatment groups were small and very wide variations in different types of abnormalities were recorded between and within treatment groups. The authors suggest that some sperm abnormalities, such as deformed head and tail, may have been artefacts of preparation of the sperm smear.

In the mouse Sanotskii (1976) found that exposure to 1 ppm or 0·1 ppm (3·5 or 0·32 mg/m^3) for two months had adverse effects on spermatogenesis, increasing the number of tubules with desquamating germinal epithelium in a dose-related way. Neither the spermatogenesis index nor the total number of spermatogonia were affected by these two doses. Exposure to 0·017 ppm (0·06 mg/m^3) was without any effects.

Conclusion

There is little doubt that high doses causing severe general toxicity are also damaging to the testes, but the reports cited above on lower doses around or below the TLV show marked discrepancies in findings both between and within laboratories. It is therefore difficult on present evidence to draw any firm conclusions on whether the male reproductive system is peculiarly sensitive to the toxic effects of low doses of chloroprene, as has been claimed by some authors. Despite the variation in no-effect level between studies (ranging from 0·014–100 ppm), the strong dose-response relationships in the positive studies at low exposure levels clearly warrants further investigation. An important confounding factor may be the degree of contamination of the chloroprene used with toxic breakdown products. In the study of Immel and Willems (1979) where the highest dose, 100 ppm, was found to be without effect, the methods used ensured exposure was to relatively pure chloroprene. In the studies of Davtyan (1972) and Davtyan *et al.* (1973) and Sanotskii (1976), where levels of 1 ppm and lower were damaging, the methodological details given are not adequate to determine whether breakdown of chloroprene could have occurred. In the study of von Oettingen *et al.* (1936) no care was taken to prevent oxidation (Clary, 1977). The problem of purity of the substance used is a recurring one in chloroprene toxicity and will be discussed later (p. 246).

Females

In one of their experiments, von Oettingen *et al.* (1936) exposed five female mice to 152 ppm (548 mg/m^3) chloroprene by inhalation for 8 h. All mated within 4–6 days of exposure, produced litters and showed normal ovarian histology at autopsy, whereas male fertility in the mouse was severely affected by a similar single 8 h exposure at concentrations as low as 11·7 ppm

(42 mg/m^3). Only one other report on ovarian function has been found; Melik-Alaverdian *et al.* (1976) exposed 90 female rats to 8·3 ppm (30 mg/m^3) for 5 h/day, 6 days/week for 6 months and mated them with untreated males at the end of the exposure period. By the third month of exposure the duration of oestrus was significantly increased from 1·1 to 1·3 days and the duration of "anoestrus" significantly decreased from 5·1 to 3·4 days when treated females were compared with 36 untreated controls. These same changes in the oestrous cycle were also seen in unexposed second and third generation offspring descended from exposed females. However fertility was comparable to controls in each generation though there was a suggestion of a reduction in litter size in the first and third generation pregnancies.

Conclusion

From the above evidence it seems likely that females are less susceptible to gonadal disruption by chloroprene than males, but more evidence is needed from chronic exposure studies employing a variety of dose levels.

C. FERTILITY

The extensive study of von Oettingen *et al.* (1936) included male reproduction tests; however, in none of these is it possible to ascertain the cause of reproductive failure, viz. failure to mate, infertile mating, or intrauterine death of offspring. Chloroprene (dose not stated) was applied cutaneously to male rats which were paired with untreated females after 34 and 44 days of treatment. The median time to successful mating was 14 days for 6 males treated for 34 days, compared with 8 days for 6 untreated controls. After 44 days of treatment, 3 of the 6 males mated after 10, 11 and 15 days but the remaining 3 did not mate successfully at all in 97 days of pairing. In those that did mate successfully, the number of young born was not affected.

The effect of administration of chloroprene by inhalation was also studied (von Oettingen *et al.*, 1936). Exposure of male rats to very high doses of 120–6250 ppm (434–22,500 mg/m^3) for 8 h as a single exposure resulted in 13/19 failing to produce young in 4 months of pairing to untreated females. The lack of any dose effect in this experiment is unusual; a similar proportion of animals were affected at each dose level and of those that did reproduce, litter size was within the normal range in all cases. It is also difficult to envisage how this experiment was carried out since another experiment in the same published study showed single 8 h exposures from 550 ppm upwards caused 100% fatalities in the rat. In the mouse, a single 8 h exposure of males to 11·7–152 ppm (43–548 mg/m^3) resulted in 6/14 producing normal-sized litters when paired with untreated females, but in 3 of these cases mating did not occur until 12–25 days after pairing. The remaining 8 males produced no litters in 2–3 months of pairing. Again, there was no dose-related effect. However, when female mice were exposed to 151 ppm (544 mg/m^3) for 8 h, 5/5 had normal-sized litters after mating within 4–6 days to untreated males, comparable to untreated controls.

The effects of longer exposure to lower concentrations of chloroprene on male and female reproduction has been studied in 2 generations in the rat by Appelman and Dreef-van der Meulen (1979) on behalf of the Joint Industry Committee on Chloroprene. Groups of 25 weanling Fo-generation males and females were exposed to 0, 10, 33 or 100 ppm for 6 h/day, 5 days/week for 13 weeks, then paired with untreated animals with no further exposure of the Fo rats. From the F_1 generation produced by these pairings, groups of 20 males and females were selected randomly and exposed to the same dose as their treated parent for 10 weeks from 4 weeks of age. There were no effects on Fo fertility, intrauterine mortality or litter size amongst either treated males or treated females. Postnatal mortality and general condition of the F_1 generation was unaffected. However, in the F_1 generation, body weight from birth to 4 weeks was significantly lower in litters from Fo females exposed to 100 ppm chloroprene. It should be noted that this group of Fo females were the most growth retarded from chloroprene exposure before mating. Relative organ weights of the liver, ovaries and testes were elevated in some groups of F_1 animals at the end of their exposure to chloroprene but this may be of little toxicological significance since no histological changes were detected in any of these organs.

Culik *et al.* (1978) have also studied the effects of exposure of male rats to a similar dose level but for a relatively short period of time only. Males were exposed to 0 or 25 ppm for 4 h/day for 22 consecutive days and then paired with 3 untreated females for the next 8 weeks, receiving no further treatment during this time. Mated females were allowed to deliver their pups and raise them to weaning. No adverse effects were noted on fertility, litter size or postnatal survival of the offspring.

Several dominant lethal studies in rodents have been reported. Davtyan *et al.* (1973) exposed male rats, 12 per treatment group, to 0, 1·1 or 11 ppm (0, 3·8 or 39 mg/m^3) by inhalation for 4 h/day for 48 days, which is slightly short of the recommended 8–10 weeks needed to cover the whole of the sperm cycle. Each male was then paired with 2 untreated females. No other details of methods were given. Fertility was said to be unaffected (no data presented), but offspring mortality, assessed at 21 days gestation, was increased from 13% in controls to 30–32% in the treated groups, largely due to pre-implantation losses. There was no clear dose-response relationship.

Sanotskii (1976) exposed male rats, 10 per treatment group, to 0, 0·016 or 0·039 ppm (0, 0·057, 0·14 mg/m^3) for 2·5 months (daily duration of exposure not given) and then mated them to untreated females. The embryonic death rate was increased from 10% at 0 and 0·016 ppm to 21% at 0·039 ppm, the majority of deaths occurring after implantation.

In two studies by Immel and Willems (1978a, 1978b) on behalf of the Joint Industry Committee on Chloroprene, groups of 12 male rats were exposed to 0 or 50 ppm or 0 or 100 ppm for 6 h/day for 5 days and then caged with 2 untreated females a week for the next 8 weeks. Females were killed 15 days after the mid-week of their caging with the males, and scored for pregnancy, numbers of corpora lutea, live and dead implants. There were no adverse effects on fertility or survival of offspring at either exposure level.

In a study of similar design, Immel and Willems (1978c) have exposed groups of 12 outbred, Swiss, male mice to 0, 10 or 100 ppm chloroprene for 6 h/day for 5 days/week for 2 weeks with subsequent pairing to untreated females for 8 weeks. At 100 ppm 8/12 males died during the first 3 days of treatment and 1 further male was excluded due to poor reproductive performance before treatment, leaving only 3 males for assessment. No mice died in the 10 ppm group. There were no effects on fertility or embryo-mortality in survivors.

Sanotskii (1976), however, has obtained positive results in the dominant lethal test with groups of 8–15 inbred C57BL/6 mice using exposure levels of 0·014–0·97 ppm (0·05–3·5 mg/m^3) for 2 months. After exposure males were mated to 2 or 3 untreated females. Fertility was said to be unaffected but embryonic death rates were increased. In the first experiment, total embryonic mortality increased from 29% in controls to 52, 50 and 63% at 0·017, 0·089 and 0·97 ppm respectively. In the second experiment, it increased from 19% in controls to 33, 36 and 42% at 0·014, 0·036 and 0·51 ppm respectively. Sanotskii also gave data on the breakdown between pre- and postimplantation losses which must have been derived from corpora lutea and resorption counts rather than mean litter size and resorption counts. The major difference between control and treated groups was said to be in pre-implantation losses. However, the validity of this data is questionable since accurate corpora lutea counts are not possible in the mouse.

Conclusion

As with effects on the gonads discussed previously, very high doses close to the lethal level have been shown to affect male fertility in the rat and mouse though the sporadic nature of these effects and the lack of any dose-response relationships in the study of von Oettingen *et al.* (1936) again suggest the possibility of variable exposure to toxic contaminants. In those studies where the purity of the chloroprene exposure is not known, exposures from 0·016–11 ppm in the rat were claimed not to affect male fertility (though it should be noted that the higher level exposures were inadequate in duration), but after mating increased intrauterine mortality was observed from doses of 0·039–11 ppm. Of those studies in the rat where the chloroprene was known to be uncontaminated, fertility and intrauterine mortality were unaffected up to 100 ppm for chronic exposure in males or females. Thus dominant lethal effects have only been reported where the purity of the chloroprene is in question.

None of the mouse studies reported above were methodologically acceptable.

D. PREGNANCY

Salnikova and Fomenko (1973, 1975) have investigated the effect of chloroprene exposure during pregnancy on prenatal and postnatal development in the rat. Exposure by inhalation to 1·1 ppm (4 mg/m^3) at different stages during embryogenesis (Salnikova and Fomenko, 1975) caused meningoencephalocoele (peak incidence of 23% after exposure on days 5–6) and hydrocephaly (peak incidence of 34% after exposure on days 11–12). These abnormalities were not seen in controls. The findings of malformations after exposure on days 5–6 is unusual since implantation is barely complete.

In an earlier study by Salnikova and Fomenko (1973) specific malformations were not reported with exposure to 1·1 ppm for 4 h/day throughout pregnancy. However, intrauterine mortality was significantly increased at 32% compared with 11% in controls. Both pre- and post-implantation losses were reported. There was also significant decrease in fetal weight and a very high incidence of internal haemorrhages observed in histological sections of fetuses from treated dams. No significant effects were seen with lower doses of 0·17 or 0·04 ppm (0·6 or 0·13 mg/m^3). However, these lower concentrations did affect postnatal development of the offspring, studied up to 2 months of age. Mortality in the first 3 weeks of life was increased at both doses and weight gain was lower at 0·17 ppm. Postnatal assessment of the nervous system, liver, kidney and metabolic functions on a battery of tests produced variable, non-dose-related significant differences from controls. The extent of the variability suggests that these particular changes may not be of any biological significance. Exposure to 0·016 ppm (0·056 mg/m^3) throughout pregnancy was found to have no effect on prenatal or postnatal development.

Culik *et al.* (1978) have studied the effect of inhalation exposure to 0, 1, 10 or 25 ppm for 4 h/day during pregnancy in the rat. Animals were exposed in groups of 50 from days 1–12 for assessment of embryotoxicity, and in groups of 25 from days 3–20 of pregnancy for teratology. Acceptable teratological methods were used. In the teratology study, the number of dams with resorptions was increased to 62% ($p < 0·05$) and 59% (not significant) at 10 and

25 ppm respectively compared with 29% at 0 or 1 ppm. However, this effect was not observed in the embryotoxicity test where 50–53% of dams had resorptions in all groups. This variability in resorption rate and lack of any clear dose-related effect suggest the results of the teratology study may be a chance finding. However, the possibility remains that the additional exposure during the second half of pregnancy may have caused a small increase in fetal deaths. The only other significant finding was a dose-related increase in fetal weight and crown-rump length, in the absence of any effect on live litter size. Since reduction in body weight is often one of the most sensitive indicators of toxicity to the embryo and fetus, then provided the increase in weight observed by Culik *et al.* is not due to oedema, these results, together with their finding of no significant increases in soft tissue or skeletal abnormalities, provide some reassurance that exposure to pure chloroprene up to 25 ppm is not toxic.

Conclusion

Where the purity of chloroprene is in question, exposure to 1·1 ppm has been shown to be embryo-lethal and markedly teratogenic, whilst lower doses down to 0·04 ppm adversely affect post-natal survival and development, with a no-effect level of 0·016 ppm. Exposure to pure chloroprene up to 25 ppm during pregnancy is without effect.

General discussion

As authors such as Culik *et al.* (1978) have pointed out, the results obtained from studies where adequate precautions were taken to prevent the break-down of chloroprene are markedly at variance with the studies from the U.S.S.R., the reported no-effect levels varying by as much as four orders of magnitude in some instances. Unfortunately the methodological descriptions in the Russian papers are not sufficiently detailed to determine whether or not exposure to breakdown products occurred, though it most certainly did in the early American study of von Oettingen *et al.* carried out in 1936. At ambient temperatures, chloroprene readily dimerises to form several cyclic compounds and oxidises into polyperoxides, acids and other products. Ideally, chloroprene should be distilled under vacuum and stored under nitrogen at not more than −10°C before use. Nystrom (1948) has demonstrated that chloroprene stored for several days at room temperature in the presence of air is about four times more toxic than pure chloroprene.

However, in the context of hazard evaluation, it may be more relevant to take into account the toxic effects of chloroprene contaminated by its breakdown products, since in some industrial situations, conditions of storage and use of chloroprene may not conform to the highest standards. From the animal data presented, there is clearly sufficient cause for concern that impure chloroprene may be hazardous to male fertility, the germ cells and to the embryo and fetus exposed *in utero* at very low exposure levels. More information is now needed on the reproductive toxicity of chloroprene contaminants together with information on their likely levels in the working situation. Since free chloroprene is also present in manufactured neoprene latex (Sanotskii, 1976) it is quite likely that workers using pre-manufactured latex may be exposed not only to pure chloroprene but to its oxidation products, dimers and small polymers. Thus epidemiological studies are required not only of workers manufacturing neoprene but also of fabricators using neoprene rubbers.

E. MUTAGENICITY

IARC Monograph Vol. 19 (1979) reports that chloroprene is mutagenic in the Ames test, and its mutagenicity is further enhanced by metabolic activation. Reports of dominant lethal studies are given in section C.

F. CARCINOGENICITY

IARC Monograph Vol. 19 (1979) stated that there were no adequate carcinogenicity studies in animals available.

HUMAN STUDIES

A. RELEVANT PHARMACOLOGY AND TOXICOLOGY

No relevant data found.

B. ENDOCRINE AND GONADAL EFFECTS

Volkova *et al.* in 1976, quoted in the N.I.O.S.H. Criteria Document on chloroprene (U.S. Department of Health, Education and Welfare, 1977), surveyed 65 workers in a neoprene rubber glove factory. She stated that 47% of the women (actual number of women not stated) had menstrual disorders compared with 10% of a control population. The major disorder was decreased blood flow and the incidence increased with length of exposure.

C. FERTILITY

Males

In a review of the Russian literature on the toxicity of chloroprene, Sanotskii (1976) referred to an unavailable study on male workers. Reproductive function was studied in 143 male chloroprene workers and compared with 118 controls. Examination showed decreased sperm motility after 6–10 years exposure and changes in morphology after 11 years exposure to chloroprene. There was also a 3-fold increase in the abortion rate in the wives of chloroprene workers. Levels of exposure of 0·3–1·9 ppm in the environment were mentioned but it is not clear if this refers to the actual working conditions of the male workers studied above. No further details were given in the paper so it is impossible to assess the significance of this report.

The N.I.O.S.H. Criteria Document on chloroprene (U.S. Department of Health, Education and Welfare, 1977) refers to a study of male workers in a polychloroprene factory in France 1969. One hundred of 130 workers exposed to chloroprene in unknown amounts showed evidence of gross over-exposure with chemical burns. In some of these there was also conjunctivitis, hair loss and sexual impotency involving both libido and sexual dynamics (no other details were given in the original report). All symptoms disappeared when the workers were relocated.

Females

In the review mentioned above by Sanotskii (1976) a study was referred to which showed that sterility incidence was 6·1% in 147 women chloroprene workers compared with 2% in 100 controls. No other details were given.

D. PREGNANCY

Teratogenicity

Davtyan *et al.* (1973) in the introduction to a paper on the effects of chloroprene in rat pregnancy, refer to observations made in the early 1940s in Russia of babies with physical and mental defects being born to women in the chloroprene rubber industry. No details were given and reference is made only to a "candidate dissertation, 1969".

Effect on lactation

Vanuni (1974) reported that there was a reduction of amino acid content of the milk of mothers sampled on the eighth day of lactation, in mothers exposed to chloroprene compared with controls. The total protein content of the milk of 12 mothers working with chloroprene was only 87% of that of a group of 25 control mothers in Northern Yerevan not exposed to chloroprene; 18 other mothers not working with chloroprene but living in the same commune as the exposed mothers had the same protein content of the milk as the chloroprene workers. Four other groups of women were studied living at various distances 500 m to 3000 m from the factory and in a town 25 km distant, and the protein in the milk increased with distance from the factory combine. It is suggested by the author that the effects on protein and amino-acid content are related to chloroprene pollution. No atmospheric values of chloroprene are given and, without much other information on nutritional status etc. of the women, it is difficult to be sure what the cause of the differences in milk composition may be due to, especially since the women working with chloroprene in the factory did not show any difference in total protein content from other women not directly exposed but working in the grounds of the combine. No milk chloroprene analysis was carried out.

E. MUTAGENICITY

Infante (1977) quoted a personal communication from Bochkov (Director of the Institute of Medical Genetics, Moscow) of a significant excess of chromosomal aberrations in workers exposed to chloroprene or chloroprene latexes. A similar effect was also reported by Sanotskii (1976) in women workers exposed to 1–2 ppm chloroprene. The N.I.O.S.H. Criteria Document (U.S. Department of Health, Education and Welfare, 1977) briefly refers to two other Russian studies reporting increased chromosomal aberrations in the blood cells of chloroprene-exposed workers. It concludes that although no single study provides conclusive evidence of mutagenicity, the consistency of the positive mutagenic responses in a wide range of tests establishes a clear need to control chloroprene as a mutagenic agent.

F. CARCINOGENICITY

IARC Monograph Vol. 19 (1979) reports that there is insufficient evidence from which to draw any conclusion about the possible carcinogenicity of chloroprene in humans.

SUMMARY AND EVALUATION

EXPERIMENTAL STUDIES

High doses causing severe general toxicity are also damaging to the testes in the rat and cat. The reports on lower doses however, show marked discrepancies both between and within laboratories. It is therefore impossible to draw any firm conclusion as to whether the testis is particularly sensitive to the toxicity of chloroprene. Two studies have shown dose response relationships with reduction in sperm count and testicular pathology with no effect levels around 0·01 ppm. However other studies have shown no effects at up to 100 ppm. The contamination with toxic breakdown products of chloroprene which occurs readily at ambient temperatures was an important variable which may account for the differences observed.

The ovary appears to be less sensitive than the testis to the toxic action of chloroprene but the studies to date have been inadequate to define a no effect level.

With pure chloroprene no effects on fertility were observed in male or female rats exposed to 100 ppm by inhalation. In studies where the purity was not confirmed, adverse effects were reported in males but the numbers of animals studied were inadequate for assessment. No dominant lethal effects were observed in rats exposed to 100 ppm pure chloroprene, but probable positive effects were observed when impure material was used at 0·04 ppm in rats and at 0·014 ppm in mice.

Exposure to pure chloroprene up to 25 ppm in one large study in rats produced no embryolethal, fetotoxic or teratogenic effects. However, in two somewhat conflicting studies from another laboratory, where the purity of the chloroprene used is not known, embryolethal and marked teratogenic effects were seen following exposure to 1 ppm with increased postnatal mortality and reduced weight gain at doses down to 0·04 ppm.

It is mutagenic in bacterial systems. Conflicting reports of dominant lethality in mammals are discussed above. There are no adequate studies on carcinogenicity and no reports on transplacental carcinogenicity.

HUMAN STUDIES

There is one report of menstrual disorders, mainly decreased flow, in women exposed to chloroprene in neoprene glove manufacture. One study in male chloroprene workers showed decreased sperm motility and changes in sperm morphology after 6 or more years exposure. A 3-fold increase in abortion rate in the wives of the workers was also reported. Another study of grossly overexposed males reported various toxic effects including reduced libido and impotence which disappeared on removal from exposure. Other anecdotal reports have appeared suggesting adverse effects on pregnancy and lactation, but the data do not support such a conclusion.

There is limited evidence that it may be mutagenic as assessed by chromosomal aberrations in the blood cells of exposed workers. There is insufficient evidence to assess the carcinogenic risk for humans.

EVALUATION

Evaluation is complicated by the ready breakdown of chloroprene to form toxic products. This more toxic material is damaging to the testis and shows embryolethal and teratogenic effects in animals at doses around 1 ppm or below by inhalation. Pure chloroprene however does not show such effects even at the maximum concentrations tested of 100 ppm. There is anecdotal evidence of adverse effects on reproduction in both men and women exposed to chloroprene industrially, but these claims are not supported by adequate data.

Attention is drawn to the lack of satisfactory data on the reproductive effects in humans.

References

Appelman, L. M. and Dreef-van der Meulen, H. C. (1979). Reproduction study with β-chloroprene vapour in rats. Central Institute for Nutrition and Food Research, Report No. R 6225.

Clary, J. J. (1977). Toxicity of chloroprene, 1,3-dichlorobutene-2, and 1,4-dichlorobutene-2. *Environmental Health Perspectives* **21**, 269–274.

Culik, R., Kelly, D. P. and Clary, J. J. (1978). Inhalation studies to evaluate the teratogenic and embryotoxic potential of β-chloroprene (2-chlorobutadiene-1,3)1,2. *Toxicology and Applied Pharmacology* **44**, 81–88.

Davtyan, R. M. (1972). Toxicological characteristics of the action of chloroprene on the reproductive function of male rats. *In* "Toxicology and Hygiene of the Products of Petroleum Chemistry and Petrochemical Productions", pp. 95–97. All Union Conference, Yaroslave, USSR, 1971. Yaroslavskii Meditsinskii Institut.

Davtyan, R. M., Fomenko, V. N. and Andreyeve, G. P. (1973). On the question of the effect of chloroprene on the generating function of mammals (males). *Toksikologiya Novykh Promyshlennykh Khimicheskikh Veschestv* **13**, 58–62.

IARC Monographs on the Evaluation of the Carcinogenic Risk of Chemicals to Humans: Some monomers, plastics and synthetic elastomers, and acrolein (1979). Volume 19, Lyon, France.

Immel, H. R. and Willems, M. I. (1978a). Dominant lethal assay with β-chloroprene in male albino rats. Central Institute for Nutrition and Food Research, Report No. R 5626.

Immel, H. R. and Willems, M. I. (1978b). Dominant lethal assay with β-chloroprene in male albino rats. Central Institute for Nutrition and Food Research, Report No. R 5762.

Immel, H. R. and Willems, M. I. (1978c). Dominant lethal assay with β-chloroprene in male mice. Central Institute for Nutrition and Food Research, Report No. R 5756.

Immel, H. R. and Willems, M. I. (1979). Effect of β-chloroprene exposure of rats on sperm concentration and sperm abnormalities. Central Institute for Nutrition and Food Research, Report No. R 6006.

Infante, P. F. (1977). Mutagenic and carcinogenic risks associated with halogenated olefins. *Environmental Health Perspectives* **21**, 251–254.

Melik-Alaverdian, N. O., Kagramanian, R. G., Kalatarova, Y. C. and Krupskaia, N. K. (1976). Reproductive function and sexual maturation in third generation rats born from mothers intoxicated with chloroprene. *Zhurnal Eksperimentalnoi I Klinicheskoi Meditsiny-A N Armyanskoi SSR* **16**, 54–59.

Nystrom, A. E. (1948). Health hazards in chloroprene rubber industry and their prevention. A clinical and experimental study, with special reference to chloroprene and its oxidation and polymerisation products. *Acta Medica Scandinavica* **132**, Supplement 219, 1–125.

Oettingen, W. F. von, Hueper, W. C., Deichmann-Gruebler, W. and Wiley, F. H. (1936). 2-Chloro-butadiene (chloroprene): its toxicity and pathology and the mechanism of its action. *Journal of Industrial Hygiene and Toxicology* **18**, 240–270.

Salnikova, L. S. and Fomenko, V. N. (1973). Experimental investigation of the influence produced by chloroprene on the embryogenesis. *Gigiena Truda i Professional 'nye Zabolevaniya* **(8)**, 23–26.

Salnikova, L. S. and Fomenko, V. N. (1975). Comparative characterization of the embryotropic effect produced by chloroprene, depending upon the mode of its action with different routes of entrance. *Gigiena Truda i Professional 'nye Zabolevaniya* (7), 30–33.

Sanotskii, I. V. (1976). Aspects of the toxicology of chloroprene: immediate and longterm effects. *Environmental Health Perspectives* **17**, 85–93.

U.S. Department of Health, Education and Welfare (1977). Criteria Document for a recommended standard: Occupational exposure to Chloroprene. DHEW (NIOSH) Publication No. 77–210.

Vanuni, S. O. (1974). Comparative characteristics of individual and total amino acids in the breast milk of working new mothers and women living in surrounding villages at various distances from a synthetic chloroprene rubber combine. *Zhurnal Eksperimentalnoi i Klinicheskoi Meditsiny* **14**, (1), 96–101.

14. Dibromochloropropane (DBCP)

TECHNICAL DATA

Formula	$ClCH_2CHBrCH_2Br$
CAS registry number	None
Chemical abstracts name	1,2-Dibromo-3-chloropropane
Synonyms	3-Chloro-1,2-dibromopropane, dibromochloropropane.
Uses	Soil fumigant; nematocide.
TLV	None (U.S. Emergency Temporary Standard 0·01 ppm).

ANIMAL STUDIES

A. RELEVANT PHARMACOLOGY AND TOXICOLOGY

Torkelson *et al.* (1961) have noted sex differences in general toxicity when DBCP was fed in the diet to male and female rats. In females, increased kidney weight was seen from 20 ppm upwards, but not at 5 ppm, and decreased weight gain from 150 ppm upwards. In the males, effects on the kidney were not seen until 1350 ppm and effects on weight gain only from 450 ppm. There was some mortality in both males (4/14) and females (2/14) at 1350 ppm.

Placental transfer of DBCP has been shown in the rat. Ruddick and Newsome (1979) gave 25 mg/kg/day on days 6–15 of pregnancy. Females were killed at intervals of 1–24 h after the last dose on day 15 and DBCP levels in the dam and fetus were measured. Limited transfer of DBCP was seen with 0·008–0·030 ppm in the whole fetus 1–6 h after dosing. By 12 h none was detectable. Maternal blood levels were highest at 3 h at 0·104 ppm and the highest maternal tissue level was in the fat (5·38 ppm at 6 h). By 12 h after dosing, levels in all maternal tissues were falling.

B. ENDOCRINE AND GONADAL EFFECTS

Males

The first observations of DBCP's marked effects on the testes were published by Torkelson *et al.* (1961). Groups of 20 rats, 10 guinea pigs and 3 rabbits were exposed to 12 ppm DBCP by inhalation for 7 h/day, 5 days/week for 10–13 weeks. Forty per cent of the rats died, largely due to lung infections. At autopsy the most striking observation in all 3 species was severe atrophy and degeneration of the testes. In the rats, this was characterized by degenerative changes in the seminiferous tubules, an increase in Sertoli cells, reduction in the number of spermatozoa, and abnormally formed spermatozoa. In another experiment, where groups of 15 rats were exposed to 5, 10 or 20 ppm for 7 h/day, 5 days/week for 10 weeks, the severity of testicular atrophy may be judged from the relative testis weights (g/100 g body weight) of 0·83, 0·53 and 0·52 in 5, 10 and 20 ppm groups, compared with 1·02 in controls. Histological changes in the testes were seen in the 5 ppm group, the lowest dose level studied, though they were less severe than at higher exposures. At 5 ppm there was no mortality, at 10 ppm 13% died, and at 20 ppm 67% died before the end of the experiment.

Rakhmatullaev (1971) has confirmed the adverse effects of DBCP on the rat testis. Groups of 10 males were given daily oral doses of 17·5, 35 or 70 mg/kg for 10 weeks. At 70 mg/kg there was 50% mortality and survivors showed haematological changes and necrosis of parenchymatous organs and the testes. The effects of the lower doses used are not reported. The same group, Faidysh *et al.* (quoted in the Federal Register, Department of Labor, 1977a) also showed testicular necrosis within 45 days of dosing with 70 mg/kg/day. The effects of lower doses given over longer periods were also studied (Rakhmatullaev, 1971); groups of 7 rats were given daily oral doses of 0·005, 0·05, 0·5 or 5 mg/kg for 8 months beginning when the animals were still sexually immature. In the 5 mg/kg group the weight of the testes was increased by 15–30%, spermatozoa showed reduced motility and histological changes were seen in the testis (unspecified). These males were infertile (see section C for details). At 0·5 mg/kg, changes in the testis were not mentioned but the males in this group were subfertile. There were no adverse effects at 0·05 mg/kg.

Reznik and Sprinchan (1975) have confirmed the testicular toxicity of similar doses of DBCP in the rat. Males were given orally a single, large dose of 100 mg/kg or daily doses of 10 mg/kg for 4–5 months. With the single dose, males showed acute signs of toxicity for a few days and reduced weight gain. By 3 weeks after dosing, there was a significant increase in the spermatogenesis index (not defined). By 5 weeks after dosing, there was increased desquamation of spermatogenic epithelium, and the numbers of spermatogonia were decreased. Sperm count and motility however were sharply reduced within 1 week of dosing, suggesting it is the late phases of spermatogenesis that are most severely affected. After chronic dosing with 10 mg/kg similar changes were seen; by the second month of dosing significant decreases in sperm count and motility were seen, progressively worsening as dosing continued. Significant changes also occurred in the spermatogenesis index, numbers of spermatogonia (no details given), and degenerating cells appeared in the ducts of the seminiferous tubules. Biochemical changes were also seen in the testis and ejaculate.

Burek *et al.* (1979) have shown a no-effect-level for inhalation exposure to DBCP in the rat and the rabbit. Males were exposed to 0, 0·1, 1·0 or 10 ppm DBCP for up to 14 weeks (daily duration of exposure not specified). Rats exposed to 10 ppm showed a 50% decrease in testicular weight and a "patchy" decrease in spermatogenesis. One or 0·1 ppm had no effect in the rat. In the rabbit, 10 ppm caused almost complete atrophy by 8 weeks; all stages of spermatogenesis were absent and seminiferous tubules were lined only by relatively normal Sertoli cells. There were no germinal cells. In this group, exposure was stopped after 8 weeks, but by 14 weeks they were still infertile. At 1 ppm in the rabbit, there was a 50% reduction in testicular size by 14 weeks, reduced spermatogenesis and abnormal spermatocytes in the tubules. There was no effect at 0·1 ppm. This study is reported in abstract only.

Females

Reznik and Sprinchan (1975) have given female rats 100 mg/kg orally as a single dose or 10 mg/kg/day orally for 4–5 months. After the single high dose, 95% developed atypical oestrous cycles. Cycles were lengthened, particularly the oestrous and dioestrous stages, and if administration coincided with oestrus, there was a marked prolongation of this phase. It is not known how long the cycles remained disturbed. With chronic administration of 10 mg/kg/day, 24% developed atypically prolonged cycles within the first month of dosing. By the third month some females showed complete cessation of cyclic changes and by the fifth month 57% were not cycling at all and 13% had prolonged cycles.

Conclusion

Disturbances in testicular function in the rat have been shown at doses which are otherwise non-toxic with chronic administration (5 ppm by inhalation, 0·5 mg/kg orally). In the rabbit adverse effects have been seen with chronic exposure to 1 ppm by inhalation. With higher doses in the rat and rabbit, causing some general toxicity, severe atrophy of the testes and complete arrest of spermatogenesis are seen. No-effect-levels (including fertility) are 0·1 ppm by inhalation in the rabbit, and 1·0 ppm by inhalation or 0·05 mg/kg orally in the rat. Female rats dosed orally with 10 mg/kg/day show rapid onset of abnormal oestrous cycles.

C. FERTILITY

Males

DBCP has been shown to affect fertility in the rat and the rabbit. Rakhmatullaev (1971) gave young male rats 0·05, 0·5 or 5 mg/kg/day orally for 10 weeks. They were then mated with untreated females. In the females mated with males given 5 mg/kg/day no pregnancies occurred. It is not clear whether mating actually took place. Seventy per cent of females that mated with males given 0·5 mg/kg/day became pregnant, compared with 80% in control × control matings, and had only 3–5 young/litter, compared with an average of 8/litter in controls. Males dosed with 0·05 mg/kg/day were unaffected.

In the male rabbit, Rao *et al.* (1979) have shown complete infertility in animals exposed to 10 ppm by inhalation for 8 weeks and placed with females 6 weeks after the end of the exposure period. It is not clear whether mating took place, but this dose caused severe atrophy of the testes (see section B).

Rao *et al.* (1979) also carried out a dominant lethal test in male rats. Exposure to 10 ppm DBCP by inhalation for 14 weeks significantly increased post-implantation deaths in control females mated to exposed males. Teramoto *et al.* (1980) have confirmed the dominant lethal effect of DBCP in the rat, but failed to find any effect in the mouse. Groups of 15 rats were given 10 or 50 mg/kg/day orally by gavage on 5 successive days and then mated with 1 untreated female/week for 10 weeks. Ethyl methane sulphonate, used as positive control, caused a significant increase in dead implants/dam in the first few weeks after dosing. DBCP had no effect on ability to mate, number of pregnancies or total implants/dam, but significantly increased post-implantation deaths in weeks 1–5 at 50 mg/kg and in weeks 4 and 5 at 10 mg/kg. The peak effect was seen in weeks 4 and 5 (early spermatid stage) when 43 and 55% of implants died in the 50 mg/kg group. In the mouse experiment, groups of 7–9 males were given 5 daily doses of 50 or 150 mg/kg DBCP orally by gavage and then each mated with 2 untreated females/week for 6 weeks. The experiment was replicated once. There were no effects on mating, number of pregnancies, implants/dam or post-implantation deaths in comparison with controls. Ethyl methanesulphonate showed positive dominant lethal effects.

Females

The effect of oral DBCP on female rats was also investigated by Rakhmatullaev (1971). Females were given 5 mg/kg/day orally for 10 weeks and mated with control males. Sixty per cent became pregnant compared with 80% in control × control matings, suggesting some decrease in fertility. Lower doses were not tested.

Conclusion

In the rat, infertility or subfertility has been shown in males with doses similar to those known to affect testicular function, viz. 10 ppm by inhalation or 0·5–5·0 mg/kg orally with chronic dosing. Dominant lethal effects were also seen in the rat, but not the mouse, with similar doses. A no-effect-level is indicated for chronic, oral dosing and fertility in the male rat (0·05 mg/kg). Effects in the female have been less thoroughly studied but seem to be less marked than those in the male.

D. PREGNANCY

The effect of DBCP administration during embryogenesis has been investigated in the rat. Ruddick and Newsome (1979) gave groups of 15 females 0, 12·5, 25 or 50 mg/kg/day orally by gavage on days 6–15 of pregnancy. Acceptable teratological methods were used. Maternal weight gain was reduced in the 25 and 50 mg/kg groups and 1 female in the 50 mg/kg group died. The LD50 for chronic oral dosing is around 350 mg/kg (Rakhmatullaev, 1971). There was no effect on implants/dam or increase in malformations in comparison with controls; however, fetal weight was reduced significantly at 50 mg/kg and decreased, but not significantly, at 25 mg/kg. Details of resorption rates were not given but there was evidence of complete resorption in 3/4 females in the 50 mg/kg group which were not carrying fetuses at term. No fetotoxicity was seen at 12·5 mg/kg, a maternally non-toxic dose. Thus there appears to be no adverse effects of DBCP except fetal weight reductions at high doses which is probably secondary to maternal toxicity.

E. MUTAGENICITY

DBCP is mutagenic in the Ames test (Rosenkranz, 1975), however, Biles *et al.* (1978) have shown that when technical grade DBCP is used, the mutagenicity in assays performed without metabolic activation is largely due to a contaminant, epichlorohydrin, which may be present in quantities as large as 3%. Pure DBCP is not mutagenic in the Ames test unless metabolically activated first.

Kapp (1979) has carried out cytogenetic analysis of spermatogonia and bone marrow cells after DBCP treatment. Groups of 20 male rats were given 0·73, 7·3 or 73 mg/kg/day orally by gavage for 5 days. Twenty-six hours after the last dose they were killed and examined. There was a dose-related increase in aberrant cells in both spermatogonia and bone marrow cells. The study is reported in abstract only and no further details are given.

F. CARCINOGENICITY

IARC Monograph Vol. 20 (1979) reports that there is sufficient evidence that DBCP is carcinogenic in mice and rats.

HUMAN STUDIES

A. RELEVANT PHARMACOLOGY AND TOXICOLOGY

No relevant data found.

B. ENDOCRINE EFFECTS

Whorton *et al.* (1977) in a study of workers in a DBCP formulation plant showed that 11 men with oligo- or azoospermia who had been exposed to DBCP for 3 years or more, had raised serum FSH and LH values compared with 11 other men who had been exposed for less than 3 months. In the affected group the FSH level was 11·3 ± 1·8 mIu/ml (control 2·6 ± 0·4, $P < 0{\cdot}001$), and the LH level was 28·4 ± 3·3 mIu/ml (control 14·0 ± 2·8, $P < 0{\cdot}01$). The serum testosterone levels were not different in the two groups, 459 ± 35 ng/dl and 463 ± 31 ng/dl in the affected and control groups respectively. The raised serum FSH was presumed to be due to the impaired spermatogenesis but the cause of the LH rise is not known.

Three women were also exposed (duration not stated) and had normal menstrual cycles and fertility and two, who were not using oral contraceptives, had normal FSH and LH levels. Thyroid function was not affected by DBCP.

In a study by Potashnik *et al.* (1979) of 23 exposed male workers in an Israeli factory, 10 of 12 azoospermic men had raised plasma FSH levels (mean 2·5 ± 1·8 mIu/ml) but all except one had normal LH and testosterone levels. On the other hand, of 6 oligospermic men 5 had normal FSH levels (one was 11·0 mIu/ml) and all had normal LH and testosterone levels. High FSH levels were also reported among severely affected, exposed field operators by Glass *et al.* (1979) and Sandifer *et al.* (1979), who felt that measurement of FSH levels in blood might have some value as a screening test, but only if high levels were found, since most men with high levels were oligospermic; though the converse was not true, viz. not all oligospermic men had high FSH levels.

C. EFFECTS ON THE TESTIS AND FERTILITY

Infertility in male workers exposed to DBCP was first described by Whorton *et al.* (1977). The study was carried out in a California pesticide factory involved in formulation of pesticides using 100 different chemical substances. For 15 years, DBCP had been formulated in a special agricultural chemical division and the men in that division had gradually become aware of a lack of fertility among those employed there. This led to a detailed examination of all the workers (36 men and 3 women) in the division.

All workers were examined thoroughly and semen samples collected from the 25 non-vasectomized men, which were examined for count, motility and morphology. Blood and urine were also examined and levels of T3, T4, testosterone, FSH and LH measured. Testicular biopsies were also carried out on 9 of the men who volunteered.

None of the men had loss of libido, difficulty with erection or ejaculation, effects on facial and body hair, testicular atrophy, epididymal abnormalities, gynaecomastia, or abnormalities of the prostate. Seven of the 36 men had never fathered children.

A striking relationship was found between duration of exposure and sperm count. The 25 non-vasectomized male workers could be divided into 3 groups, A—exposed for more than 3 years, B—exposed for less than 3 months and C—exposed for 1–3 years. The average duration of exposure of group A was $8{\cdot}0 \pm 1{\cdot}2$ years; 9 of them were azoospermic and the other 2 had a sperm count of 1×10^6 per ml with reduced motility and increase in abnormal forms. In group B the mean sperm count was $93 \pm 18 \times 10^6$ per ml and in group C the total sperm counts were $10\text{–}30 \times 10^6$. There was thus a clear relationship between duration of exposure and the incidence of oligo- and azoospermia. Preliminary examination of the biopsy samples of the severely affected men showed loss of spermatogonia with no inflammation or severe fibrosis.

Detailed examination of the total DBCP exposure for each person was impossible but the airborne concentrations of DBCP in the factory was believed to be less than the recommended limit of 1 ppm. Measurement in the division at the time of the study in 1977 using personal air samplers was 0·4 ppm averaged for an 8 hour day.

A subsequent paper by Whorton and his colleagues (Biava *et al.*, 1978) described in detail the histology of the testicular biopsies. In all, biopsies from

10 individuals were studied, 7 of whom had oligo- or azoospermia. The two most severely affected cases with azoospermia had the longest durations of exposure to DBCP (10, 10·5 years). The seminiferous tubules were devoid of germ cells when examined by light and electron microscopy. There was no evidence of cell necrosis and Sertoli cells were normal. Five individuals with oligospermia with a shorter duration of exposure of 1–5 years showed moderate to marked diminution of sperm production, and spermatogenic cells were observed in only a minority of seminiferous tubules or in only a few short segments of tubules. Sertoli cells were normal. The remaining 3 individuals had normal or slight reduction in sperm production and no abnormalities were detected in the biopsy specimens. Two of the subjects had short exposure times to DBCP (0·25, 1·75 years) and the third had been exposed for 3·5 years followed by 3 years with no exposure. The interstitial (Leydig) cells appeared normal in all specimens.

No indications were found concerning the mechanism of action of DBCP on the spermatogenic cells. None of the characteristic changes produced by cytotoxic drugs were observed, nor interstitial or vascular lesions like those produced by cadmium in animals. There was no evidence of effects such as could be found with a mitotic inhibitor or alkylating agent.

A more complete study of the Californian pesticide workers referred to above was reported by Whorton *et al.* (1979), in which an attempt was made to study testicular function in all male employees at the plant. The men were questioned about their reproductive history including libido, erections, children, genito-urinary infections or problems, other diseases, etc. Sperm counts and gonadotrophin levels were measured. Actual exposure levels to DBCP could not be clearly established. Exposure could occur at several points in the plant, and movement of labour within the plant led to problems in assessing the duration of exposure in individuals. However best estimates were made for each worker of the total number of months of potential exposure to DBCP.

The total male population at risk was 310, of which 196 agreed to be examined. In addition 5 women workers were examined and no effects observed. Of the 114 workers who would not agree to be examined, 62 did respond anonymously to a questionnaire. Of the 196 examined, 154 were considered to be potentially exposed to DBCP and 42 not exposed. The total amounts of DBCP formulated each year between 1969–1977 were between 1·5–3 million pounds. The results of this study confirmed those of the original smaller study, i.e. that there was a clear relationship between duration of exposure and sperm count. Of the 196 examined, 142 had semen samples tested, and of 107 "ever" exposed workers the median sperm count was 46×10^6 per ml whereas of 35 workers "never" exposed the median count was 79×10^6 per ml. Oligospermia, defined as less than 20 million sperm per ml was present in 1 of 35 unexposed compared with 29 of 91 exposed (16 workers with unquantifiable exposure were excluded). In all, 13·1% of the exposed non-vasectomized workers were azoospermic, 16·8% were oligospermic and 15·8% had low normal counts (20–39 × 10^6 per ml).

Serum levels of FSH, LH and testosterone were examined to see if one or more could act as an indicator of impaired spermatogenesis without the need for taking a semen sample. FSH alone was as good as any combination of the three, provided that a high proportion of the workers had azoospermia, as in the present study. However, if the azoospermics are excluded then FSH is of no value in detecting oligospermia. FSH assays alone cannot therefore be regarded as a satisfactory screen for effects on sperm production unless a significant number of those exposed have complete azoospermia. Thus, despite its obvious disadvantages, a sperm count remains the best clinical laboratory test of testicular function.

The most recent publication of Whorton and colleagues (Whorton and Milby, 1980) addresses the question of recovery of testicular function after removal from exposure. The authors attempted to re-assess the affected workers of the 1977 study (Whorton *et al.*, 1977). Of the original 25 exposed workers with azoospermia or oligospermia, 21 agreed to take part in the re-assessment 1 year later, i.e. 12 of the 13 azoospermics and 9 of the 12 oligospermics. Semen and blood samples were collected. None of the 12 azoospermics showed any improvement in sperm count. Of 4 with a 1977 sperm count of more than zero but less than 1 × 10^6 per ml, 3 showed improvement—2 were normospermic (> 20 × 10^6 per ml) in 1978. Of the 5 with a 1977 sperm count of 10–19 × 10^6 per ml, 4 were normospermic and the other unchanged in 1978. With regard to the effect of duration of exposure, 11 of the 12 men exposed for 4 or more years were azoospermic in 1977 and remained so 1 year later, and the other still remained oligospermic. Of the 9 men exposed for less than 4 years, 7 showed some degree of recovery. Since it was impossible to assess the actual intensity of exposure, this 4-year criterion may not apply to greater or less degrees of exposure. Since experience with cytotoxic drugs has shown that testicular recovery may take 3 to 6 years, further studies will be required to assess whether any recovery occurs in the most severely affected cases. Between July 1977 and August 1978, 4 children were born to the wives of the 9 oligospermic men. Three of the children were normal and one had several defects (hypospadias and umbilical hernia). The significance of this defect for such a small sample is unknown.

Studies in workers exposed to DBCP have also been reported from Israel. An original report was published by Potashnik *et al.* (1978) on 6 male workers who presented with infertility or loss of libido or impotence. A larger, more detailed report was later published (Potashnik *et al.*, 1979) which included the original 6 cases. They investigated testicular function in 23 workers exposed to

DBCP during production in a local factory. All were given a complete physical examination and 2 semen samples from each were examined for volume, pH and count. All azoospermic and two oligospermic men had bilateral testicular biopsies. Exposure to DBCP and date of last contact were obtained from plant records. No estimate of environmental DBCP concentrations were available.

No relevant effects were found on physical examination or routine laboratory tests including haematology, liver and renal function tests. Semen volume and pH were all normal but marked effects were observed on sperm counts. The workers could be classified into 3 groups. Group A consisted of 12 workers all with azoospermia who were directly involved in DBCP production and with exposure times of 100 to 6726 hours. In 5 of these the last exposure had been 1 to 5 years previously. Fertility had been confirmed in 8 of them on the basis of pregnancies in their wives, and normal karyotypes were found in the others. Group B consisted of 6 employees with oligospermia of $0{\cdot}5\text{–}10 \times 10^6$ per ml with exposure times of 34 to 95 hours. Three of the workers had their last exposure 1–2 years previously. Group C consisted of 5 employees with normal sperm counts of $20\text{–}65 \times 10^6$ per ml and all were involved only in the packing process with duration of exposure of 10–30 hours in 4 and 60 hours in the fifth. Histological examination of the group A biopsies all showed complete atrophy of the seminiferous tubules with Sertoli cells only. Leydig cells were present in all. The two group B biopsy specimens showed a similar picture but with some evidence of active spermatogenesis. The reason for the impotence (1 case) and loss of libido (3 cases) is uncertain since they were in good general health, capable of providing semen samples for analysis and their plasma testosterone levels were normal. The authors suggest that the worry of the revelation of the sterilizing effect of the chemical was the most likely cause.

There was clearly a close correlation between duration of exposure and sperm count, azoospermia being present in all those exposed for more than 100 hours. All of the most severely affected were actual production workers and all the unaffected were packers, but no quantitative measurement of DBCP was possible. The question of recovery remains open, but 3 of the azoospermic workers had not been directly exposed for 5 years. In confirmation of the results reported above by Whorton *et al.* (1979), the serum FSH levels were raised in the azoospermic men but was unaffected in men with oligospermia. It would therefore be of limited value as a screening procedure. The LH and testosterone levels were normal in all the affected workers.

Sperm count depression in pesticide applicators using DBCP in the fields has also been reported (Glass *et al.*, 1978). They studied applicators employed by professional firms in 5 counties of California which had all reported heavy DBCP use during the year 1976–77. Twenty of the 22 firms reporting DBCP use agreed to participate. Because of the variable quality of record-keeping, accurate quantification of exposure was impossible, though those heavily exposed could be identified as well as those with no or low exposure. They had originally hoped to identify 50 matched pairs of heavy versus no exposure of the same age and in the same area. This however proved impossible so that the men were eventually classified on the basis of number of days of DBCP use during the current year. Eventual analysis of the results of 31 matched pairs proved to be the same as for the total cohort but no details of this are given.

Of 112 men originally approached, 96 men were interviewed for medical histories and physical examination, haematology and clinical chemistry and serum FSH and LH. A semen sample was obtained from all men and a second sample from those with counts of less than 20×10^6 per ml. Samples were analysed for count and morphology. For analysis the men were grouped in 4 classes, i.e. exposure in the current year of >2 months, >2 weeks–2 months, 1 day–2 weeks, zero. There was a significant trend of sperm count against degree of exposure ($P = 0{\cdot}018$). However, only the sperm count of those exposed for more than 2 months was significantly lower than the rest. This was accounted for by 14 men with a sperm count of less than 40×10^6 per ml, of whom 4 were azoospermic. Six men with exposures of 2 weeks–2 months had counts of less than 10×10^6 per ml, of whom 1 was azoospermic. The effect of previous years' exposure was difficult to assess since men with long term exposure also tended to be heavy current users, but 5 of 40 men with 5 or more years exposure were azoospermic. There was no relationship between abnormal sperm morphology and DBCP use. There was a significant trend towards raised FSH levels with DBCP exposure but individual values were not shown so this data could not be analysed further. No other effects on blood or physical examination related to DBCP use. The men involved with spraying grapes, calibrating equipment, irrigation and supervision were most affected though the actual extent and route of exposure was unknown. It is however interesting that as well as the factory workers previously reported, intermittent, seasonal open air workers like pesticide operators were also affected by DBCP.

These results were supported by another study of agricultural workers, including formulators, applicators, farmers, researchers and salesmen who were all potentially exposed to DBCP (Sandifer *et al.*, 1979). Seventy-three workers from six states of the U.S.A. participated. All filled in a questionnaire, had a medical examination and blood (for FSH, LH and testosterone) and semen samples examined. The frequency distribution of sperm counts among 6 sperm densities of <10, 10–20, 20–40, 40–60, 60–100 and >100 millions per ml indicated highly significant differences between the exposed workers and published values for 9000 control males with no known occupational exposure to toxic chemicals. Six of 8 formulators and 13 of 43 users had counts below 20×10^6 per ml and so would be classed as oligospermic. The lowest counts were found in formulators, applicators and farm workers, and were all significantly lower than the control data. Exposure was assessed by dividing the total number of pounds of DBCP used by the number of days in which it was used. This is obviously a fairly crude estimate but the sperm counts were significantly negatively correlated with this index of exposure. Three of the 8 formulators had counts below 10^6 per ml and 11 of the other 45 non-vasectomized men had counts of less than 10^6 per ml, 2 of them being azoospermic. In the control data on 9000 men, less than 9% had counts below 10^6/ml. No effects on sperm morphology were observed.

The serum FSH and LH levels were negatively correlated with sperm count and one third of the men had FSH levels above their accepted normal high of 17 mIu/ml; only 3 of these 17 men with FSH levels above 17 mIu/ml had sperm counts over 30×10^6 per ml.

We are not aware of detailed reports published by Dow Chemical Co. or Shell Chemical Co., the only two U.S.A. producers of DBCP. However, the Department of Labor (1977b) reported a letter from Dow Chemical Co. stating that in their plant in Magnolia, Arkansas, 86 of a total of 150 workers possibly exposed to DBCP had been examined. Of these 24% had aspermia (? azoospermia) and 46% had oligospermia. No other details were given. The same publication refers to a telegram from Shell Chemical Co. stating that 7 of 11 employees from one plant had sperm counts of 40×10^6/ml or less and 29 of 39 employees in a second plant had sperm counts of less than 40×10^6. Shell estimated that exposure levels were from less than 100 ppb to 600 ppb during the past 3 years. No other details were given and it is uncertain what the exposure data refers to, since one of the plants discontinued production of DBCP 2 years previously.

A later report (Department of Labor, 1978) stated that during DBCP production at the Dow plant, the 8 hour TWA exposures were measured to range between 0·04 and 0·4 ppm, and there was a negative correlation between degree of exposure and sperm count. The final results from Shell Chemical Co. were also reported from the Denver and Mobile plants. At Mobile, of 80 workers tested, 2 were azoospermic and 11 were oligospermic, rates which they claim do not differ from control values. The duration of DBCP production at Mobile was about 15 months. At the Denver plant however where production continued from 1955 to 1976, of 49 workers tested 5 were azoospermic and 7 were oligospermic which Shell maintained were comparable to some published control data. This however was disputed at the O.S.H.A. hearing and not accepted. The 8 hour TWA values measured at the Denver plant ranged from 0·2–0·4 ppm.

D. PREGNANCY

No relevant data found.

E. MUTAGENICITY

Kapp *et al.* (1979) studied the sperm of 18 workers exposed to DBCP to look for evidence of Y-chromosomal non-disjunction as assessed by the presence of 2 quinacrine fluorescent spots within the sperm (YFF). Neither the origin of the workers nor details of the exposure were given except a statement that the average exposure was 15·2 months (range 6–18 months) to environmental levels less than 1 ppm. Results were compared with 15 controls without known exposure to mutagens and with the same average age (33·0 years) as the exposed group (33·8 years). A minimum of 400 sperm per sample of normal appearance were scored and 2 separate fluorescent bodies had to be present within the membrane to score YFF. The average YF (single body) frequency in the control group was 41·5% (range 36·7–46·3) and the average YFF frequency was 1·2% (range 0·8–1·8). The exposed workers had an average YF frequency of 41·8% (range 36·3–46·3), i.e. similar to that for the controls, but a YFF frequency of 3·8% (range 2·0–5·3) which was significantly higher than the control values. The background frequency of YFF observed by the authors in their laboratory from analysis of 262 semen samples was 1·3%. Thus 16 of 18 exposed workers had a frequency of Y chromosomal non-disjunction above their normal limit of 2%, indicating an aberrance in meiotic anaphase II. The authors state that since XYY individuals are born with a frequency of 1 per 1000 male births it may be advisable for exposed individuals to have available genetic counselling or amniocentesis in the event of pregnancy.

The authors state, without giving details, that conventional cytogenetic analysis on peripheral lymphocytes of these exposed workers did not indicate any structural aberrations or karyotypic changes.

E. CARCINOGENICITY

IARC Monograph Vol. 20 (1979) stated that there is sufficient evidence of carcinogenicity of DBCP in animals and in the absence of adequate data in humans it is reasonable, for practical purposes, to regard DBCP as if it presented a carcinogenic risk to humans.

SUMMARY AND EVALUATION

EXPERIMENTAL STUDIES

Limited placental transfer has been shown to occur in rats. Reduced testicular weight and depression of all stages of spermatogenesis has been found in several studies in the rat with doses of DBCP which were otherwise non-toxic, i.e. 5 ppm by inhalation or 0·5 mg/kg orally. No effect levels in the rat were 1 ppm by inhalation and 0·05 mg/kg orally. Similar changes have also been shown in rabbits with inhalation of 1 ppm and above, the no effect level was 0·1 ppm. Females seem less sensitive to the gonadotoxic effect but one study reported that 10 mg/kg daily produced disturbances in the oestrous cycle in about half of the treated rats.

In a fertility study in rats, treatment of males with 5 mg/kg daily orally produced complete infertility, 0·5 mg/kg daily produced reduced fertility as evidenced by reduced litter size but 0·05 mg/kg was without effect. Exposure of rabbits to 10 ppm by inhalation produced infertility.

One study in which female rats were treated with 5 mg/kg orally showed only a slight effect on fertility.

Two studies in rats have shown dominant lethal activity from 10 ppm by inhalation or 10 mg/kg orally. The effect was particularly noticeable at the early spermatid stage. One study in mice dosed with 150 mg/kg for 5 days showed no dominant lethality.

One study in rats showed no embryolethality or teratogenicity at doses up to 50 mg/kg orally. Reduced fetal weight was observed with the top dose level only which was also toxic to the dam.

It is mutagenic in bacterial systems with activation. DBCP may be contaminated with epichlorohydrin which is mutagenic without activation. Dominant lethality has also been demonstrated in rats but not mice. One study has also claimed an increase in chromosomal aberrations in spermatogonia and bone marrow cells in DBCP treated rats. It is carcinogenic in mice and rats. There are no reports of transplacental carcinogenicity.

HUMAN STUDIES

Studies of men involved in DBCP manufacture and also of exposed field workers have shown reduction in sperm count and evidence of testicular damage. There is a clear relationship between the degree of testicular damage and the duration and degree of exposure. In the most severely affected cases there is a loss of spermatogonial stem cells with no sign of recovery even after an interval of 5 years. Less severely affected workers show oligospermia with some signs of recovery. All of the above effects occur in the absence of any other signs of toxicity and without loss of libido or potency. High FSH levels have been found in blood samples of men with oligo- or azoospermia as a result of exposure to DBCP. LH levels are occasionally also raised but not consistently. There is no effect on testosterone levels.

No studies were found on the effect of DBCP in pregnancy. A mutagenicity study carried out on exposed workers reported an increased incidence in the frequency of Y chromosomal non-disjunction as assessed by the presence of 2 quinacrine fluorescent spots within the sperm. No increase in chromosomal abnormalities were found in the peripheral lymphocytes of these workers.

It is regarded as a potential carcinogen for humans.

EVALUATION

There is clear evidence in both animals and man that DBCP exerts a specific toxic effect on the testes. All parts of the seminiferous tubule including the spermatogonia, but excluding the Sertoli cells and Leydig cells, are affected. The extent of damage is proportional to the degree of exposure, and in the most severely affected subjects, recovery has not been shown to occur. Plasma FSH levels were only consistently altered in the most severely affected men. Semen examination is the most reliable method for the detection of the effects.

Attention is drawn to the lack of adequate information on the offspring of men who have been partially affected. The possible mutagenic effect in men also requires further study.

References

Biava, C. G., Smuckler, E. A. and Whorton, D. (1978). The testicular morphology of individuals exposed to dibromochloropropane. *Experimental and Molecular Pathology* **29**, 448–458.

Biles, R. W., Connor, T. H., Trieff, N. M. and Legator, M. S. (1978). The influence of contaminants on the mutagenic activity of dibromochloropropane (DBCP). *Journal of Environmental Pathology and Toxicology* **2**, (2), 301–312.

Burek, J. D., Murray, F. J., Rao, K. S., Crawford, A. A., Beyrer, J. S., Albee, R. R. and Schwetz, B. A. (1979). Pathogenesis of inhaled 1,2-dibromo-3-chloropropane (DBCP) induced testicular atrophy in rats and rabbits. *Toxicology and Applied Pharmacology* **48**, A 121.

Department of Labor (1977a). Occupational exposure to 1,2-dibromo-3-chloropropane (DBCP). *Federal Register* **42**, (7), 45537–45549.

Department of Labor (1977b). Occupational exposure to 1,2-dibromo-3-chloropropane (DBCP). *Federal Register* **42**, (210), 57266–57283.

Department of Labor (1978). Occupational exposure to 1,2-dibromo-3-chloropropane (DBCP). *Federal Register* **43**, (53). 11517–11533.

Glass, R., Lynes, R., Mengle, D., Powell, K. and Kahn, E. (1978). The gonadal toxicity of DBCP among male pesticide applicators. *American Journal of Epidemiology* **108**, (3), 242.

Glass, R. I., Lynes, R. N., Mengle, D. C., Powell, K. E. and Kahn, E. (1979). Sperm count depression in pesticide applicators exposed to dibromochloropropane. *American Journal of Epidemiology* **109**, (3), 346–351.

IARC Monographs on the Evaluation of the Carcinogenic Risk of Chemicals to Humans: Some halogenated hydrocarbons (1979). Volume 20, Lyon, France.

Kapp, R. W., Jr. (1979). Mutagenicity of 1,2-dibromo-3-chloropropane (DBCP): *In vivo* cytogenetics study in the rat. *Toxicology and Applied Pharmacology* **48**, (1), A46.

Kapp, R. W., Jr., Picciano, D. J. and Jacobson, C. B. (1979). Y-Chromosomal nondisjunction in dibromochloropropane-exposed workmen. *Mutation Research* **64**, 47–51.

Potashnik, G., Ben-Aderet, N., Israeli, R., Yanai-Inbar, I. and Sober, I. (1978). Suppressive effect of 1,2-dibromo-3-chloropropane on human spermatogenesis. *Fertility and Sterility* **30**, 444–447.

Potashnik, G., Yanai-Inbar, I., Sacks, M. I. and Israeli, R. (1979). Effect of dibromochloropropane on human testicular function. *Israel Journal of Medical Science* **15**, (5), 438–442.

Rakhmatullaev, N. N. (1971). Hygienic characteristics of the nematocide Nemagon in relation to water pollution control. *Hygiene and Sanitation* **36**, 344–348.

Rao, K. S., Murray, F. J., Crawford, A. A., John, J. A., Potts, W. J., Schwetz, B. A., Burek, J. D. and Parker, C. M. (1979). Effects of inhaled 1,2-dibromo-3-chloropropane (DBCP) on the semen of rabbits and the fertility of male and female rats. *Toxicology and Applied Pharmacology* **48**, (1), A 137.

Reznik, Ya. B. and Sprinchan, G. K. (1975). Data of Experiments on the gonadal effects of 1,2-dibromo-3-chloropropane. *Gigiena i Sanitariya* **6**, 101–102.

Rosenkranz, H. S. (1975). Genetic activity of 1,2-dibromo-3-chloropropane, a widely-used fumigant. *Bulletin of Environmental Contamination and Toxicology* **14** (1), 8–12.

Ruddick, J. A. and Newsome, W. H. (1979). A teratogenicity and tissue distribution study on dibromochloropropane in the rat. *Bulletin of Environmental Contamination and Toxicology* **21**, 483–487.

Sandifer, S. H., Wilkins, R. T., Loadholt, C. B., Lane, L. G. and Eldridge, J. C. (1979). Spermatogenesis in agricultural workers exposed to dibromochloropropane (DBCP). *Bulletin of Environmental Contamination and Toxicology* **23**, 703–710.

Teramoto, S., Saito, R., Aoyama, H. and Shirasu, Y. (1980). Dominant lethal mutation induced in male rats by 1,2-dibromo-3-chloropropane (DBCP). *Mutation Research* **77**, 71–78.

Torkelson, T. R., Sadek, S. E., Rowe, V. K., Kodama, J. K., Anderson, H. H., Loquvam, G. S. and Hine, C. H. (1961). Toxicologic investigation of 1,2-dibromo-3-chloropropane. *Toxicology and Applied Pharmacology* **3**, 545–559.

Whorton, D., Krauss, R. M., Marshall, S. and Milby, T. H. (1977). Infertility in male pesticide workers. *Lancet* **ii**, 1259–1261.

Whorton, D. and Milby, T. H. (1980). Recovery of testicular function among DBCP workers. *Journal of Occupational Medicine* **22**, (3), 177–179.

Whorton, D., Milby, T. H., Krauss, R. M. and Stubbs, H. A. (1979). Testicular function in DBCP exposed pesticide workers. *Journal of Occupational Medicine* **21**, (3), 161–166.

15. Dichlorobenzene

TECHNICAL DATA

(a) *o-Dichlorobenzene*

Formula

CAS registry number 95–50–1

Chemical abstract name o-Dichlorobenzene

Synonyms DCB; 1,2-dichlorobenzene; o-dichlorobenzene; o-dichlorobenzol; ODB; ODCB; orthodichlorobenzene; orthodichlorobenzol.

Uses Solvent for waxes, gums, resins, tars, rubbers, oils, asphalts, insecticide for termites and locust borers; removing sulfur from illuminating gas; as degreasing agent for metals, leather, wool; as ingredient of metal polishes; as heat transfer medium; as intermediate in the manufacture of dyes.

TLV 50 ppm

(b) *p-Dichlorobenzene*

Formula

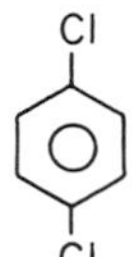

CAS registry number	106–46–7
Chemical abstracts name	p-Dichlorobenzene
Synonyms	1,4-Dichlorobenzene; p-dichlorobenzene; p-dichlorobenzol; paradichlorobenzene; paradichlorobenzol; PDB; PDCB.
Uses	Insecticidal fumigant. Popular for domestic use against clothes moths.
TLV	75 ppm

ANIMAL STUDIES

A. RELEVANT PHARMACOLOGY AND TOXICOLOGY

No relevant data found.

B. ENDOCRINE AND GONADAL EFFECTS

No relevant data found.

C. FERTILITY

No relevant data found.

D. PREGNANCY

No relevant data found.

E. MUTAGENICITY

No relevant data found.

F. CARCINOGENICITY

IARC Monograph Vol. 7 (1974) reported that at that time no adequate studies on which to base an evaluation of its animal carcinogenicity were available.

HUMAN STUDIES

A. RELEVANT PHARMACOLOGY AND TOXICOLOGY

No relevant data found.

B. ENDOCRINE AND GONADAL EFFECTS

No relevant data found.

C. FERTILITY

No relevant data found.

D. PREGNANCY

No relevant data found.

E. MUTAGENICITY

No relevant data found.

F. CARCINOGENICITY

IARC Monograph Vol. 7 (1974) reported there was one study suggesting an association between leukaemia and exposure to dichlorobenzenes, but this was insufficient evidence from which to assess the carcinogenic risk of the compound.

SUMMARY AND EVALUTION

EXPERIMENTAL STUDIES

No studies were found on any aspect of reproductive toxicity, mutagenicity or carcinogenicity.

HUMAN STUDIES

No studies were found on any aspect of reproductive toxicity or mutagenicity. One study reporting an association between leukaemia and exposure to dichlorobenzenes was regarded as insufficient evidence to assess carcinogenic risk.

EVALUATION

No evaluation is possible. Attention is drawn to the lack of animal and human data.

References

IARC Monographs on the Evaluation of Carcinogenic Risk of Chemicals to Man: Some anti-thyroid and related substances, nitrofurans and industrial chemicals (1974). Volume 7, Lyon, France.

16. 1,1-Dichloroethane

TECHNICAL DATA

Formula CH_3CHCl_2

CAS registry number 75–34–3

Chemical abstracts name 1,1-Dichloroethane

Synonyms Ethylidene chloride, ethylene dichloride.

Uses Cleansing agent; degreaser; solvent for plastics, oils and fats; grain fumigant; chemical intermediate.

TLV 200 ppm

ANIMAL STUDIES

A. RELEVANT PHARMACOLOGY AND TOXICOLOGY

No relevant data found.

B. ENDOCRINE AND GONADAL EFFECTS

No relevant data found.

C. FERTILITY

No relevant data found.

D. PREGNANCY

Schwetz *et al.* (1974) have studied the effect of exposure to 1,1-dichloroethane by inhalation in pregnant rats. The material used was 99·7% pure, containing minute amounts of ethyl chloride, butylene oxide, trichloroethylene, ethylene dichloride and other unknown contaminants. Groups of 20 rats were exposed to 3800 or 6000 ppm 1,1-dichloroethane for 7 h/day on days 6–15 of pregnancy. Acceptable teratological methods were used. Maternal food consumption and body weight were significantly reduced in comparison with controls in both exposed groups during the exposure period but some catch-up had occurred by day 21, especially in the 6000 ppm group. There were no signs of maternal liver toxicity or other signs of general toxicity. There were no significant effects on implants/dam, live fetuses/dam, resorptions/dam or fetal body weight in comparison with air-exposed controls. There were no effects on abnormalities or anomalies except for a significant increase in delayed ossification of sternebrae in the 6000 ppm group and a significant decrease in bipartite centra in the 3800 ppm group in comparison with controls. Thus exposure to high levels of 1,1-dichloroethane may cause slight retarded development in rat fetuses, which is in accordance with the small but non-significant reduction in fetal body weight also observed.

E. MUTAGENICITY

No relevant data found.

F. CARCINOGENICITY

No relevant data found.

HUMAN STUDIES

No relevant data found.

SUMMARY AND EVALUATION

EXPERIMENTAL STUDIES

No studies were found on endocrine or gonadal effects, or of effects on fertility. A limited study in rats has shown that exposure to up to 6000 ppm for 7 h daily during embryogenesis had no adverse effects on pregnancy except for slight retardation of development of the fetuses possibly secondary to reduced food intake in the dams. No studies on mutagenicity or carcinogenicity were found.

HUMAN STUDIES

No data on any aspect of reproductive toxicity were found.

EVALUATION

Only very limited evaluation is possible. Attention is drawn to the small amount of animal data and lack of data on endocrine and gonadal effects and on fertility. There is limited evidence that it is not teratogenic in rats. Attention is drawn to the complete absence of data in humans.

Reference

Schwetz, B. A., Leong, B. K. J. and Gehring, P. J. (1974). Embryo- and fetotoxicity of inhaled carbon tetrachloride, 1,1-dichloroethane and methyl ethyl ketone in rats. *Toxicology and Applied Pharmacology* **28**, 452–464.

17. Dichloromethane

TECHNICAL DATA

Formula	CH_2Cl_2
CAS registry number	75–09–2
Chemical abstract name	Dichloromethane
Synonyms	Methane dichloride; methylene bichloride; methylene chloride, methylene dichloride.
Uses	Solvent for cellulose acetate; degreasing and cleaning fluids.
TLV	200 ppm (1980 Intended change 100 ppm).

ANIMAL STUDIES

A. RELEVANT PHARMACOLOGY AND TOXICOLOGY

Dichloromethane is metabolized to carbon monoxide in both rodents and man, and whilst extensive tissue storage of dichloromethane does not seem to occur, there may be prolonged carboxyhaemoglobinaemia after exposure in both animals and man (Schwetz *et al.*, 1975; Hardin and Manson, 1980). In mice and rats carboxyhaemoglobin levels ranged from 7–13% immediately following a 7 h exposure to 1250 or 4500 ppm dichloromethane. The no-effect level for raised carboxyhaemoglobin is not known.

B. ENDOCRINE AND GONADAL EFFECTS

No relevant data found.

C. FERTILITY

No relevant data found.

D. PREGNANCY

Schwetz *et al.* (1975) have exposed mice and rats to dichloromethane at 1250 ppm for 7 h/day from days 6–15 of pregnancy. Acceptable teratological methods were used but the data is reported on a per litter basis only. The number of fetuses affected is not given.

At term, in the 13 mice exposed, mean maternal body weight gain and absolute, but not relative, liver weights were increased significantly in comparison with 24 controls exposed to filtered air. In the 19 rats exposed, only absolute liver weight was significantly increased in comparison with 25 controls. Maternal carboxyhaemoglobin levels immediately after exposure were between 9 and 13% compared with 0·4–2·6% in controls in both rats and mice. They had returned to within control levels by 24 h after the last exposure.

There were no effects on implantation sites, live fetuses, resorptions or fetal body weight in either mice or rats. When examined for teratogenic effects, the only anomaly significantly increased in the treated mice was extra sternebrae, occurring in 50% of treated litters compared with 14% of controls. Cleft palate (2 affected litters) and rotated kidney (2 affected litters) were also seen in the treated mice and not in controls, but the difference was not statistically significant. In the rats, there were significant increases in litters affected by dilated renal pelvis and delayed ossification of sternebrae and a significant decrease in lumbar ribs or spurs (extra or rudimentary 14th rib(s)). The question of whether these increases in minor anomalies were due to the parent compound, dichloromethane, or the rise in maternal carboxyhaemoglobin levels, cannot be answered by the data of Schwetz *et al.* (1975).

Manson and her colleagues have assessed the reproductive toxicity of dichloromethane exposure before as well as during pregnancy, thus maximizing the effect of prolonged exposure and therefore of prolonged carboxyhaemoglobinaemia (Hardin and Manson, 1980; Bornschein *et al.*, 1980). Groups of 30 rats were exposed to 4500 ppm for 6 h/day, 7 days/week before mating only, before mating and during pregnancy, or during pregnancy. The premating exposure period was approximately 3 weeks and during pregnancy exposure was from days 1–17. Approximately two-thirds of the rats were killed for teratology on day 21 of pregnancy and the remainder allowed to litter out for postnatal evaluation. Acceptable teratological methods were used.

Absolute and relative liver weights at term were increased in the groups exposed before and during pregnancy, and during pregnancy only, but maternal body weights were unaffected. During exposure to dichloromethane, maternal carboxyhaemoglobin levels ranged from 7·2–10·1% but were undetectable in controls.

In the teratology study (Hardin and Manson, 1980) there were no significant effects on implantation sites, live fetuses or resorptions but fetal body weight was significantly reduced by about 10% in the groups exposed before and during gestation or during gestation only. In contrast to the experiment of Schwetz *et al.* (1975) discussed above, there were no significant increases in dilated renal pelvis or retarded ossification, and the incidence of rudimentary 14th rib(s) was increased, rather than decreased, in some treated groups; the incidence of 14th rib(s) expressed as percentage of fetuses affected, was 13% in those exposed before and during pregnancy, 10% in those exposed before pregnancy only, 3% in those exposed during pregnancy only and $<1\%$ in controls. The difference between the first group and controls is significant on a Chi-square test. Since the major effect appeared to be with pre-mating exposure, these data are not entirely incompatible with those of Schwetz *et al.* (1975). There were no other significant differences in Hardin and Manson's study in individual or total soft tissue or skeletal anomalies.

In the postnatal part of the study (Bornschein *et al.*, 1980) there were no significant effects on birth weight or postnatal growth rate up to 400 days of age, though there was a trend, especially amongst the female offspring, towards lower body weights in the groups exposed before mating. This contrasts with the prenatal part of the study, described above, where significant reductions in fetal weight were seen only in those groups exposed during gestation.

General activity at 5 days of age and subsequently locomotor activity in novel environments, wheel running activity, and avoidance learning ability were assessed at intervals up to 5 months of age. A number of measures were significantly affected in the offspring of all dichloromethane-exposed groups relative to controls on one or more tests. At 10 days of age the group exposed before and during pregnancy and the group exposed during pregnancy only habituated more slowly to the test environment. Amongst male offspring in these 2 groups, alterations in habituation persisted up to 5 months of age but at this time they habituated more rapidly and were significantly less active than controls during the last part of the testing period. At 15 days of age, it was the groups exposed before and during pregnancy and the groups exposed before pregnancy only which deviated significantly from controls, habituating more slowly to the test environment. There were no significant effects on wheel running activity or performance in a one-way avoidance learning task.

In general, the significant behavioural changes indicate an alteration in orientation, reactivity and/or habituation to novel environments. These findings, where the relationship between treated and control groups varied considerably at different ages, may at first sight seem confusing. However, it is not uncommon in behavioural teratology studies to obtain results that are age and task specific. It is unlikely that these are chance findings since the design of the experiment was such that behavioural observations were carried out on 2 replicate groups, separated by 2 months in time, and the same behavioural changes were observed in each cohort.

A further complicating factor is the possibility of differential responses to the direct effects of dichloromethane exposure and the indirect effects of the carboxyhaemoglobinaemia, induced at 2 different times, i.e. before and during pregnancy, which may have resulted in a complex pattern of interacting behavioural changes.

Conclusion

From these 3 studies involving both prenatal and postnatal evaluation, it can be seen that whilst dichloromethane caused no gross teratogenic effects at the exposure levels used, there may be more subtle effects of slight fetotoxicity and persistent behavioural alterations in the offspring resulting from premating or gestational exposure. There is clearly a need for studies involving lower doses to establish a no-effect level. The conversion of dichloromethane to carbon monoxide and the known effects of carbon monoxide on the embryo and fetus (see page 182) suggest that this substance should be viewed with concern.

E. MUTAGENICITY

IARC Monograph Vol. 20 (1979) reported studies showing dichloromethane was mutagenic in the Ames test with or without metabolic activation.

F. CARCINOGENICITY

IARC Monograph Vol. 20 (1979) reported on the only available study in mice, where results suggested an increase in lung tumours, but did not draw any conclusions on its carcinogenicity in animals.

HUMAN STUDIES

A. RELEVANT PHARMACOLOGY AND TOXICOLOGY

Dichloromethane is metabolized to carbon monoxide in the human, as in animals. In man, levels of 10% carboxyhaemoglobin have been recorded 1 h after the end of a 2 h exposure to 1000 ppm (quoted by Schwetz *et al.*, 1975).

One study provides evidence that dichloromethane crosses the placenta and passes into breast milk. Mukhametova and Vozovaya (1972) have measured dichloromethane levels in the blood, embryonic and fetal tissues and membranes in female glueing operatives undergoing termination of pregnancy (see section B of Benzene, human studies for full description). Levels of $0{\cdot}66 \pm 0{\cdot}21$ mg/kg were found in maternal blood, $0{\cdot}34 \pm 0{\cdot}10$ mg/kg in fetal membranes and $1{\cdot}15 \pm 0{\cdot}20$ mg/kg in fetal tissue. The higher levels in fetal tissue than maternal blood suggest that dichloromethane is readily transferred across the placenta. They also analysed the breast milk of 40 of the glueing operatives who were nursing their infants. The average level of chlorinated hydrocarbons (dichloromethane and dichloroethane) was given as $0{\cdot}074 \pm 0{\cdot}046$ mg/kg. Separate values for the individual chemicals were not given. It was also stated that chlorinated hydrocarbons were found in breast milk 17 h after the last contact with these substances at work.

B. ENDOCRINE AND GONADAL EFFECTS

See details of the study by Mukhametova and Vozovaya (1972) in section B of Benzene, human studies for effects on menstrual function and gynaecological disorders. It is not possible to determine whether dichloromethane exposure or the other chemicals were causally related to the disorders observed.

C. FERTILITY

As detailed in section C of Benzene, human studies, there were no significant differences in infertility rates in exposed and control groups in the study of Mukhametova and Vozovaya (1972).

D. PREGNANCY

The outcome of pregnancies in the study of Mukhametova and Vozovaya (1972) has already been described in detail in section D of Benzene, human studies. It is not possible to ascertain what contribution, if any, dichloromethane may have made to the increases in pregnancy and labour complications observed.

E. MUTAGENICITY

No relevant data found.

F. CARCINOGENICITY

IARC Monograph Vol. 20 (1979) reports that no case studies or epidemiological studies were available for evaluation of the carcinogenic risk of dichloromethane.

SUMMARY AND EVALUATION

EXPERIMENTAL STUDIES

No studies were found on endocrine or gonadal effects or effects on fertility.

One study in rats and mice exposed during embryogenesis to 1250 ppm by inhalation showed no adverse effects other than increases in anomalies, mostly indicative of retarded development. Another study in which rats were exposed before and during pregnancy to 4500 ppm by inhalation showed no adverse effects or increase in anomalies, but there was some decrease in fetal weight. Behavioural variations were observed, however, in some of the offspring when examined up to 5 months of age. Neither of the above exposure levels caused significant maternal toxicity. Maternal carboxyhaemoglobin levels of 7–13% produced by metabolism of dichloromethane were observed during the exposure periods. It is mutagenic in bacterial systems with and without activation. There are inadequate data to assess its carcinogenicity. No reports on transplacental carcinogenicity were found.

HUMAN STUDIES

Dichloromethane crosses the placenta and has also been found in breast milk of women occupationally exposed to a glue.

No adequate studies were found on endocrine or gonadal effects or of effects on fertility, pregnancy, mutagenicity or carcinogenicity.

EVALUATION

There is limited evidence that it is not teratogenic or embryolethal in maternally sub-toxic doses in animals. There is some evidence of increase in anomalies and of postnatal behavioural changes. The significance of these is unknown.

Attention is drawn to the lack of data on reproductive effects in humans.

References

Bornschein, R. L., Hastings, L. and Manson, J. M. (1980). Behavioural toxicity in the offspring of rats following maternal exposure to dichloromethane. *Toxicology and Applied Pharmacology* **52**, 29–37.

Hardin, B. D. and Manson, J. M. (1980). Absence of dichloromethane teratogenicity with inhalation exposure in rats. *Toxicology and Applied Pharmacology* **52**, (1), 22–28.

IARC Monographs on the Evaluation of the Carcinogenic Risk of Chemicals to Humans: Some halogenated hydrocarbons (1979). Volume 20, Lyon, France.

Mukhametova, I. M. and Vozovaya, M. A. (1972). Reproductive power and the incidence of gynecological effects in female workers exposed to the combined effect of benzene and chlorinated hydrocarbons. *Gigiena Truda i Professional'nye Zabolevaniya* **16**, (11), 6–9.

Schwetz, B. A., Leong, B. K. J. and Gehring, B. J. (1975). The effect of maternally inhaled trichloroethylene, perchloroethylene, methyl chloroform, and methylene chloride on embryonal and fetal development in mice and rats. *Toxicology and Applied Pharmacology* **32**, 84–96.

18. Dioxane

TECHNICAL DATA

Formula

CAS registry number 123–91–1

Chemical abstracts name Dioxane

Synonyms Diethylene dioxide; 1,4-diethylene dioxide; diethylene ether; di(ethylene oxide); 1,4-dioxacyclohexane; dioxan; 1,4-dioxam; para-dioxan; dioxane; para-dioxane; dioxyethylene ether; glycol ethylene ether; tetrahydro-1,4-dioxin; tetrahydro-para-dioxin.

Uses Solvent for cellulose acetate, ethyl cellulose, benzyl cellulose, resins, oils, waxes, oil and spirit-soluble dyes, and many other organic as well as some inorganic compounds.

TLV 50 ppm (skin) (1980 Intended change to 25 ppm).

ANIMAL STUDIES

A. RELEVANT PHARMACOLOGY AND TOXICOLOGY

No relevant data found.

B. ENDOCRINE AND GONADAL EFFECTS

No relevant data found.

C. FERTILITY

No relevant data found.

D. PREGNANCY

Dioxane has been shown to cause a small increase in malformation rates in the chick embryo after injection into the egg (Salzgeber and Salaün, 1965) and to arrest growth of chick embryo limb bud cultures (Franceschini, 1964). However no studies using mammals have been carried out.

E. MUTAGENICITY

No relevant data found.

F. CARCINOGENICITY

IARC Monograph Vol. 11 (1976) reported that dioxane is carcinogenic in the rat and the guinea pig after oral administration.

HUMAN STUDIES

A. RELEVANT PHARMACOLOGY AND TOXICOLOGY

No relevant data found.

B. ENDOCRINE AND GONADAL EFFECTS

No relevant data found.

C. FERTILITY

No relevant data found.

D. PREGNANCY

No relevant data found.

E. MUTAGENICITY

Six employees in a dioxane production plant and 6 controls had lymphocyte cultures examined for chromosome gaps and other aberrations. No difference between the groups was detected. Exposure details of the subjects were not given (Thiess, A. M., Tress, E. and Fleig, L., 1976, *Arbeits Sozialmed Preventivmed* **11**, 35–46, quoted by the U.S. Department of Health, Education and Welfare (1977), original paper not seen by us).

F. CARCINOGENICITY

IARC Monograph Vol. 11 (1976) reported that no case reports of epidemiological studies were available for evaluation.

SUMMARY AND EVALUATION

EXPERIMENTAL STUDIES

No studies were found on endocrine or gonadal effects or on fertility or pregnancy in mammals. Two studies reported adverse effects on chick embryos. No studies on mutagenicity were found. Dioxane is carcinogenic in the rat and guinea pig, but no studies on transplacental carcinogenicity were found.

HUMAN STUDIES

No studies were found on any aspect of reproductive toxicity. No mutagenic effect was observed in a small study of lymphocyte cultures from exposed workers. There are no studies on carcinogenicity.

EVALUATION

Since the chick embryo is not regarded as a satisfactory model for prediction of teratogenic hazard, no evaluation is possible. Attention is drawn to the lack of data on animals and humans.

References

Franceschini, M. (1964). The influence of dioxane and thalidomide on the growth of chick-embryotibial buds in organotropic cultures. *Sperimentale* **114**, (1), 1–17.

IARC Monographs on the Evaluation of the Carcinogenic Risk of Chemicals to Man: Cadmium, nickel, some epoxides, miscellaneous industrial chemicals and general considerations on volatile anaesthetics (1976). Volume 11, Lyon, France.

Salzgeber, B. and Salaün, J. (1965). The action of thalidomide on the fowl embryo. *Journal of Embryology and Experimental Morphology* **13**, (2), 159–170.

U.S. Department of Health, Education and Welfare (1977). Occupational exposure to dioxane: Criteria for a recommended standard DHEW (NIOSH) Publication No. 77–226.

19. Epichlorohydrin

TECHNICAL DATA

Formula

$$CH_2\underset{O}{\text{—}}CHCH_2Cl$$

CAS registry number 106–89–8

Chemical abstracts name Chloromethyloxirane

Synonyms 1-Chloro-2,3-epoxypropane; 3-chloro-1,2-epoxypropane; (chloromethyl)ethylene oxide; 2-(chloromethyl)oxirane; chloropropylene oxide; γ-chloropropylene oxide; 3-chloro-1,2-propylene oxide; epichlorhydrin; α-epichlorohydrin; (DL)-α-epichlorohydrin; 1,2-epoxy-3-chloropropane; 2,3-epoxypropyl chloride.

Uses Solvent for natural and synthetic resins, gums, cellulose esters and ethers, paints, varnishes, nail enamels and lacquers, cement for Celluloid.

TLV 2 ppm (skin).

ANIMAL STUDIES

A. RELEVANT PHARMACOLOGY AND TOXICOLOGY

Tissue distribution and excretion of epichlorohydrin have been studied in male and female rats by Weigel *et al.* (1978). Epichlorohydrin, 10 mg/kg, was administered orally. The relative distributions in the different organs were similar in both sexes, but peak tissue levels were higher and occurred earlier after dosing (2 h compared with 4 h) in males than females. Peak tissue levels in the testes of 0·5% of the dose and in the ovaries of 0·07% of the dose were not suggestive of any selective concentration of epichlorohydrin in these organs.

B. ENDOCRINE AND GONADAL EFFECTS

Cooper *et al.* (1974) have studied the effect of a large dose of epichlorohydrin on testicular histology. They gave a single dose of 100 mg/kg orally to rats and killed them (numbers not given) at intervals during the next 20 weeks. Effects were apparent by 8 weeks; small spermatocoeles were seen in the ductuli efferentes and fertility was low (see section C). By 12 weeks these had progressed to large retention cysts in the ductuli efferentes and proximal caput causing sterility in 4/5 test animals.

Hahn (1970) gave a lower dose, 15 mg/kg, orally to rats for 12 successive days (numbers not given). This dose caused infertility within one week of dosing but no histological changes could be seen in the testes, epididymides, prostate or seminal vesicles on the 12th day of dosing.

Inhalation toxicity studies sponsored by the Manufacturing Chemists Association (1979a, 1979b) have shown changes in the epididymides of rats. After exposure to 100 ppm epichlorohydrin for 7 h/day, 5 days/week for 12 days the epididymides contained not only their normal sperm content but also increased numbers of nucleated cells and/or amorphous eosinophilic-staining material of unknown origin. There was no evidence of testicular damage nor of the type of epididymal damage found by Cooper *et al.* (1974) following oral dosing. No epididymal or testicular changes were seen in the one strain of mouse tested after similar exposure to 100 ppm. In the 90-day study (Manufacturing Chemists Association, 1979a) rats and mice were exposed to 5, 25 or 50 ppm for 6 h/day, 5 days/week. Epididymal changes similar to those found in the 12-day study were seen only at 50 ppm in one of the 2 strains of rat tested and not in the one strain of mouse tested.

C. FERTILITY

Epichlorohydrin has been shown to induce infertility in male rats similar in mechanism to that caused by the structurally-related α-chlorohydrin, but less severe on a dose for dose basis (Jones *et al.*, 1969; Hahn, 1970; Cooper *et al.*, 1974). α-Chlorohydrin has antifertility activity in a number of species including primates. In the rat, there is evidence that epichlorohydrin may be hydrolysed *in vivo* to α-chlorohydrin (Jones *et al.*, 1969).

In rats, Cooper *et al.* (1974) found the effects of repeated doses of epichlorohydrin given over several days differ from the effects of the same total dose given on a single day. They gave 20 or 50 mg/kg/day orally for 5 successive days, or a single oral dose of 100 mg/kg, and monitored fertility for 10 weeks after dosing. Twenty mg/kg × 5 resulted in complete infertility in the first 2 weeks after dosing but a return to full fertility by the third week, suggesting epididymal effects on late spermatids and spermatozoa only. Fifty mg/kg × 5 caused complete infertility in all test animals in the 10 weeks after dosing. The single oral dose of 100 mg/kg also caused complete infertility in the majority of test animals in the 10 weeks after dosing. Histological changes in the epididymides were also seen in this group (see section B).

Hahn (1970) studied the effect of a lower dose in the rat with subchronic administration. Fifteen mg/kg/day orally for 12 days caused infertility within one week of commencing dosing, but it was reversible, fertility returning within one week of the last dose being given Libido and ejaculatory ability of the males was normal. There were no histological changes.

Thus lower doses have an immediate but reversible effect on fertility, probably affecting post-testicular stages of spermatogenesis, without interfering with mating ability or causing histological changes, whereas higher doses cause obstructive histological changes in the epididymides, resulting in permanent sterility.

The studies just described, by reason of design or inadequate reporting of data, do not distinguish between dominant lethal effects and true infertility. However, studies in mice indicate that whilst epichlorohydrin may reduce fertility, it is not mutagenic in the dominant lethal assay. Epstein *et al.* (1972) showed that a single i.p. dose of 150 mg/kg given to 10 male mice had no effect on pregnancy rate, early fetal deaths or total implantations when they mated subsequently to 3 untreated females per week for 8 weeks. Šrám *et al.* (1976a) gave male mice (20 per treatment group) single i.p. doses of 5, 10 or 20 mg/kg, or single oral doses of 20 or 40 mg/kg. These had no effect on intrauterine deaths when they were mated subsequently to 2 untreated females per week for 8 weeks, but there was a suggestion of reduced fertility in the 20 mg/kg i.p. group; the weekly proportion of females pregnant ranged from 52·5–65% compared with 65–85% in controls. In the same study (Šrám *et al.*, 1976a), after repeated doses over 5 successive days of 1–5 mg/kg/day i.p. or 4–20 mg/kg/day p.o., no dominant lethal effects were found. However, there was a variable reduction in fertility, seen, for example, in the 5 × 1 mg/kg i.p. group, but not in the 5 × 4 mg/kg i.p. group. The absence of a dose-response relationship in this mouse study and the lack of studies in rats employing doses lower than 15 mg/kg do not permit any estimation of a no-effect-level on fertility. However, it is clearly some way below overtly toxic doses, the oral LD50 being 240–260 mg/kg and the i.p. LD50 being 120–170 mg/kg in mice and rats (IARC Monograph Vol. 11, 1976). These data suggest a selective effect on male fertility is a possible hazard with this compound.

In a single inhalation study by the Manufacturing Chemists Association, U.S.A. (1979a) exposure to 50 ppm for 10 weeks produced transient infertility in male rats but not male rabbits during the exposure period. Recovery of fertility occurred in the rats by the second week following termination of exposure. Exposure of male rats to 25 ppm did not affect the pregnancy rate when they were mated to untreated females but there was a marked pre-implantation loss, suggesting reduced fertilizing ability of the spermatozoa.

D. PREGNANCY

In a study sponsored by the Manufacturing Chemists Association, U.S.A. (1979c) the effects of inhalation exposure to epichlorohydrin during pregnancy in rats and rabbits have been studied. In a preliminary tolerance study groups of 5 or 6 rats and 5 rabbits were exposed to 0, 25, 50 or 100 ppm for 7 h/day on days 6–15 (rats) or 6–18 (rabbits) of pregnancy. In the rats, exposure to 50 or 100 ppm decreased maternal body weight gain. At 100 ppm 3/6 animals on day 16 contained only resorbed implantation sites, 1/6 had normal live fetuses, and 2/6 had no evidence of any implantation sites. At 25 or 50 ppm no such adverse effects were seen. In the rabbits, 3/5 dams died at 100 ppm, and 1/5 at 50 ppm. Maternal body weight gain was decreased at both 50 and 100 ppm and there was evidence of pneumonia in nearly all animals at these dose levels. Rabbits that died during the course of exposure contained resorbed fetuses only. Surviving dams all contained viable fetuses at all dose levels.

In the subsequent large-scale study, groups of 43–46 rats and 20–25 rabbits were exposed to 0, 2·5 or 25 ppm for 7 h/day on days 6–15 (rats) or 6–18 (rabbits) of pregnancy as before. Acceptable teratological methods were used.

In the rat study, there was little evidence of maternal toxicity except for a slight decrease in body weight gain on the first day of exposure, and decreased food consumption with increased water consumption during the treatment period, in the 25 ppm group. No evidence of adverse effects on implantation, numbers of live fetuses, resorption rate or fetal body weight were seen at either dose level. Similarly there were no significant increases in major or minor malformations. However, the value of this study is somewhat diminished by the fact that the timing of the pregnancies was known to be erroneous in 9 cases where the dams delivered spontaneously up to 9 days before Caesarian section was done on designated day 21 of pregnancy, and possibly erroneous in an unknown number of the remaining rats. Thus the dams may have been exposed on days other than the true days 6–15 and killed on days other than the true day 21. This latter possibility calls into question the reliability of the fetal weight data in particular.

In the rabbit study, the only suggestion of maternal toxicity was seen in the 25 ppm group where one rabbit died of pneumonia. There were no adverse effects at either 2·5 or 25 ppm on implantation sites, resorptions, fetal weight or malformations. In this study pregnancy timing was known accurately because artificial insemination was used.

E. MUTAGENICITY

Epichlorohydrin is mutagenic in bacterial systems *in vitro* with or without metabolic activation (Elmore *et al.*, 1976; Biles *et al.*, 1978). Šrám *et al.* (1976a) found that epichlorohydrin caused dose-related mutagenic changes in female mouse bone-marrow cells, predominantly breaks and exchanges, after single doses from 1–50 mg/kg i.p. or 5–100 mg/kg p.o., effects being noted from the lowest doses. Repeated doses over 5 successive days induced a higher frequency of abnormal cells and a higher frequency of breaks per cell than the same total dose given in a single administration. In the same study, they noted the absence of dominant lethal effects in male mice of the same strain. They suggested this could be due to rapid biotransformation of epichlorohydrin. However, epichlorohydrin or its possible active metabolite α-chlorohydrin clearly reach the testes and epididymides in sufficient quantities to cause infertility and one study (Jones *et al.*, 1969) has specifically shown the absence of dominant lethal mutation with doses of α-chlorohydrin between that causing sterility and that having no effect on fertility.

F. CARCINOGENICITY

IARC Monograph Vol. 11 (1976) reported that epichlorohydrin is carcinogenic in mice. There have been no studies of the possible transplacental carcinogenicity of epichlorohydrin.

HUMAN STUDIES

A. RELEVANT PHARMACOLOGY AND TOXICOLOGY

No relevant data found.

B. ENDOCRINE AND GONADAL EFFECTS

No relevant data found.

C. FERTILITY

Although epichlorohydrin has been shown to cause infertility in rats there are no published studies on its effects in humans. Rose and Lane (1979) in a N.I.O.S.H. Current Intelligence Bulletin on epichlorohydrin, refer to an unpublished report of the Shell Oil Company on a study of testicular function among epichlorohydrin workers. The study concluded that exposure did not decrease sperm counts or affect hormonal activity in the workers. The data were not analysed statistically. No other details are given.

D. PREGNANCY

No relevant data found.

E. MUTAGENICITY

Epichlorohydrin was positive in human lymphocytes *in vitro* (Šrám *et al.*, 1976a and 1976b; Kučerová, 1976; Kučerová *et al.*, 1976).

Kučerová *et al.* (1977) published the results of an interesting study on 35 workers aged 23 to 54 years of age (sex not stated) who had blood samples taken for analysis just before they started work in a new epichlorohydrin factory in Czechoslovakia. One and 2 years later they were all healthy and not exposed to irradiation or other known mutagens including drugs. They were exposed in the factory to epichlorohydrin 0·0–5·0 mg/m^3 (0·13–1·3 ppm). The peripheral lymphocytes were cultured for 56–58 h and 4 slides prepared per donor and coded. Two slides with different code numbers were scored independently in each of 2 laboratories, one in Prague and one in Moscow. Fifty cells per slide were scored when possible for chromatid breaks and exchanges and chromosome breaks and exchanges. Cells with only gaps were not counted as aberrant. The percentage of cells with chromosome aberrations was 1·37% before exposure, 1·91% after the first year and 2·69% after the second year. This increase was significant after the first year ($P=0{\cdot}025$) and highly significant ($P<0{\cdot}0001$) after the second year. The second year was significantly higher ($P<0{\cdot}005$) than after the first year. The increase was mostly due to chromatid and chromosomal breaks, and exchanges were rare. The authors conclude that epichlorohydrin, at the concentration to which the workers were exposed, has a significant mutagenic effect.

This study was supported by a report of Picciano (1979) of O.S.H.A., U.S.A. He studied 93 workers exposed in 2 centres to epichlorohydrin and compared the results with those from 75 pre-employment individuals. Blood samples were taken and peripheral lymphocytes cultured and 200 metaphase spreads per individual were examined for chromatid and chromosome breaks, marker chromosomes, severely damaged cells (≥ 10 aberrations of any type) and total abnormal cells. The controls were matched for sex, time of lymphocyte culture and partly for age. The numbers of each sex are not stated, and the duration and degree of exposure is not stated, but thought to be within the Federal standard of 5 ppm. He found that the exposed workers had significantly increased incidences of all types of aberration studied compared with the controls. For example, more than 4 chromosome breaks were found in cells from 11·8% of exposed workers compared with 1·3% of controls. The types of aberrations found were the same as those reported by Kučerová *et al.* (1977), and the author concludes that this leaves little doubt about the mutagenic effect of epichlorohydrin exposure in man.

F. CARCINOGENICITY

IARC Vol. 11 (1976) reported that no case reports or epidemiological studies were available at that time. A N.I.O.S.H. Current Intelligence Bulletin (Rose and Lane, 1979) refers to an unpublished study by Shell Oil Company which is suggestive of an increase in respiratory cancer in exposed workers.

SUMMARY AND EVALUATION

EXPERIMENTAL STUDIES

Large single doses of 100 mg/kg orally or 50 mg/kg daily for 5 days may cause complete infertility in male rats with no sign of recovery up to 12 weeks. This is accompanied by production of large epididymal cysts. Lower doses of 15–20 mg/kg daily orally cause rapid onset of sterility but recovery occurs within 2 to 3 weeks of stopping treatment. No histological changes are produced in the testes or epididymis at these doses and the effect must be on the late spermatids and sperm.

Inhalation of 50 or 100 ppm repeatedly in rats but not in mice caused the appearance of nucleated cells in the epididymis with transient infertility but no histological evidence of damage to the testes or epididymis. No effects were observed at 25 ppm or below. No no-effect level has been demonstrated for oral administration in rats.

No dominant lethal effects were demonstrated in male mice following oral administration up to 40 mg/kg or intra-peritoneally up to 150 mg/kg in single doses, though some reduction in fertility was seen in some of the treated groups. Inhalation of 50 ppm repeatedly by male rabbits produced no effect on fertility. Limited studies of inhalation of 2·5 or 25 ppm by rats and rabbits during pregnancy produced no adverse effects on litter size, resorptions, fetal weights or malformation rates.

It is mutagenic in bacterial systems with and without activation and causes chromosomal damage to bone marrow cells in mice. Dominant lethal studies are difficult to assess because of the anti-fertility effect of the substance.

It is carcinogenic in mice. No reports of transplacental carcinogenicity were found.

HUMAN STUDIES

No studies were found on endocrine or gonadal effects. No data have been published on effects on fertility but reference is made in a N.I.O.S.H. Current Intelligence Bulletin (Rose and Lane, 1979) to an unpublished report of the Shell Oil Company of no decrease in sperm count or hormonal activity among epichlorohydrin exposed workers. No details were available. No studies were found of effects in pregnancy. It is mutagenic to human lymphocytes in culture. Two studies have reported that it is mutagenic in workers as assessed by chromosomal damage in peripheral lymphocytes. The exposure level in one case was reported to be 1·3 ppm or less.

An unpublished Shell Oil Company study has produced suggestive evidence that there may be an increase in respiratory cancer in exposed workers.

EVALUATION

Epichlorohydrin has antifertility activity in male rats and no no-effect level has been established for oral administration. The no-effect level in limited studies is 25 ppm by inhalation. It is less effective in mice and rabbits. It is not embryolethal or teratogenic in rabbits at doses not toxic to the dam. In rats there is limited evidence that it is embryolethal at doses toxic to the dam but is not embryolethal or teratogenic at lower doses. Attention is drawn to the lack of published data on effects on fertility in man. It is mutagenic in bacteria, and mammalian systems including exposed workers. There are unpublished data suggestive of a respiratory carcinogenic effect in exposed workers. Attention is drawn to the need for further human studies.

References

Biles, R. W., Connor, T. H., Trieff, N. M. and Legator, M. S. (1978). The influence of contaminants on the mutagenic activity of dibromochloropropane (DBCP). *Journal of Environmental Pathology and Toxicology* **2**, (2), 301–321.

Cooper, E. R. A., Jones, A. R. and Jackson, H. (1974). Effects of α-chlorohydrin and related compounds on the reproductive organs and fertility of the male rat. *Journal of Reproduction and Fertility* **38**, 379–386.

Elmore, J. D., Wong, J. L., Lumbach, A. D. and Streps, U. N. (1976). Vinyl chloride mutagenicity via the metabolites chlorooxirane and chloroacetaldehyde monomer hydrate. *Biochimica et Biophysica Acta* **442**, (3), 405–419.

Epstein, S. S., Arnold, E., Andrea, J., Bass, W. and Bishop, Y. (1972). Detection of chemical mutagens by the dominant lethal assay in the mouse. *Toxicology and Applied Pharmacology* **23**, 288–325.

Hahn, J. D. (1970). Post-testicular antifertility effects of epichlorhydrin and 2,3-epoxypropanol. *Nature* **226**, 87.

IARC Monographs on the Evaluation of the Carcinogenic Risk of Chemicals to Man: Cadmium, nickel, some epoxides, miscellaneous industrial chemicals and general considerations on volatile anaesthetics (1976). Volume 11, Lyon, France.

Jones, A. R., Davies, P., Edwards, K. and Jackson, H. (1969). Antifertility effects and metabolism of α- and epi-chlorhydrins in the rat. *Nature* **224**, 83.

Kučerová, M. (1976). Cytogenic analysis of human chromosomes and its value for the estimation of genetic risk. *Mutation Research* **41**, (1), 123–130.

Kučerová, M., Polivkova, Z., Šrám, R. and Matousek, V. (1976). Mutagenic effect of epichlorhydrin. I. Testing on human lymphocytes in vitro in comparison with TEPA. *Mutation Research* **34**, 271–278.

Kučerová, M., Zhurkova, V. S., Polivkova, Z. and Ivanova, J. E. (1977). Mutagenic effect of epichlorhydrin. *Mutation Research* **48**, (3–4), 355–360.

Manufacturing Chemists Association (1979a). Epichlorhydrin – Subchronic studies. I. A 90-day inhalation study in laboratory rodents. Manufacturing Chemists Association, Washington, D.C., U.S.A.

Manufacturing Chemists Association (1979b). Epichlorhydrin – Subchronic studies. II. A 12-day inhalation study in laboratory rodents. Manufacturing Chemists Association, Washington, D.C., U.S.A.

Manufacturing Chemists Association (1979c). Epichlorhydrin – Subchronic studies. IV. The effects of maternally inhaled epichlorhydrin on rat and rabbit embryonal and fetal development. Manufacturing Chemists Association, Washington, D.C., U.S.A.

Picciano, D. (1979). Cytogenic investigation of occupational exposure to epichlorhydrin. *Mutation Research* **66**, 169–173.

Rose, D. and Lane, J. M. (1979). Epichlorhydrin. *American Industrial Hygiene Association Journal* **40**, (6), A48–A58.

Šrám, R. J., Černá, M. and Kučerová, M. (1976a). The genetic risk of epichlorhydrin as related to the occupational exposure. *Biologisches Zentralblatt* **85**, (4), 451–462.

Šrám, R. J., Černá, M. and Kučerová, M. (1976b). Investigation and evaluation of mutagenic activity of epichlorhydrin. *Ceskoslovenska Hygiena* **21**, (8), 353–360.

Weigel, W. W., Plotnick, H. B. and Conner, W. L. (1978). Tissue distribution and excretion of 14C-epichlorhydrin in male and female rats. *Research Communications in Chemical Pathology and Pharmacology* **20**, (2), 275–287.

20. Ethylene Dibromide (dibromoethane)

TECHNICAL DATA

Formula	$BrCH_2CH_2Br$
CAS registry number	106–93–4
Chemical abstracts name	1,2-Dibromoethane
Synonyms	α,β-Dibromoethane; sym-dibromoethane; EDB; ethylene bromide, glycol bromide.
Uses	Fumigant; in anti-knock gasolines.
TLV	None

ANIMAL STUDIES

A. RELEVANT PHARMACOLOGY AND TOXICOLOGY

A sex difference in the acute oral LD50 for dibromoethane, commonly known as ethylene dibromide (EDB), has been observed by Rowe *et al.* (1957) in the rat. The LD50 in 60 male rats averaged 146 mg/kg (95% confidence limits 126–170 mg/kg) and that in 40 female rats averaged 117 mg/kg (108–126 mg/kg). However, an oral LD50 test in guinea pigs, in the same study, showed no significant difference between the sexes.

B. ENDOCRINE AND GONADAL EFFECTS

Males
The structural similarity of EDB (dibromoethane) to dibromochloropropane necessitates detailed consideration of its possible effects on testicular function.

It has been shown that EDB reaches the testis. Edwards *et al.* (1970) injected radiolabelled EDB i.p. into the mouse (40 mg/kg). One to 3 h after injection, 1·0–1·5% of the dose/g of wet tissue was found in the testis. By 24 h after injection 0·23% of the dose/g remained in the testis, much higher concentrations being found in the small intestine, kidney and liver. Short *et al.* (1979) gave 10 or 100 mg/kg radiolabelled EDB p.o. to rats. Four hours after administration significant amounts were found in the testis (1·7 μg/g tissue), but concentrations in the liver, kidney and stomach were higher. The relative tissue distribution of EDB in the rat 4 h after administration (Short *et al.*, 1979) was very similar to that seen in the mouse 3 h after i.p. injection (Edwards *et al.*, 1970). Amir (1973) has shown in the bull that radiolabelled EDB given orally or by i.p. injection appears within a day in seminal plasma and in 2–5 days in spermatozoa.

A number of studies have investigated the effect of chronic inhalation exposure to EDB on testicular weight, histology and function. Short *et al.* (1979) exposed male rats to 0, 19, 39 or 89 ppm for 7 h/day, 5 days/week for 10 weeks. At 89 ppm 7/33 males died and body weight gain and food consumption in survivors were significantly reduced compared with controls throughout the treatment period. At the end of the 10-week exposure period 9 or 10 males in each group were killed and examined. Mean testicular weight and serum testosterone levels were markedly reduced to 0·5 g and 0·48 μg/100 ml respectively in the 89 ppm group compared with 3·4 g and 1·04 μg/100 ml in controls. At the end of the exposure 10 males from each group were paired with untreated females for fertility and dominant lethal testing and two weeks later killed for histological examination of the reproductive organs. Males in the 89 ppm group, which did not impregnate any females (see section C for details), all showed moderate to severe atrophy of the testis, epididymis, prostate and seminal vesicles. The incidence of calcification of the testis (8/10) and prostatitis (6/10) were also significantly increased in this group. Males exposed to 19 or 39 ppm showed no adverse effects at all except lower weight gain in the 39 ppm group. It is doubtful whether such severe testicular weight loss and atrophy seen at 89 ppm can be attributed solely to the effect of EDB on food consumption and body weight, but, as with the effects on female rats discussed later, it is not possible in the presence of such severe general toxicity (20% mortality) to say whether EDB has a primary effect on the reproductive organs.

Rowe *et al.* (1957) exposed male rats to 0 or 50 ppm for 7 h/day, 5 days/week for 13 weeks. Ten out of 20 animals died from respiratory infections, including pneumonia, in the exposed group. In survivors, body weight did not differ significantly from controls, but relative lung, liver and kidney weights were increased and testicular weights decreased by around 10%. Histological examination of these organs showed pneumonic changes in the lungs but no lesions elsewhere. Exposure of 8 guinea pigs, 3 rabbits and one monkey to 50 ppm 7 h/day, 5 days/week for 10–12 weeks caused no testicular weight changes or histopathological changes. Similarly, exposure of further groups of 20 rats, 8 guinea pigs, 3 rabbits and one monkey to 25 ppm for 30 weeks caused no testicular changes, though mortality from respiratory infections was again high in the rats (10/20 died).

Amir and co-workers have investigated in some detail the effect of EDB on bull semen. In their first experiment (Amir and Volcani, 1965), EDB was given orally to 4 calves from 4 days of age to 12 months at 2 mg/kg/day and from 12 months onwards at 4 mg/kg every other day. Semen collections were made weekly from 14–16 months of age onwards. Growth, general health and libido (reaction time to ejaculation) were unaffected in comparison with controls, but sperm density was low, sperm motility very poor and sperm morphology abnormal throughout the 8–10 months of collections. At $17\frac{1}{2}$ and $22\frac{1}{2}$ months of age, 2 of the bulls were unilaterally castrated and treatment discontinued. The testes removed showed gross abnormalities (Amir and Volcani, 1967). The seminiferous tubules showed little spermatogenic activity and their lumens were filled with cell debris or were empty. There were no spermatozoa in the epididymis and the vas deferens was surrounded by thick connective tissue. Following discontinuation of the treatment, semen samples with normal sperm density, motility and morphology were obtained by 10 days in one bull and by $3\frac{1}{2}$ months in the other (Amir and Volcani, 1965). Restoration of treatment to one of these recovered bulls and initiation of treatment to a fresh 16-month-old bull resulted in semen and sperm abnormalities after 2 weeks of treatment. After withdrawal of treatment from this latter bull, recovery again took 2–3 months. All the treated bulls were killed 8 months after withdrawal of treatment and histology of the testis showed normal spermatogenesis.

Amir (1973) has further established, through timed morphological and radioactive labelling studies in bulls, that EDB does not act directly on spermatozoa but probably acts on spermiogenesis, producing sperm with mishapen heads, and on epididymal maturation, producing sperm with acrosomal defects. The mechanism by which this occurs may be through alteration of the testicular and epididymal fluids. This hypothesis fits well with findings in young bulls 15–24 months old, where sperm morphology and viability returned to normal by 3–4 weeks after cessation of dosing (10 doses of 4 mg/kg every other day), the duration of spermiogenesis being around 3 weeks and epididymal transit 11 days in this species (Amir, 1975; Amir *et al.*, 1977). However, the possibility also remains that EDB may affect earlier stages of spermatogenesis since recovery of normal morphology took around 15 weeks in adult bulls similarly treated (10×4 mg/kg) (Amir, 1975).

Females

The possibility that EDB might affect gonadotrophin levels has been suggested by Alumot and co-workers following their observations that relatively low doses (5–7·5 ppm) in the feed of laying hens decreased egg size and impaired ovarian follicular growth, whilst higher doses (90 ppm) caused irreversible cessation of egg laying (Alumot and Mandel, 1969). However, they found that pituitary FSH levels in 3-month-old pullets or mature hens were unaffected by EDB in the feed for 1–2 months at levels which eventually stop egg laying (10 mg/animal/day). Neither did injections of chicken pituitary extract or ovine FSH increase the weight of eggs laid by hens fed 10 mg EDB/day. Thus, the mechanism by which EDB affects follicle growth is not known and the possibility of a direct effect on the ovary cannot be ruled out.

In the rat, reversible changes in the oestrous cycle have been observed at high doses. Short *et al.* (1979) exposed female rats to 0, 20, 39 or 80 ppm EDB by inhalation for 7 h/day, 7 days/week for 3 weeks. Each treatment group comprised 50 rats. Body weight and food consumption were significantly reduced throughout the exposure period in the 80 ppm group and 20% of these animals died. There were no deaths at 20 or 39 ppm and food consumption and body weight were only significantly reduced in the first week of exposure at these dose levels. No numerical or graphical data on oestrous cycles were given but the authors stated that at the end of the 3-week exposure period all females in the 0, 20 and 39 ppm groups had normal cycles and those in the 80 ppm group were all in dioestrus. In this group normal cycles resumed 3 or 4 days after exposure had ended. Only 8/20 females in the 80 ppm group paired with males mated in the 10 days following the end of exposure compared with 19/20 in each of the 0, 20 and 39 ppm groups (see section C for further details). In view of the severe toxicity caused by exposure to 80 ppm it is not possible to say whether the oestrous cycle and mating disturbances seen in this group were a primary effect of EDB exposure or secondary to the general toxicity observed.

Conclusion

In the male, studies in the rat suggest that gross testicular effects are only seen at doses that are lethal to a high proportion of animals and further suggest that the rat may be particularly susceptible to the toxic effects of EDB. However, studies in the bull raise the possibility that doses of EDB which are not generally toxic may have selective effects on testicular function, at least at the stage of spermiogenesis, and are in accordance with findings from a dominant lethal study in the rat indicating a selective effect on spermatids (see section C for details). There is limited evidence from the bull suggesting the effects of EDB on testicular function may be reversible.

In the female, one inhalation study in the rat has shown disruption of the oestrous cycle at a dose causing severe general toxicity but no effect below that dose.

In both male and female rats adverse effects on endocrine and gonadal function are accompanied by infertility (see section C).

C. FERTILITY

Males

A number of studies have investigated the effects of EDB given by various routes on male fertility. Short *et al.* (1979) exposed male rats to 0, 19, 39 or 89 ppm by inhalation for 7 h/day, 5 days/week for 10 weeks. Nine or 10 males from each group were housed for 2 weeks with 2 unexposed females/week from the end of the 10-week treatment period. The adverse effects of exposure to 89 ppm on survival, weight gain and testicular appearance have already been described (see section B). None of the males exposed to 89 ppm succeeded in impregnating any females. It was not recorded whether this was due to a failure to mate or infertile matings. The females were killed around mid-gestation and no adverse effects on fertility (number pregnant and total implants/dam) nor dominant lethal effects (post-implantation losses) were seen in those mated with males exposed to 19 or 39 ppm, in comparison with controls.

Two studies have looked at the effects of EDB injected i.p. Epstein *et al.* (1972), using the mouse, gave a single i.p. dose of 18 mg/kg to 7 males and 90 mg/kg to 9 males with 10 concurrent controls. They were housed with 3 untreated females/week for 8 consecutive weeks and the females killed 13 days after the midweek of being caged with the males. There were no male deaths, no effects on pregnancy rate or dominant lethal effects. Edwards *et al.* (1970), however, have found adverse effects from i.p. doses in the rat. They gave 6 rats a total of 50 mg/kg in 5 divided doses on successive days. The rats were then mated for the next 10 weeks to untreated females and the females killed during the third week after mating. Data, given as average litter sizes only, indicated reduced litter size in the fourth week and no litters in the fifth week, suggesting a selective effect on spermatids, though data on resorptions would be required to confirm this. No indication was given of whether the males showed any other signs of toxicity at the dose level used.

Epstein *et al.* (1972) have also given EDB orally to mice, 50 or 100 mg/kg/day for 5 days, 10 mice per treatment group. At 50 mg/kg/day one male died and at 100 mg/kg/day two died. Survivors were mated with 3 untreated females/week for 8 consecutive weeks, but no adverse effects on fertility or dominant lethal effects were observed.

These studies suggest that EDB may have an adverse effect if given i.p., when presumably higher concentrations reach the testis. EDB is rapidly removed from the circulation and rapidly metabolized (Short *et al.*, 1979; Edwards *et al.*, 1970) which may reduce its testicular toxicity. In the mouse, the primary metabolite of EDB, S-(2-hydroxyethyl)-cysteine, was not found to affect fertility when given p.o., 1 g/kg/day for 5 days (Edwards *et al.*, 1970). However, the results of the mouse studies discussed in this section suggest that this species may be particularly resistant to the effects of EDB on reproductive function, no adverse effects on the testes being found even at lethal doses (Epstein *et al.*, 1972). Thus it would be premature to infer from the above study of Edwards *et al.* (1970) that it is EDB and not its metabolite that has antifertility activity.

Females

The effect of inhaled EDB on female fertility has been investigated by Short *et al.* (1979). Female rats were exposed to 0, 20, 39 or 80 ppm for 7 h/day, 7 days/week for 3 weeks. The adverse effect of exposure to 80 ppm on the oestrous cycle in these rats has already been described (see section B). At the end of the exposure period 20 females in each group were paired with untreated males for 10 days. In the 20 and 39 ppm groups, 19/20 mated and all those that mated were pregnant when killed in the third week following pairing. Total implants/dam, viable implants/dam and resorptions/dam did not differ significantly from controls. At 80 ppm however, a dose which caused 20% mortality, decreased food consumption and body weight, and disrupted oestrous cycles, only 8/20 mated. Those that mated were all pregnant at mid-gestation. Total implants/dam and viable implants/dam were reduced while resorptions/dam were increased in comparison with controls, but not significantly so since these differences were largely due to one female with complete resorptions.

Conclusion

From the inhalation studies of Short *et al.* (1979) it is evident that doses of 80 ppm and above, which cause generalized toxicity, including death, markedly affect fertility in the male and female rat. These results are not surprising in view of the disturbances of testicular and ovarian function also observed at these dose levels. At a lower level of 50 ppm, Rowe *et al.* (1957) have shown a questionable reduction in testicular weight in rats (and not in three other species), and it is not known if testicular function is affected at this dose level. Exposure to 39 or 20 ppm is without effect in male or female (Short *et al.*, 1979).

Oral dosing at 50 or 100 mg/kg/day for 5 days is without effect in the mouse as are single i.p. doses of 18 or 90 mg/kg (Epstein *et al.*, 1972). However,

10 mg/kg/day for 5 days in the rat damages spermatids (Edwards *et al.*, 1970) as does oral administration in the bull (Amir, 1973). These two latter studies are the only ones which suggest that EDB affects male fertility at doses below those affecting general health, and further work is needed to clarify this point.

D. PREGNANCY

Short and co-workers have investigated the teratogenic potential of inhaled EDB in rats and mice. In an initial study animals were exposed to 0 or 32 ppm for 23 h/day from days 6–15 of pregnancy (Short *et al.*, 1976). Acceptable teratological methods were used. Numbers of animals used were 13–18/treatment group.

There was no maternal mortality due to the treatment but food consumption during treatment was decreased in both species. In the rats body weight decreased by an average of 27 g during treatment compared with an increase of 49 g in controls. In the mice, body weight increased by only 1 g during treatment compared with 14 g in controls.

In rats exposed to EDB there was a significant decrease in implants/dam and consequently a decrease in live fetuses/dam at term. However, since EDB exposure commenced after implantation this is unlikely to be a treatment-related effect, unless very early resorptions were missed (the authors do not mention if the uteri were stained to reveal very early resorptions). Early resorptions were increased from 1% in controls to 8% in EDB exposed rats, but this increase was not significant and was largely due to one animal with complete resorptions. There was no effect on fetal body weight. Only one major abnormality was found (one fetus with limb reduction deformities in the EDB exposed group). Total numbers of malformed fetuses in each group are not given and cannot be ascertained from the data published where anomalies are given on a mean percentage litter effect basis. However, eleven different types of anomaly were found in treated litters compared with only six in controls, and in every category except one (extra 14th ribs), more treated fetuses and litters are affected than controls. Statistically significant increases in individual types of anomaly were seen in EDB-exposed fetuses for hydrocephalus of the fourth ventricle and wavy ribs. However, the biological significance of the findings on hydrocephalus is difficult to assess. True hydrocephalus is rare in the strain of rat used (Charles River CD-1), yet 9/18 control litters and 11/17 treated litters were said to be affected. As prenatal development proceeds, the ventricles become smaller and so slight retardation of development can give the appearance of hydrocephalus. A higher, non-significant, proportion of fetuses in the treated group had incomplete ossification of the skull bones, suggesting slight retardation. Indeed the absence of any cases of hydrocephalus in either control or treated CD-1 rats (exposed to 20 or 38 ppm 23 h/day, days 6–15) in the follow-up experiment of Short *et al.* (1978), detailed below, together with the very variable incidence of hydronephrosis (0%, 7·3% and 9·7%), a common defect in this strain of rat, suggest there may have been considerable observer bias in the examination of fetuses for anomalies in these two studies of Short *et al.* (1976, 1978).

In mice there was no effect on implants/dam but early resorptions were increased from 15% to 32% and late resorptions from 2% to 7% in control and EDB-exposed groups respectively. These rates are largely due to three dams with complete resorptions in the treated group compared with two in controls and so are probably of no biological significance. Fetal body weight was reduced from 1·24 g in controls to 0·93 g in the treated group. There was only one major malformation (one control fetus with exencephaly). Hydrocephalus of the third and fourth ventricles was increased but not significantly (no fetuses affected in controls). Incomplete ossification of the supraoccipitals, incus and sternebrae was markedly increased in treated litters ($p < 0{\cdot}01–0{\cdot}05$).

In order to control for the effects of EDB exposure on food consumption and body weight change, groups of rats and mice were food restricted on days 6–15 of pregnancy. The results indicated that food restriction in the mouse produced similar effects to EDB (increased resorptions, decreased fetal weight, increased hydrocephalus and poor ossification), but it did not account for the increase in anomalies in EDB exposed rats.

In a later study, Short *et al.* (1978) exposed rats and mice to 0, 20, 38 or 80 ppm for 23 h/day, from days 6–15 of pregnancy. In the rats there were 15–17 animals/treatment group and in the mice 18–22/treatment group. Concurrent unexposed, food restricted controls as well as unrestricted, unexposed controls were run.

The highest dose (80 ppm) was toxic, killing 8/16 rats and 22/22 mice. At 38 ppm 7/20 mice died. In the food restricted control mice 8/18 died due to cannibalism. There was no maternal mortality in any of the other groups. Food consumption was significantly reduced in a dose-related manner in all EDB-exposed groups during treatment and remained so after exposure in the rats exposed to 80 ppm and the mice exposed to 38 ppm. In both rats and mice there was an adverse, dose related effect on body weight gain during EDB exposure, and comparison with the food restricted controls showed that these effects were only partially due to the reduced food consumption.

In the rats there were no significant effects on implants/dam, live fetuses/dam or resorptions/dam at 20 or 38 ppm. At 80 ppm 7/8 surviving dams had complete early resorptions only and the remaining dam contained only dead fetuses. Fetal body weight was significantly reduced to a mean of 3·6 g at 38 ppm compared with 4·0 g in untreated controls but there was a similar reduction to 3·4 g in the food restricted controls. In this study, unlike the previous one using 32 ppm (Short *et al.*, 1976), there were no significant effects on anomaly rates, except for a reduction in normally ossified centra from 69% in untreated controls to 47% (mean percentage litter effect) in the 20 ppm group. However, this is probably of no biological significance since 55% of centra were normally ossified at the higher dose of 38 ppm.

In the mice, there was no effect on implants/dam but there were significant increases in late resorptions/dam at 20 and 38 ppm. At 38 ppm, only 35% fetuses were viable compared with 90% at 20 ppm and 94% in controls. At 38 ppm 6/10 dams had complete resorptions, but 5/6 dams in the food restricted group also had complete resorptions with the remaining dam having only one viable fetus. Fetal body weight was significantly reduced to a mean of 0·63 g at 38 ppm and 1·09 g at 20 ppm compared with 1·35 g in untreated controls. There were no fetuses from food restricted dams for comparison. There were no significant effects on anomaly rates except for a dose-related increase in incomplete ossification of the skull, incus, hyoid, sternebrae and digits, similar to the findings in the food restricted control mice in the previous study (Short *et al.*, 1976).

Conclusion

Taking the results of these two studies of Short *et al.* (1976, 1978) together, EDB does not appear to cause any increase in the incidence of major malformations in either rats or mice. However at doses severely toxic to the dam there is a marked effect on intrauterine mortality and fetal weight in rats and mice, which are partially, and possibly wholly, attributable to the maternal toxicity and its effect on food consumption. Retarded ossification in the mouse also seems likely to be due to the decrease in food consumption. In the rat the possibility of a direct effect of EDB on anomalies remains equivocal. Anomalies found in the first study at 32 ppm (hydrocephalus, wavy ribs) were not found in the second study at 20 or 38 ppm, perhaps for the reasons already discussed. However, there remains the overall increase in anomaly rates seen at 32 ppm, which was not seen in food restricted controls.

There is clearly a need to look at the effects of lower doses again and to investigate whether doses which are non-toxic to the dam, below 20 ppm, have any effect on prenatal or postnatal development.

E. MUTAGENICITY

IARC Monograph Vol. 15 (1977) reports on studies showing EDB is mutagenic in the Ames test without metabolic activation. Results from host-mediated tests are equivocal.

F. CARCINOGENICITY

IARC Monograph Vol. 15 (1977) reports EDB is carcinogenic in mice and rats.

HUMAN STUDIES

A. RELEVANT PHARMACOLOGY AND TOXICOLOGY

No relevant data found.

B. ENDOCRINE AND GONADAL EFFECTS

No relevant data found.

C. FERTILITY

One study of reproductive performance of workers exposed to dibromoethane has been published (Wong *et al.*, 1979). Four chemical plants manufacturing dibromoethane or ethylene dibromide (EDB) located in Southern U.S.A. (Arkansas and Texas) were surveyed. The exposure level in all of the plants was at or less than 5 ppm. Since it was felt that it would be too difficult to examine the fertility of the men directly, it was decided to approach the problem by studying the fertility of their wives in the hope that this would at least reveal if there was a major fertility problem. All single men were excluded but otherwise all exposed males in the plants were included in the study. The following information was collected from each man: name, age, race, dates of marriage and divorces, wife's ages, ages of all children, details of adoptions, history of vasectomy or sterilization, dates of exposure to EDB and estimated level of exposure. For each of the four cohorts a computation was made of the standardized birth ratio between the observed number of children born to each couple from 9 months following the onset of exposure and the expected number of children derived from national fertility tables published for successive birth cohorts of U.S.A. women by the National Centre for Health Statistics. Account was taken of maternal age, race, parity and calendar year on birth rates. The ratio of observed to expected births was used as the measure of fertility and a statistical analysis based on the Poisson distribution was used to detect any significant departure from unity at the 0·05 level.

A total of 297 couples with 1092 person-years of exposure was included in the study covering the period 1958–1977. The average age of the observed person-years fell in the 30–34 age group. For plants A, B and C there were total births observed of 17, 13 and 19 with expected values of 17·22, 13·64 and 20·81 respectively. No significant differences were found between the observed and expected values either overall or when compared as sub-groups (a) exposure $<0{\cdot}5$ ppm, (b) exposure 0·5–5 ppm, (c) all whites, or (d) all non-whites.

In plant D exposure data was not available for individual workers. Among the white workers there were only 11 births compared with 22·2 expected ($p<0{\cdot}05$). For non-whites there were 2 births compared with 3·32 expected which was not significant possibly because of the large statistical variation in such a small sample. For all workers pooled in plant D, the ratio was 0·51 ($P<0{\cdot}05$).

If data from all plants are summed, a total of 62 births were observed with 77·18 expected with a ratio of 0·80 ($P>0{\cdot}05$ i.e. not significant). A computation of the statistical power of the study at $\alpha=0{\cdot}05$, showed a 90% chance of detecting a 20% reduction in fertility in the complete study.

The authors discuss at some length the many assumptions and limitations of this study, including such factors as employment status of the wives, educational attainments of the couples, income levels, etc., which were not taken into account. Also the role of sterilization as a method of birth control was difficult to assess in computing the expected birth rates. In plant D for example which had the highest sterilization rate, i.e. 22 of 67 couples, 33% of the sterility was known to be unrelated to EDB exposure. The regional differences in birth rate were also not taken into account, and since the West South Central Region which includes Arkansas and Texas had the second highest birth rate in 1969–71, the numbers of expected births is slightly underestimated. Comparison of exposed with unexposed workers in the same plants would have overcome some of these problems but this was not done.

In conclusion, this study has produced an inconclusive result. For the four plants taken together the standardized birth ratio is close to unity, suggesting that EDB has no antifertility effect at these exposure levels. Where high and low exposures could be compared, i.e. 0·5–5 ppm vs $<0{\cdot}5$ ppm, no dose related effect was observed. For plant D however, the birth ratio was significantly low suggesting an antifertility effect, although the average exposure level was below 5 ppm. The conclusion must be that EDB does not produce any major antifertility effect at exposures below 5 ppm, but that the methodology used in this study was inadequate to detect effects on sub-groups of workers who may have had higher individual exposures.

D. PREGNANCY

No relevant data found.

E. MUTAGENICITY

Only one report on studies utilizing human cells has been found. This consists only of a brief abstract by Kristoffersson (1974) who reported that no chromosome breaks or effects on satellite association were observed from EDB in human lymphocyte cultures. No other details were given.

F. CARCINOGENICITY

IARC Monograph Vol. 15 (1977) reported that no case studies or epidemiological studies on carcinogenicity in humans were available for evaluation at that time.

SUMMARY AND EVALUATION

EXPERIMENTAL STUDIES

Inhalation studies in rats showed atrophy of the testis and secondary sex organs only at 89 ppm daily which was lethal to 20% of the animals. No effects were observed at 39 ppm daily which was non-toxic. Very limited studies at 25 and 50 ppm by inhalation showed no adverse effects on the testes in rats, guinea pigs, rabbits or monkeys. Oral administration to calves or bulls at 2–4 mg/kg however produced rapid reduction in sperm count and motility and with abnormal morphology in the absence of other signs of toxicity. Prolonged administration resulted in severe testicular damage to the seminiferous tubules. The effects however were rapidly reversible. The primary effect appears to be on spermiogenesis.

In female rats, effects were only seen on the oestrous cycle at 80 ppm which was lethal to 20% of the animals, but no effect was seen at the non-toxic dose of 39 ppm.

No effects were seen on fertility in male or female rats exposed to non-lethal doses. No effects were observed in dominant lethal studies in mice given doses up to 90 mg/kg i.p. or 100 mg/kg orally for 5 days. However, one study in male rats did report infertility 4 and 5 weeks after 10 mg/kg i.p. for 5 days suggesting an effect on spermatids.

Exposure by inhalation of pregnant rats or mice to toxic doses caused increases in resorptions and reduced fetal weight and ossification, which are largely related to reduced food intake of the dams. In one study in rats at 32 ppm, which was toxic to the dams, there was an increase in congenital anomalies that was not seen in food-restricted controls.

It is mutagenic in bacterial systems without activation. It is carcinogenic in mice and rats. No studies on transplacental carcinogenicity were found.

HUMAN STUDIES

No studies were found on endocrine or gonadal effects in humans. One study of pregnancies in wives of exposed workers was carried out at 4 manufacturing plants in Southern U.S.A. with exposure levels at or less than 5 ppm. No difference was found between the observed and expected numbers of children when compared with national fertility data, in 3 of the plants. In the fourth plant however, only 11 births were observed compared with 22·2 expected ($P < 0{\cdot}05$). No explanation could be found for this difference.

No adequate studies on mutagenicity and no studies on carcinogenicity were found.

EVALUATION

Ethylene dibromide has an antifertility effect in bulls at otherwise non-toxic doses, around 2–4 mg/kg orally. Similar effects have not been seen in limited studies in rats, mice, guinea pigs, rabbits or monkeys. There is inadequate data to assess its embryotoxicity and teratogenicity at non-toxic doses. It is mutagenic in bacteria and carcinogenic in mice and rats. Although a possible effect on fertility was observed in exposed workers in one of 4 factories studied, further studies are needed to confirm this effect. Attention is drawn to the lack of adequate studies on fertility, pregnancy, mutagenicity and carcinogenicity in humans.

References

Alumot, (Olomucki) E. and Mandel, E. (1969). Gonadotropic hormones in hens treated with ethylene dibromide. *Poultry Science* **48**, (3), 957–960.

Amir, D. (1973). The sites of spermicidal action of ethylene dibromide in bulls. *Journal of Reproduction and Fertility* **35**, 519–525.

Amir, D. (1975). Individual and age differences in the spermicidal effect of ethylene dibromide in bulls. *Journal of Reproduction and Fertility* **44**, 561–565.

Amir, D. and Volcani, R. (1965). Effect of dietary ethylene dibromide on bull semen. *Nature* **206**, (4979), 99–100.

Amir, D. and Volcani, R. (1967). The effect of dietary ethylene dibromide (EDB) on the testes of bulls. *Fertility and Sterility* **18**, (1), 144–148.

Amir, D., Esnault, C., Nicolle, J. C. and Courot, M. (1977). DNA and protein changes in the spermatozoa of bulls treated orally with ethylene dibromide. *Journal of Reproduction and Fertility* **51**, 453–456.

Edwards, K., Jackson, H. and Jones, A. R. (1970). Studies with alkylating esters. II. A chemical interpretation through metabolic studies of the antifertility effects of ethylene dimethanesulphonate and ethylene dibromide. *Biochemical Pharmacology* **19**, 1783–1789.

Epstein, S. S., Arnold, E., Andrea, J., Bass, W. and Bishop, Y. (1972). Detection of chemical mutagens by the dominant lethal assay in the mouse. *Toxicology and Applied Pharmacology* **23**, 288–325.

IARC Monographs on the Evaluation of the Carcinogenic Risk of Chemicals to Man: Some fumigants, the herbicides 2,4-D and 2,4,5-T, chlorinated dibenzodioxins and miscellaneous industrial chemicals (1977). Vol. 15, Lyon, France.

Kristoffersson, U. (1974). Genetic effects of some gasoline additives. *Hereditas* **78**, 319.

Rowe, V. K., Spencer, H. C., McCollister, D. D., Hollingsworth, R. I. and Adams, E. M. (1957). Toxicity of ethylene dibromide determined on experimental animals. *American Medical Association Archives of Industrial Hygiene and Occupational Medicine* **6**, 158–163.

Short, R. D., Minor, J. L., Ferguson, B., Unger, T. and Lee, C. C. (1976). The developmental toxicity of ethylene dibromide inhaled by rats and mice during organogenesis. U.S. National Technical Information Service EPA 560/6–76–018 PB 256 659.

Short, R. D., Minor, J. L., Winston, J. M., Seifter, J. and Lee, C.-C. (1978). Inhalation of ethylene dibromide during gestation by rats and mice. *Toxicology and Applied Pharmacology* **46**, 173–182.

Short, R. D., Winston, J. M., Hong, C.-B., Minor, J. L., Lee, C.-C. and Seifter, J. (1979). Effects of ethylene dibromide on reproduction in male and female rats. *Toxicology and Applied Pharmacology* **49**, 97–105.

Wong, O., Utidjian, H. M. D. and Karten, V. S. (1979). Retrospective evaluation of reproductive performance of workers exposed to ethylene dibromide. *Journal of Occupational Medicine* **21**, (2), 98–102.

21. Ethylene Dichloride

TECHNICAL DATA

Formula	$ClCH_2CH_2Cl$
CAS registry number	107–06–02
Chemical abstract name	1,2-Dichloroethane
Synonyms	1,2-Bichloroethane; α,β-dichloro-ethane; symdichloroethane; dichloroethylene; EDC, ENT 1,656; ethylene chloride; ethylene dichloride; glycol dichloride.
Uses	Solvent for fats, oils, waxes, gums, resins and particularly for rubber; manufacture of acetyl-cellulose, tobacco extract.
TLV	10 ppm

ANIMAL STUDIES

A. RELEVANT PHARMACOLOGY AND TOXICOLOGY

No relevant data found.

B. ENDOCRINE AND GONADAL EFFECTS

Vozovaya (1974) exposed 28 sexually mature female rats to $14 \pm 2{\cdot}5$ ppm (57 ± 10 mg/m^3) ethylene dichloride vapour by inhalation for 4 h/day, 6 days/week for 6 months. She noted an increase in the average length of their oestrous cycle due to prolongation of dioestrus, beginning after about one month of exposure and continuing through the rest of exposure, when compared with 26 air-exposed controls (no further details given). However, these females were not infertile as they did mate when paired with males twice, once for 6 days then a second time for 10–12 days (see section C for further details).

C. FERTILITY

In the experiment of Vozovaya (1974) mentioned above, female rats exposed to $14 \pm 2{\cdot}5$ ppm ethylene dichloride for 4 h/day, 6 days/week for 6 months prior to mating took more pair-days to become pregnant than controls (details not given). Of those that mated, the proportion carrying to term was similar in treated and control groups, but fewer pups were born in the treated group, where average litter size was $6{\cdot}5 \pm 1{\cdot}1$ compared with $9{\cdot}7 \pm 0{\cdot}6$ in controls ($p < 0{\cdot}05$). However, since exposure to ethylene dichloride was continued throughout pregnancy, and dams were allowed to deliver and rear their young, it is not known whether this reduction in litter size at birth was due to reduced fertility in the females or due to pre- and post-implantation losses.

Alumot *et al.* (1976) have studied growth, fertility and reproduction in rats fed on mash fumigated with ethylene dichloride to a level of 250 ± 30 ppm or 500 ± 40 ppm. Groups of 18 male and female rats were treated. After 6 weeks on the diet, treated females were mated with untreated males and then at 2-monthly intervals, the females were bred with treated males. Treatment was continued throughout the pregnancies, lactation and until termination of the experiment after 2 years. There were no significant effects on numbers mating, numbers carrying to term, mean litter size, stillbirths, postnatal mortality, or body weight of young at birth or weaning in any of the pregnancies, suggesting that ethylene dichloride up to 500 ppm in the diet has no effect on reproduction in male or female rats.

D. PREGNANCY

In the experiment of Vozovaya (1974) 28 female rats were exposed to ethylene dichloride at 14 ppm for 4 h/day, 6 days/week for 6 months before mating to untreated males, and exposed during the entire course of pregnancy. No significant maternal toxicity could be detected. Litter size at birth was significantly reduced (see section C for details). Stillbirths were significantly increased from 5·1% in controls to 23·1% in treated dams, and birth weight was significantly reduced from 6·4 g in controls to 5·1 g in treated pups. Mortality in the first month of life was significantly increased from 3% in controls to 20% in the treated group. By weaning, the weights of treated and control offspring were similar, possibly due to the smaller numbers of pups to be suckled in the treated group, giving treated pups a growth advantage. After weaning, however, growth of female offspring from treated dams was slower than controls. Males' growth rates were unaffected. Those pups which survived in the treated group did not show any difference from controls in time of eruption of incisors, growth of hair, or opening of the ears and eyes during the preweaning period. At 2, 4 and 6 months of age leukocyte counts and neutrophil phagocytic activity was assessed along with functional tests of the central nervous system, liver and muscular endurance, but no differences were found between treated and control groups. However, study of the oestrous cycle in female offspring showed regular cycles but significantly prolonged oestrus in females from treated dams ($1{\cdot}32 \pm 0{\cdot}07$ days) compared with controls ($1{\cdot}02 \pm 0{\cdot}01$ days). Histology of the ovaries, uterus and tubes carried out at 6 months of age revealed no pathology in the treated group. The female progeny of the first generation, which had been exposed *in utero*, and first generation controls were mated to control males at 3 months of age to produce a second generation. Fertility was not affected, but postnatal mortality was significantly increased from 7% in controls to 18% in the treated group in the first month of life, suggesting an adverse effect on the reproductive capacity of female rats exposed *in utero* only to ethylene dichloride. Larger studies are needed to confirm this.

E. MUTAGENICITY

Ethylene dichloride is mutagenic in bacterial systems with or without metabolic activation, the mutagenic effect being enhanced by metabolic activation, and it has produced single-strand breaks in DNA of hamster cells (studies reviewed by Nylander *et al.*, 1978; IARC Monograph Vol. 20, 1979).

F. CARCINOGENICITY

IARC Monograph Vol. 20 (1979) concluded that there was sufficient evidence that ethylene dichloride is carcinogenic in mice and rats after oral administration.

HUMAN STUDIES

A. RELEVANT PHARMACOLOGY AND TOXICOLOGY

Mukhametova and Vozovaya (1972) have measured the concentration of 1,2-dichloroethane (ethylene dichloride) in blood, fetal tissues and breast milk of female gluing operatives exposed to benzene and chlorinated hydrocarbons, chiefly dichloroethane and methylene chloride, through their work in a mechanical-rubber products factory. The details of the study have been described in section B of Benzene. The concentrations of chlorinated hydrocarbons in the air exceeded the maximum permissible levels (not stated) by 1·2–2·4-fold in 41·5% of measurements. Skin contact also occurred. Unfortunately, the results of the 1,2-dichloroethane measurements in blood and fetal tissues of exposed workers undergoing termination of pregnancy were not given. In women carrying to term, samples of breast milk were analysed in 40 gluing operatives nursing their infants. Both chlorinated hydrocarbons were found and the average level was $0{\cdot}074 \pm 0{\cdot}046$ mg/kg (separate values for methylene chloride and 1,2-dichloroethane not given). Chlorinated hydrocarbons were still found in breast milk 17 h after exposure to them had ceased. Disturbances of lactation (unspecified) were found in 56% of exposed workers compared with 21% of controls and early refusal of the breast was found in an unspecified proportion of the exposed workers' babies, mostly not related to hypogalactia. Thus there is limited evidence that 1,2-dichloroethane passes into the breast milk. The cause(s) of the lactational problems and the babies' refusal to suckle is difficult to ascertain from this study.

B. ENDOCRINE AND GONADAL FUNCTION

In the same study, detailed in section B of Benzene, Mukhametova and Vozovaya (1972) also studied menstrual function and gynaecological disorders in the female gluing operatives. The outcome of these studies has also already been described in section B of Benzene. They indicated an increase in the incidence of menstrual and gynaecological disorders in the gluing operatives compared with controls. However, it is not possible to identify which component(s), if any of the glue were causal factors.

C. FERTILITY

As detailed in section C of Benzene, there were no significant differences in infertility rates in exposed and control groups in the study of Mukhametova and Vozovaya (1972).

D. PREGNANCY

The course and outcome of pregnancies in the study of Mukhametova and Vozovaya (1972) has already been described in detail in section D of Benzene. It is not possible from this study to ascertain what contribution, if any, ethylene dichloride may have made to the increase in "toxicoses", spontaneous abortions and labour complications observed in the exposed group.

E. MUTAGENICITY

No relevant data found.

F. CARCINOGENICITY

IARC Monograph Vol. 20 (1979) reported there were no case studies or epidemiological reports available for evaluation, but since there is sufficient evidence that ethylene dichloride is carcinogenic in rodents, then it is reasonable, for practical purposes, to regard it as if it presented a carcinogenic risk to humans.

SUMMARY AND EVALUATION

EXPERIMENTAL STUDIES

Exposure of female rats to 14 ppm by inhalation daily for 6 months produced some lengthening of the oestrous cycle but did not affect fertility, although litter size and postnatal survival were reduced. Diet containing up to 500 ppm fed to rats over a period of 2 years did not affect fertility, litter size or postnatal development. No studies on teratogenicity were found.

It is mutagenic *in vitro* with and without activation, and is carcinogenic in mice and rats after oral administration. No studies on transplacental carcinogenicity were found.

HUMAN STUDIES

There is limited evidence that ethylene dichloride passes into the breast milk. There are inadequate data to assess the effects on endocrine or gonadal function in exposed women, or on pregnancy. No data were found on mutagenicity or carcinogenicity in humans.

EVALUATION

Evaluation is impossible due to lack of data. Attention is drawn to the lack of teratogenicity data in animals and to the lack of any adequate data on the reproductive effects in humans.

References

Alumot, E., Nachtami, E., Mandel, E. and Holsten, P. (1976). Tolerance and acceptable daily intake of chlorinated fumigants in the rat diet. *Food and Cosmetics Toxicology* **14**, 105–110.

IARC Monographs on the Evaluation of the Carcinogenic Risk of Chemicals to Humans: Some halogenated hydrocarbons (1979). Vol. 20, Lyon, France.

Mukhametova, I. M. and Vozovaya, M. A. (1972). Reproductive power and the incidence of gynecological affections in female workers exposed to the combined effect of benzine and chlorinated hydrocarbons. *Gigiena Truda i Professional'nye Zabolevaniya* **16**, (11), 6–9.

Nylander, P., Olofsson, H., Rasmuson, B. and Svahlin, H. (1978). Mutagenic effects of petrol in Drosophila melanogaster. 1. Effects of benzene and 1,2-dichloroethane. *Mutation Research* **57**, (2), 163–167.

Vozovaya, M. A. (1974). Development of posterity of two generations obtained from females subjected to the action of dichloroethane. *Gigiena I. Sanitariya* **(7)**, 25–28.

22. Ethylene Oxide

TECHNICAL DATA

Formula	(epoxide ring: O bridging H_2C—CH_2)
CAS registry number	75–21–8
Chemical abstracts name	Oxirane
Synonyms	Dihydrooxirene; dimethylene oxide; 1-2-epoxyethane; ethylene oxide, ETO; oxacyclopropane; oxane; oxidoethane; α,β-oxidoethane.
Uses	Fumigant for foodstuffs and textiles. To sterilize surgical instruments. Agricultural fungicide. In organic syntheses, especially in the production of ethylene glycol. Starting material for the manufacture of acrylonitrile and nonionic surfactants.
TLV	50 ppm (1980 Intended change to 10 ppm).

ANIMAL STUDIES

A. RELEVANT PHARMACOLOGY AND TOXICOLOGY

Appelgren *et al*. (1977) have studied the distribution of intravenously injected or inhaled ^{14}C-ethylene oxide by whole body radioautography in the mouse. There was no quantitative difference in distribution of radioactivity between the 2 routes of administration with the exception of the lung mucosal membranes which showed a marked accumulation by the inhalational route only. This suggests that i.v. injection permitting more accurate dosing might be an acceptable route for toxicity studies in terms of reaching the same tissues, though the pharmacokinetics following bolus injection might be markedly different from steady inhalation over a long period of time. This work indicated that the concentration of ethylene oxide and/or its metabolites in the testis and epididymis was higher than that in the blood 20 min–4 h after i.v. injection. However, quantitative studies by Ehrenberg *et al.* (1974) have shown that testis tissue concentrations of radioactivity up to 3·5 h after inhalation are close to the expected average assuming uniform distribution, whereas liver and kidney levels are much higher than average.

B. ENDOCRINE AND GONADAL EFFECTS

Hollingsworth *et al.* (1956) exposed a number of species to various concentrations of ethylene oxide by inhalation for 7 h/day, 5 days/week for 25 weeks. The highest dose used, 841 ppm, was lethal to most species within a few days. At 357 ppm, in the guinea pig, they observed degeneration of testicular tubules with replacement fibrosis, accompanied by general growth depression. In the rat, exposure to 357 ppm caused death within 6 weeks, and it is not clear whether the testes were examined. In the rabbit and monkey testicular effects were not reported at 357 ppm but exposures were for shorter periods of 9–12 weeks. At 204 ppm there was slight testicular tubal degeneration in the rat, accompanied by other signs of toxicity such as growth depression, increased kidney and liver weights, and secondary respiratory infections which resulted in over 50% mortality. At this dose level there was also a small but non-significant decrease in testicular weights in guinea pigs and rats. At lower dose levels of 113 and 49 ppm there was no effect on the testes in rats, guinea pigs or rabbits.

Strekalova *et al.* (1975) exposed male rats to 2 or 62 ppm (3·6 or 112 mg/m^3) for 66 days. The duration of daily exposure was not specified. After mating with untreated females for assessment of dominant lethal effects (see section C) the males were killed and functional tests carried out on the spermatozoa as well as testicular histology and biochemistry. There were no significant effects on sperm number, motility, viability, morphology, osmotic or acid resistance. Histologically, there were no reductions in the spermatogenesis index, number of spermatogonia, number of tubules with seminiferous epithelium or number of tubules with the twelfth stage of meiosis. There was a reduction in RNA but not DNA content of testicular homogenate in both exposed groups relative to controls, but the difference was only just significant and was not dose related.

C. FERTILITY

A number of dominant lethal studies have been reported in rodents. Appelgren *et al.* (1977) gave single i.v. injections of 25, 50 or 100 mg/kg to groups of 5 male mice. A negative control group (i.v. saline) and a positive control group (i.v. cyclophosphamide) were also included. Following injection, each male was mated with 3 fresh females a week for 8 weeks and the females killed 17 days after placing with the males. Total implantation sites, dead fetuses and resorptions were counted. Only random, non dose-related significant differences were found occasionally between ethylene oxide and negative control groups and pregnancy rate was unaffected. The positive controls showed a significant, dose dependent increase in dead implants. Injection of 200 mg/kg interfered with the ability to mate and was lethal to some animals within 2–3 days. Others have reported an LD50 of 260 mg/kg for i.v. ethylene oxide in the mouse (see review by Glaser, (1979)).

In the rat, dominant lethal effects have been found following inhalation exposure. Embree *et al.* (1977) exposed 15 male rats to 1000 ppm ethylene oxide for 4 h. A group of 10 rats exposed to filtered air for 4 h and given i.p. olive oil served as negative controls, and 10 rats given i.p. triethylenemelamine as positive controls. Twenty-four hours after treatment the males were mated with 2 fresh females/week for 10 weeks. The females were killed 17 days after placing with the males and scored for corpora lutea, total implants, early and late fetal deaths. In the first 5 weeks after treatment, significant reductions in fertility and/or significant increases in post-implantation deaths were seen in the ethylene oxide group in comparison with negative controls. Fertility ranged from 47–67% in ethylene oxide treated rats, compared with 67–100% in controls, and the proportion of dead implants from 10–30% in the ethylene oxide group compared with 2–10% in controls. There was no effect on pre-implantation losses and fertility and mutagenic indexes were not affected in weeks 6–10, suggesting that ethylene oxide only affects sperm stages following meiotic division. Positive controls showed the expected increase in pre- and post-implantation losses, with no significant reduction in fertility, in weeks 1–5. It should be noted that all rats exposed to ethylene oxide showed signs of general toxicity, viz. central depression, diarrhoea, ocular and respiratory irritation, but they recovered within 24 h and no deaths occurred. Some have reported death in the rat following 8 h exposure to 1,100 ppm whereas others have reported no deaths after 4 h exposure to 4000 ppm but 100% lethality after 4 h exposure to 8000 ppm (see review by Glaser, (1979)).

The effects of much lower exposures for longer periods in the rat have also been reported. Strekalova *et al.* (1975) exposed males to 0 (n = 21), 2 (n = 24) or 62 (n = 14) ppm (3·6 or 112 mg/m^3) for 66 days, sufficient to cover the whole sperm cycle. The males were mated once during the last 4 days of exposure to ethylene oxide, the females being killed on day 21 of pregnancy and scored for corpora lutea, total implants and dead implants. After mating, the males were killed and a functional study of the spermatozoa, histology and biochemistry of the testes were carried out (see section B). Fertility and post-implantation losses were unaffected but pre-implantation losses were 11% in controls, 36% at 2 ppm and 48% at 62 ppm.

As part of a single generation reproduction study, Snellings *et al.* (1979) exposed male and female weanling rats to 10, 33 or 100 ppm for 6 h/day, 5 days/week for 12 weeks. They were then mated, but the report (in abstract only) does not make it clear whether treated rats were mated to other treated rats or to untreated rats. Fertility was stated to be reduced in females exposed to 100 ppm but no details were given. No conclusions may be drawn about dominant lethal effects since exposure to ethylene oxide was continued during pregnancy. (The outcome of pregnancy in this study is reported in section D.)

Conclusion

In view of the difficulties in assessing the data from long-term exposure and the marked effects seen at a high dose after only 4 h exposure to ethylene oxide, further fertility and dominant lethal studies employing a range of doses is needed in order to establish a no-effect level.

D. PREGNANCY

Two teratology studies on ethylene oxide have been reported, both in abstract only. Kimmel and Laborde (1979) gave 75 or 150 mg/kg ethylene oxide by i.v. injection to mice in 3 day periods during the first half of pregnancy. Preliminary work showed that a higher dose of 200 mg/kg caused high maternal mortality and so was not used in the full teratology study. At 75 and 150 mg/kg the dams showed general signs of ethylene oxide toxicity especially at the higher dose, but maternal body weight was not affected. Treatment on days 4–6 or 10–12 of pregnancy caused a significant increase in resorptions at both dose levels, whilst treatment on days 6–8 or 8–10 significantly increased malformations at 150 mg/kg only. No details were given of the incidence of these effects. Malformations reported were fused vertebral arches, fused and branched ribs, scrambled sternebrae and a low incidence of exencephaly.

Snellings *et al.* (1979) reported absence of embryotoxicity and teratogenicity with inhalational exposure to 10, 33 or 100 ppm in the rat exposed for 6 h/day from days 6–15 of pregnancy. However, there was a significant reduction in fetal body weight at 100 ppm. In a single generation study, Snellings *et al.* (1979) exposed male and female weanling rats to 10, 33 or 100 ppm for 6 h/day 5 days/week for 12 weeks, then mated them, with exposure continuing to day 19 of gestation and from day 5–21 of lactation. It is not clear whether treated animals were mated to other treated animals or to controls. Effects were seen at 100 ppm where exposed females had reduced fertility, prolonged gestation and smaller litters compared with controls. Postnatal survival of pups was unaffected.

Conclusion

Ethylene oxide in the mouse has been shown to be embryotoxic at 75 and 150 mg/kg i.v. and possibly teratogenic at 150 but not 75 mg/kg i.v. and embryo- and fetotoxic in the rat at 100 ppm but not 33 ppm. Further studies are required to establish no-effect levels for different routes of administration.

E. MUTAGENICITY

Ethylene oxide is mutagenic in bacterial systems. Mutagenic effects have also been observed in rodents following inhalational exposure to ethylene oxide. Fomenko and Strekalova (1973) exposed rats to 0·55–1·67 ppm or 16·7–33·3 ppm for 2, 4, 8 and 30 day periods and carried out aberration and mitotic index counts in bone marrow cells. With exposure to the lower range of concentrations, chromosome aberrations were not increased at 2, 4 or 8 days but were significantly increased at 30 days (9·8% compared with 3% in controls). At the higher concentrations, chromosome aberrations were increased significantly on the second (7·1%), fourth (8·4%), eighth (11·3%) and thirtieth (11·6%) days. Chromosome breaks were the principle aberration seen.

In a similar study, Strekalova *et al.* (1975) have also exposed rats to 2 or 62 ppm for 66 days and found an increase in chromosome aberrations from 2·6% in controls to 7·6% at 2 ppm and 9·4% at 62 ppm at the end of the exposure period. These exposures also caused a significant increase in pre-implantation losses in the dominant lethal test (see section C). In neither of the above experiments was the daily duration of inhalation exposure stated.

Appelgren *et al.* (1978) have found mutagenic effects in the micronucleus test in rats and mice following i.v. injection of doses of 50–200 mg/kg 30 h and 6 h before the animals are killed. The percentage of bone marrow cells with micronuclei was significantly increased at 150 mg/kg (1/3 of the LD50) in mice and at 100 mg/kg (1/5 of the LD50) in rats.

F. CARCINOGENICITY

IARC Monograph Vol. 11 (1976) reported that the data available at that time did not permit evaluation of the carcinogenicity of ethylene oxide in animals.

HUMAN STUDIES

A. RELEVANT PHARMACOLOGY AND TOXICOLOGY

No relevant data found.

C. FERTILITY

Other than the Russian study referred to below, no data were found on the reproductive effects of ethylene oxide. In an extensive review of the toxicology and hospital use of ethylene oxide by Glaser (1979) prepared for N.I.O.S.H., and which concentrated on its mutagenic, teratogenic and carcinogenic potential, it is stated that no human data is available on which to assess the teratogenicity of ethylene oxide.

B. & D. ENDOCRINE AND GONADAL EFFECTS/PREGNANCY

There is one study of the effects of working in an ethylene oxide production plant on the health of women workers (Yakubova *et al.*, 1976). They studied the incidence of gynaecological disorders and also pregnancy outcome in women employed at the Kazanskii organic synthesis factory. In all 541 women workers were studied, 282 in ethylene oxide production and 259 co-workers in plant management. A control group of 100 other women, probably from another part of the town and without contact with chemicals, was included. Many important details about the selection of the sample populations, their age distributions, previous reproductive histories, socio-economic status, actual exposure to ethylene oxide, etc., are not recorded so that it is very difficult to assess the paper critically. Furthermore, the actual disease states mentioned are difficult to understand and no definitions or criteria of severity are included. In addition, the women involved in ethylene oxide synthesis were exposed to sudden changes in temperature and pressure and a high frequency noise of 75–90 decibels from the equipment as well as the ethylene oxide in the atmosphere which was below the MAC of 1 mg/m^3. It is uncertain which of the effects observed related directly to the ethylene oxide.

Yakubova *et al.* (1976) reported that the incidence of gynaecological disorders was 55/282 (19·5%) in the production workers compared with 20/259 (7·7%) in plant management and 6/100 (6%) of the controls. The commonest condition was erosion of the cervix in about 8–16% of the production workers depending in which part of the process they were involved compared with 1% of management staff and control groups. Inflammatory disease of the uterus was also about 3 times more common in the production workers compared with the others.

The pregnancy data are difficult to assess also because of lack of details, but they reported on pregnancies in 95 production workers, 65 plant management workers and 50 controls. Eighty-nine per cent of the first group were aged 20–29 compared with 65% and 68% in the other 2 groups, the majority of the rest being 30–39 years of age. There was a history of a higher incidence of spontaneous abortions (15/95) in the production workers compared with management (6/65) but no details are given of this in relation to prior exposure to ethylene oxide. In the study pregnancies, treatment for threatened abortion was required in 23 production workers (related also to duration of service) compared with 4 management and no controls. Abortions occurred in 9 of the production workers compared with 5 in management. Anaemia was more common (6/95) in production staff than in management (1/65), as well as "toxicosis" in the second half of pregnancy affecting 30% of production workers compared with 5% and 8% in management and controls. No other significant effects were observed. It is impossible to assess these data critically because of the paucity of details. No indication is given of the time scale over which the pregnancy data was collected nor of the relative numbers of married and unmarried women in the different groups. so no inference of any effects on fertility can be made. The data on abortions and threatened abortions, however, do indicate a possible difference between the production workers and the others, but whether this relates to the ethylene oxide or to other environmental factors cannot be assessed.

E. MUTAGENICITY

Ehrenberg and Hällström (1967) investigated 8 workers exposed to a high (unmeasured) concentration of ethylene oxide for about 2 hours following an accidental tube burst in a factory. The exposure was high enough for 2 of the workers to require hospital treatment for respiratory difficulties. Eighteen months after the accident, chromosomal aberrations were studied in lymphocyte preparations (details of method not described) of 7 of the men with an average of 20 (range 6–26) metaphases per person, and the results compared with 10 control, unexposed workers from the same factory. A clear increase in gross aberrations, i.e. breaks, exchanges and supernumerary chromosomes was detected from the control level of 4·3% to 17·5% ($p<0{\cdot}05$). The authors calculated that the breaking effect of ethylene oxide at the exposure level of this accident was equivalent to the action of 50–100 rad of acute total body γ-irradiation.

In a subsequent publication, Ehrenberg *et al.* (1974) discuss a possible method of assessing the genetic risk from alkylating agents like ethylene oxide in terms of their radiation dose equivalent. They calculate, from data on mouse exposures, that ethylene oxide workers exposed to 5 ppm for a 40-hour week receive a weekly gonadal dose amounting to 4 rad-equivalents. This is about 40 times the maximum permissible dose to radiological workers of 0·1 rad/week.

F. CARCINOGENICITY

IARC Monograph Vol. 11 (1976) reported at that time that no data on the carcinogenicity of ethylene oxide in humans was available. Hogstedt *et al.* (1979) reported 3 cases of leukaemia, 2 female, 1 male, between 1972 and 1977 in a small group of Swedish workers exposed to ethylene oxide at a time-weighted average of 20 ± 10 ppm. The expected number of cases from such a group size was 0·2. However, larger studies are required to confirm whether ethylene oxide is carcinogenic in humans.

SUMMARY AND EVALUATION

EXPERIMENTAL STUDIES

Studies in rats, rabbits and monkeys have not shown any specific testicular damage at otherwise non-toxic doses, i.e. less than 200 ppm. Negative results have been obtained in dominant lethal studies in mice injected i.v. with 100 mg/kg, but decreased fertility and increase in dead implants has been reported in rats exposed to a toxic dose of 1000 ppm. The effect persisted for 5 weeks after exposure. Reduced litter size has also been reported following exposure of rats to 2 and 62 ppm for 2 months. Abstracts only have been published of 2 teratology studies in mice and rats. At doses toxic to the dams, embryo and fetal toxicity were observed with some malformations at 150 mg/kg i.v. in mice. In rats, exposure to 100 ppm by inhalation caused reduction in fetal body weight but was not teratogenic. Mutagenic effects have been observed both *in vitro* and *in vivo*.

HUMAN STUDIES

An increased incidence of gynaecological disorders and abortions has been reported in workers in an ethylene oxide production plant but the data is inadequate to determine if these effects related to exposure to ethylene oxide. No other studies were found on effects on fertility or on pregnancy. Chromosomal damage has been reported in exposed workers and it has been calculated that occupational exposure to 5 ppm is almost equivalent to a radiation dose of 4 rad-equivalents per week. Only one report on the possible association of exposure to ethylene oxide with leukaemia has been published.

EVALUATION

The available data are inadequate to assess the reproductive toxicity of ethylene oxide in animals or humans. There is sufficient evidence, however, that it is mutagenic *in vitro* and *in vivo*, but the data on carcinogenicity is inadequate for evaluation.

References

Appelgren, L. E., Eneroth, G. and Grant, C. (1977). Studies on ethylene oxide: whole-body autoradiography and dominant lethal tests in mice. *Proceedings of the European Society for Toxicology* **18**, 315–317.

Appelgren, L. E., Eneroth, G., Grant, C., Landstrom, L. E. and Tenghagen, K. (1978). Testing of ethylene oxide for mutagenicity using the micronucleus test in mice and rats. *Acta Pharmacologica et Toxicologica* **43**, (1), 69–71.

Ehrenberg, L. and Hällström, T. (1967). Haematologic studies on persons occupationally exposed to ethylene oxide. *International Atomic Energy Report*, SM-92/26, 327–334.

Ehrenberg, L., Hiesche, K. D., Osterman-Golkar, S. and Wennberg, I. (1974). Evaluation of genetic risks of alkylating agents: tissue doses in the mouse from air contaminated with ethylene oxide. *Mutation Research* **24**, 83–103.

Embree, J. W., Lyon, J. P. and Hine, C. H. (1977). The mutagenic potential of ethylene oxide using the dominant lethal assay in rats. *Toxicology and Applied Pharmacology* **40**, 261–267.

Fomenko, V. N. and Strekalova, E. E. (1973). Mutagenic action of some industrial poisons as a function of concentration and exposure time. *Toksikologiya Novykh Promyshlennykh Khimicheskikh Veshchestvh* **13**, 51–57.

Glaser, Z. R. (1979). Ethylene oxide: toxicology review and field study results of hospital use. *Journal of Environmental Pathology and Toxicology* **2**, (5), 173–207.

Hogstedt, C., Malmqvist, N. and Wadman, B. (1979). Leukemia in workers exposed to ethylene oxide. *Journal of the American Medical Association* **241**, 1132–1133.

Hollingsworth, R. L., Rowe, V. K., Oyen, F., McCollister, D. D. and Spencer, H. C. (1956). Toxicity of ethylene oxide determined on experimental animals. *American Medical Association Archives of Industrial Health* **13**, 217–227.

IARC Monographs on the Evaluation of the Carcinogenic Risk of Chemicals to Humans: Cadmium, nickel, some epoxides, miscellaneous industrial chemicals and general considerations on volatile anaesthetics (1976). Vol. 11, Lyon, France.

Kimmel, C. A. and Laborde, J. B. (1979). Teratogenic potential of ethylene oxide. *Teratology* **19**, 34A–35A.

Snellings, W. M., Pringle, J. L., Dorko, J. D. and Kintigh, W. J. (1979). Teratology and reproduction studies with rats exposed to 10, 33 or 100 ppm of ethylene oxide. *Toxicology and Applied Pharmacology* **48**, (1), A84.

Strekalova, E. E., Chirkova, E. M. and Holubovich, E. (1975). On the mutagenic action of ethylene oxide on the reproductive and somatic cells of male white rats. *Toksikologiya Novykh Promyshlennykh Khimicheskikh Veshchestvh* **14**, 11–16.

Yakubova, Z. N., Shamova, N. A., Miftakhova, F. A. and Shilova, L. F. (1976). Gynecological disorders in workers engaged in ethylene oxide production. *Kazanskii Meditsinskii Zhurnal* **57**, (6), 558–560.

23. Fluorocarbons

TECHNICAL DATA

(a) *Trichlorofluoromethane*

Formula CCl_3F

Synonyms Trichloromonofluoromethane; fluorotrichloromethane; fluorocarbon 11; Freon 11; Refrigerant 11; Arcton 9.

Uses Refrigerant; aerosol propellant; solvent.

TLV 1000 ppm

(b) *Dichlorodifluoromethane*

Formula CCl_2F_2

Synonyms Difluorodichloromethane; fluorocarbon 12; Freon 12; Refrigerant 12; Arcton 6.

Uses Refrigerant; aerosol propellant.

TLV 1000 ppm

(c) *Dichlorofluoromethane*

Formula $CHFCl_2$

Synonyms Dichloromonofluoromethane; fluorodichloromethane; fluorocarbon 21; Freon 21; Refrigerant 21; Arcton 7.

Uses	Refrigerant; aerosol propellant.
TLV	10 ppm

(d) *Chlorodifluoromethane*

Formula	$CHClF_2$
Synonyms	Fluorocarbon 22; Freon 22; Refrigerant 22.
Uses	Refrigerant
TLV	1000 ppm

(e) *1,1,2-trichloro-1,2,2-trifluoroethane*

Formula	$FCCl_2CClF_2$
Synonyms	Fluorocarbon 113; Freon 113; Refrigerant 113; TCTFE.
Uses	Refrigerant; solvent.
TLV	1000 ppm

(f) *1,2-dichloro-1,1,2,2-tetrafluoroethane*

Formula	$ClCF_2CClF_2$
Synonyms	Fluorocarbon 114; Freon 114; Refrigerant 114; Arcton 33; cryofluorane.
Uses	Refrigerant; aerosol propellant.
TLV	1000 ppm

ANIMAL STUDIES

A. RELEVANT PHARMACOLOGY AND TOXICOLOGY

The reproductive toxicity of several fluorocarbons has been studied by the Haskell Laboratory of Du Pont, U.S.A. and by I.C.I. Ltd., Mond Division, U.K. both major manufacturers of fluorocarbons, but only summaries of the results have been released. These and other available published data on fluorocarbons are reviewed below. Wherever possible, the chemical name of the fluorocarbon studied as well as its identification has been given.

B. ENDOCRINE AND GONADAL EFFECTS

No relevant data found.

C. FERTILITY

In a large study by Epstein *et al.* (1972) investigating 174 different test agents, fluorocarbon-112 and fluorocarbon-113 (1,1,2-trichloro-, and 1,2,2-trifluoroethane) were found to have no dominant lethal effects in the mouse. Males were given i.p. doses of 200 mg/kg (7 mice) or 1000 mg/kg (9 mice) and then caged with 3 virgin females per week for 8 consecutive weeks. The females were killed 13 days after the midweek of being caged with the males and scored for pregnancy, total implantation sites, live implants, early and late intrauterine deaths. There were no deaths of treated males and no dominant lethal effects or reduction in pregnancy rate in comparison with results from 10 concurrent untreated controls.

In a study reported in abstract only, Coate *et al.* (1979) exposed male rats and monkeys to fluorocarbon-31 (monochloromonofluoromethane), 0·5% for 6 h/day for 20 days. They noted "minimal to slight hypospermatogenesis" in rats but not monkeys. At 0·1% there was no effect after 20 days exposure, but after 13 weeks hypospermatogenesis, which did not reverse with a 4 week recovery period and occurred in the absence of any other toxic effects, was again evident in rats. Male rats exposed to 0·1% for 10 weeks, then mated to untreated females over the next 16 weeks showed reduced fertility (lower pregnancy rate) during the whole of this time, but no dominant lethal effects were seen.

D. PREGNANCY

The teratogenicity of fluorocarbon-12 (dichlorodifluoromethane) has been investigated as part of a study on triamcinolone acetate administered as an aerosol to pregnant rabbits (Brar *et al.*, 1976). The study is reported in abstract only. Rabbits (number not stated) were restrained and exposed by inhalation to fluorocarbon-12 (concentration and duration of exposure not stated) from days 6–18 of pregnancy and killed on day 30. A low incidence of cleft palate and/or hydrocephalus was seen in all treatment groups (triamcinolone plus fluorocarbon-12, fluorocarbon-12 alone and restrained unexposed controls). In the fluorocarbon-12 group one litter was affected. However, there is insufficient data presented to evaluate the teratogenicity of fluorocarbon-12.

As part of a study on isoproterenol aerosol by Vogin *et al.* (1970), a mixture of fluorocarbon-12 (dichlorodifluoromethane) and fluorocarbon-114 (dichlorotetrafluoroethane) was administered to pregnant rats and rabbits. Rats were exposed by inhalation, twice daily for 15 min/exposure on days 5 or 6 to 16 or 17 of pregnancy or day 15 or 16 of pregnancy until weaning and rabbits were similarly exposed on days 6–16 of pregnancy. The concentration of fluorocarbons was not stated. The rats exposed during embryogenesis were killed on day 20 or 21 of pregnancy and the fetuses examined by adequate teratological methods. The numbers of implantation sites, live fetuses, intrauterine deaths and fetal weight did not differ significantly between treatment groups (isoproterenol plus fluorocarbons, fluorocarbons alone and placebo). The study however is unusual in that no soft tissue or skeletal malformations were recorded in a total of 494 fetuses from the various treatment groups, although in the discussion the authors state that: "the usual variations often seen in animals submitted to teratogenic investigation . . . were also evident. . . ." There were no differences in "variations" between groups. Delayed ossification was seen in 80–90% of the fetuses from 3 of the 4 treatment groups including fluorocarbons alone and placebo. However, these data were impossible to evaluate since the exact gestational age composition of the fetuses in each group was not stated, some dams being killed on day 20, others on day 21 of pregnancy.

In the same study by Vogin *et al.* (1970) rats exposed to fluorocarbons 12 and 114 from the third week of pregnancy through to weaning had high offspring mortality; only 4/7 litters born were still alive at 4 days of age. However, the 3 litters lost were very small, comprising only 6 pups altogether, and in the isoproterenol plus fluorocarbons group postnatal mortality was low and did not differ from the placebo group. There were no significant effects on offspring mortality between 4 and 21 days of age, or on body weights at birth and 21 days of age. No gross abnormalities were seen from external observation of the pups, but neither detailed autopsies nor specific developmental and behaviour tests were carried out.

In the rabbit teratology part of this same study by Vogin *et al.* (1970) on fluorocarbons 12 and 114, dams were killed on day 30, the pups placed in an incubator for 12 h for assessment of viability, then killed and examined. There were no significant differences between groups in survival, implantation rates, live litter size, intrauterine mortality or fetal weight. No malformations were recorded in a total of 247 fetuses from the 4 treatment groups. Retarded ossification was seen in all groups and attributed to the trauma of the exposure conditions (restraint with inhalation from a face-mask).

Three other fluorocarbons have been examined for teratological effects in the rat by Kelly *et al.* (1978) from Du Pont. The results have been reported in abstract only. Groups of 25 rats were exposed by inhalation for 6 h/day to fluorocarbon-142b (chlorodifluoroethane) at 1000 or 10,000 ppm on days 4–15 of pregnancy or to 10,000 ppm of fluorocarbon-123 (2,2-dichloro-1,1,1-trifluoroethane) or fluorocarbon-21 (dichlorofluoromethane) on days 6–15 of pregnancy. No embryotoxic or teratogenic effects were observed with fluorocarbons 142b or 123. Fluorocarbon-21 reduced maternal body weight gain and caused pre-implantation loss of all fertilized ova in 15/25 dams, but was not teratogenic to surviving embryos. In a study by Anan'ina (1972), where rats were exposed continuously to fluorocarbon-21 from days 1–21 of pregnancy, it was reported that DNA levels were reduced in liver and brain of the dams and their fetuses, and in the ovaries and placentae. No further details of exposure levels, numbers of animals, or DNA levels were given. The TLV for fluorocarbon-21 has recently been lowered from 1000 ppm to 10 ppm (Threshold Limit Values for 1980, Health and Safety Executive, U.K., October 1980).

In a study reported in abstract only (Coate *et al.*, 1979), where only brief experimental methods and results were mentioned, rats were exposed to fluorocarbon-31 at 0·1% for 6 h/day from days 6–15 of pregnancy. The authors noted an incidence of cervical ribs in 8/208 treated fetuses but no control rates were given and the significance level was not stated. No other teratological effects were found.

Teratology studies on fluorocarbon-22 (chlorodifluoromethane) have been carried out by the Haskell Laboratory, Du Pont, U.S.A. and by I.C.I., Mond Division, U.K. The results are available in summary only in statements issued by these 2 companies. In the I.C.I. study, a significant increase in anophthalmia was seen in rat offspring at an exposure level of 50,000 ppm (numbers affected not stated). Anophthalmia was seen also at lower levels but the incidence did not differ significantly from that seen in controls. No cases of anophthalmia were seen in rabbits, even at 50,000 ppm (Anonymous, 1979). Similar work on fluorocarbons 11 (trichlorofluoromethane) and 12 showed no teratogenic effects (Anonymous, 1979). However, in the experiments conducted by Du Pont, anophthalmia and microphthalmia has been found in rats at several exposure levels down to as low as 500 ppm (Anonymous, 1977a). The appearance of the same specific eye defects in 2 separate studies at considerably different dose levels clearly warrants further investigation. In view of their data, Du Pont have taken the precautionary measures of equipping women employees of childbearing age with respirators where practicable or excluding them from exposure (Anonymous, 1977a). I.C.I. have recommended minimizing exposure to fluorocarbon-22 and ensuring good ventilation with "no need, on the basis of evidence so far, to take additional precautions" (Anonymous, 1977b; 1978).

E. MUTAGENICITY

Screening for mutagenicity using short-term tests has been carried out by Du Pont (Anonymous, 1979). Fluorocarbon-22 (chlorodifluoromethane) was positive in the Ames test but negative in 4 other (unspecified) tests. Fluorocarbons 11 (trichlorofluoromethane) and 12 (dichlorodifluoromethane) were negative in the same 5 tests, and fluorocarbon-115 was negative in the 2 most reliable test systems used (not tested in the other 3). I.C.I. (Anonymous, 1976) have themselves tested fluorocarbon-22 in 6 different short-term tests and confirmed that it is positive in the Ames test. Of the remaining tests, 4 were negative and one gave uncertain results. Cell transformation tests (Anonymous, 1978) on fluorocarbon-22 have been found to be negative, but in other studies (details not given) on rats and mice a "weak mutagenic effect" has been observed which was not dose related.

F. CARCINOGENICITY

No relevant data found.

HUMAN STUDIES

No relevant data found on any aspect of reproductive toxicity, mutagenicity or carcinogenicity (but see end of section D in Animal Studies).

SUMMARY AND EVALUATION

EXPERIMENTAL STUDIES

No studies were found on endocrine or gonadal effects. FC112 (1,1,2,trichloroethane) and FC113 (1,2,2,trifluoroethane) did not produce dominant lethal mutations in mice given 200 or 1000 mg/kg i.p. in one study. FC31 (monochloromonofluoromethane) has been reported to cause reduced sperm count and reduced fertility in rats chronically exposed to 0·1% by inhalation daily, but not in monkeys exposed to 0·5%. Recovery was not observed in the rat study over 4 months, but details of this study have not been published.

Although teratogenicity studies involving FC12 (dichlorodifluoromethane), FC114 (dichlorotetrafluoroethane), FC142b (chlorodifluoroethane), FC123 (2,2 dichloro-1,1,1-trifluoroethane), FC21 (dichlorofluoromethane) and FC31 have been published, the studies have either been inadequately performed or inadequately reported so that no conclusions about effects in pregnancy can be reached.

Studies carried out by two laboratories, but reported only in summary, have demonstrated teratogenic effects from FC22 (chlorodifluoromethane) in rats. Studies from one laboratory reported anophthalmia and microphthalmia at exposure levels as low as 500 ppm. The second laboratory reported the same defects but only significantly increased at 50,000 ppm. The defect was not seen in rabbits exposed to 50,000 ppm. Negative mutagenicity results have been reported for FC11, FC12 and FC115 in a variety of unspecified tests. FC22 has been reported positive by two laboratories in the Ames test but negative or equivocal in other tests.

No data on carcinogenicity were found.

HUMAN STUDIES

No studies were found on endocrine or gonadal effects or of effects on fertility, pregnancy, mutagenicity or carcinogenicity.

EVALUATION

Limited studies have shown that FC31 may reduce the sperm count and fertility of rats. Unpublished studies have reported that FC22 is teratogenic in rats but not rabbits, producing microphthalmia and anophthalmia. Since this is a very rare defect in rats and has been reported by two different groups of workers, this must be considered as a specific teratogenic effect. In the absence of published data it is impossible to assess the hazard to man.

Attention is drawn to the lack of adequate experimental data on the other fluorocarbons and to the absence of carcinogenicity data on FC22 which is positive in the Ames test. Attention is also drawn to the lack of any human data on the reproductive effects of fluorocarbons. Because of the reported specific teratogenicity of FC22, a risk evaluation with regard to exposure of women is required.

References

Anan'ina, T. (1972). Effect of aliphatic and halogenated hydrocarbons on the concentration of nucleic acids in animal tissues during embryogenesis. *Trudy-Permskogo Gosudarstvennogo Meditsinskogo Instituta* **110**, 69–71.

Anonymous. (1976). Test results on chlorodifluoromethane (R 22). I.C.I. Ltd., Mond Division.

Anonymous. (1977a). Statement on fluorocarbon 22. Du Pont Information Service.

Anonymous. (1977b). Refrigerant 22. I.C.I. Ltd., Mond Division.

Anonymous. (1978). Refrigerant 22. I.C.I. Ltd., Mond Division.

Anonymous. (1979). Safety aspects of chlorofluorocarbon refrigerants. I.C.I. Ltd., Mond Division.

Brar, B. S., Jackson, B. A., Traitor, C. E., Rodwell, D. E., Boshart, C. R. and Noble. J. F. (1976).Triamcinolone acetonide (1,4-pregnadiene-3,20-dione, 9a-fluoro-11b, 21 dihydroxy 16a, 17a-(isopropylidenedioxy)); aerosol inhalation and teratology studies in rabbits. *Toxicology and Applied Pharmacology* **37**, 151–152.

Coate, W. B., Voelker, R. and Kapp, R. W. (1979). Inhalation Toxicity of Monochloromonofluoromethane. *Toxicology and Applied Pharmacology* **48**, A109.

Epstein, S. S.., Arnold, E., Andrea, J., Bass, W. and Bishop, Y. (1972). Detection of chemical mutagens by the dominant lethal assay in the mouse. *Toxicology and Applied Pharmacology* **23**, 288–325.

Kelly, D. P., Culik, R., Trochimowicz, H. J. and Fayerweather, W. E. (1978). Inhalation teratology studies on three fluorocarbons. *Toxicology and Applied Pharmacology* **45** (1), 293.

Vogin, E. E., Goldhamer, R. E., Scheimberg, J., Carson, S. and Boxill, G. C. (1970). Teratology studies in rats and rabbits exposed to an isoproterenol aerosol. *Toxicology and Applied Pharmacology* **16**, 374–381.

24. Formaldehyde

TECHNICAL DATA

Formula	HCHO
CAS registry number	50–00–0
Chemical abstracts name	Formaldehyde gas, solution
Synonyms	Methanal; oxomethane; oxymethylene; methylene oxide; formic aldehyde; methyl aldehyde.
Uses	Ionizing solvent; manufacture of formic esters, resins, leather, rubber, metals and woods.
TLV	2 ppm

ANIMAL STUDIES

A. RELEVANT PHARMACOLOGY AND TOXICOLOGY

Sanotskii *et al.* (1976) have compared the toxicity of inhaled formaldehyde in the pregnant and non-pregnant rat. Females were exposed for 20 days (in the case of pregnant rats, from days 1–20 of pregnancy), for 4 h/day to 0, 0·33 or 5 ppm (0, 0·4 or 6·0 mg/m^3). The number of rats in each treatment group was not specified but was within the range 8–32. Fifteen different measures of toxicity were assessed on days 16 and 20 of exposure. In non-pregnant rats exposed to 5 ppm, 4 measures differed significantly from controls; altered kidney function was evident from the decreased urinary volume and chloride content, and increased urinary albumin content; altered liver function was evident from the reduction in hippuric acid excretion in the urine following a sodium benzoate load. In pregnant rats exposed to 5 ppm, the only sign of toxicity was reduced haemoglobin content of the blood. There were no signs of toxicity in non-pregnant or pregnant rats exposed to 0·33 ppm. This study suggests non-pregnant rats may be more susceptible to formaldehyde toxicity than pregnant rats.

B. ENDOCRINE AND GONADAL EFFECTS

Females

Injections of formalin,* given s.c., induce pseudopregnancy in the rat, possibly by altering gonadotrophin secretion (Chatterjee, 1965). However, injection of formalin provokes a marked stress response (Solem, 1966) and is frequently used as a non-specific "stressor" in animal experiments. Thus the oestrous cycle disturbances observed may be secondary to the numerous hormonal and metabolic changes induced by stress, particularly high ACTH secretion. Support for this possibility comes from a study showing normal oestrous cycles can be restored in rats injected with formalin by giving cortisone, which suppresses ACTH secretion (Chatterjee, 1965).

It is not known whether exposure to non-stressful levels of formaldehyde, say by inhalation, affect gonadotrophin levels directly. However, Hagino (1968) exposed female rats to "strong" formalin vapour (concentration not stated) for 4 min, 4 times/day and found 8/10 developed prolonged dioestrus around day 26 of exposure. Laparotomy of 4 of the affected rats showed corpora lutea present in only 2 of them, but all 4 mated subsequently, even though vaginal smears showed they were still in dioestrus. Two of these 4 rats became pregnant, one from those with corpora lutea and one from those without. The author assumed mating induced ovulation. Apart from the small numbers of animals used, it is not possible in this study to separate the effects of formaldehyde *per se* from the possible secondary effects of stress (the author was using formaldehyde exposure as a "stressor"). However, other stressors used in the study (noise and constant illumination) induced persistent oestrus rather than dioestrus, suggesting formaldehyde may have a specific effect.

Males

Guseva (1972) has studied the effects of exposure to formaldehyde given simultaneously in water and by inhalation in the male rat. Rats were exposed to formaldehyde for 4 h/day, 5 days/week for 6 months at the following doses in water and by inhalation respectively; 0·1 mg/l and 0·4 ppm (0·5 mg/m^3), 0·01 mg/l and 0·2 ppm (0·25 mg/m^3), or 0·005 mg/l and 0·1 ppm (0·12 mg/m^3). The number of males in each treatment group was not stated, nor is it clear exactly how it was given in water (? drinking water). At the end of the exposure

*Formaldehyde in solution, 40%w/v, with alcohol added as preservative.

period, pituitary gonadotrophin levels were measured by bioassay; pituitary gland homogenates were injected s.c. for 3 days into immature females which were then killed 4 days after the first injection and uterine and ovarian weights measured. No significant differences in weight were found between females injected with homogenates from test males and those injected with homogenates from control males. Whilst this suggests there is no large change in pituitary gonadotrophin levels following exposure to low levels of formaldehyde in males, the bioassay technique used is not highly sensitive and no information on numbers of animals used nor numerical results was given. Testicular nucleic acid levels were also measured in the males at the end of the treatment period and significant reductions were seen from 816 μg/100 g tissue in unexposed males to 751 μg/100 g in the middle dose group (0·01 mg/l and 0·2 ppm) and 719 μg/100 g in the highest dose group (0·1 mg/l and 0·4 ppm). Reproductive function in these same males was also assessed before autopsy and no reduction in fertility was seen (see section C for details).

Gofmekler and Bonashevskaya (1969) studied the effect of exposure to inhaled formaldehyde on testicular histology in the rat. Males were exposed to 0 or 0·8 ppm (1 mg/m^3) for 24 h/day for 10 consecutive days, but no differences were found in the histological appearance of exposed and control rat testes. The number of rats used was not stated.

Conclusion

None of the inhalation studies to date where the exposure level has been stated have employed exposures above 0·8 ppm and there is clearly a need for further experiments on exposure levels around the TLV (2 ppm). Studies employing injections of formalin are particularly unsuitable since it is difficult to separate the effects of formaldehyde itself from the non-specific stress responses induced.

C. FERTILITY

Males

During the course of investigations into the preservation of spermatozoa for artificial insemination, Dott *et al.* (1976) have shown that dilution of sheep and pig semen *in vitro* with low concentrations of formaldehyde (0·025% HCHO) in a 40% solution (v/v) with saline or Krebs-Ringer, renders the spermatozoa immotile but does not affect their subsequent fertilizing capacity. However, the significance of such *in vitro* findings for industrial exposures is hard to assess.

Guseva (1972) has investigated the effects on male fertility in the rat of chronic exposure to formaldehyde simultaneously in the drinking water and by inhalation. Males were exposed 4 h/day, 5 days/week for 6 months at the following dose levels in drinking water and by inhalation respectively, 0·1 mg/l and 0·4 ppm, 0·01 mg/l and 0·2 ppm, or 0·005 mg/l and 0·1 ppm, with a fourth group of unexposed rats. At the end of the treatment period 3 males/treatment group were each mated with 2 unexposed females with normal oestrous cycles. Some females in each group were killed on day 20 of pregnancy. The rest were allowed to litter out and the development of the pups followed up to one month of age by measurement of body weight, opening of ears, eyes and hair growth. No numerical data are given. However, the author stated that there was no effect on fertility, all the females becoming pregnant. Litter size, fetal and newborn body weights and postnatal development were said to be unaffected, and no anomalies were seen in the offspring. Whilst this study indicates there are no gross effects on fertility or induction of dominant lethal effects from such exposures (the highest dose was the threshold dose for chronic toxicity), the numbers of males and females used were grossly inadequate for fertility and teratology studies.

Epstein *et al.* (1972) have carried out a dominant lethal study in male mice given single i.p. doses of formaldehyde at 16–40 mg/kg. A number of deaths occurred (3/12 at 16 mg/kg, 2/16 at 20 mg/kg, 2/5 at 32 mg/kg and 5/5 at 40 mg/kg) but no effects on pregnancy rate or dominant lethal effects were seen when survivors were mated to 3 untreated females/week for 8 weeks after the injection.

Females

No studies found.

D. PREGNANCY

Observations that formaldehyde is antimitotic at concentrations below those that fix cells (Sentein, 1975) suggest that it may have teratogenic potential.

In a study of a variety of contragestational agents, Conner *et al.* (1976) have injected formaldehyde into the uterine horn of pregnant rats. On day 3 or day 7 of pregnancy, 0·05 ml of formaldehyde solution, at varying concentrations between 0·005% and 40%, was injected into one uterine horn and 0·9% saline into the other. The stock formaldehyde solution was 40% v/v and contained 12–15% methanol as preservative. On day 15 of pregnancy the rats were killed, the corpora lutea counted and the contents of the uterus examined. After injection on day 3, pre-implantation survival was not affected by injection of 0·005% formaldehyde, but 0·05% reduced viable fetuses from 70–90% of the total number of corpora lutea found in saline controls to around 35%. Concentrations from 0·5%–40% reduced viable fetuses to 2% or less.

Concentrations of 10% and above produced maternal toxicity and death. Injections of formaldehyde of day 7 had no significant effect on post-implantation survival at any concentration.

Marks *et al.* (1980) have studied the teratogenic potential of formaldehyde in mice. Formaldehyde 1% (w/v), containing 12–15% of methanol as preservative, was given orally by gavage on a body weight basis at doses of 74, 148 or 185 mg/kg/day from days 6–15 of pregnancy. There were 29–35 mice/treatment group and 76 controls given vehicle (distilled water) only by gavage. Acceptable teratological methods were used.

The highest dose, 185 mg/kg, was toxic to the dam, 22/34 dying before day 18 of pregnancy. The methanol may have contributed to toxicity, its concentration at this dose being equivalent to 60–75 mg/kg/day. Weight gain was significantly reduced at the lowest dose of 74 mg/kg, but this is unlikely to be biologically significant since weight gain was unaffected at higher doses. There were no significant effects on implantations/dam, live fetuses/dam, resorptions, fetal deaths or fetal weights. There was no significant effect on the overall incidence of malformations; the average % malformed fetuses was 0·4% in controls and 1·0–1·3% in treated groups. Neither were there any significant differences in any individual malformations. Thus formaldehyde caused no significant embryolethality or teratogenicity, even at doses which were clearly toxic to the dam.

Gofmekler and co-workers have carried out a series of studies on rats exposed to formaldehyde by inhalation at concentrations of 0·01 ppm (0·012 mg/m^3) and 0·8 ppm (1·0 mg/m^3), for 24 h/day for 10–15 days before fertilization and throughout pregnancy. However in none of the reports of this work (Gofmekler, 1968; Gofmekler *et al.*, 1968; Pushkina *et al.*, 1968; Gofmekler and Bonashevskaya, 1969) is any information given about the day on which the dams were killed, or the methods used for teratological and biochemical examinations. In some of their studies, it is not known whether the offspring were examined at the fetal stage or after birth. Such numerical results as are presented are frequently inadequate in detail. The dams exposed to 0·8 ppm showed involution of lymphoid tissue, indicating there was an elevation in corticosteroid hormone levels, probably stress-induced. Gofmekler reported that at both concentrations the mean duration of pregnancy was prolonged by 14–15%. However, the paper stated that the duration of pregnancy was determined from the day the males were introduced into the females' cages and not from the day of fertilization. It is also not clear whether "pregnancy" was prolonged in relation to control animals, or in relation to reports from other workers. The average number of fetuses/dam was stated to be reduced in a dose-related manner but numerical data given in the paper are confusing. From 12 dams in each group they reported 135 offspring were obtained from controls, 235 from the 0·01 ppm group, and 208 from the

0·5 ppm group. An unknown number of dams in each group did not carry to term. Fetal body weights were significantly increased from 5·6 g in controls to 6·0 g at 0·01 ppm and 6·3 g at 0·8 ppm. This would be compatible with a true increase in the length of pregnancy. Fetal organ weights were different; at 0·01 ppm adrenal weight was significantly increased and at 0·8 ppm adrenal, thymus and kidney weights were significantly increased. At both 0·01 and 0·8 ppm liver and lung weights were significantly decreased (Gofmekler, 1968). There was no evidence of malformations. However, histological examination of fetal organs revealed changes in those exposed to 0·8 ppm (Gofmekler and Bonashevskaya, 1969). In the liver, there was epithelial proliferation in the common bile ducts and extramedullary haematopoietic centres were occasionally larger and more numerous than in controls. In the kidney, nuclei of renal epithelial cells sometimes showed polymorphism and there were occasionally cast-off cells in the tubular lumens. Measurements of ascorbic acid and nucleic acid levels (Pushkina *et al.*, 1968) showed significant dose-related falls in ascorbic acid contents of maternal liver and whole fetus (reductions in the placenta were not significant), and significant dose-related falls in the DNA contents of maternal and fetal liver.

Sheveleva (1971) exposed rats to 4 ppm (0·005 mg/l) or 0·4 ppm (0·0005 mg/l) formaldehyde by inhalation for 4 h/day from days 1–19 of pregnancy. Fifteen dams/group were killed on day 20 for examination of the uterine contents, and 6/group allowed to litter out. In tests for maternal toxicity carried out on day 17 of pregnancy, those exposed to 4 ppm were found to have significantly lowered threshold for "neuromuscular excitability", higher activity, lower rectal temperature and lower haemoglobin concentrations. Reduced haemoglobin concentrations have also been reported by Sanotskii *et al.* (1976) in pregnant rats exposed to 5 ppm formaldehyde by inhalation. At both 4 and 0·4 ppm there was a significant dose-related increase in the leucocyte count. There were no significant effects on numbers of corpora lutea/dam, live fetuses/dam, pre- or post-implantation loss rates, or fetal weight. Fetuses were examined for external malformations only and none were observed, which is unusual in a group of approximately 575 fetuses.

In those allowed to litter out, Sheveleva reported that all births occurred on day 22 of pregnancy, which does not support Gofmekler's reported prolongation of gestation at lower exposures (Gofmekler, 1968). However Sheveleva exposed rats to 4 and 0·4 ppm for only 4 h/day, whereas Gofmekler exposed rats to 0·8 and 0·01 ppm for 24 h/day. Sheveleva reported litter sizes ranging from 10–14. Opening of ears, eruption of incisors, hair growth and opening of the eyes proceeded "normally" (no numerical data given). One male and one female in each litter were weighed and tested for neuromuscular excitability, activity and oxygen consumption, at one and 2 months of age.

Spontaneous activity was significantly decreased at one month of age in both groups of treated female offspring in a dose-related manner and in males exposed to 0·4 ppm but not in those exposed to 4 ppm. At 2 months of age, the following significant changes were seen. Activity was increased in the high-dose females, peripheral haemoglobin levels decreased in low-dose males and high-dose females and blood leucocytes decreased in high-dose males. Bearing in mind the small numbers of animals tested (6 of each sex/treatment group), the lack of any clear dose-response relationships, and the inconsistency between ages and sexes in these postnatal observations, the statistically significant differences reported may not be of any biological significance.

A number of workers using formaldehyde as a "stressor" in late pregnancy have observed changes on the placenta and fetus. De Almeida (1968) gave rats 2 s.c. injections of formaldehyde, 12 h apart, on day 15 or day 18 of pregnancy. Each injection was 0·5 ml of one part 40% formaldehyde solution to 3 parts distilled water. There was no effect on placental glycogen levels, but placental acid and neutral lipids were increased. However, these same effects were obtained using cold or hypoxia as stressors and so it is likely that the effects of formaldehyde are secondary to the stress it induces.

Cohen and co-workers have shown that direct injections of formalin s.c. into fetal rats causes adrenal ascorbic acid depletion at 20·5 days gestation (Cohen *et al.*, 1968), but not if injected earlier at 17–18 days (Cohen, 1972). Thus a fetal stress response to formaldehyde does not mature until late pregnancy and it is dependent on the integrity of the hypothalamo-pituitary-adrenal axis (Cohen *et al.*, 1968). However, it is not known whether formaldehyde reaching the fetus indirectly, via placental transfer, can trigger a similar stress response in late gestation, nor whether such responses *in utero* have any long-term effects on fetal or postnatal development.

The effect of formaldehyde on reproduction in the dog has been studied by Hurni and Ohder (1973). Beagle bitches were fed on diet containing 0, 125 or 375 ppm formaldehyde (10 or 11 dogs/group) from days 4–56 after mating, equivalent to an intake of 0, 3·1 and 9·4 mg/kg/day. There was no effect on pregnancy rate, litter size or stillbirths. No malformations were found in any stillbirths or in a proportion of the live births killed at 9 months of age. Mean body weight of the treated pups was reduced by 5–13% in a dose-related manner from birth to 8 weeks of age (no data given after 8 weeks), but the authors do not state whether the reductions were significant (means only given). Observation of the dogs indicated normal behaviour, appearance, motility and muscular co-ordination, but the nature of these observations were not specified. A small number of dogs (sex not specified) were transferred to the breeding colony and have produced normal litters.

Conclusion

Considering the fertility and pregnancy studies to date, there have been no inhalation studies on male or female fertility or teratogenicity studies that have employed a wide range of exposure levels or adequate methods. The one adequate teratology study by Marks *et al.* (1980) in the mouse suggests that formaldehyde given orally is not embryolethal or teratogenic at doses around or below those toxic to the dam. However, further inhalation studies are required.

E. MUTAGENICITY

No relevant data found.

F. CARCINOGENICITY

IARC Monograph Volume 29 (1982 in press) reported that there is sufficient evidence for the carcinogenicity of formaldehyde gas in rats.

No reports on transplacental carcinogenicity have been found.

HUMAN STUDIES

A, RELEVANT PHARMACOLOGY AND TOXICOLOGY

No relevant data found.

B. ENDOCRINE AND GONADAL EFFECTS

Menstrual function in workers exposed to urea-formaldehyde resins, in the First Moscow Print works and in the Moscow "Three Mountain Fabric" cotton combine, was studied by Shumilina (1975). Free formaldehyde is released from these resins and gynaecologists studied 446 women workers, comprising 130 shop trim finishers exposed to a high environmental level of formaldehyde of 1·2–3·6 ppm (1·5–4·5 mg/m^3) (MAC=0·4 ppm or 0·5 mg/m^3), 316 warehouse inspectors exposed to lower levels of 0·05–0·7 mg/m^3, and a third group of 200 women (industrial sales staff) not exposed to chemicals at all who were examined as controls. Both groups of exposed workers work standing up all day and move around very little during a work shift, with ambient temperature of 25–30°C and humidity of 63–76%.

Seventy percent of the subjects were under 40 years of age and 55–65% of them had worked for 10 years or more.

Menstrual disorders were found in 47·5% of the exposed women compared with 18·6% of the controls, with dysmenorrhoea being the commonest disorder—24% of finishers, 20% of inspectors and 9% of controls; this was frequently found in the older (30–40 year) women. The actual age distributions are not clear in the paper. It was also stated that there was a decrease in oestrogen levels in women with menstrual disorders, but no details of the levels or how these were measured or on which workers the tests were carried out are given. The incidence of inflammatory disease of the genital tract was significantly higher in the finishers than in the warehouse staff (38% versus 25%, $P<0.05$) and this was associated with a higher rate of secondary infertility (15% in finishers compared with 7% in controls, no figure given for warehouse staff).

C. FERTILITY

No other relevant data found.

D. PREGNANCY

The outcome of pregnancy in women exposed to formaldehyde vapour from urea-formaldehyde resins was reported as part of the same study referred to above by Shumilina (1975). A total of 446 women exposed to formaldehyde and 200 controls were studied but no details of the number of pregnancies, number of women involved, age distributions, or other pregnancy histories are given; however, the percentage distribution of age and parity seemed similar in the 2 groups. Anaemia was the most frequent complication and was observed in twice as many exposed workers as in controls, with haemoglobin levels below 10 g% in 10% of exposed versus 4·6% of controls. Threatened abortion was recorded in 31% of exposed versus 18% of controls (no statistical analysis). Details of the outcome of pregnancy are unclear, though 91·3% and 90·5% are reported to have ended in term births in the exposed and control groups respectively. The risk of intra-uterine asphyxia was reported in the exposed group as double that in controls (no figures given). Operative deliveries (? Caesarian sections) were used in 5·3% of exposed women and in no controls. The reasons for this were not stated. Weight distributions of the babies were recorded and there seemed to be a tendency for the exposed mothers to have babies of lower birth weight. For example, 26·9% of the "exposed" babies weighed 2500–2990 g compared with 11·3% of control babies ($P < 0{\cdot}05$). It is impossible to critically evaluate this study because of the lack of data recorded. The authors conclude however that pregnant women should not be subject to formaldehyde exposure.

E. MUTAGENICITY

No relevant data found.

F. CARCINOGENICITY

IARC Monograph Volume 29 (1982 in press) reported that epidemiological studies provide inadequate evidence to assess the carcinogenicity of formaldehyde in man.

SUMMARY AND EVALUATION

EXPERIMENTAL STUDIES

Very limited studies in male rats exposed chronically to doses up to 0·1 mg/l in water and simultaneously to 0·4 ppm by inhalation, have shown no effect on fertility or on the subsequent pregnancies. A dominant lethal study in mice with single doses of 16–40 mg/kg i.p. (all of which produced some fatalities) showed no effects on fertility or dominant lethality. No satisfactory studies on fertility in females were found. Administration of doses of 74, 148 and 185 mg/kg orally daily to pregnant mice showed no adverse effects on number of implants, resorptions, fetal weight or malformations, although the top dose was lethal to a high proportion of the dams. Dogs fed 125 or 375 ppm in the diet, equivalent to 3·1 and 9·4 mg/kg/day, during gestation, showed no effect on pregnancy, litter size or stillbirths. No satisfactory studies in rats have been carried out.

No data on mutagenicity were found.

HUMAN STUDIES

There is one report of menstrual disorders, mainly dysmenorrhoea, in women workers occupationally exposed to environmental levels of formaldehyde of 1·2–3·6 ppm. There was also reported to be a higher than control level of inflammatory disease of the genital tract and infertility. The same authors also reported a higher incidence of anaemia in pregnancy and of threatened abortion in exposed women, and also an excess of low birth weight babies.

No data on mutagenicity or carcinogenicity were found.

EVALUATION

Very few satisfactory studies on the reproductive toxicity of formaldehyde have been carried out. The limited available data suggest that there is no adverse effect on male fertility or on pregnancy at otherwise non-toxic doses. Limited studies in women occupationally exposed to levels around the TLV, suggest an effect on menstrual function and on pregnancy. Due to lack of adequate data these cannot be evaluated. Attention is drawn to the lack of data on the reproductive effects of formaldehyde in both animals and humans.

References

Chatterjee, A. (1965). The role of cortisone in the prevention of formalin induced pseudopregnancy in rats. *Naturwissenschaften* **52**, (23), 643–644.

Cohen, A. (1972). Response of rat foetal adrenal glands to the harmful effects of formol at different stages of development. *Comptes Rendus-Academie des Sciences-Paris-Series* D **275**, (8), 921–924.

Cohen, A., Pernod, J-C. and Jost, A. (1968). Role of the hypothalamus in the rat adrenal response of the rat foetus to formol aggression. *Comptes Rendus des Sceances—Societe de Biologie* **162**, (12), 2070–2073.

Conner, E. A., Blake, D. A., Parmley, T. H., Burnett, L. S. and King, T. M. (1976). Efficacy of various locally applied chemicals as contragestational agents in rats. *Contraception* **13**, (5), 571–582.

De Almeida, P. A. M. (1968). Effects of cold, formaldehyde and anoxia on the lipids and glycogen in placentas of pregnant rats (Rattus norvegicus albinus, Rodentia, Mammalia). *Maternidade E Infancia* **27**, (3), 237–262.

Dott, H. M., Moor, R. M. and Polge, C. (1976). Artificial insemination with spermatozoa in formaldehyde. *Journal of Reproduction and Fertility* **46**, (1), 277.

Epstein, S. S., Arnold, E., Andrea, J., Bass, W. and Bishop, Y. (1972). Detection of chemical mutagens by the dominant lethal assay in the mouse. *Toxicology and Applied Pharmacology* **23**, 288–325.

Gofmekler, V. A., Pushkina, N. N. and Kletsova, G. N. (1968). Various biochemical shifts during a study of the embryotropic effect of benzene and formaldehyde. *Gigiena I Sanitariya* **33**, (7), 96–98.

Gofmekler, V. A. (1968). The embryotropic action of benzene and formaldehyde in experimental administration by inhalation. *Gigiena I Sanitariya* **33**, (3), 12–16.

Gofmekler, V. A. and Bonashevskaya, T. I. (1969). Experimental studies of teratogenic properties of formaldehyde, based on pathological investigations. *Gigiena I Sanitariya* **37**, (5), 92–94.

Guseva, V. A. (1972). Study of the gonadotropic effect in male rats exposed to the action of formaldehyde simultaneously present in the air and water. *Gigiena I Sanitariya* **37**, (10), 102–103.

Hagino, N. (1968). Ovulation and mating behavior in female rats under various environmental stresses or androgen treatment. *Japanese Journal of Physiology* **18**, (3), 350–355.

Hurni, H. and Ohder, H. (1973). Reproduction study with formaldehyde hexamethylenetetramine in beagle dogs. *Food and Cosmetic Toxicology* **11**, (3), 459–462.

Marks, T. A., Worthy, W. C. and Staples, R. E. (1980). Influence of formaldehyde and Sonacide® (potentiated acid glutaraldehyde) on embryo and fetal development in mice. *Teratology* **22**, 51–58.

Pushkina, N. N., Gofmekler, V. A. and Klevisova, T. N. (1968). Changes in the ascorbic acid titer and in the nucleic acids following action of benzol and formaldehyde. *Byulleten Eksperimental Noi Biologii I Meditsiny* **66**, (8), 51–53.

Sanotskii, I. V., Fomenko, V. N., Sheveleva, G. A., Salnikova, L. S., Nakoryakova, M. V. and Pavlova, T. E. (1976). A study on the effect of pregnancy upon the sensitivity of animals to chemical agents. *Gigiena Truda I Professional 'Nye Zabolevaniya* **1**, 25–28.

Sentein, P. (1975). Action of glutaraldehyde and formaldehyde on segmentation mitoses. *Experimental Cell Research* **95**, (2), 233–246.

Sheveleva, G. A. (1971). Specific action of formaldehyde on the embryogeny and progeny of white rats. *Toksikologiya Novykh Promyshlennykh Khimicheskikh Veshchestv* **12**, 78–86.

Shumilina, A. V. (1975). Menstrual and child-bearing functions of female-workers occupationally exposed to the effects of formaldehyde. *Gigiena Truda I Professional 'Nye Zabolevaniya* **12**, 18–21

Solem, J. H. (1966). Plasma corticosteroids in mice, with special regard to sex differences in adrenocortical responsiveness to exogenous corticotrophin. *Scandinavian Journal of Clinical and Laboratory Investigations* **18**, (Suppl. 93).

25. Formamides

TECHNICAL DATA

(a) *Formamide*

Formula	$HCONH_2$
CAS registry number	75–12–7
Chemical abstracts name	Formamide
Synonyms	Methanamide
Uses	As ionizing solvent, manufacture of formic esters, hydrocyanic acid by catalytic dehydration, as softener for paper, animal glues, water-soluble gums.
TLV	20 ppm

(b) *N-Methyl-Formamide*

Formula	$HCONHCH_3$
CAS registry number	None
Chemical abstracts name	None
Synonyms	Monomethylformamide
Uses	None known
TLV	None

(c) *N,N-Dimethylformamide*

Formula	$HCON(CH_3)_2$
CAS registry number	68–12–2
Chemical abstracts name	N,N-dimethylformamide
Synonyms	DMF, DMFA
Uses	Solvent for liquids and gases; in synthesis of organic compounds; solvent for Orlon and similar polyacrylic fibres.
TLV	10 ppm (skin)

ANIMAL STUDIES

A. RELEVANT PHARMACOLOGY AND TOXICOLOGY

Chanh *et al.* (1971) have investigated sex differences in the toxicity of a series of formamides in the rat and mouse. No sex differences in LD_{50} were found following i.p. injection of formamide, N-methylformamide, N,N-dimethylformamide, N-ethylformamide or N,N-diethylformamide in either species.

Sheveleva *et al.* (1977) have studied placental transfer of N,N-dimethylformamide following inhalation of 3·4 ppm (10·2 mg/m^3) or 63·3 ppm (189·4 mg/m^3) in rats from days 1–20 of pregnancy. At both exposure levels significant amounts of dimethylformamide reached the fetus.

Sheveleva *et al.* (1979) have compared the effects of N,N-dimethylformamide in pregnant and non-pregnant rats. Groups of 8–32 rats were exposed in 4h/day for 20 days (in the case of pregnant animals, on days 1–20 of pregnancy) to 3·6 ppm (10·7 mg/m^3) or 0·77 ppm (2·3 mg/m^3). Fourteen difference indices of toxicity were assessed on days 16 and 20 of exposure. At 3·6 ppm in non-pregnant rats there was an increase in urinary chloride content and a decrease in hippuric acid excretion following sodium benzoate loading, indicating alterations in kidney and liver function respectively. In pregnant rats exposed to 3·6 ppm a similar decrease in hippuric acid excretion was observed. At 0·77 ppm, the change in kidney function was still present in the non-pregnant rats, but no significant changes were seen in the pregnant animals. The authors, however, point out that whilst the aforementioned differences between exposed and control groups were statistically significant, all values obtained in pregnant and non-pregnant exposed animals were within the normal physiological range for that species. There appears to be no substantial difference in the toxicity of dimethylformamide between pregnant and non-pregnant rats.

B. ENDOCRINE AND GONADAL EFFECTS

Chanh *et al.* (1971) investigated the toxicity of a series of formamides in the rat and the mouse. Injection of a single dose of formamide, 5·0–5·4 g/kg i.p., caused testicular atrophy with complete disruption of the seminiferous epithelium and hyperplasia of interstitial tissue in rats which died as a result of the injection. Similar, but less severe lesions, with the presence of multinucleated giant cells, necrotic spermatogonia and spermatocytes were seen following i.p. injections of N-methylformamide lethal to some animals (exact dose not stated) in both rats and mice. However these lesions are presumably reversible, since they were not seen at all in rats or mice surviving to one month after injection of formamide or N-methylformamide. Testicular lesions were not found following i.p. administration of N,N-dimethylformamide, N-ethylformamide or N,N-diethylformamide to rats and mice in doses up to the LD_{50}.

Sheveleva *et al.* (1979) reported that exposure of male rats to N,N-dimethylformamide at 206–195 ppm (616–584 mg/m^3) or 17–16 ppm (51–49 mg/m^3) for 2, 4 or 8 days caused no changes in the spermatogenic epithelium. Numbers of animals used, daily duration of exposure and details of methods and results were not given.

In the same study Sheveleva *et al.* (1979) also looked at the effect of N,N-dimethylformamide on the oestrous cycle. Non-pregnant female rats were exposed to 3·6 ppm (10·7 mg/m^3) or 0·77 ppm (2·3 mg/m^3) for 4 h/day for 20 days, with 7–15 rats/group. Oestrous cycles were followed during exposure and during recovery after a 10-day exposure-free interval. Rats exposed to 3·6 ppm showed a significant lengthening of the inter-oestrous interval to a mean of 4·0 days compared with 3·1 days in controls, which was still present at 10 days after the last exposure; the inter-oestrous interval being 3·4 days compared with 3·0 days in controls. There was also a significant lengthening of oestrus itself from 1·1 days in controls to 1·3 days in those exposed to 3·6 ppm. However, the authors state that there were no changes in the total numbers of cycles observed nor in the total duration of cycles. The latter information is difficult to reconcile with the significant changes claimed for duration of oestrus and the inter-oestrus interval. At 0·77 ppm no significant changes in the cycle were observed. In some females in this study gonadotropic activity of the pituitary gland was studied and it is reported that no changes were seen. However, no further details are given.

D. PREGNANCY

Formamide

In vitro experiments have shown that formamide (F) disturbs microtubule structure in a number of cell systems, affecting for example the mitotic apparatus and chromosome structure in sea urchin eggs and cell elongation and neurulation in the chick embryo (Messier, 1976). F is also cytotoxic (Oettel and Frohberg, 1964). Thus it is a potential teratogen in higher animals.

Thiersch (1962) has studied the effect of F given orally to rats. The LD_{50} for this route of administration was 6 g/kg. Administration of 2 g/kg on day 7 of pregnancy caused resorption of half the implanted embryos and stunting of 26% of survivors. No malformations were seen in survivors. Administration of 3 × 2 g/kg after day 7 of pregnancy (days not stated) caused complete destruction of the litters. This study is reported in abstract only and no further details were given.

Gleich (1974) gave F i.p. to mice on days 6–15 of pregnancy. At a dose of 0·076 ml/kg/day, fetal losses were 13% and 4% of survivors were malformed. At 0·19 ml/kg/day fetal losses were 27% and malformations 25%. This study is reported in abstract only and no further details, including the types of malformation, are given.

Von Kreybig (1968) reported that F was teratogenic in the rat when injected s.c. at doses above 3 g/kg on day 13 of pregnancy. The LD_{50} for this route was above 4 g/kg. No further details were given and the abnormalities were not described.

Oettel and Frohberg (1964) have shown that percutaneous absorption of F is teratogenic in the mouse. When 0·1 ml was dropped onto the skin on day 11 of pregnancy, 50% of fetuses were resorbed, and in survivors, 50% had cleft palate, with isolated cases of exomphalos and phocomelia. Application of 2 × 0·1 ml drops onto the skin caused 80% fetal resorptions and amelia. No further details were given. The above doses correspond to $\frac{1}{4}$ (0·1 ml) and $\frac{1}{2}$ (0·2 ml) the LD_{50} (Von Kreybig, 1968).

Similar findings following percutaneous absorption of F in the mouse have been reported by Gleich (1974). Two applications of 0·076 ml were made on days 10 and 11 of pregnancy, resulting in 61% fetal resorptions and 36% malformations. Applications of lower doses of 0·008 ml (1/50 of the LD_{50}) on days 10 and 11 caused 8% fetal resorption but no malformations. No control data and no further details were given.

In the rat, percutaneous absorption of low doses (1/28 of the average lethal dose*) is reported to be weakly embryotoxic. Stula and Krauss (1977) gave groups of 6 or 7 rats 600 mg/kg F applied on one or 2 days between days 9–13

*Average lethal dose determined by using a variety of doses, with a factor of 1·5 between dose levels. One animal/dose level was treated on day 11 of pregnancy for rats and day 15 of pregnancy for rabbits.

of pregnancy. Adequate teratological methods were used. Embryomortality in controls was 2%, and in treated groups 5%, except those treated on days 11 and 12 where it was 13%. From their historical control data the authors suggest that mortality in excess of 10% is treatment related, but significance levels were not presented. Average fetal weights were 2·4 g in controls and were reduced to 2·1 g in some treated groups, but only averages are given and no significance levels are stated. No abnormalities were seen in controls and in treated groups the abnormalities were similar to those seen in historical controls (1/53 with distorted face after F on days 10 and 11, and 4/60 s.c. haemorrhage after F on days 12 and 13, with no abnormalities after F on day 9 or days 11 and 12).

N-Methylformamide

Roll and Bär (1967) have reported that oral administration of N-methylformamide (MMF) to mice on day 11 of pregnancy is teratogenic at doses of 5 and 10 mg/animal (about 150–300 mg/kg). There were 25–31 mice/group. Maternal weight gain was significantly reduced by both doses but there were no other signs of toxicity in the dams. Resorptions occurring in mid-pregnancy increased significantly in a dose-related manner from 1% in controls to 11% at 5 mg (3% of litters totally resorbed) and 67% at 10 mg (53% of litters totally resorbed). Fetal weight was significantly reduced from 1·24 g in controls to 1·05 g at 5 mg and 0·80 g after 10 mg. All surviving fetuses at 10 mg had multiple defects including exencephaly (100%), kyphosis (95%), spina bifida (95%), cleft palate (68%), neck and chest (79%), rib (79%) and sternebral (100%) defects. At 5 mg these same abnormalities were present in 11–37% of surviving fetuses. Exencephaly (0·4%) was the only abnormality seen in controls.

Roll and Bär (1967) also investigated postnatal survival and weight gain following single oral administrations of MMF on day 11 of pregnancy of 0 mg (24 mice), 2·5 mg (23 mice), 5 mg (33 mice) or 10 mg (11 mice). There were significant dose-related increases in stillbirths form 0% in controls to 8% at 2·5 mg, 28% at 5 mg and 86% at 10 mg. Postnatal deaths up to the third week of life brought total mortality to 12% in controls, 21% at 2·5 mg, 53% at 5 mg, and 98% at 10 mg. Birth weight was significantly reduced in a dose-related manner in the 5 and 10 mg groups, as was weaning weight in the 5 mg group (no results given for 10 mg because of poor survival). Maternal weight gain was not affected in the 2·5 mg group but was significantly reduced in the 5 and 10 mg groups.

Oettel and Frohberg (1964) also gave mice MMF orally and obtained malformations similar in type to those reported by Roll and Bär (1967), including general retardation, exencephaly, cleft palate, spina bifida, rib malformations and exomphalos. However, no information on dosages was given except that they were non-toxic to the dam and maximal teratogenic effects were obtained after administration on days 11–12 of pregnancy.

Thiersch (1962) gave MMF orally and by i.p. injection to rats. A single dose of 1 g/kg (oral or i.p. route not specified) on day 7 or 11 of pregnancy killed 90% of fetuses, whilst repeated oral doses of 0·4 g/kg or repeated i.p. doses of 0·1 g/kg given "after day 7" led to "extensive fetal loss and malformations in the survivors". No further details are given including the type(s) of malformation.

Gleich (1974) injected i.p. various doses of MMF into mice on days 6–15 of pregnancy. Following 0·1 ml/kg/day, fetal losses were 25%, and 74% of fetuses were malformed. At 0·05 ml/kg/day there were 11% fetal losses and 28% malformations. No further details were given.

Von Kreybig (1968) gave mice single i.p. doses of 250 mg/kg (1/10th of the LD_{50}) on day 11 of pregnancy and obtained malformations, including hypoplasia of the epidermis, aplasia of the cranial and sternal bones and haemorrhagic oedema. No information on numbers affected or fetal losses were reported.

Oettel and Frohberg (1964) have given MMF to rats i.p. on days 4–8, 11–12 or 14–15 of pregnancy, obtaining maximal teratogenic effects after administration on days 11–12. Two i.p. injections of 0·1 ml/kg (1/25th of the LD_{50}) caused, in addition to general retardation of the fetuses, severe exencephaly, cleft jaw and cleft palate, spina bifida, rib malformations and exomphalos in about 50% of surviving fetuses. Fetal loss rates were not reported and no further details were given. Larger doses (not specified) on days 10–11 of pregnancy, which were still not toxic to the dam, caused 100% fetal resorption.

Pfiefer and Von Kreybig (1974) injected MMF s.c. in doses of 250–1000 mg/kg on day 13 of pregnancy in the rat. There were 3–6 rats/group. At the lowest dose, 250 mg/kg (1/10th of the LD_{50}) only 1/35 implantations were resorbed and there were no malformations. Dose-related increases in resorption rate were seen at 500 mg/kg (17%), 750 mg/kg (22%) and 1000 mg/kg (83%). No surviving fetuses were normal at 500–1000 mg/kg and the severity of malformations (including cranial and sternal hypoplasia and aplasia, exencephaly, short jaw and haemorrhagic oedema) increased with increasing doses. No control data and no further details are given.

Percutaneous absorption of MMF is also teratogenic. Stula and Krauss (1977) applied various doses to groups of 4–8 rats on days 10 and 11, 11 and 12, or 12 and 13 of pregnancy. Acceptable teratological methods were used. In untreated and vehicle-treated controls embryomortality ranged from 1–3% and no malformations were found in fetuses from a total of 19 dams. At a daily dose of 600 mg/kg (1/18th of the average lethal dose) embryomortality ranged from 25–72% and malformations from 4–100%, the proportion of malformed fetuses increasing the later in gestation MMF was applied. Malformations found were umbilical hernia and encephalocoele. When the dose was increased to 2400 mg/kg on the most sensitive days (12 and 13), all embryos died. Lowering the dose to 200 mg/kg on days 12 and 13 caused 2% embryomortality and 20% encephalocoele, 2% umbilical hernia and 8% s.c. haemorrhage. Average fetal weights were lower than controls in most treated groups, but no significance levels are given.

Tuchmann-Duplessis and Mercier-Parot (1965) have reported similar findings in the rat from percutaneous application. An unspecified quantity of MMF (3 drops) was applied to the skin of the back or the tail for 1–6 days at different times in gestation. The numbers of animals used is not given. No evidence of maternal toxicity was seen but body weight measurements are not given. With application to the skin of the back, on days 8, 9, 9 and 10, 9–11, 11–14 and 11–16 all embryos were resorbed; with application on days 10 and 11 75% of embryos died and the remainder were all malformed; with application on days 11 and 12, 25% of embryos died and 42% were malformed. With applications on the tail, a lower incidence of resorptions and malformed survivors was seen. The frequency of individual malformations was not given but they were described as varied, involving the nervous system, viscera and skeleton; occasional exencephaly and more frequent encephalocoele of varying degrees were seen, together with generalized oedema and haemorrhage. No abnormalities were seen in controls. Fetal weights were not reported.

Gleich (1974) has reported teratogenic effects in the mouse from percutaneous application of MMF. A dose of 0·01 ml/animal was applied on days 10 and 11 of pregnancy resulting in fetal losses of 54% and 37% malformations. The type(s) of malformation were not specified.

Oettel and Frohberg (1964) using the same strain of mouse as Gleich (1974) reported similar findings after application of 0·01 ml/animal on day 11 of pregnancy; 50% of surviving fetuses were malformed (exencephaly, spina bifida, cleft palate, rib malformations and exomphalos).

Roll and Bär (1967) applied 5, 10 or 20 mg percutaneously on day 11 of pregnancy in the mouse. There were 23–29 mice/group. Resorption rates were slightly increased at 10 and 20 mg; 89% of fetuses were alive in control and 5 mg groups (no litters with complete resorptions), 81% at 10 mg (3% of litters completely resorbed), and 40% at 20 mg (26% of litters completely resorbed). Fetal weights were reduced from 1·24 g in controls to 1·16 g at 5 mg, 0·96 g at 10 mg and 0·97 g at 20 mg. Malformations were seen at 5 mg (7% cleft palate, 8% encephalocoele) and multiple dose-related malformations (encephalocoele, kyphosis, spina bifida, cleft palate, neck, chest, rib and sternebral defects) at 10 and 20 mg affecting 7–89% of the fetuses. In groups of mice allowed to litter out (25 or 26 animals/group), stillbirths were increased from 0% in controls to 2·5% at 5 mg and 42% at 10 mg. Birth weights and weaning weights were also reduced in a dose-related manner.

Stula and Krauss (1977) have applied MMF to 2 rabbits percutaneously at a dose of 200 mg/kg (1/18 of the average lethal dose) on days 8–16 of pregnancy. Embryomortality was 100% compared with 3% in 4 vehicle control rabbits.

N,N-dimethylformamide

N,N-dimethylformamide (DMF) is the only formamide on which a number of inhalational studies have been carried out.

Kimmerle and Machemer (1975) have exposed rats to 0, 18 or 172 ppm for 6 h/day on days 6–15 of pregnancy. There were 22–23 animals/group. Acceptable teratological methods were used. There were no signs of maternal toxicity. There were no significant effects at any dose level on numbers carrying to term, implants/dam, live fetuses/dam, resorptions/dam or placental weight. Fetal weight was significantly reduced at 172 ppm to 3·78 g compared with 4·07 g in controls. There were no effects on malformations; one control fetus was abnormal (wavy ribs) and 2 from each of the treated groups (umbilical hernia, multiple malformations, split sternum and wavy ribs). There were no effects on ossification, even at 172 ppm.

Sheveleva *et al.* (1979) have exposed groups of 7–15 rats to 3·6 ppm (10·7 mg/m^3) or 0·77 ppm (2·3 mg/m^3) for 4 h/day from days 1–20 of pregnancy in the rat. They reported increased embryomortality at 3·6 ppm but not at 0·77 ppm. Fetal abnormalities and functional changes in the offspring were also mentioned, the threshold for these effects being 1·3 ppm (4 mg/m^3). However no further details nor incidence rates were given for any of these parameters. Signs of maternal toxicity (altered kidney function) have been noted in pregnant rats exposed to 3·6 ppm but not at 0·77 ppm on days 1–20 of pregnancy (see section A for details).

Gofmekler *et al.* (1970) have exposed rats to a range of concentrations of inhaled DMF from 167–0·003 ppm (500–0·01 mg/m^3) from days 1 to 20 or 22 of pregnancy. The highest dose used, 167 ppm, was toxic, killing 5/12 dams with none of the remaining animals showing any signs of pregnancy at term. At the second highest dose, 6·7 ppm, 1/12 dams died and only 4/11 carried to term. There was no significant effect on length of gestation at any dose. There was a significant reduction in mean fetuses/dam at 6·7 ppm to 43% of the control mean, and also at 0·003 ppm to 35% of the control value, but no reductions at intermediate dose levels of 0·33 or 0·01 ppm. There were sporadic significant effects on fetal weight and fetal organ weights but none showed any dose-related trend. Measurements of maternal and fetal ascorbic acid, nucleic acid and DNA levels in liver and brain tissue revealed some significant differences between treated and control groups, but again no dose-response relationships were evident. Gross structural changes were not seen at 0·01 ppm or 0·003 ppm. Findings at higher exposures were not specifically mentioned. Histological examination of tissues from fetuses and dams was carried out and a number of changes reported in lungs and blood vessels but the authors failed to differentiate between dams and fetuses or between treatment groups in their descriptive report of these effects.

An effect of inhaled DMF in late pregnancy in the rat has been investigated by Filomonov *et al.* (1974). They have shown that slowing of the fetal heart rate in response to maternal asphyxia is significantly greater in rats exposed beforehand to 134 ppm (400 mg/m^3) on days 15–20 of pregnancy.

Thiersch (1962) has given DMF orally or i.p. to rats on day 7 of pregnancy or after. The report in abstract only noted that there was no "differential toxicity" between mother and fetus and that no malformations were seen. Presumably, fetal losses were not seen except at doses which killed the dams. In this study the oral LD_{50} was given as 3 g/kg and the i.p. LD_{50} as 2·5 g/kg. No further information was given.

Oettel and Frohberg (1964) reported that DMF given orally, i.p. or percutaneously was not teratogenic in mice even at doses which killed the dams. No further details were given.

Von Kreybig (1967, 1968) has also noted the absence of teratogenicity of DMF when given s.c. in the rat or i.p. in the mouse, even at lethal doses ($>$2·5 g/kg). Similarly, Gleich (1974) has reported that 1·24 ml/kg DMF given i.p. in the mouse was not teratogenic.

Finally, Stula and Krauss (1977), applying DMF percutaneously in rats and rabbits have found no effect on embryomortality except at doses which killed the dam, and no effect on fetal weight or malformations. Groups of 4–8 rats were given 600–2400 mg/kg (1/28–1/7 of the average lethal dose) on one, 2 or 3 of days 9–13 of pregnancy. Significant increases in embryomortality were seen only after 2400 mg/kg on days 10 and 11 (26% resorptions) 6 × 200 mg/kg on days 11–13 (43% resorption), and 6 × 400 mg/kg on days 11–13 (30% resorptions). The incidence of s.c. haemorrhages was higher than in simultaneous controls but no different from historical controls. DMF was applied to 5 rabbits at 200 mg/kg/day (1/17 of the average lethal dose) on days 8–16 of pregnancy. No significant differences in embryomortality, fetal weight or malformations (none found) were seen in comparison with the 4 control dams.

Conclusion

Both F and MMF are highly embryolethal and teratogenic at doses below those lethal to the dam when given by a variety of routes including percutaneous administration. In the case of MMF effects are seen in the absence of any overt signs of toxicity in the dam such as weight loss, and abnormalities produced in rats and mice are similar in type. There is some evidence that the toxicity of formamides increases with increasing molecular weight (Thiersch, 1962; Chanh *et al.*, 1971). However, although MMF is clearly more embryolethal and more teratogenic than F (about 5–10 times more on a dose/kg basis, Thiersch, 1962; Gleich, 1974) DMF has been reported to be non-teratogenic in 5 studies employing one or more of the inhalational, oral, i.p., s.c. and percutaneous routes, and only embryolethal at doses which may also kill the dam. Two inhalational studies, where there is inadequate reporting of teratological methods and results, claim embryolethal and teratogenic or histopathologic effects at low doses. Sheveleva *et al.* (1979) report a threshold for effects of 1·3 ppm and Gofmekler *et al.* (1970) claim effects were seen at doses as low as 0·003 ppm, though their reported data only shows convincing effects at 6·7 ppm. These data are incompatible with the study of Kimmerle and Machemer (1975), who used large treatment groups, acceptable comprehensive teratological methods and full reporting of results but found no effects at 18 or 172 ppm apart from a 7% reduction in fetal weight at 172 ppm.

The lack of teratogenicity of DMF is at first sight surprising since it is metabolized to the highly teratogenic MMF. However it has been shown in the rat and in human subjects that this metabolite is very rapidly eliminated from the body (Kimmerle and Machemer, 1975), and this may account for the findings of most workers. Gleich (1974), for example, has shown that even a dose of DMF 20 times greater on a molar basis than a known teratogenic dose of MMF, causes no abnormalities in the mouse.

It is interesting also to note that testicular lesions have been found in rats and mice after F or MMF administration, but not after DMF (see section B). Thus it is these 2 compounds in the formamide series which may pose a reproductive hazard. However, it should be noted that compounds of higher molecular weight than DMF have not been systematically investigated for effects on reproduction.

E. MUTAGENICITY

No relevant data found.

F. CARCINOGENICITY

No relevant data found.

HUMAN STUDIES

A. RELEVANT PHARMACOLOGY AND TOXICOLOGY

No relevant data found.

B. & C. ENDOCRINE AND GONADAL EFFECTS/FERTILITY

There has been a single report by Richardson and Sadleir (1967) on the effects of N-methylformamide (MMF) and N,N-dimethylformamide (DMF) on sperm motility *in vitro*. Samples of semen with normal motility from healthy male volunteers were diluted 1:5 with solutions of MMF or DMF ranging in concentration from 2·5–10% in 0·9% saline. Both agents decreased sperm motility in a dose-related manner, but DMF had a greater effect, reducing motility by 78% at the 10% concentration compared with 33% in 10% MMF. The reduction in motility seen with MMF was equivalent to that obtained with glycerol, an agent used to protect spermatozoa during freezing when preserved for artificial insemination.

D. PREGNANCY

A question about possible health hazards from felt-tipped pens containing 40–50% formamide was raised in the European Parliament in 1974 (Anonymous, 1974). In reply it was stated that a major manufacturer had indicated in its technical sales literature that formamide could have teratogenic effects (presumably, in animals) and that in West Germany there was an agreement between the Ministry of Health and the appropriate trade association that formamide should not be used in fibre-tipped pens. The European Economic Commission had not at that time been notified of any "accidents to pregnant women or other individuals resulting from normal use of felt-tipped pens" (Anonymous, 1974).

E. MUTAGENICITY

No relevant data found.

F. CARCINOGENICITY

No relevant data found.

SUMMARY AND EVALUATION

EXPERIMENTAL STUDIES

Limited studies have shown that near lethal doses of formamide and N-methylformamide (MMF) can cause reversible damage and atrophy of the testes in rats. However, doses up to the i.p. LD_{50} of N,N-dimethylformamide (DMF) N-ethylformamide (MEF) and N,N-diethylformamide (DEF) in rats and mice did not cause testicular damage.

Limited studies with DMF in rats exposed to 3·6 ppm daily showed slight prolongation of all phases of the oestrous cycle. This was not observed at 0·77 ppm daily.

A number of studies with formamide in rats and mice have been reported as showing embryolethal and teratogenic effects when given parenterally or percutaneously but none of them are adequately reported.

A number of teratogenicity studies in mice and rats have demonstrated that MMF given by a variety of routes, i.p., s.c., orally or percutaneously is embryolethal and highly teratogenic. The malformations observed were similar in both species involving primarily the central nervous system (exencephaly and spina bifida), the thorax and palate. These have been observed at doses around 150–500 mg/kg which were often non-toxic to the dams. In most studies the range of doses was too restricted to define a no-effect level. In one study in which mice were given a single oral dose of MMF and allowed to litter down, there was an increase in stillbirths and post-natal mortality down to the lowest dose of about 75 mg/kg studied. One very small study in rabbits given 200 mg/kg percutaneously showed complete resorptions only.

DMF has been reported in several studies in rats and mice exposed by a variety of routes, inhalation, oral, s.c., i.p. and percutaneous not to be teratogenic and embryolethality was seen in some studies only at doses lethal to the dam. Two studies reported embryolethal and teratogenic effects at very low doses down to 0·003 ppm by inhalation but lack of data make these studies impossible to assess. One small study in rabbits exposed to 200 mg/kg DMF percutaneously during embryogenesis showed no adverse effects.

No studies were found on mutagenicity or carcinogenicity.

HUMAN STUDIES

No relevant studies were found on endocrine or gonadal effects or of effects on fertility, pregnancy, mutagenicity or carcinogenicity of any of the formamides.

EVALUATION

Formamide and more clearly, MMF have been shown to be both embryolethal and highly teratogenic in rodents and to a limited extent, embryolethal in rabbits. DMF is much less active in this regard in animals and the majority of studies suggest that it is not teratogenic, but may be embryolethal in high doses. This is surprising since DMF is metabolized to MMF and further studies are required to clarify the reasons for this difference. Attention is drawn to the fact that MMF is embryolethal and teratogenic when given by a variety of routes, including percutaneously and that no "no-effect level" has been established.

Attention is drawn to the lack of data in humans on any of the formamides.

References

Anonymous. (1974). Formamide hazard from felt-tipped pens? *Bibra Bulletin* **13**, (9), 509.

Chanh, P. H., Xuong, N. D. and Azum-Gelade, M.-C. (1971). Etude toxicologique de la formamide et de ses dérives N. Méthylés et N. Ethylés. *Thérapie* **26**, 409–424.

Filomonov, V. G., Finikova, L. S. and Sheveleva, G. A. (1974). On the mode of embryotropic action of dimethylformamide inhaled in low concentrations. *Farmakologiya i Toksikologiya* **37**, (2), 208–210.

Gleich, J. (1974). The influence of simple acid amides on fetal development of mice. *Naunyn-Schmiedeberg's Archives of Pharmacology* **282**, R25.

Gofmekler, B. A., Pushkina, H. H., Bonashevskaya, T. I. and Klevtsova, O. N. (1970). Effect of Dimethylformamide on embryogenesis in experiments with entry into the organism by inhalation. *Trudy-Permskogo Gosudarstvennogo Meditsinskogo Instituta* **82**, 168–173.

Kimmerle, G. and Machemer, L. (1975). Studies with N,N-Dimethylformamide for embryotoxic and teratogenic effects on rats after dynamic inhalation. *Internationales Archiv für Arbeitsmedizin* **34**, 167–175.

Messier, P.-E. (1976). Effects of formamide on neuroepithelial cells and on interkinetic nuclear migration in the chick embryo. *Journal of Embryology and Experimental Morphology* **35**, (1), 197–212.

Oettel, H. and Frohberg, H. (1964). Teratogene Wirkung einfacher Säureamide in Tierversuch. *Archiv fuer Experimentalle Pathologie und Pharmakologie* **247**, 363–364.

Pfiefer, G. and Von Kreybig, T. (1974). Chemisch Erzeugte Missbildungen des Kausschaedels bei Versuchstieren. III. Die Teratogenitaet verschiedener Formamidderivate bei der Ratte. *Deutsche Zahn-, Mund-, und Kieferheilkunde* **62**, 32–42.

Richardson, D. W. and Sadleir, R. M. F. S. (1967). The Toxicity of various non-electrolytes to human spermatozoa and their protective effects during freezing. *Journal of Reproduction and Fertility* **14**, 439–444.

Roll, R. and Bär, F. (1967). Teratogenic effect of monomethylformamide in pregnant mice. *Arzneimittel Forschung* **17**, (5), 610–614.

Sheveleva, G. A., Sivochalova, O. V., Osina, S. A. and Salkinova, L. S. (1977). Permeability of the placenta for dimethylformamide. *Akusherstvo i Ginekologiya (Moskva)* (5), 44–45.

Sheveleva, G. A., Strekalova, E. E. and others. (1979). A study of the embryotropic, mutagenous and gonadotropic effect of dimethylformamide with exposure by inhalation. *Toksikologiya Novykh Promyshlennykh Khimicheskikh Veshchestv* **15**, 21–25.

Stula, E. F. and Krauss, W. C. (1977). Embryotoxicity in rats and rabbits from cutaneous application of amide-type solvents and substituted ureas. *Toxicology and Applied Pharmacology* **41**, 35–55.

Thiersch, J. B. (1962). Effects of acetamides and formamides on the rat litter "*in utero*". *Journal of Reproduction and Fertility* **4**, 219–220.

Tuchmann-Duplessis, H. and Mercier-Parot, L. (1965). Production of anomalies in the rat after cutaneous applications of an industrial solvent: mono-methyl formamide. *Comptes Rendus de l'Academie des sciences (Paris)* **261**, 241–243.

Von Kreybig, T. (1967). Chemische Konstitution und teratogene Wirkung in einigen Verbindungsgruppen. *Archiven fuer Pharmakologie und experimentelle Pathologie* **257**, 296–298.

Von Kreybig, T. (1968). Experimentalle Prenatal-Toxocologie. *Arzneimittel-Forschung* **17**, 134–135.

26. Lead (Organic)

TECHNICAL DATA

(a) *Tetraethyl lead*

Formula $Pb(C_2H_5)_4$

CAS registry number 78–00–2

Chemical abstracts name Tetraethyl lead

Synonyms Plumbane, tetraethyl-; lead tetraethyl; TEL; tetraethylplumbane.

Uses Component of antiknock mixes for motor petrol.

TLV 0·1 mg/m^3

(b) *Tetramethyl lead*

Formula $Pb(CH_3)_4$

CAS registry number 75–74–1

Chemical abstracts name Tetramethyl lead

Synonyms Plumbane, tetramethyl-; lead tetramethyl; TML; tetramethylplumbane.

Uses Component of antiknock mixes, especially for aviation and premium grade petrols with high aromatic content.

TLV 0·15 mg/m^3

ANIMAL STUDIES

A. RELEVANT PHARMACOLOGY AND TOXICOLOGY

The major metabolic products of tetra-alkyl lead compounds are tri-alkyl lead compounds, and it is the tri-alkyl lead compounds which are thought to be mainly reponsible for the toxicity of tetra-alkyl lead compounds (Cremer, 1965).

The tetra-alkyl lead compounds are highly lipid soluble and would be expected to cross the placental membranes into the fetus without difficulty. McClain and Becker (1972) have measured the placental transfer of one of the metabolites, trimethyl lead, on day 20 of pregnancy in the rat. When trimethyl lead chloride was infused into the maternal artery at a rate of 1 mg/kg/min, none could be detected in the fetus 32 min after the start of infusion despite a linear increase in maternal blood levels during this time. At 64 min after the start of the infusion fetal levels were 7·9 μg/g and maternal whole blood and plasma concentrations 943 and 36 μg/ml respectively. At a higher rate of infusion, 2·5 mg/kg/min, trimethyl lead was detected in the fetus after 16 min of infusion, and had reached 70 μg/g by 64 min when maternal whole blood and plasma concentrations were 1482 and 68 μg/ml respectively. A sharp deviation from a linear increase in maternal whole blood concentration was seen between 32 and 64 min. These results suggest that trimethyl lead is initially bound to maternal erythrocytes, but at high infusion rates the binding sites become saturated and trimethyl lead then passes across to the fetus in substantial quantities.

B. ENDOCRINE AND GONADAL EFFECTS

No relevant data found.

C. FERTILITY

Kennedy *et al.* (1971) have carried out a dominant lethal test in mice with tetraethyl lead (TEL). TEL was administered as a single dose (unspecified), orally or i.p. and each male mated with 4 females/week for 6 weeks. At mid-pregnancy the females were killed and the contents of the uterus examined. There was no significant increase in early resorptions, suggesting no dominant lethality. The study is reported in abstract only and no further details are given.

D. PREGNANCY

McClain and Becker (1972) have investigated the teratogenicity of tetraethyl lead (TEL), tetramethyl lead (TML) and its metabolite trimethyl lead (TriML) in the rat. Acceptable teratological methods were used except for the small group sizes. With each of the 3 compounds, slight to severe, dose-related organolead toxicity was seen in the dams.

TEL was given orally by gavage in doses of 2·5, 5 or 10 mg/kg/day on days 9, 10 and 11, or 12, 13 and 14 of pregnancy to groups of 3–7 animals. All the dams died in the highest dose level groups given 10 mg/kg/day, and 1/5 died in those given 5 mg/kg/day on days 12–14. There was no effect on implants/dam. Resorption rate was increased from 1·5% in controls to 18% in the group given 5 mg/kg/day on days 9–11 and to 15% in those given 2·5 mg/kg/day on days 12–14. Fetal body weight was significantly reduced in a dose-related manner at all doses and times of administration. No gross malformations of external appearance, soft tissue or skeletal system were seen in any group. There was no evidence of increased retarded ossification in treated groups.

TML was given orally by gavage in doses of 13·3, 26·6, 37·3 or 53·3 mg/kg/day on days 9, 10 and11, or 26·6, 37·3 or 53·3 mg/kg/day on days 12, 13 and 14 of pregnancy, to groups of 4–8 animals. All the dams died in the 53·3 mg/kg/day groups and 4/6 died in those given 37·3 mg/kg/day on days 12–14. There was no effect on implants/dam and resorption rate was increased only in those given 37·3 mg/kg on days 9–11 from 1·5% in controls to 25%. Fetal body weight was significantly reduced in a dose-related manner at all doses and times of administration. The reduction in the group given 37·3 mg/kg/day on days 9–11 was particularly severe, fetuses weighing only 50% of controls. No gross malformations were seen but there was a significant increase in retarded ossification in all groups except those given 13·3 mg/kg/day on days 9–11.

TriML was given orally by gavage in doses of 5, 10 or 12·7 mg/kg/day on days 9–11 of pregnancy, or 10 or 12·7 mg/kg/day on days 12–14 of pregnancy, to groups of 3–5 animals. On days 9–11 all dams in the 12·7 mg/kg/day group died. On days 12–14, 2/4 in the 12·7 mg/kg/day group died and 1/5 in the 10 mg/kg/day group. There was no effect on implants/dam, but 34% of full-term fetuses were dead in those given 10 mg/kg/day on days 12–14, compared with none in controls. Fetal body weight was significantly reduced in a dose-related manner in all groups, but particularly in those dosed on days 12–14, fetuses weighing 50–60% less than controls. No gross malformations were seen but there was a significant increase in retarded ossification, affecting 22–100% of fetuses in different dose groups compared with 8% in controls.

In a second experiment by McClain and Becker (1972), TriML was given as a single i.v. injection in doses of 20, 28, 33 or 40 mg/kg on one of days 8–15 of pregnancy to groups of 1–7 rats. All dams given 40 mg/kg died and some rats died in a number of the 28 and 33 mg/kg groups. There was no effect on implants/dam but resorptions were increased in those given 33 mg/kg on day 8 or day 10. Fetal body weight was significantly reduced in 4/8 of the 33 mg/kg groups but a clear dose-response relationship was not seen on all days of dosing. There was a dose-related reduction in skeletal ossification.

McClain and Becker (1972) also gave direct intra-amniotic injections of TriML on day 15 of pregnancy in doses of 0, 10, 50 or 100 μg/fetus in groups of 3–5 rats. There was a dose-related increase in fetal mortality (assessed on day 22 of pregnancy) of 51–96% compared with control rates of 19–41% in vehicle-injected sacs.

Despite the small numbers of animals in each treatment group in this series of experiments, the large numbers of treated groups allow some firm conclusions to be drawn. TEL, TML andTriML given to the dam do not appear to cause malformations, and dose-related effects on fetal weight and ossification may well be secondary to the dose-related maternal toxicity seen in all treated groups. Some severely affected dams that carried to term were paralysed and unable to eat or drink for 2 or more days after organolead administration. Under these circumstances, 50% reductions in fetal weight are not surprising.

Kennedy *et al.* (1975) have investigated the teratogenicity of lower doses of TEL in the rat and mouse. Acceptable teratological methods were used. Groups of 20 animals were given 0, 0·01, 0·10, 1·0 and 10·0 mg/kg/day orally on days 5–15 of pregnancy in the mouse or days 6–16 of pregnancy in the rat. Overt toxicity (hypoactivity, tremors and convulsions) was seen in rats and mice after 3 daily doses of 10 mg/kg and further dosing was discontinued. The numbers pregnant at term in these groups were only 5/20 in mice and 7/20 in rats. In lower dose groups, the only sign of maternal toxicity was at 1 mg/kg where mice showed 25% less weight gain and rats 70% less weight gain than controls. There were no effects on implants/dam, live fetuses/dam, resorptions/dam or fetal weight at 0·01 or 0·10 mg/kg/day in rats or mice. But resorptions/dam were significantly increased in both species at 1·0 mg/kg, from 0·8% in vehicle control mice to 2·1% in treated mice, and from 0·8% in vehicle control rats to 2·3% in treated rats. Mean fetal weight was significantly reduced in a dose-related manner in 1·0 and 10·0 mg/kg/day groups by 30–60% in the mouse and by 12–25% in the rat compared with vehicle controls. A few malformed fetuses (not more than 3/group) were seen in some treated and control groups of rats and mice but there were no treatment-related effects. Delayed ossification was seen in fetuses from 1·0 and 10·0 mg/kg groups of mice and in the 10 mg/kg group of rats. These findings of increased resorption and decreased fetal weight with retarded ossification at maternally toxic doses are similar to those of McClain and Becker (1972).

Conclusion

In general, organolead compounds have a small embryolethal effect and a substantial effect on fetal weight and ossification at doses which are severely toxic to the dam. It seems likely that these effects are secondary to the maternal toxicity. At doses which are not toxic to the dam, no embryolethal or fetotoxic effects are seen. Teratogenicity is not seen, even at doses close to the maternal lethal dose.

These studies, together with the results of direct intra-amniotic injections of TriML and placental transfer studies (see section A for details), suggest that when tetra-alkyl lead compounds cross the placenta they are not readily converted into tri-alkyl compounds, presumably because the appropriate hepatic microsomal enzyme capacity does not develop until some time after birth in rodents. TriML, which is produced by maternal metabolism after administration of TML, only crosses the placenta in toxic amounts when maternal blood concentrations are very high and all maternal erythrocyte binding sites have become saturated. By these mechanisms, the embryo and fetus may be relatively "protected" from organolead toxicity.

E. MUTAGENICITY

No relevant data found, other than the abstract of the negative dominant lethal study in mice mentioned above.

F. CARCINOGENICITY

IARC Monograph Vol. 23 (1980) reported on a single study in neonatal mice injected s.c. with tetraethyl lead. An increased incidence of lymphomas occurred in female animals only. They commented that additional studies are needed before an evaluation of the carcinogenicity of this compound can be made.

HUMAN STUDIES

A. RELEVANT PHARMACOLOGY AND TOXICOLOGY

Poisoning by organic lead produces a clinical picture, primarily involving the central nervous system, which is distinguishable from that produced by inorganic lead poisoning. Thus the toxicity of organic lead would seem to be due to the molecular species as a whole rather than the metallic constituent alone (reviewed by Cremer, 1965; Boeckx *et al.*, 1977). In children, however, poisoning by either organic or inorganic lead may lead to encephalopathy. Organic lead is much more rapidly absorbed than inorganic lead salts by all routes including the skin and has a high lipid solubility, rapidly penetrating into the brain. Kehoe (quoted by Vurdelja *et al.*, 1967) has stated that organic lead absorbed by the body is broken down into inorganic lead in 3–14 days, but others have stated that the amounts of inorganic lead produced are minute (IARC Monograph Vol. 23, 1980). The lack of clear improvement in symptoms in cases of tetraethyl lead poisoning treated with metal chelators BAL or EDTA, normally effective in inorganic lead poisoning (Cremer, 1965; Vurdelja *et al.*, 1967) also implies that much of the toxicity is due to the organic parent compound rather than breakdown into metallic lead. Others, however, have reported a lowering of blood lead levels in tetraethyl lead poisoning with BAL and EDTA therapy (Boeckx *et al.*, 1977). This review however will be confined to those studies where organic lead specifically has been absorbed and will not cover those studies where effects have been noted in relation to elevated inorganic lead levels in tissues or resulting from inorganic lead poisoning.

Since organic lead is highly lipid soluble it is likely that it crosses the placenta; however no epidemiological studies or case reports are available on organic lead. A number of studies, reviewed by Roels *et al.* (1978) have found total lead concentrations (source not known) in the placenta ranging from 7–40 μg/100 g wet weight in pregnant women living in urban and rural environments. Roels *et al.* (1978) found significant correlations between placental and maternal blood levels, and placental and newborn blood levels, but maternal and cord blood levels were much more closely correlated (Lauwerys *et al.*, 1978).

B. ENDOCRINE AND GONADAL FUNCTION

There have been 2 reports concerning sexual function and spermatogenesis in man poisoned by petrol containing tetraethyl lead. Vurdelja *et al.* (1967) have reported on 14 cases of poisoning, 8 female and 6 male, where absorption of tetraethyl lead from petrol used to degrease metal objects caused admission to hospital. The workers came from 2 different industrial establishments. Poisoning was categorized as "discreet" (3 males), "manifest" (2 males) and "severe" (1 male). In the discreet form there were subjective complaints of tiredness, headaches, loss of appetite, insomnia, irritability, inner tension, reduced sexual potency or impotence. Clinically they showed tremor and spasms in the hands, slight dysarthric disturbances resembling stuttering, lively symmetrical tendon reflexes and painful sensitivity in the testis. In the manifest form there were similar signs and symptoms but more strongly marked and in the severe form excitation of the central nervous system was most noticeable. Symptoms began to recede about 14 days after the onset of clinical poisoning. Blood and urinary lead levels were measured but full details were not given. All lead levels were stated to be considerably above normal but it is not clear from the data given what the mean values were for these parameters.

During the acute phase of poisoning semen samples were taken for analysis. In 3 cases the sperm count was below normal, in one case there was azoospermia and in another case the sperm were of low motility. No quantitative details were given. Five months later there was improvement in the semen sample in only one male though potency was said to have returned in all 6 cases and only subjective symptoms remained. Urinary lead levels at this time were still above normal in all cases (96–410 $\mu g\%$).

Neshkov (1971) has published findings on 66 males aged 24–49 with sexual disturbances attending the sexological unit at a regional hospital, in whom exposure to ethyl benzine containing tetraethyl lead was thought to be the aetiological factor. Other aetiological factors were excluded by careful history-taking. The men had been in contact with ethyl benzine containing 0·82, 3·3 or 2·5 g/kg tetraethyl lead for 4–8 years. Besides sexual disturbances they also reported tiredness, feeling generally unwell, loss of appetite, occasional nausea, excessive salivation and perspiration, absentmindedness, loss of memory, disturbed sleep, excessive dreaming, vertigo and headache, a similar spectrum of complaints to that reported by Vurdelja *et al.* (1967).

The main complaints of all 66 patients were about decreases of potency, with poor or absent erection in 58, premature ejaculation in 41, reduced orgasm in 12 and reduced libido in 9. These effects developed gradually in the majority of cases, but were sudden in onset in 7 men whose history revealed they had swallowed ethyl benzine and who were suffering from chronic poisoning. Semen analysis and measurement of urinary 17-ketosteroids were carried out in all 66 patients. Semen volume was reduced (<2 ml) in 23 patients, semen viscosity increased in 28 patients and time of dilution of sperm increased in 32 patients. Semen pH was normal. In 22 patients sperm counts were normal (60–80 millions/ml) but in the remaining 44 they were below normal and the proportion of non-motile spermatozoa was around 20%. Abnormal sperm morphology was found in 6 patients. Androgenic activity as assessed by urinary 17-ketosteroids was within normal variations in 50 patients, but decreased to a mean of 6·2 mg/day in 16 patients. Following therapy (stopping contact with ethyl benzine, treatment with drugs and physiotherapy), after several weeks non-sexual symptoms disappeared and potency was fully restored in 42 patients and significantly improved in 22, with no improvement in 2 men. However, semen analysis at this time showed no significant improvements.

Whilst both of these studies have methodological problems, such as lack of control and quantitative data, the qualitative picture is strikingly similar. From the nature of the clinical signs and symptoms described it is likely that poisoning was due to the tetraethyl lead component of the petrol. The recovery of potency alongside disappearance of other neurological disturbances, following removal from exposure and therapy, but the persistence of low sperm counts and low motility up to 5 months after exposure, suggest that spermatogenesis may be particularly sensitive to organic lead poisoning. It is not clear whether androgenic activity may also be affected. Longer term follow-up was not available and so it is not known whether the effects on spermatogenesis are ultimately reversible.

C. FERTILITY

Robinson (1976) has studied the health of a group of 153 men with occupational exposure to lead, chiefly in the form of tetraethyl lead. The men selected for study had had 20 years or more of occupational exposure. Urinary and blood lead levels, averaged from measurements taken over 8–10 years of employment, were 0·089 mg lead/l and 0·043 mg lead/100 g respectively. However, the blood lead levels were not representative since they were only measured when urinary levels were high, blood lead levels not being a sensitive indicator of tetraethyl lead absorption. Body weight, blood pressure, haemoglobin, electrocardiogram and absences for non-occupational illness or injury did not differ in the tetraethyl lead-exposed group when compared with matched controls with no recognized occupational exposure to lead. Similarly, the average number of children/man was 2·6 in both exposed and control groups. However, little significance can be attached to this study since many of the children were born prior to the employees commencing work with lead or were born fairly shortly thereafter, and in studying those who had been occupationally exposed for 20 years or more, the "healthy worker" effect would be maximized.

D. PREGNANCY

No relevant data found.

E. MUTAGENICITY

A number of cytogenetic studies have been carried out on lead-exposed workers, summarized in IARC Monograph Vol. 23 (1980), but none related solely to workers exposed to organic lead only and most related to inorganic lead exposure.

F. CARCINOGENICITY

IARC Monograph Vol. 23 (1980) reported one study showing a slight but not significant excess of skin cancer in workers exposed to tetraethyl lead, but stated that available experimental and epidemiological data was insufficient to evaluate the carcinogenicity of organic lead compounds.

SUMMARY AND EVALUATION

EXPERIMENTAL STUDIES

Trialkyl lead is largely bound to erythrocytes in blood and only the small amount of the free organic lead in plasma crosses the placenta. No studies were found on endocrine or gonadal effects of alkyl lead, nor any adequate study of effects on fertility.

Studies using toxic doses of tetraethyl lead (TEL), tetramethyl lead (TML) and trimethyl lead (TriML) orally in rats have shown that these are not teratogenic. When embryolethality and fetotoxicity were observed, these were probably secondary to toxicity to the dams. Studies in rats and mice with lower doses of TEL of 0·01 and 0·1 mg/kg per day which were not toxic to the dams, showed no adverse effects on pregnancy.

No adequate data were found on mutagenicity, and studies are inadequate to assess its carcinogenic potential. No data on transplacental carcinogenicity were found.

HUMAN STUDIES

Although there is evidence that lead crosses the placenta into the fetus, there is no direct evidence that organic lead crosses the placenta although from its lipid solubility it would be expected to do so. There are two reports of toxicity in groups of workers from exposure to tetraethyl lead in petrol. In both studies there were complaints of reduced libido and potency in men with reduced semen volume, sperm count, motility and abnormal morphology. In the majority of those studied, urinary androgens were normal. On removal from exposure, potency soon returned but the sperm counts remained low, and there was inadequate follow-up to assess sperm recovery. No studies were found of effects on fertility, on pregnancy or on mutagenicity. Evidence is insufficient to assess effects on carcinogenicity.

EVALUATION

Only limited evaluation is possible. There is evidence that TEL, TML and TriML are not teratogenic in rats or mice and are embryolethal only at doses toxic to the dams. There is limited evidence that exposure to petrol containing TEL causes impotence and depresses spermatogenesis in men.

Attention is drawn to lack of adequate animal data on fertility, pregnancy, mutagenicity and carcinogenicity. Attention is drawn to the lack of adequate data on the levels of exposure required to adversely affect spermatogenesis in men and on the reversibility of this effect. The lack of data on effects on fertility, pregnancy, mutagenicity and carcinogenicity is also notable with such a wide-spread environmental contaminant.

References

Boeckx, R. L., Postl, B. and Coodin, F. J. (1977). Gasoline sniffing and tetraethyl lead poisoning in children. *Pediatrics* **60**, (2), 140–145.

Cremer, J. E. (1965). Toxicology and biochemistry of alkyl lead compounds. *Occupational Health Review* **17**, 14–19.

IARC Monographs on the Evaluation of the Carcinogenic Risk of Chemicals to Humans: Some metals and metallic compounds. (1980). Vol. 23, Lyon, France.

Kennedy, G., Arnold, D., Keplinger, M. L. and Calandra, J. C. (1971). Mutagenic and teratogenic studies with lead acetate and tetraethyl lead. *Toxicology and Applied Pharmacology* **19**, 370.

Kennedy, G. L., Arnold, D. W. and Calandra, J. C. (1975). Teratogenic evaluation of lead compounds in mice and rats. *Food and Cosmetics Toxicology* **13**, 629–632.

Lauwerys, R., Buchet, J. P., Roels, H. and Hubermont, G. (1978). Placental transfer of lead, mercury, cadmium, and carbon monoxide in women. 1. Comparison of the frequency distributions of the biological indices in maternal and umbilical cord blood. *Environmental Research* **15**, (2), 278–289.

McClain, R. M. and Becker, B. A. (1972). Effects of organolead compounds on rat embryonic and fetal development. *Toxicology and Applied Pharmacology* **21**, 265–274.

Neshkov, N. C. (1971). The influence of chronic intoxication of ethylated benzene on the spermatogenesis and sexual function of man. *Gigiena Truda i Professional 'nye Zabolevaniya* **13**, (2), 45–46.

Robinson, T. R. (1976). The health of long service tetraethyl lead workers. *Journal of Occupational Medicine* **18**, (1), 31–40.

Roels, H., Hubermont, G., Buchet, J. P. and Lauwerys, R. (1978). Placental transfer of lead, mercury, cadmium and carbon monoxide in women. *Environmental Research* **16**, 236–247.

Vurdelja, N., Farago, F., Nikolic, V. and Vuckovic, S. (1967). Clinical experience with intoxications of fuel containing lead-tetraethyl. *Folia Facultatis Medicae, Universitas Comenianae* **5**, (1), 133–138.

27. Manganese and its Compounds

TECHNICAL DATA

(a) *Manganese*

Formula Mn

CAS registry number 7439–96–5

Chemical abstracts name Manganese

Synonyms None

(b) *Manganese compounds* (Reviewed by IARC)

Formula	CAS registry number	Chemical abstracts name
$Mn(CH_3COO)_2$	638–38–0	Manganese acetate
$MnB_4O_7.8H_2O$ Appr.	12228–91–0	Manganese borate
$MnBr_2$	13446–03–2	Manganese bromide
$MnCO_3$	598–62–9	Manganese carbonate
$Mn_2(CO)_{10}$	10170–69–1	Manganese carbonyl
$MnCl_2$	7773–01–5	Manganese chloride
MnF_2	7782–64–1	Manganese difluoride
MnO_2	1313–13–9	Manganese dioxide
$Mn(H_2PO_2)_2$	10043–84–2	Manganese hypophosphite
MnI_2	7790–33–2	Manganese iodide
$Mn(NO_3)_2$	10377–66–9	Manganese nitrate
$Mn(C_{18}H_{33}O_2)_2$ Appr.	23250–73–9	Manganese oleate
MnC_2O_4	640–67–5	Manganese oxalate
Mn_3O_4	1317–35–7	Manganese oxide
$MnHPO_4$	7782–76–5	Manganese phosphate, dibasic
MnP_2O_7	53731–35–4	Manganese pyrophosphate
MnSe	1313–22–0	Manganese selenide
Mn_2O_3	1317–34–6	Manganese sesquioxide
$MnSiO_3$ Appr.	7759–00–4	Manganese silicate

$MnSO_4$	7785–87–7	Manganese sulphate
MnS	18820–29–6	Manganese sulphide
MnF_3	7783–53–1	Manganese trifluoride

Uses Manufacture of steel; for rock crushers, railway points and crossings, waggon buffers; constituent of several alloys; manufacture of dry cell batteries, glass, ink, ceramics, paints, welding rods, rubber and wood preservatives.

TLV 5 mg/m^3 (as manganese).

ANIMAL STUDIES

A. RELEVANT PHARMACOLOGY AND TOXICOLOGY

Excessive intake of manganese (Mn) has been shown to disturb the storage and metabolism of other essential trace metals such as iron, copper and zinc (Järvinen and Ahlström, 1975) and so the toxic effects of high doses of Mn may, in part, be mediated through such changes.

The effects of Mn on mineral metabolism may differ in the pregnant and the non-pregnant rat, despite similar relative tissue distribution of Mn given to pregnant and non-pregnant rats (Kaur *et al.*, 1980). Järvinen and Ahlström (1975) fed rats Mn in the diet at 4, 24, 54, 154, 504 and 1004 ppm from the time of weaning. After 8 weeks on the diet 10 females from each group were mated with untreated males. On day 21 of pregnancy they were killed and maternal liver Mn, copper, iron and zinc levels compared with those of non-pregnant females on the same diet. At all dietary levels, liver Mn content was higher in pregnant than non-pregnant animals, and increased as the dietary Mn level increased, whereas it did not increase in non-pregnant animals. Similarly, liver copper levels increased in pregnant rats with increasing dietary Mn levels, but did not change in non-pregnant rats. As might be expected liver iron levels were depleted in pregnant compared with non-pregnant rats, and in the pregnant animals, increasing dietary Mn levels did not cause any significant fall in liver iron content as it did in non-pregnant rats. Liver zinc levels were unaffected by dietary Mn. Thus pregnancy appears to enhance disturbances in liver copper and Mn levels in response to increasing Mn intake.

In these same groups of pregnant animals Järvinen and Ahlström (1975) have also shown increasing concentrations of Mn in the fetal liver at 21 days' gestation with increasing maternal dietary Mn intake, suggesting that placental transfer of Mn occurs. Fetal liver iron levels showed a marked tendency to decrease and copper levels a slight tendency to decrease with increasing maternal intake of Mn. Fetal liver zinc levels were also increased in the 1004 ppm group. The changes in fetal liver Mn, iron and zinc levels were most marked between 504 and 1004 ppm groups.

Clear demonstrations of the placental transfer of Mn have been obtained in experiments using radio-labelled $^{54}MnCl_2$. Onoda *et al.* (1978) injected $^{54}MnCl_2$ i.v. into pregnant rats on days 10, 13, 17, or 19 of gestation and tissue ^{54}Mn distribution was examined 3 h after injection and on day 20 in all groups. Two doses were injected, a low dose of 0·5 mg/kg, which is lower than the calculated daily intake of Mn from laboratory chow, and a high dose of 10 mg/kg, the maximum tolerated dose by single i.v. injection. Each group comprised 4 rats. The relative distribution of Mn in maternal tissues did not differ with different stages of pregnancy and tissue levels reflected the difference in high and low doses. Placental levels ranged from 78–215 ng/g tissue in low-dose animals and from 783–3495 ng/g tissue in high-dose animals, levels being highest in both groups on day 17 of pregnancy. Levels in the fetus (whole body) ranged from 65–73 ng/g at the low dose and 822–1258 ng/g at the high dose and did not differ significantly with different stages of gestation.

Retention of Mn in the dam and fetus was also shown from radioactivity measurements on day 20 after i.v. injection on days 10, 13, 17 or 19 of pregnancy. With the low dose retention in the dam ranged from 74% to 22% of the total dose and in the fetus from 0·90% to 0·12% of the total dose, with increasing interval between injection and day 20. At the high dose retention was 55% to 13% and 0·72% to 0·03% of the total dose in the dam and fetus respectively. On day 20, concentrations in the whole fetus were always higher than in the placenta. In the fetal tissues the highest concentrations of Mn were found in the liver, bone and brain, the concentrations in bone and brain being higher than the equivalent maternal concentrations.

Kaur *et al.* (1980) have also shown placental transfer in the rat after i.v. injection of $^{54}MnCl_2$ on day 18 of pregnancy. Eighteen hours after injection mean liver, kidney and brain levels in fetuses from 6 rats were 6·2%, 0·30% and 0·27% of the total dose/g tissue respectively. Levels in fetal liver and brain were 22-fold and 6-fold higher respectively than in the tissues of the dams.

Hanlon *et al.* (1975) have shown placental transfer of Mn in the hamster. Twenty-four hours after i.v. injection of $^{54}MnCl_2$ at a dose of 1·4 mg/kg Mn^{++} into 12 dams on day 8 of pregnancy, concentrations in the embryo and placenta were approximately 17% and 64% respectively of maternal liver concentrations and several-fold higher than maternal blood levels.

Gamble *et al.* (1971) have also shown placental transfer of Mn in the pig. $^{54}MnCl_2$ was injected i.v. into 13 pregnant sows at 103 days of gestation and the sows killed at intervals of 3, 6, 120 and 168 h after dosing. At 3 h, 12% of the total dose was in the placenta and 0·34% in the fetus, but by 168 h, 3% was in the placenta and 23% in the fetus. Fetal levels were high in the pancreas and liver, but brain levels were not measured. The relative distribution, metabolism and retention of Mn was similar in pregnant and non-pregnant pigs.

Transfer of Mn to suckling rats in the milk has also been demonstrated, with preferential concentration in the neonatal brain. Husain *et al.* (1977) gave groups of 6 rats 0 or 15 mg/kg/day $MnCl_2$ orally by gavage from the second day of lactation for up to one month. At 15 days of age the Mn concentrations in the brain, ovary and testis of the offspring were significantly higher in treated compared with control pups and at 30 days of age still higher. The concentrations in brain and ovary in the offspring at 30 days of age were higher than in the equivalent tissues in the dam. In the brain they were 2–3-fold higher.

Cotzias *et al.* (1976) have demonstrated absence of excretion of Mn given either i.p. or through the dam's milk, during the first 17 days of life in the mouse and rat and during the first 45 days of life in the cat. It is this absence of excretion of Mn which may account for the increasing concentrations of Mn in the liver and brain of the neonates also seen at this time. However, some protection is afforded to the neonate which does show premature excretion of Mn if massive levels ($>280\ \mu g/ml$) are given in the dam's milk diet.

Conclusion

These studies show that placental transfer of Mn can occur very rapidly in a variety of species with differing types of placenta and that Mn may be retained in the fetus for some time. After placental or lactational transfer fetuses and neonates show a preferential concentration of Mn in the brain in comparison with adult animals, probably due to a combination of a poorly-developed blood-brain barrier and inability to excrete Mn, except at high doses, in the early neonatal period. The demonstration of similar findings in a wide variety of species suggests that similar effects may occur in humans. Indeed, with an essential trace element for growth and development such as Mn, it would be remarkable if it did not reach the fetal and neonatal brain in humans. The known toxic effects of Mn on the brain of adults suggest that Mn exposure may be a particular hazard during development. The effects on developing brain in animals will be reviewed in section D.

B. ENDOCRINE AND GONADAL EFFECTS

Males

A number of studies in the mouse, rat and rabbit have shown that Mn adversely affects the male reproductive organs, and can do so at doses which do not have any other toxic effects.

Gray and Laskey (1980) have shown significantly retarded growth of the testes, seminal vesicles and preputial glands in male mice fed on standard diet with an additional 1050 ppm Mn, as Mn_3O_4, from 15 days of age, compared with males fed on standard diet containing 50 ppm Mn, as $MnSO_4$, at 58, 73 and 90 days of age. Subjects were taken from 26 litters of treated and control mice. General appearance, body, liver and kidney weights were unaffected by treatment, though locomotor activity measured at 70 days of age was significantly reduced in treated males.

Chandra and co-workers have carried out a series of studies on testicular effects in the rat. Administration of $MnCl_2$ at 8 mg/kg/day i.p. for 180 days to male rats averaging 120 g at the start of treatment, causes gradual histopathological changes in the testis (Chandra, 1971). Groups of 10 treated and 5 control males were killed at 30-day intervals for examination. No changes were evident at 90 days but by 120 days there was oedema in the interstitial tissue and vascular engorgement. By 150 days, there was degeneration of spermatids in about one-third of the tubules and a reduction in the number of spermatocytes. By 180 days about 50% of tubules were affected and numerous degenerating spermatocytes and spermatids and multinucleate cells were seen. Interstitial tissue, Leydig cells and blood vessels were generally unchanged. Only mild histological changes were seen in liver and brain of these rats.

Biochemical changes in the testis appear earlier than histological changes after dosing with $MnCl_2$ at 8 mg/kg/day i.p. in the rat. Kar *et al.* (1972) showed Mn levels in the testis increased 4-fold after 30 days of dosing and 9-fold after 60 days, by which time significant increases were seen in alanine, cysteine, leucine, proline, phenylalanine and glutamine levels in the testis. Saxena *et al.* (1977) showed significant decreases in succinic dehydrogenase, lactic dehydrogenase, phospholipid, cholesterol and glycogen levels of the testes after 60 days of dosing.

A further demonstration of the particular vulnerability of the testis by Chandra's group was seen in the study of Singh *et al.* (1974) in the rat. Administration of 6 mg Mn/kg/day as manganese sulphate i.p. for 25 days and comparison of Mn levels, enzyme activities and histopathological changes in testis, liver and brain, showed a 316% increase in testicular Mn levels, compared with 216% in liver and 155% in brain, accompanied by maximum biochemical changes and degeneration of 10% of seminiferous tubules. In the liver there were few enzymatic or histological changes and in the brain there were marked enzyme changes but no histological alterations.

Protection from Mn-induced testicular damage has been shown by Chandra *et al.* (1975) with simultaneous administration of zinc. Administration of chelating agents to rats treated previously with Mn reduces testicular Mn levels consistently, but has a variable effect on biochemical and histological changes induced by Mn, some of which may be irreversible (Tandon *et al.*, 1975; Singh *et al.*, 1975).

Similar Mn-induced testicular changes have been shown in the rabbit by Chandra *et al.* (1973). Twenty mature, male rabbits were given a single intra-tracheal injection of 250 mg/kg manganese dioxide and 10 given a vehicle injection. They were killed 4 or 8 months later. At 4 months the testes showed interstitial tissue oedema and vascular engorgement and 30% of seminiferous tubules showed epithelial degeneration. Spermatids and spermatocytes were considerably reduced in number and degenerating. At 8 months more extensive degeneration was seen and calcification observed in about 20% of tubules. Succinic dehydrogenase, acid phosphatase and adenosine triphosphatase levels were significantly reduced at 8 months. The testes were small and these animals proved sterile when paired with fertile females 8 months after dosing, before autopsy. Subsequent work by Seth *et al.* (1973) showed that the biochemical changes paralleled the histopathological changes and occurred as early as 2 months after injection of manganese dioxide. They preceded the development of encephalopathy, evident from lethargy appearing 6 months after dosing. The progressive development of testicular damage, the authors suggest, may be due to transfer of Mn from the lung to the testes over time.

These studies in the rat and rabbit did not determine whether the biochemical changes were a cause or an effect of the histopathological changes. However, subsequent work by Imam and Chandra (1975) showed decreased activity of succinic dehydrogenase in the seminiferous tubules of rabbits given 3·5 mg Mn/kg/day i.v. after only 5 days of dosing, whereas morphological changes were not seen up to the 10th day of dosing. By 15 days however degenerative changes were present with no evidence of spermatogenesis. This experiment suggests that the primary effect of Mn may be inhibition of succinic dehydrogenase in the mitochondria of the seminiferous epithelium with a consequent disturbance of energy metabolism, causing cell death. It is known that Mn is localized in the mitochondria where it has a high turnover (Ferm, 1972). If this is the case, however, the early vulnerability of testicular succinic dehydrogenase remains to be explained.

Conclusion

A number of studies in the mouse, rat and rabbit have shown that Mn adversely affects the testes and accessory organs and can do so at doses which do not have any other toxic effects; thus the testes may be particularly vulnerable to Mn toxicity. Oral, i.p., i.v. and intra-tracheal routes have all been shown to be effective. Biochemical changes generally precede histological changes and effects on spermatogenesis.

The demonstration in the rabbit that intra-tracheal administration, like i.v. or i.p. administration, still causes testicular damage may be of relevance to occupational exposure in humans, since inhalation of manganese dioxide is one of the commonest sources of exposure.

There have been no studies on effects on the endocrine system and gonads in females.

C. FERTILITY

Females

Exposure to Mn in the diet has not been found to significantly affect fertility in the female rat. Järvinen and Ahlström (1975) fed rats on diet containing 4, 24, 54, 154, 504 or 1004 ppm Mn from weaning. After 8 weeks on the diet 10 or 11 females/group were mated with untreated males and continued on the Mn diet during pregnancy. There were no significant effects on maternal weight gain, implants/dam, resorptions/dam or dead fetuses/dam. No gross external malformations were seen, which is unusual in an overall number of approximately 600–700 fetuses from all groups. No skeletal malformations were observed either but only 5 fetuses/group were examined, which is not adequate for a teratology study.

Males

Epstein *et al.* (1972) have carried out a dominant lethal study in male mice given single i.p. doses of manganese chloride. Nine were injected with 20 mg/kg and 7 with 100 mg/kg, and 10 males were concurrent controls. Each male was caged with 3 untreated females/week for 8 weeks. The treatment did not cause any male deaths and there was no effect on pregnancy rate amongst the females and no dominant lethal effects.

The study carried out by Chandra *et al.* (1973) on male rabbits has been mentioned in section B. Eight months after intra-tracheal injection of a single dose of 250 mg/kg manganese dioxide the males were placed with healthy females, but no pregnancies occurred though interstitial tissue was more or less intact. Under these circumstances testosterone could still have been produced but it is not known whether the males failed to mate or had infertile matings.

Conclusion

A single, large dose of Mn in the rabbit, but not in the mouse, affects male fertility. In view of the severe effects of Mn on the testes it is unlikely that fertility would be normal after chronic dosing of male rodents, but no such experiments have been carried out. Chronic dosing in females with high doses in the diet (up to 1000 ppm) would appear to be without effect in the rat, though no other work on different species has been carried out.

D. PREGNANCY

Mn deficiency is teratogenic in a number of species, causing skeletal abnormalities and irreversible ataxia due to defective otolith development in the middle ear (Ferm, 1972). However, much less work has been done on the effects of Mn excess during pregnancy.

The possible teratogenic effect of Mn in the rat has been examined by Kimmel *et al.* (1974). A dose of 10 mg/kg/day manganous sulphate was given i.p. on days 8–10 of pregnancy to 6 rats. Acceptable teratological methods were used. Mn had no significant effect on implants/dam, resorptions/dam, fetal weight or malformations in comparison with controls.

A comprehensive teratogenicity study on manganese sulphate monohydrate has been carried out in the mouse, rat, hamster and rabbit by Food and Drug Laboratories, Inc., on behalf of the F.D.A. in the U.S.A. (1973). In mice, doses of 1·25, 5·81, 27 and 125 mg/kg were given orally by gavage to groups of 25 animals on days 6–15 of pregnancy. There were no significant effects on maternal body weight, implants/dam, live fetuses/dam, resorptions/dam or fetal weight. Skeletal abnormalities did not differ significantly between groups and only 2 soft tissue abnormalities were seen, both at 125 mg/kg, one fetus having exophthalmos and another meningoencephalocoele.

In rats, doses of 0·783, 3·63, 16·9 and 78·3 mg/kg were given orally by gavage to groups of 25 animals on days 6–15 of pregnancy. There were no significant effects on maternal body weight, implants/dam, live fetuses/dam, resorptions/dam, fetal weight or skeletal abnormalities. No soft tissue abnormalities were seen except in positive controls given aspirin. The absence of any abnormalities of this type in Mn groups that would have yielded approximately 1000 fetuses is unusual.

In hamsters, doses of 1·36, 6·32, 29·3 and 136 mg/kg were given orally by gavage to groups of 25 animals on days 6–10 of pregnancy. There were no significant effects on maternal body weight, implants/dam, live fetuses/dam, resorptions/dam, fetal weight or skeletal anomalies. The only soft tissue abnormality reported was meningoencephalocoele in one fetus at 29·3 mg/kg.

In rabbits, doses of 1·12, 5·2, 24·2 and 112 mg/kg were given orally by gavage to groups of 15 does on days 6–18 of pregnancy. There were no significant effects on maternal body weight, implants/doe, live fetuses/doe, resorptions/doe, skeletal or soft tissue abnormalities. The only malformation seen was in a positive control group given 6-aminonicotinamide.

This F.D.A. study is remarkable for the very small number of soft tissue abnormalities reported in all the species tested. According to the methods, all fetuses were examined by dissection under a $\times 10$ microscope. The few abnormalities which were reported would all have been visible externally to the naked eye. It must be concluded that the internal examination was inadequate or under-reported, and that while Mn is clearly not a gross teratogen, further studies are needed to ascertain whether it might be a mild teratogen.

Confirmation of absence of teratogenicity in the hamster comes from experiments carried out by Ferm and his colleagues. Manganese chloride, given i.v. at a dose of 1·36 mg/kg on day 8 of pregnancy to 6 hamsters was not embryolethal or teratogenic (Hanlon *et al.*, 1975). $MnCl_2$ i.v. at doses of 10, 20, 30 or 35 mg/kg on day 8 of pregnancy, given to groups of 3 or 7 animals, however, did have embryolethal effects (Ferm, 1972). There was a dose-related increase in resorptions from 2·6% at 10 mg/kg to 19% at 20 mg/kg and 38% at 30 mg/kg, but no increases in malformations in survivors; 1/37 was malformed at 10 mg/kg, 2/73 at 20 mg/kg, 2/56 at 30 mg/kg and 0/9 at 35 mg/kg. Of the 3 dams injected with 35 mg/kg, 2 died immediately after injection.

Injection of $MnCl_2$ during late gestation in the pig affects the offspring. Wade (1972) gave 1, 2 or 3 weekly doses of 1·0 mg Mn^{++}/kg or one or 2 weekly doses of 0·5 mg Mn^{++}/kg i.p. during the last month of pregnancy. Live births, 35-day survival and 35-day-old weights of the piglets were lower in treated than control groups. The study is reported in abstract only and no further details are given.

The effects of Mn in newborns, particularly on the brain where Mn concentrates, have been extensively studied. Absorption and retention of heavy metals in general by neonates appears to be higher than in older animals (Kostial *et al.*, 1978). The transfer of Mn to suckling offspring from the dam's milk has already been discussed in section A. Exogenously administered Mn behaves in a similar manner to that passed into the offspring in the mother's milk. Kostial *et al.* (1978) have shown much higher absorption and retention of Mn given orally in cow's milk or i.p. in 1-week-old rats compared with 6-week-old rats. Both age and the nature of the diet influence absorption, a milk diet enhancing the effect of age. Retention of Mn in the brain 6 days after i.p. injection was much higher in those injected at one week of age (7%) than at 6 weeks of age (0·26%).

Cotzias *et al.* (1976) have shown a reduction in body weight at 30 days of age of mice suckled by dams given Mn in a basal diet of evaporated milk throughout lactation. Significant dose-related effects on offspring body weight were seen in those whose mothers received $>40\ \mu g/ml$ of diet, reaching only 50% of control weight when the dams consumed 400 μg/ml of diet. Above 1000 μg/ml early death of the young occurred.

Seth *et al.* (1977) have followed the development of rat pups exposed to Mn through the mother's milk. The dams were given 15 mg/kg $MnCl_2.4H_2O$ orally by gavage from day 2 of lactation. There were 6 treated and 6 control dams, each with a litter of 8 pups. The mean Mn content of the pups' brains was

3·94 ppm at 15 days of age and 6·93 ppm at 30 days of age, compared with control values of 2·40 ppm and 2·25 ppm at 15 and 30 days respectively. These levels in brains of Mn pups were 2–3-fold higher than in the brains of the treated dams. The brains of the pups showed no gross or histopathological changes, but enzyme activities were changed; at 15 days, adenosine triphosphatase, adenosine deaminase and acetyl cholinesterase were decreased, and at 30 days these enzymes were further decreased and succinic dehydrogenase was decreased while monoamine oxidase was increased. There were no significant effects on offspring body weight or on developmental landmarks such as opening of the eyes, growth of body hair and "walking movements".

Antonova (1978) gave manganese sulphate orally by gavage in doses of 7·5, 10·0, 12·5, 17·5, 30·0 and 42·5 mg/kg/day to rats throughout pregnancy and lactation. "Controls" received 4 mg/kg/day by gavage. In addition all rats had a dietary intake of 0·7–1·0 mg/day, equivalent to 4–5 mg/kg/day. Mean litter size was higher by 0·2–1·8 pups in dams given 7·5–42·5 mg/kg/day compared with those given 4 mg/kg. At 7·5–17·5 mg/kg/day the weight of the pups at birth and up to 28 days of age was higher than controls. At 30·0 and 42·5 mg/kg/day postnatal weight gain was lower than in controls and survival at 28 days was 79% and 59% respectively, compared with around 93% in control and lower Mn groups. Times of opening of ears and eyes, and appearance of hair and teeth in the pups were also noted according to the methods, but the results were not reported. At 28 days of age immunological reactivity was assessed in terms of the phagocytic index and content of non-specific agglutinins in serum. It was generally stimulated at 7·5–17·5 mg/kg/day compared with 4, 30 or 42·5 mg/kg/day.

In the guinea pig, dircct administration of manganese chloride to the pup in the neonatal period alters brain amine levels. Shukla and Chandra (1979) gave 0 or 10 mg/kg/day i.p. from 2–30 days of age to groups of 12 pups. At the end of dosing there were significant reductions in serum tryptophan, serum tyrosine, brain tryptophan, brain 5-hydroxytryptamine (5-HT) and brain 5-hydroxyindoleacetic acid, and significant increases in brain dopamine (DA) and Mn levels in Mn-treated pups compared with controls. The changes in 5-HT levels and turnover most probably are a consequence of a decrease in the precursor, tryptophan. Increases in brain DA levels indicate earlier maturation of dopaminergic pathways, but elevated DA levels have also been noted in early Mn toxicity in adults.

Conclusion

There is evidence that Mn is not teratogenic at doses not toxic to the dam in the mouse, rat, hamster and rabbit. However, it may cause some embryolethality at doses just below those toxic to the dam and is definitely embryolethal in the hamster at doses near to maternally lethal doses.

There is evidence that Mn may have more marked postnatal than prenatal effects. Adverse effects on postnatal weight gain and survival have been seen after administration of Mn in late pregnancy in the pig and neonatally in mice and rats. Alterations in brain enzyme and neurotransmitter levels have also been found in rats and guinea pigs after neonatal administration of Mn. These latter observations are particularly notable in view of the preferential concentration of Mn in the brain. The behavioural consequences, if any, of such biochemical changes in the brain are not yet known.

E. MUTAGENICITY

Mn and its salts are probably the best-known metal mutagens. It is mutagenic in bacteria (Flessel, 1977).

Mn does not alter the frequency of chromosomal aberrations in bone marrow cells or spermatogonia of rats. Dikshith and Chandra (1978) gave groups of 10 male rate $MnCl_2.4H_2O$ orally at a dose of 0 or 50 μg/kg/day for 180 days. Bone marrow cells and spermatogonial cells were collected at the end of the dosing period. No cytogenetic changes were seen in spermatogonia or in bone marrow cells. The only aberrations seen were chromatid gaps or breaks, the incidence of which did not differ between treated and control rats.

F. CARCINOGENICITY

No relevant data found.

HUMAN STUDIES

A. RELEVANT PHARMACOLOGY AND TOXICOLOGY

Leonov *et al.* (1971) measured the blood levels of manganese (Mn) as well as nickel, copper, chromium and molybdenum in mothers and newborn babies at some unspecified time in relation to pregnancy. They stated that in 25 mothers with toxicosis in the first half of pregnancy no change in the amount of these elements was observed (no details given). However, when 120 new mothers with late pregnancy toxicosis were compared with a control group of 110 mothers with normal pregnancy, higher levels of Mn were found in the "toxic" mothers and babies (27·5 ± 1·5 (mother), 28·0 ± 2·2 (baby)) compared with the controls (17·0 ± 0·52, 17·5 ± 0·51). The levels of nickel and copper were also elevated in late pregnancy toxicosis. (The units of measurements were not stated. They were possibly μg/100 ml, but see values below.) The authors suggest that the changes are part of the adaptive mechanism of the mother to the anoxia caused by the toxicosis, but no other details are given.

Hambidge and Droegemueller (1974) studied plasma levels of zinc, copper, chromium and Mn in 20 normal, young, well nourished women in the U.S.A. during the third to fifth months of pregnancy and again in the last month of pregnancy. No alteration was found in Mn level, which was the same as their stated control non-pregnant level of 1·5 to 2·0 ng/ml.

B. ENDOCRINE AND GONADAL EFFECTS

Mena *et al.* (1967) studied 13 chronically Mn-poisoned miners, 12 of whom had been pensioned off from a Chilean mine 2–25 years prior to examination (median 5 years) and whose ages ranged from 18–56 years (median age 50 years). All were severely affected and the disease consisted of a limited period of severe psychiatric disorder followed by a permanent crippling neurological disease, with disorder of gait, speech and postural reflexes. Eight of the men also complained of sexual impotence. This symptom was not recorded as present in a group of 14 healthy miners, with approximately the same age range, who were studied at the same time.

Similar psychiatric and neurological symptoms had previously been reported by Schuler *et al.* (1957) in a detailed study of 15 severely affected Chilean workers. They also reported diminution or abolition of libido in 4 of the men, with a delay in ejaculation in 3 of these. Penalver (1955), in a review of Mn poisoning, states that impotence is one of the commonest manifestations of the disease although the mechanism is unknown. Rodier (1955) reported that in the early stages of the disease, during the "psychotic" period, nearly 80% of cases report impotence. With a background of such severe and widespread psychological, psychiatric and neurological disturbances, a central cause seems possible. Rodier (1955) reported in his study of Mn poisoning in Moroccan workers a clear reduction in urinary 17-ketosteroids in 81% of the cases (no values given), suggesting reduced testosterone secretion.

C. FERTILITY

No relevant data found.

D. PREGNANCY

No relevant data found.

E. MUTAGENICITY

No relevant data found.

F. CARCINOGENICITY

No relevant data found.

SUMMARY AND EVALUATION

EXPERIMENTAL STUDIES

Placental transfer of manganese has been shown to occur rapidly in several species, with retention in the fetal tissues. Transfer also occurs via the milk and manganese tends to show a preferential concentration in the fetal and neonatal brain. Neonates do not excrete manganese unless massive doses are given, so that cumulation can occur. Studies in mice, rats and rabbits have shown that manganese adversely affects the seminiferous tubules in the testes at doses producing no other toxic effects. Fertility in female rats was unaffected by doses up to 1000 ppm in the diet chronically.

Manganese is an essential element and deficiency has been shown to be teratogenic in several species causing skeletal defects and ataxia due to defective otolith development in the middle ear. Manganese excess has been less well studied but several studies in a variety of species have shown that it is not teratogenic even at high doses. Embryolethality is observed at doses toxic to the dam. Postnatal growth and survival may however be affected and alterations have been shown in neurotransmitter levels in the brain. It is mutagenic *in vitro* but limited studies have not shown effects *in vivo*. No data on carcinogenicity were found.

HUMAN STUDIES

Chronic manganese poisoning in male miners produces a variety of neurological deficits and impotence is common. Decreased libido is also reported and may be related to reduced testosterone secretion. No other relevant data were found on reproductive effects or on mutagenicity or carcinogenicity.

EVALUATION

There is sufficient evidence that manganese can cause specific testicular damage in animals at otherwise non-toxic doses. There is sufficient evidence that it is not teratogenic in several species but may be embryolethal at toxic doses. Attention is drawn to the lack of adequate data on postnatal development in animals treated during pregnancy or during lactation. Human data is inadequate for evaluation except for effects in grossly contaminated men where impotence is a common symptom. Attention is drawn to the lack of human data on fertility and pregnancy after moderate exposure.

References

Antonova, M. V. (1978). The influence of different amounts of manganese in the daily ration on the growth and development of albino rats offsprings. *Voprosy Pitaniya* **1**, 65–68.

Chandra, S. V. (1971). Cellular changes induced by manganese in the rat testis—preliminary results. *Acta Pharmacologica et Toxicologica* **29**, 75–80.

Chandra, S. V., Ara, R., Nagar, N. and Seth, P. K. (1973). Sterility in experimental manganese toxicity. *Acta Biologica et Medica Germanica* **30**, 857–862.

Chandra, S. V., Saxena, D. K. and Hasan, M. Z. (1975). Effect of zinc on manganese induced testicular injury in rats. *Industrial Health* **13**, (1–2), 51–56.

Cotzias, G. C., Miller, S. T., Papavasiliou, P. S. and Tang, L. C. (1976). Interactions between manganese and brain dopamine. *Medical Clinics of North America* **60**, (4), 729–738.

Dikshith, T. S. S. and Chandra, S. V. (1978). Cytological studies in albino rats after oral administration of manganese chloride. *Bulletin of Environmental Contamination and Toxicology* **19**, 741–746.

Epstein, S. S., Arnold, E., Andrea, J., Bass, W. and Bishop, Y. (1972). Detection of chemical mutagens by the dominant lethal assay in the mouse. *Toxicology and Applied Pharmacology* **23**, 288–325.

Ferm, V. H. (1972). The teratogenic effects of metals on mammalian embryos. *Advances in Teratology* **5**, 51–75.

Flessel, C. P. (1977). Metals as mutagens. *Advances in Experimental Medicine and Biology* **91**, 117–128.

Food and Drug Laboratories, Inc. (1973). Teratologic evaluation of FDA 71–71 (manganese sulphate monohydrate). Prepared for the FDA May 1973 NTIS P8–223 813.

Gamble, C. T., Hansard, S. L., Moss, B. R., Davis, D. J. and Lidvall, E. R. (1971). Manganese utilization and placental transfer in the gravid gilt. *Journal of Animal Science* **32**, (1), 84–87.

Gray, L. E. and Laskey, J. W. (1980). Multivariate analysis of the effects of manganese on the reproductive physiology and behaviour of the male house mouse. *Journal of Toxicology and Environmental Health* **6**, (4), 861–867.

Hambidge, K. M. and Droegemueller, W. (1974). Changes in plasma and hair concentrations of zinc, copper, chromium and manganese during pregnancy. *Obstetrics and Gynecology* **44**, (5), 666–672.

Hanlon, D. P., Gale, T. F. and Ferm, V. H. (1975). Permeability of the Syrian hamster placenta to manganous ions during early embryogenesis. *Journal of Reproduction and Fertility* **44**, 109–112.

Husain, R., Mushtaq, M., Seth, P. K. and Chandra, S. V. (1977). The effect of maternally administered manganese on neonatal rat brain. *In* "Environmental Pollution and International Health—Proceedings of the International Symposium on Industrial Toxicology", pp. 725–735. Toxicology Research Centre, Lucknow, India.

Imam, Z. and Chandra, S. V. (1975). Histochemical alterations in rabbit testis produced by manganese chloride. *Toxicology and Applied Pharmacology* **32**, 534–544.

Järvinen, R. and Ahlström, A. (1975). Effect of the dietary manganese level on tissue manganese, iron, copper and zinc concentrations female rats and their fetuses. *Medical Biology* **53**, 93–99.

Kar, P. P., Mustafa, S. J. and Satya, V. C. (1972). Amino acid changes in rat testis in manganese poisoning. *Arhiv za Higijenu Rada I Toksikologiju* **23**, (4), 307–310.

Kaur, G., Hasan, S. K. and Srivastava, R. C. (1980). The distribution of manganese-54 in fetal, young and adult rats. *Toxicology Letters* **5**, 423–426.

Kimmel, C. A., Butcher, R. E., Vorhees, C. E. and Schumacher, H. J. (1974). Metal-salt potentiation of salicylate-induced teratogenesis and behavioral changes in rats. *Teratology* **10**, 293–300.

Kostial, K., Kello, D., Jugo, S., Rabar, I. and Maljkovio, T. (1978). Influence of age on metal metabolism and toxicity. *Environmental Health Perspectives* **25**, 81–86.

Leonov, A., Gurskaya, I. K., Medvedeva, V. I. and Chichko, M. V. (1971). Disturbances in Mn, Ni, Cr, Cu and Mo exchange between mother and fetus in late pregnancy toxicoses. *Proceedings of the Academy of Sciences BSSR* **XV**, (7), 656–657.

Mena, I., Marin, O., Fuenzalida, S. and Cotzias, G. C. (1967). Chronic manganese poisoning. Clinical picture and manganese turnover. *Neurology* **17**, 128–136.

Onoda, K., Hasegawa, A., Tanaka, S., Takanaka, A., Omori, Y. and Urakubo, G. (1978). Studies on the fate of poisonous metals in experimental animal. VII. Distribution and transplacental passage of manganese in pregnant rat and fetus. *Journal Food Hygienic Society of Japan* **19**, (2), 208–215.

Penalver, R. (1955). Manganese Poisoning. The 1954 Ramazzini Oration. *Industrial Medicine and Surgery* **24**, 1–7.

Rodier, J. (1955). Manganese poisoning in Moroccan miners. *British Journal of Industrial Medicine* **12**, 21–35.

Saxena, D. K., Husain, R., Chandra, S. V. and Seth, P. K. (1977). Manganese induced biochemical alterations in rat seminiferous tubules. *Industrial Health* **14**, (1–2), 15–20.

Schuler, P., Oyanguren, H., Maturana, V., Valenzuela, A., Cruz, E., Plaza, V., Schmidt, E. and Haddad, R. (1957). Manganese poisoning. Environmental and Medical Study at a Chilean mine. *Industrial Medicine and Surgery* **26**, 167.

Seth, P. K., Nagar, N., Husain, R. and Chandra, S. V. (1973). Effects of manganese on rabbit testes. *Environmental Physiology and Biochemistry* **3**, (6), 263–267.

Seth, P. K., Husain, R., Mushtap, M. and Chandra, S. V. (1977). Effect of manganese on neonatal rat: manganese concentration enzymatic alterations in brain. *Acta Pharmacologica et Toxicologica* **40**, (5), 553–560.

Shukla, G. S. and Chandra, S. V. (1979). Species variation in manganese induced changes in brain biogenic amines. *Toxicology Letters* **3**, 249–253.

Singh, J., Husain, R., Tandon, S. K., Seth, P. K. and Chandra, S. V. (1974). Biochemical and histiopathological alterations in early manganese toxicity in rats. *Environmental Physiology and Biochemistry* **4**, 16–23.

Singh, J., Chandra, S. V. and Tandon, S. K. (1975). Chelation in metal intoxication II: *In vitro* and *in vivo* effect of some compounds on brain, liver, and testis of rats treated with manganese sulphate. *Bulletin of Environmental Contamination and Toxicology* **14**, (4), 497–504.

Tandon, S. K., Chandra, S. V., Singh, J., Husain, R. and Seth, P. K. (1975). Chelation in metal intoxication. I. In vivo effect of chelating agents on liver and testis of manganese administered rats. *Environmental Research* **9**, (1), 18–25.

Wade, D. A. (1972). Effects of manganese chloride on gravid gilts and newborn pigs. *Dissertation Abstracts International* B **33**, (7), 2872–2873.

28. Mercury and its Compounds (Inorganic)

TECHNICAL DATA

(a) *Mercury*

Formula Hg

CAS registry number 7439–97–6

Chemical abstracts name Mercury

Synonyms Hydrargyrum; liquid silver; quicksilver.

(b) *Mercury compounds*

Formula	CAS registry number	Chemical abstracts name
$Hg(CH_3COO)_2$	1600–27–7	Mercuric acetate
$HgHAsO_4$	7784–37–4	Mercuric arsenate
$HgBr_2$	7789–47–1	Mercuric bromide
$HgCl_2$	7487–94–7	Mercuric chloride
HgNHCl	10124–48–8	Mercuric chloride, ammoniated
$Hg(CN)_2$	592–04–1	Mercuric cyanide
$HgCr_2O_7$	7789–10–8	Mercuric dichromate
HgF_2	7783–39–3	Mercuric fluoride
$Hg(IO_3)_2$	7783–32–6	Mercuric iodate
HgI_2	7774–29–0	Mercuric iodide
$Hg(NO_3)_2$	10045–94–0	Mercuric nitrate
HgO	21908–53–2	Mercuric oxide, red
$HgO.Hg(CN)_2$	1335–31–5	Mercuric oxycyanide
$HgSO_4.2HgO$	1312–03–4	Mercuric subsulphate
$HgSO_4$	7783–35–9	Mercuric sulphate
HgS	1344–48–5	Mercuric sulphide, red
$Hg(SCN)_2$	592–85–8	Mercuric thiocyanate
$Hg_2(CH_3COO)_2$	631–60–7	Mercurous acetate

Hg_2Br_2	10031–18–2	Mercurous bromide
$Hg_2(ClO_3)_2$	10294–44–7	Mercurous chlorate
Hg_2Cl_2	10112–91–1	Mercurous chloride
Hg_2F_2	13967–25–4	Mercurous fluoride
Hg_2I_2	15385–57–6	Mercurous iodide
$Hg_2(NO_3)_2$	10415–75–5	Mercurous nitrate
Hg_2SO_4	7783–36–0	Mercurous sulphate

Uses Barometers, thermometers, hydrometers, pyrometers; mercury arc lamps; switches, fluorescent lamps; mercury boilers; manufacture of all mercury salts, mirrors; catalyst in oxidation of organic compounds; gold and silver extraction from ores; manufacture of amalgams, electric rectifiers, mercury fulminate; dentistry; in Kjeldahl nitrogen determination method, Millon's reagent; cathode in electrolysis, electroanalysis and many other uses; in pharmaceuticals, agricultural chemicals, antifouling paints.

TLV 0·05 mg/m^3 (as mercury vapour) (skin).

ANIMAL STUDIES

A. RELEVANT PHARMACOLOGY AND TOXICOLOGY

In adult animals, inorganic mercury is generally less toxic than organic mercury, at least in part because the inorganic form is much more poorly absorbed through the gastro-intestinal tract. Toxicity of inorganic mercury to the embryo and fetus is also much less than that of organic mercury; even with parenteral administration to the dam, placental transfer of inorganic mercury compounds is lower than that for the lipid-soluble organic mercury compounds. The marked embryolethal, teratogenic and fetotoxic effects of prenatal exposure to organic mercury, with marked adverse effects postnatally on survivors, has been well documented in a number of species, including humans, and will not be further considered.

Placental transfer

Placental transfer of inorganic mercury has been studied in a number of species. Berlin and Ullberg (1963) first showed very limited transfer of inorganic mercuric chloride to the mouse fetus with marked uptake by the yolk sac epithelium, using autoradiography. Suzuki *et al.* (1967) compared the placental transfer of s.c. injections of radiolabelled mercuric chloride, phenyl mercuric acetate and methyl mercuric acetate, given on day 14 of pregnancy in the mouse. Fetuses were removed on day 18. Each fetus contained around 0·1% of the injected dose of mercuric chloride, compared with 1% in the case of methyl mercuric acetate and 0·07% in the case of phenyl mercuric acetate. (There is some evidence that phenyl mercuric compounds are metabolised to inorganic mercuric compounds in the body.) In contrast with the 2 organic compounds, large amounts of inorganic mercuric chloride (0·6% of the dose) were retained in the placenta and amniotic membrane. With injection of mercuric chloride, the ratios of mercury concentration in the maternal blood, placenta and fetus were 1:19:0·4.

Dencker (1976) injected mice with radiolabelled mercuric chloride i.v. on one of days 8–17 of pregnancy, and killed them 4, 8 or 24 h after injection. Whole body radioautography showed uptake of mercury to be high in the visceral yolk sac endoderm at all stages and increasing with advancing gestation. Uptake was also very high in the chlorioallantoic placenta in the later stages of pregnancy. However, uptake by the embryo and fetus was low, with no uptake observed after injection on days 9–11, though the low sensitivity of the method used might have missed some transfer. In the embryo there was uptake into the gut, but only traces were found in other tissues. In the fetus, uptake increased 2·5-fold between days 12 and 18 of gestation, but the ratio of concentrations in whole homogenised fetus compared to maternal serum did not exceed 0·075.

Experiments by Dencker (1976) in the hamster revealed a very similar pattern of distribution to that in the mouse. Gale and Hanlon (1976) have also found high placental levels but low embryonic levels in the hamster after i.v. injection of mercuric nitrate or mercuric acetate on day 8 of pregnancy, with sacrifice on day 9 or 12.

Similar findings have been reported by several workers in the rat. Garrett *et al.* (1972) gave radiolabelled mercuric chloride by intracardiac injection on day 16 of pregnancy in the rat. Thirty minutes after injection there were high concentrations in the chorioallantoic and yolk sac placentae but little transmission to the fetus. Concentrations in the chorioallantois and yolk sac were 73 and 36 times greater than in the fetus. Intracellular partitioning studies showed uptake of mercury in the stromal fraction of the placenta, suggesting a strong binding of mercury to the placental cell surface.

Clarkson *et al.* (1972) have compared the placental transfer of elemental mercury and mercuric chloride. On one of days 18–20 of pregnancy, rats were injected i.v. with radiolabelled mercury or mercuric chloride and killed 2·5 mins after injection, or exposed to mercury vapour by inhalation for

2·5 mins, then killed. Transfer to the fetus of elemental mercury after injection was around 10-fold greater than that of mercuric chloride, whilst placental content of mercuric chloride was much greater than that of elemental mercury. With inhalation of elemental mercury vapour placental transfer to the fetus was around 40-fold greater than i.v. injection of mercuric chloride despite lower maternal body mercury levels. Maternal blood levels declined more rapidly following elemental mercury than mercuric chloride as more elemental mercury was exhaled and taken up by the tissues.

Mansour *et al.* (1973) compared maternal retention and placental transfer of mercuric nitrate and methyl mercuric chloride in the rat after s.c. injection on day 16, 18 or 20 of pregnancy. Whole body retention in the dam of mercuric nitrate (half-life approximately 16 days) was longer than that of the organic compound (half-life around 8 days). With injection on day 12 of pregnancy, the ratio of placental:newborn concentrations for organic mercury was around 1 and the pups contained 1·2% of the dose. But for mercuric nitrate, the placental levels were 6–17-fold higher than levels in the newborn pup which took up about 0·07% of the dose. In a later study by Mansour *et al.* (1974) using the same compounds, injected on day 15 or 20 of pregnancy, in the rat, similar findings were obtained, with the additional observation of high levels of inorganic mercury in the yolk sac placenta, which exceeded those in the chorioallantoic placenta by 24 h after injection.

Kelman (1977) has looked at inorganic mercury transfer across the perfused guinea pig placenta *in situ* to determine whether it is the placenta which restricts passage of inorganic mercury or whether there is a fetal "resistance" to uptake. The dams were injected i.v. with radiolabelled mercuric chloride at approximately 62 days of pregnancy. Clearance across the placenta into the perfusate was small, and was only about 1/12 of that measured using organic mercury under identical conditions. Since in the rat, fetal contents of organic mercury are around 5–17 times greater than those of inorganic mercury following maternal administration of the same body load of mercury, Kelman has suggested that the restriction in the placental transfer may entirely account for the lower fetal uptake, though measurements of fetal uptake in the guinea pig would be needed to confirm this hypothesis.

Interactions between inorganic mercury and other substances at the placental level have been shown. Goodman *et al.* (1978) have noted that mercuric chloride reduces amino acid transport across placental membranes *in vitro*. The presence of other metals may also interfere with the passage of mercury across the placenta. Selenium given as sodium selenite decreases the passage of mercuric chloride into the fetus in late pregnancy in the rat (Pařízek *et al.*, 1969), despite increasing maternal blood levels and unchanged placental levels of mercury. Similarly, mercuric chloride and mercuric acetate will decrease the placental transfer of selenium in late pregnancy in the rat (Pařízek *et al.*, 1971). These interactions may be explained by the formation of a mercury-selenium-protein complex in the blood that is known to occur, which prevents transfer to the fetus of both metals (Nordberg *et al.*, 1978).

Transfer in the milk

Mansour *et al.* (1973) have shown transfer of inorganic mercury in the milk of the rat. Dams were injected s.c. with mercuric nitrate or methyl mercuric chloride 24 h post-partum. At 3 weeks after birth, the dams contained similar amounts of organic or inorganic mercury (16–20% of the administered dose) and the pups contained 0·2–0·3% of the dose, with highest concentrations in the kidney and liver. Thus, while there are marked differences in placental transfer of organic and inorganic mercury, transfer to suckling pups in the milk is similar.

Whilst oral absorption of inorganic mercury is generally poor in adult animals, in neonates it may be higher. Kostial *et al.* (1978) showed a 5-fold greater retention of radiolabelled mercuric chloride in 1-week-old rats compared with 18-week-old rats, 6 days after dosing orally with mercury in cows' milk. Relative retention of inorganic mercury in the brain was 19-fold higher in 2-week-old pups than in 21-week-old adult rats.

Passage of mercuric chloride into milk in the goat has been studied by Howe *et al.* (1972). Goats were given radiolabelled mercuric chloride i.v. or orally. Little was absorbed orally, around 95% appearing in the faeces and 0·006–0·039% in the milk. With i.v. administration, around 25% appeared in the faeces and 0·9% was recovered from the milk.

Conclusion

Inorganic mercury compounds have been shown to cross the placenta in very small, but measurable quantities in all species so far investigated, viz. the mouse, rat, hamster and guinea pig. However, transfer of inorganic mercury salts is much less than the transfer of organic compounds such as methyl mercuric salts. The high placental:fetal ratios of inorganic mercury suggest that the chorioallantoic placenta may act as a barrier to transfer, perhaps by binding mercury to cell surfaces. Retention in the yolk sac placenta, which may in time exceed that of the chorioallantoic placenta, may also protect the embryo and fetus in those species where it persists throughout pregnancy.

The much more rapid placental transfer of elemental mercury, particularly following exposure to mercury vapour by inhalation, suggests that this route of occupational exposure may pose a particular hazard to the fetus.

Postnatally, the relative protection afforded by the placenta disappears and organic and inorganic compounds both enter the milk in a similar way. Levels in milk do not appear to be very high (up to 1% of the dose) and are considerably lower than maternal blood levels. However, there is some evidence that neonates may be able to absorb and/or retain more inorganic mercury by oral absorption from milk than adults and retain more in the brain. Thus, the neonatal period may be one of particular vulnerability to inorganic mercury toxicity.

B. ENDOCRINE AND GONADAL EFFECTS

Males

Lee and Dixon (1975) have compared the effects of organic and inorganic mercury compounds on spermatogenesis in the mouse. Uptake of radiolabelled methyl mercuric chloride by the testes was initially 4 times greater than that of radiolabelled mercuric chloride, with a peak level around 12 h for organic mercury and 24 h for inorganic mercury. However, the half-life of the inorganic compound, of around 55 days, was much longer than that of around 3·4 days for the organic compound. Both organic and inorganic mercury *in vitro* and *in vivo* (1 mg Hg/kg i.p.) inhibited the uptake of tritiated thymidine, uridine and L-leucine into selected spermatogenic cells, suggesting that they inhibit DNA, RNA and protein synthesis. However, the effects of the inorganic compound were less marked than those of the organic compound. Similarly, uptake of organic mercury into spermatogonial cells and spermatids was about 3 times greater than the uptake of the inorganic compound. In this same study, it was found that fertility was adversely affected after i.p. injection of 1 mg Hg/kg (see section C for details).

Females

The effect of inorganic mercury on the oestrous cycle has been investigated in the mouse, rat and hamster. Lach and Srebro (1972) gave groups of 10 female mice with normal cycles mercuric nitrate by s.c. injection, in doses of 0·1 mg/day for 8 days, or 0·2 mg/day for 12 days. In the 0·1 mg/day group, 3/10 showed no oestrus period at all and none had more than one oestrus period, during the 8 days of treatment. Cycles returned to normal in the 12 days after treatment ended. In the 0·2 mg/day group, 4/10 showed no oestrus period and 3/10 only one oestrus period, during the 12 days of treatment. Days in dioestrus were significantly increased from 30% before treatment to 70% during treatment. In the 15 days after the end of treatment, 4/10 failed to show any oestrus period, only one of these 4 having been anoestrus during treatment. Total days in dioestrus in the 15-day post-treatment period were 45%.

Baranski and Szymczyk (1973) exposed groups of 24 rats to air or mercury vapour at 0·3 ppm (2·5 mg/m^3) for 6 h/day for 21 days and found a significant increase in the length of the oestrous cycle in mercury-exposed rats, from a mean of 4·3 days before exposure to a mean of 6·7 days at the end of exposure, compared with equivalent means of 4·5 and 5·1 days in the controls.

Lamperti and Printz (1973, 1974) have also found absence of ovulation in the hamster after treatment with inorganic mercury. Females were given s.c. injections of mercuric chloride at doses of 0·2 mg/day for 8 days or 1 mg/day for 2, 3 or 4 days, beginning on day 1 of the cycle. In the hamster there is normally a regular 4-day cycle and day 1 is marked by a characteristic post-ovulatory vaginal discharge. The lower dose of 0·2 mg/day had no effect on ovulation or on ovarian or uterine histology. In those receiving 1 mg/day, marked histological differences had appeared by the third day of the cycle in comparison with controls; corpora lutea failed to regress, follicular development was retarded, and there was no uterine hypertrophy. Ovulation did not occur in the second cycle and only then did the corpora lutea of the first cycle begin to regress. In the third cycle, 60% did not ovulate and their ovaries contained atretic follicles only. Plasma progesterone levels were low on the second day of the first cycle and on the first day of the second cycle in comparison with controls. Radioautography studies of the ovary following injection of radiolabelled mercuric chloride showed concentration of mercury in the corpora lutea rather than the follicles, suggesting there may be a direct effect of mercury on the ovary to prolong the life of the corpus luteum. However, mercury was found in the hypothalamus and anterior pituitary too, and a further experiment showed that normal ovulation and normal ovarian and uterine histology could be obtained by also giving mercury-treated animals PMS on the first day of treatment, suggesting that the ovaries were responsive to pituitary hormones. It thus seems more likely that the primary effect of mercury is at the hypothalamic and/or pituitary levels.

C. FERTILITY

Males

Lee and Dixon (1975) gave groups of 10 male mice 1 mg Hg/kg i.p. as a single injection of mercuric chloride or methyl mercuric chloride. Fertility was followed up afterwards by pairing each male with one untreated female/week for 7 weeks. Females were considered pregnant if they contained 4 or more viable fetuses when examined approximately 12·5 days after conception. Fertility in untreated controls was 90–100%. In those given inorganic mercury, fertility began to decline by the third week and was lowest at 50% by the fifth week, recovering to 90–100% by the ninth and tenth weeks, indicating adverse effects on spermatocytes and spermatogonia. There were no effects on spermatids or mature spermatozoa, and no dominant lethal effects as judged by resorption rates in the pregnant females. Gross and histological examination of the testes showed no abnormalities. The effects of organic mercury were more pronounced than those of inorganic mercury, with complete infertility at 6 weeks and additional effects on early spermatids. These differences in extent and types of cell populations affected, following inorganic and organic mercury, reflected differences seen in mercury uptake by these cells and inhibition of DNA, RNA and protein synthesis seen in the same study (see section B for details).

Females

Baranski and Szymczyk (1973) exposed female rats to 0 or 0·3 ppm (2·5 mg/m^3) metallic mercury vapour for 6 h/day for 6–8 weeks before mating. It is not clear whether all exposed females succeeded in mating. Of the 18 treated and 23 control females that did mate, all became pregnant. There were no effects on total pups/litter or live pups/litter at birth. However, postnatal mortality was significantly increased, particularly in the first 4 days of life when 26% of the pups from the mercury-exposed groups died compared with 1% in controls. At 2 months of age, offspring body and organ weights were measured; males were unaffected, but females from the mercury-exposed group had significantly lower kidney and liver weights and significantly higher ovary weights than controls.

Conclusion

The limited studies available indicate that inorganic mercury can affect endocrine and gonadal function with considerable reductions in fertility in both male and female rodents, but the effects of inorganic compounds are not as great as those of organic compounds. No-effect levels have not been indicated since in the one study in males, only 1 mg/kg i.p. was used, and in females, the lowest dose studied of 0·1 mg/day s.c. caused anovulation in some animals. A single study suggests 1 mg/kg i.p. does not cause dominant lethal effects in the male.

Inhalation of metallic mercury vapour at 0·3 ppm has also been shown to lengthen the oestrous cycle and increase offspring mortality after pre-conceptional exposure.

D. PREGNANCY

Baranski and Szymczyk (1973) have exposed groups of 12 female rats to 0·3 ppm (2·5 mg/m^3) metallic mercury vapour by inhalation for 6 h/day for 3 weeks before pregnancy and again on days 7–20 of pregnancy, and allowed them to litter out. Maternal weight gain was reduced, but not significantly, in the mercury-exposed group. There were no significant effects on pregnancy rates, litters born, or total litter size at birth. However, mean live litter size at birth was significantly reduced to 7·6 pups in the mercury-exposed group compared with 9·6 pups in controls, and in the first 4 days of life 96% of pups from the exposed group died; none survived to weaning. With exposure to mercury before conception only, offspring mortality was also increased but around 75% survived to weaning. In a further experiment, groups of 8 rats were similarly exposed for 3 weeks before pregnancy and on days 7–20 of pregnancy, and killed on day 20. A significant reduction in live litter size was confirmed, and found to be due to a decrease in the number of implantations, reflecting a decrease in ovulation and/or increase in pre-implantation losses.

Rizzo and Furst (1972) investigated the teratogenicity of inorganic mercury in the rat. Groups of 3–5 rats were given single doses of 2 mg Hg^{++} as mercuric oxide or vehicle alone, on day 5, 12 or 19 of pregnancy. They were killed on day 20 or 21 and fetuses examined for external defects only. A number of rats delivered spontaneously on day 19, however, suggesting inaccurate dating of the pregnancies had occurred. There was no evidence of maternal toxicity. In controls, 2/154 fetuses were abnormal (1 umbilical hernia and 1 runt). In experimental groups, the resorption rate was increased to 24% in those dosed on day 19 compared with 0% in controls, but was not increased in those dosed on day 5 or 12. Abnormality rates were 29·7%, 6·8% and 3·4% in those dosed on days 5, 12 and 19 respectively, compared with 0–2% in controls. Malformations consisted of runting and eye defects ("lack of eye pigmentation and pupil").

Pařízek *et al.* (1971) noted no effects on viability of fetuses or fetal and placental weights, after single s.c. injections of 2·5–20 μmol/kg of mercuric chloride on day 19 of pregnancy in the rat, when killed 20 h after injection.

Gale and Ferm (1971) have also shown embryolethal, teratogenic and fetotoxic effects of inorganic mercury in the hamster. Groups of 14–19 animals were given 2, 3 or 4 mg Hg^{++}/kg as a single i.v. injection of mercuric acetate on day 8 of pregnancy. The dams were killed on day 12 or 14 of pregnancy and the fetuses examined for external and rib defects only. Resorption rates were significantly increased in a dose-related manner from 4% in controls to 12, 34 and 52% in 2, 3 and 4 mg/kg groups respectively. Growth retardation of 1–2 days was seen in 16, 41 and 60% of surviving fetuses in the 2, 3 and 4 mg/kg groups respectively, and many showed s.c. oedema on the neck and back regions. In the control group 1/79 had exencephaly. In the treated groups malformations occurred in 1/152 fetuses at 2 mg/kg, 4/166 at 3 mg/kg and 7/103 at 4 mg/kg. Malformations included exencephaly, encephalocoele, anophthalmia, microphthalmia, cleft lip and palate, rib fusions and syndactyly. Injections of phenyl mercuric acetate at doses of 7·5–10 mg Hg/kg were found to produce similar lethal and teratogenic effects to inorganic mercuric acetate, possibly due to its metabolism to inorganic mercury in the liver and kidney.

Goncharuk (1971) has reported altered immunological reactivity in first and second generation offspring of rats exposed to mercury vapour or mercury compounds before and during pregnancy. No information on dosing was given, other than that initial symptoms of poisoning were seen. Offspring showed higher antibody titres in response to typhoid vaccine and lower phagocytic activity in leucocytes in comparison with controls from unexposed dams. The number of animals used was not stated.

Conclusion
There is clear evidence that metallic mercury vapour exposure or administration of inorganic mercury compounds during pregnancy can cause very high incidences of growth retardation and prenatal and postnatal mortality. No comprehensive teratology studies have been carried out, but 2 studies on external malformation rates only suggest there may be a small increase in malformation rates in the rat and hamster. No-effect levels have not been established for any of the above effects.

E. MUTAGENICITY

It is not known whether inorganic mercury is mutagenic in bacterial systems.

Jagiello and Lin (1973) have shown that *in vitro* mercuric acetate at high concentrations ($\geqslant 50$ μg/ml) can completely inhibit meiotic division in mouse ova, and at lower concentrations (25–35 μg/ml) can cause abnormalities of the chromosomes. However, *in vivo*, single i.v. doses of 2–10 mg Hg^{++}/kg given to adult females, or 3 s.c. doses of 2 mg Hg^{++}/kg given to superovulated immature females, had no effect on meiosis. Mercury can be concentrated in mammalian ovarian follicular fluid and in the walls of large follicles, so the results of the above study suggest that there may be a barrier preventing access of mercury to the nucleus or spindle of the ovum.

F. CARCINOGENICITY

No relevant data found.

HUMAN STUDIES

A. RELEVANT PHARMACOLOGY AND TOXICOLOGY

Several investigators have measured placental, maternal and fetal blood mercury levels. However, the proportion of the total body burden derived from inorganic mercury sources is likely to be small. One group of workers have assumed for the Japanese population that the ratio of methylmercury to total mercury in embryos and fetuses is around 0·8 (see Thompson, 1978). The available data indicate that almost all the methylmercury in the diet is derived from methylmercury present in fish (WHO, 1973), and the Japanese diet generally contains a higher proportion of fish, particularly shellfish, than other diets.

However, some workers have specifically studied inorganic mercury levels of workers exposed to inorganic mercury. Wannag and Skjaeråsen (1975) have compared maternal, neonatal and placental levels of total mercury at delivery in 19 women working as dentists, dentists' assistants or dental technicians with 26 controls delivering at the same hospital and not exposed occupationally to mercury. In the dental group, exposure was to elemental mercury, probably around 0·05 mg Hg/m^3, though levels were not actually measured. This would be rapidly oxidized in the body to the inorganic mercuric ion, though animal experiments indicate some may also cross the placenta whilst still in the elemental state (see Animal Studies). There were no significant differences between exposed and control groups in mercury levels in amniotic fluid, maternal or neonatal red blood cells or plasma. They did not expect to find differences in blood levels since blood mercury falls rapidly after exposure to elemental mercury. However, the exposed group had significantly higher mercury levels in placenta and fetal membranes than controls; in the exposed group, levels in placenta, chorio-allantoic membrane and amniotic membrane were 24·5, 21·6 and 14·5 ng Hg/g tissue respectively, compared with 12·0, 11·5 and 5·3 ng Hg/g tissue respectively in controls. In both exposed and control groups mercury levels in the placenta and membranes were higher than in maternal or fetal blood, suggesting that accumulation of mercury in the placenta might partially protect the fetus, though another group of workers has found no evidence of a placental barrier in terms of total mercury levels in maternal blood, cord blood and placenta (Lauwerys *et al.*, 1978; Roels *et al.*, 1978). Whilst it seems likely that the increase in mercury levels in placenta and membranes of the exposed group in the present study was largely due to inorganic mercury, this cannot be said with certainty since only total mercury was measured. Mercury in the controls was presumably derived largely from organic mercury in the diet.

Suzuki *et al.* (1977) have measured separately inorganic and organic mercury content of amniotic fluid in 57 Japanese women with gestational ages of 4 months to term, mostly undergoing therapeutic abortions. Eight women had mild or moderate toxaemia. Inorganic mercury was detected in all but 2 samples while organic mercury was found in 30/57 samples and inorganic mercury levels were significantly higher (mean 6 nmol Hg/l) than organic mercury levels (mean 2·0 nmol Hg/l). Both inorganic and organic mercury levels were highest in the seventh month of pregnancy. Mercury levels in toxaemics were not different from controls. This study provides the only firm evidence that the fetus is exposed to inorganic mercury, since the fetus swallows amniotic fluid and fetal urine contributes to amniotic fluid. The inorganic mercury in the amniotic fluid could have come directly from the mother by diffusion in the water phase across the amnion or indirectly via the fetus after placental transfer. The higher levels of inorganic compared with organic mercury in the amniotic fluid suggest the former route may be the most likely, since in animal experiments alkyl mercury is more readily transferred across the placenta than inorganic mercury (see Animal Studies). In addition, organic mercury may be more readily retained in the fetal tissues than the more water soluble inorganic form, which may preferentially accumulate in amniotic fluid.

A number of other studies have found detectable mercury levels in placenta, maternal and cord blood and breast milk in normal term deliveries of Japanese, American and Belgian women (Fujita and Takabatake, 1977; Pitkin *et al.*, 1976; Baglan *et al.*, 1974; Creason *et al.*, 1976; Lauwerys *et al.*, 1978; Roels *et al.*, 1978). Similarly, mercury has been detected in embryos and fetuses of 5–40 weeks' gestation (Nishimura *et al.*, Biol. Neonat. **24**, 197, 1974, quoted by Thompson (1978)—original paper not seen by us) and in fetal liver tissue from spontaneous and therapeutic abortions, premature deliveries and anencephalic fetuses (Robkin *et al.*, 1973). However, in all these studies, only total mercury levels were measured and, for the reasons already described, much of this is likely to be methylmercury derived from the diet.

Goodman *et al.* (1978, 1979) have shown that mercuric chloride may affect amino acid transport across the placenta. *In vitro* experiments using preparations of vesicles from human placental syncytiotrophoblast microvillous membrane have demonstrated that at 50 or 100 μM mercuric chloride there is an initial increase in γ-aminoisobutyric acid (AIB) facilitated diffusion into the vesicles, but an overall reduction in the equilibrium level of AIB uptake. Active transport of the AIB was inhibited by 43% at 200 μM mercuric chloride.

B. ENDOCRINE AND GONADAL EFFECTS

Males

McFarland and Reigel (1978) have described loss of libido in 6 men poisoned by exposure to metallic mercury vapour in an industrial accident. A thermostat containing mercury broke and more than 10 ml of mercury was vaporized in an oven at 450°C. The calculated possible concentration of mercury was 44·3 mg/m^3 and exposure was for less than 8 h. After discovery of the accident the entire night shift of 9 men were sent home but 6/9 were subsequently hospitalized and the other 3 denied illness. The 6 patients all had symptoms of acute mercury poisoning with fever, chills, chest pain and weakness and 3 had diffuse pulmonary infiltrates suggestive of chemical pneumonitis. Two excreted large amounts of mercury in their urine 2 days after exposure, following BAL therapy. All 6 cases were followed up over a number of years and their chronic symptoms differed somewhat but most complained of nervousness, irritability, lack of ambition and lack of sexual desire. In the first case, lack of interest in sex occurred when he developed a shaking tremor, wide-based gait, irritability and suspiciousness. Abnormal gait and tremor persisted for 2 years but then gradually disappeared and by 5 years handwriting had returned to normal, but he never regained interest in sexual relations. In the second case lack of interest in sexual relations lasted 2 years and in the third and fourth case for 8 years. In the fifth case, he complained he was suddenly unable to have an erection 18 months after the exposure had occurred but this cleared with time. The sixth case reported initially losing interest in sexual relations but later reported he was able to have a normal but limited sex life. The authors of this study have suggested that the persistence of nervousness, irritability, lack of ambition and lack of interest in sex following brief exposure to mercury vapour indicates chronic mercury poisoning. They also commented that the effect of mercury poisoning on sexual behaviour is rarely mentioned, perhaps due to reluctance on the part of the workers to describe these symptoms and/or physicians ascribing impotence to the depression that generally occurs in such cases. Further studies on this aspect of mercury poisoning are required.

Females

Marinova *et al.* (1973) have found an increase in menstrual cycle disturbances in 111 women working with mercury in dentistry or in mercury rectifier stations. They were compared with 30 controls who were nurses or laboratory assistants from the same polyclinic as those working in dentistry. There were no significant differences between the 2 groups in age, work experience or obstetric history. Women with endocrine or gynaecological disorders which could cause menstrual disturbances were excluded. In the mercury exposed group 28·8% had hypermenorrhoea compared with 0·3% in controls, and 15·3% had hypomenorrhoea compared with 0·6% in controls. Mercury exposure levels were not measured but preliminary tests revealed mercury on the hands of the exposed employees and on benches and floors of the workshops.

Mikhailova *et al.* (1971) have also reported menstrual disturbances in 26·8% of women working in an atmosphere polluted with mercury vapour in a "high concentration". No further details were given of sample size, exposure levels or the nature of the menstrual disturbances.

Panova and Dimitrov (1974) have studied menstrual function in women exposed to mercury in the manufacture of fluorescent lamps. Mercury levels in the environment were not specified but were said to exceed the MAC by several times, particularly in the 2 years prior to the survey, since production had increased. A total of 74 women were studied, aged 20–40 years, and they were compared with 100 controls of similar ages working in a tailoring and clothing enterprise. Questionnaires revealed an incidence of menstrual disturbances of 36·5% in women employed in lamp manufacture for more than 6 months, compared with 11·3% in controls. The commonest disturbances were oligo- and hypomenorrhoea, and less commonly, hypermenorrhoea, metrorrhagia and dysmenorrhoea. Vaginal cytology was carried out in 60 of the exposed women during 2 successive menstrual cycles, and in controls, during one cycle. The incidence of anovulatory cycles was 27% in controls and, in the exposed group, 46·7% for the first cycle and 43·3% for the second cycle. The anovulatory cycles were said to be mainly of the hypofollicular type. Stratification by age (20–25 years, 26–35 years and 36–40 years) showed abnormal cycles in all age groups but predominantly in the 20–25 year age group. Further breakdown of the data showed abnormal cycles were occurring in women employed for up to 5 years and no abnormalities with longer durations of employment. The authors suggest this may be due to adaptation or to the fact that women coming into the factory are located in the workplaces with the greatest exposure. Urinary mercury levels were highest in the exposed group with abnormal cycles (3·90 μg %/24 h) compared with exposed women with normal cycles (3·13 μg %/24 h) or controls (1·1 μg %/24 h).

Goncharuk (1977) has studied gynaecological disorders and menstrual function in women working in the preparation of mercury ore for smelting and in various jobs during and after processing of the ore. Mercury fumes were observed in all departments of the factory and levels in the air fluctuated between traces and 0·08 mg Hg/m^3. A total of 196 exposed women were compared with 204 controls who were also seen in the plant's medical clinic but did not come into contact with mercury in their work in offices, trading establishments and small businesses. There was no difference between the groups in sickness rates for gynaecological disorders but menstrual disturbances were found in 44·7% of women in the mercury plant, compared with 18·6% in controls. The commonest disturbances were dysmenorrhoea and hypermenorrhoea. The majority of disturbances (67%) occurred in women with more than 3 years' exposure.

An increased frequency of precancerous lesions of the cervix has been found in women working in dentistry exposed to up to 0·07 mg Hg/m^3 in the air (Vikshraitis and Moteyunene, 1972). In a group of 557 mercury-exposed women 11·0% had precancerous lesions of the cervix compared with 5·3% in 262 office worker controls, the frequency of lesions increasing with length of employment. However, lesion rates in other groups of workers (pharmacists 11·9%, chemical factory workers 11·4%, tinsmiths 28%) were comparable to or higher than those working with mercury. It is likely that there were differences in socioeconomic status and perhaps other variables known to be related to the development of cervical cancer between these various groups of workers, especially those in industry, and the office worker controls. No firm conclusions on the possible role of mercury can therefore be drawn.

D. PREGNANCY

It was first suggested that mercury might be toxic to the fetus when it was noted that frequent abortions occurred in women undergoing mercury treatment for syphilis (Afonso and Alvarez, 1960). From the sixteenth to mid-nineteenth century colloidal mercury and inorganic mercurial salts were used and then organomercurials for the treatment of syphilis. However, it is not known whether abortion was due to the mercury or to syphilis.

Canale (1969) has reported that women have taken mercury as an abortifacient, but its use was rare. Mercury, usually in the form of corrosive mercury sublimate, was taken by vaginal irrigation. In one such case which has been recorded in the literature, where the woman and fetus survived serious mercury poisoning, delivery at term had to be by Caesarian section since the mercury had caused scarring of the cervix.

Afonso and Alvarez (1960), reviewing the literature up to 1960, noted that there were no single proved or even well-documented cases of abortion or fetal intoxication due to mercury. In 2 cases reported in the French literature, described by Afonso and Alvarez (1960) (original papers not seen by us), the information provided was inconclusive; in one case there was a vague history of ingestion of a mercuric salt and a clinical picture suggesting maternal intoxication; the mother died after aborting. In the second case, the mother had occupational mercurial poisoning during the course of 2 pregnancies. The first resulted in neonatal death and the second in stillbirth. Both babies had hepatosplenomegaly and what the authors believed to be erythroblastosis due to mercury, but toxicological examination of the babies did not reveal any mercury. Thus in neither of these cases could it be established whether the adverse outcome of pregnancy was due to mercury directly or secondary to maternal illness.

Afonso and Aivarez (1960) have recorded a case of a 31-year-old woman, gravida 9, para 8, about 10 weeks pregnant, referred to King County Hospital, U.S.A. with acute renal failure 5 days after taking 2·5 g of mercuric chloride in an attempt to induce abortion. She had initially been treated in the community by gastric lavage and administration of BAL soon after taking the mercuric chloride. She developed severe vomiting, haematemesis, bloody diarrhoea and anuria and progressively lost weight. On admission there were no signs of abortion at a pelvic examination. Thirteen days after the ingestion of mercury uterine cramping and vaginal bleeding occurred and a 5 cm fetus and placenta were found in the vagina. The fetus was not macerated and appeared grossly normal. Histological examination of the fetus and placenta revealed no lesions but the fetal tissue contained 0·2 mg/kg mercury. Examination of 2 10-week-old control fetuses showed no mercury in one case and 0·04 mg/kg in the other. By the twentieth day after ingestion the mother had recovered and discharged herself. In view of the normal appearance of the fetus and placenta and the past obstetric history of the patient it was thought unlikely that the abortion was spontaneous. The authors considered the abortion was probably due to mercury intoxication, though the patient's uraemia could have been an important contributing factor, but again it is impossible to distinguish in this case between a direct effect of mercury and abortion secondary to severe maternal illness.

Marinova *et al.* (1973) have examined reproductive histories of women exposed to mercury through work in dentistry or mercury rectifier stations. Of 130 pregnancies occurring in 111 exposed women, 28·4% ended as normal births, 6·9% in spontaneous abortions and 63·9% in abortions carried out on request, compared with control rates of 34% normal births, 3·3% spontaneous abortions and 63% abortions on request. Thus there is a suggestion that there may be a slight increase in spontaneous abortions in the exposed group. Details of menstrual disturbances in the exposed group have been given in section B. The authors also recorded that urinary mercury levels following provocation were within normal limits except in 2 of the exposed group who had elevated values. Pregnanediol and 17-ketosteroids were decreased in 7·2% of the exposed group (no control values given) and there was a higher incidence of anaemia in the exposed group (26%) compared with controls (10%). However, it is not clear whether these various investigations were carried out on non-pregnant, pregnant or both types of women in exposed and control groups. The exposed women also complained of more gastroenteric problems than controls.

Goncharuk (1977) has also reported on reproductive histories of women exposed to mercury through work connected with the smelting of mercury ore. Menstrual disturbances in these women have already been described in section B. They analysed case histories of pregnant women who had attended the clinic attached to the mercury plant between 1968 and 1972, 168 having contact with mercury and 178 controls with no occupational exposure to mercury. Exposure levels ranged from traces to 0·08 mg Hg/m^3 in the air in the plant. The age distribution in the 2 groups was similar but they were not matched for any other variables. In the exposed group there were significant increases in threatened abortion (8·7% versus 1·7%), abortion (16·7% versus 4·9%), "toxicosis" (34·9% versus 1·9%), premature birth (6·0% versus 1·1%) and incorrect position of the fetus (2·3% versus 0·4%) compared with controls. There was no significant difference in stillbirths and death of the child (2·3% versus 1·9%). "Toxicosis" was explained as occurring predominantly in the first half of pregnancy and including nausea, vomiting, heartburn and disorders of appetite. The author stated that, comparing this data with other data in the literature, the effects on pregnancy are less marked where there is exposure to smaller concentrations of mercury fumes. Whilst mercury may well have contributed to the obstetric problems recorded in the exposed group, it is very likely that there were marked differences in other factors known to affect obstetric outcome, such as socio-economic status, between exposed and control groups in this study. Controls worked in offices, trading establishments and small businesses and thus may be poorly matched with the industrially exposed group.

However, Goncharuk's (1977) study, that of Marinova *et al.* (1973), and the anecdotal cases described earlier, all suggest an increased risk of spontaneous abortion in women exposed to inorganic mercury, but further studies are needed to confirm this. A number of authors have speculated that mercury may cause damage, especially to the placenta, by inactivation of sulphydryl groups in cellular enzymes (Marinova *et al.*, 1973; Afonso and Alvarez, 1960; Koos and Longo, 1976).

E. MUTAGENICITY

Paton and Allison (1972) cultured human lymphocytes *in vitro* in the presence of mercuric chloride at concentrations up to $3{\cdot}0 \times 10^{-8}$ M. Whilst the highest concentration was toxic to the cells, chromosome aberrations were not induced.

Verschaeve and Susanne (1979) have investigated persons involved in dentistry, exposed occupationally to mercury (abstract only available). They found a significant increase in aneuploidy in the dental group compared with 10 age-matched controls. Other chromosome aberrations were not increased. The authors suggest that aneuploidy may be caused by the action of mercury on the sulphydryl groups of the spindle apparatus, but they point out that the dental group would also be exposed to X-rays which may be responsible for the aneuploidy observed.

F. CARCINOGENICITY

No relevant data found.

SUMMARY AND EVALUATION

EXPERIMENTAL STUDIES

Studies in several species have shown that placental transfer of inorganic mercury is much less than that of organic mercury. Mercuric chloride, however, does become concentrated in the placenta in rodents, and may interfere with the transfer of amino acids and selenium across the placenta. The transfer to the fetus of elemental mercury, following exposure to mercury vapour, is much greater than the transfer of mercuric chloride. Transfer of organic and inorganic mercury to the milk are about equal, and although levels in milk are lower than plasma levels, there is some evidence that neonates absorb mercury more readily than adults and retain more in the brain.

Doses of inorganic mercury of about 3 mg/kg s.c. or exposure to 2·5 mg/m^3 (0·3 ppm) mercury vapour disrupts the oestrous cycles of rodents, possibly due to an action on the hypothalamic pituitary axis. Single doses of organic or inorganic mercury of around 1 mg/kg i.p. transiently reduced fertility of males by an action primarily on spermatogonia and spermatocytes. Fertility in females is also reduced and in one study, exposure to mercury vapour at 2·5 mg/m^3 of females prior to mating increased postnatal mortality. In animals exposed also during pregnancy, an increase in stillbirths and almost complete postnatal mortality was observed. Limited studies have shown that inorganic mercury is teratogenic in rats and hamsters. No no-effect levels have been established.

No data on adequate mutagenicity studies or on carcinogenicity studies were found.

HUMAN STUDIES

Both organic and inorganic mercury cross into the fetus and some cumulation occurs in the placenta and membranes since these have higher levels than either maternal or fetal blood. Occupational exposure in dentistry has been reported to result in double the usual levels of mercury in the placenta.

A limited study has suggested that exposure to toxic amounts of mercury vapour may reduce libido and potency in men as well as producing other signs of chronic mercury poisoning. Several studies have reported menstrual disturbances in women occupationally exposed to mercury vapour, with hypomenorrhoea, hypermenorrhoea and dysmenorrhoea being the commonest. Limited studies have also suggested a reduced ovulation rate, but no data on fertility were found.

Although commonly thought to cause abortions, the evidence is inadequate to assess the effects of mercury exposure during pregnancy.

Evidence is inadequate to assess the mutagenicity of mercury *in vivo* and no adequate data on carcinogenicity were found.

EVALUATION

There is limited evidence that inorganic mercury is teratogenic in rats and hamsters and may also affect postnatal survival. Attention is drawn to the lack of adequate data on the effects of mercury on fertility in men and women and to the absence of data on teratogenicity, mutagenicity and carcinogenicity. The limited studies on inhalation of mercury vapour indicate that this may pose a particular hazard. Attention is drawn to the need for studies on the reproductive effects of occupational exposure to this form of mercury.

References

Afonso, J. F. and Alvarez, R. R. (1960). Effects of mercury on human gestation. *American Journal of Obstetrics and Gynaecology* **80**, 145–154.

Baglan, R. J., Brill, A. B., Schulert, A., Wilson, D., Larsen, K., Dyer, N., Mansour, M., Schaffner, W., Hoffman, L. and Davies, J. (1974). Utility of placental tissue as an indicator of trace element exposure to adult and fetus. *Environmental Research* **8**, (1), 64–70.

Baranski, B. and Szymczyk, I. (1973). Effects of mercury vapours upon reproductive function on white female rats. *Medycyna Pracy* **24**, (3), 249–261.

Berlin, M. and Ullberg, S. (1963). Accumulation and retention of mercury in the mouse: I. An autoradiographic study after a single intravenous injection of mercuric chloride. *Archives of Environmental Health* **6**, 589.

Canale, M. (1969). Clinical symptoms of intoxication with chemical abortifacients. *Minerva Ginecologica* **21**, (18), 1183–1185.

Clarkson, T. W., Magos, L. and Greenwood, M. R. (1972). The transport of elemental mercury into fetal tissues. *Biology of the Neonate* **21**, 239–244.

Creason, J. P., Svendsgaard, D., Bumgarner, J., Pinkerton, C. and Hinners, T. (1976). Maternal-fetal tissue levels of 16 trace elements in 8 selected continental United States communities. *Trace Substances in Environmental Health* **10**, 53–62.

Dencker, L. (1976). Inorganic mercury: changes in the embryonic-fetal uptake throughout gestation related to placental development. *Acta Pharmacologica et Toxicologica* **39**, (Suppl. 1), 37–58.

Fujita, M. and Takabatake, E. (1977). Mercury levels in human maternal blood, hair and milk. *Bulletin of Environmental Contamination and Toxicology* **18**, 205.

Gale, T. F. and Ferm, V. H. (1971). Embryopathic effects of mercuric salts. *Life Sciences* **10**, (2), 1341–1347.

Gale, T. F. and Hanlon, D. P. (1976). The permeability of the Syrian hamster placenta to mercury. *Environmental Research* **12**, 26–31.

Garrett, N. E., Burriss Garrett, R. J. and Archdeacon, J. W. (1972). Placental transmission of mercury to the fetal rat. *Toxicology and Applied Pharmacology* **22**, 649–654.

Goncharuk, G. A. (1971). Effect of chronic mercury poisoning on the immunological reactivity of offspring. *Gigiena Truda (Kiev)* **7**, (11), 73–75.

Goncharuk, G. A. (1977). Problems relating to occupational hygiene of women in production of mercury. *Gigiena Truda i Professional'nye Zabolevaniya* (5), 17–20.

Goodman, D. L., Fant, M. and Harbison, R. D. (1978). Placental toxicity of mercury and cadmium: evidence for direct effects on placental plasma membranes. *Pharmacologist* **20**, 262.

Goodman, D. L., Fant, M. E. and Harbison, R. D. (1979). Direct effects of the heavy metals mercury and cadmium on γ-aminoisobutyric acid transport across human placental membranes. *Federation Proceedings* **38**, 535.

Howe, M., McGee, J. and Lengemann, F. W. (1972). Transfer of inorganic mercury to milk of goats. *Nature* **237**, 516–518.

Jagiello, G. and Lin, J. S. (1973). An assessment of the effects of mercury on the meiosis of mouse ova. *Mutation Research* **17**, 93–99.

Kelman, B. J. (1977). Inorganic mercury movements across the perfused guinea pig placenta in late gestation. *Toxicology and Applied Pharmacology* **41**, 659–665.

Koos, B. J. and Longo, L. D. (1976). Mercury toxicity in the pregnant woman, fetus and newborn infant. *American Journal of Obstetrics and Gynecology* **126**, 390–409.

Kostial, K., Kello, D., Jugo, S., Rabar, I. and Maljkovic, T. (1978). Influence of age on metal metabolism and toxicity. *Environmental Health Perspectives* **25**, 81–86.

Lach, H. and Srebro, Z. (1972). The oestrous cycle of mice during lead and mercury poisoning. *Acta Biologica Cracoviensia. Series Zoologia* **15**, (1), 121–130.

Lamperti, A. A. and Printz, R. H. (1973). Effects of mercuric chloride on the reproductive cycle of the female hamster. *Biology of Reproduction* **8**, 378–387.

Lamperti, A. A. and Printz, R. H. (1974). Localization, accumulation, and toxic effects of mercuric chloride on the reproductive axis of the female hamster. *Biology of Reproduction* **11**, 180–186.

Lauwerys, R., Buchet, J. P., Roels, H. and Hubermont, G. (1978). Placental transfer of lead, mercury, cadmium and cabon monoxide in women. 1. Comparison of the frequency distributions of the biological indices in maternal and umbilical cord blood. *Environmental Research* **15**, (2), 278–289.

Lee, I. P. and Dixon, R. L. (1975). Effects of mercury on spermatogenesis studied by velocity sedimentation cell separation and serial mating. *Journal of Pharmacology and Experimental Therapeutics* **194**, (1), 171–181.

Mansour, M. M., Dyer, N. C., Hoffman, L. H., Davies, J. and Brill, A. B. (1974). Placental transfer of mercuric nitrate and methyl mercury in the rat. *American Journal of Obstetrics and Gynecology* **119**, 557–562.

Mansour, M. M., Dyer, N. C., Hoffman, L. H., Schulert, A. R. and Brill, A. B. (1973). Maternal-fetal transfer of organic and inorganic mercury via placenta and milk. *Environmental Research* **6**, 479–484.

Marinova, G., Cakarova, O. and Kaneva, Y. (1973). A study on the reproductive function in women working with mercury. *Problemi na Akusherstvoto i Ginekologiyata* **1**, 75–77.

McFarland, R. B. and Reigel, H. (1978). Chronic mercury poisoning from a single brief exposure. *Journal of Occupational Medicine* **20**, (8), 532–534.

Mikhailova, L. M., Kobyets, G. P., Lyubomudrov, V. E. and Braga, G. F. (1971). The influence of occupational factors on diseases of the female reproductive organs. *Pediatriya Akusherstvo Ginekologiya* **33**, (6), 56–58.

Nordberg, G. F., Fowler, B. A., Friberg, L., Jernelov, A., Nelson, N., Piscator, M., Sanstead, H. H., Vostal, J. and Vouk, V. B. (1978). (Task Group on Metal Interaction.) Factors influencing metabolism and toxicity of metals: a consensus report by the Task Group on Metal Interactions. *Environmental Health Perspectives* **25**, 3–41.

Panova, Z. and Dimitrov, G. (1974). Ovarian function in women, having professional contact with metallic mercury. *Akusherstvoi Ginekologiya* **13**, (1), 29–34.

Pařízek, J., Babický, A., Oštádalová, I., Kalousková, J. and Pavlík, I. (1969). The effect of selenium compounds on the cross-placental passage of 203 Hg. *Atomic Energy Commission Conference*—690501 **17**, 137–143.

Pařízek, J., Oštádalová, I., Kalousková, F., Babický, A., Pavlík, L. and Bibr, B. (1971). Effect of mercuric compounds on the maternal transmission of selenium in the pregnant and lactating rat. *Journal of Reproduction and Fertility* **25**, 157–170.

Paton, G. R. and Allison, A. C. (1972). Chromosome damage in human cell cultures induced by metal salts. *Mutation Research* **16**, (3), 332–336.

Pitkin, R. M., Bahns, J. A., Filer, L. J. and Reynolds, W. A. (1976). Mercury in human maternal and cord blood, placenta and milk. *Proceedings of the Society for Experimental Biology and Medicine* **151**, 565–567.

Rizzo, A. M. and Furst, A. (1972). Mercury teratogenesis in the rat. *Proceedings—Western Pharmacology Society* **15**, 52–54.

Robkin, M. A., Swanson, D. R. and Shepard, T. H. (1973). Trace metal concentrations in human fetal livers. *Transactions—American Nuclear Society* **17**, 97–98.

Roels, H., Hubermont, G., Buchet, J. P. and Lauwerys, R. (1978). Placental transfer of lead, mercury, cadmium and carbon monoxide in women. *Environmental Research* **16**, 236–247.

Suzuki, T., Matsumoto, N., Miyama, T. and Katsunuma, H. (1967). Placental transfer of mercuric chloride, phenyl mercury acetate and methyl mercury acetate in mice. *Industrial Health* **5**, 149–155.

Suzuki, T., Takemoto, T.-I., Shishido, S. and Kani, K. (1977). Mercury in human amniotic fluid. *Scandinavian Journal of Work Environment and Health* **3**, 32–35.

Thompson, M. A. (1978). Mercurial dangers for neonates. *Food and Cosmetics Toxicology* **16**, 622–625.

Verschaeve, L. and Susanne, C. (1979). Genetic hazards of mercury exposure in dental surgery. *Mutation Research* **64**, 149.

Vikshraitis, C. J. and Moteyunene, N. P. (1972). Colposcopic recognition of the cervical precancer in females working with certain industrial poisons. *Voprosy Onkologii* **18**, (12), 41–45.

Wannag, A. and Skjaeråsen, J. (1975). Mercury in the placenta and foetal membranes as an indication of low mercury pressure. *Commission of the European Communities* (Rep) **3**, (5360), 1233–1238.

World Health Organization Expert Committee Report (1973). Trace elements in human nutrition. World Health Organization Technical Report Series No: 532, Geneva.

29. Methyl n-Butyl Ketone

TECHNICAL DATA

Formula	$CH_3COC_4H_9$
CAS registry number	591–78–6
Chemical abstracts name	2-Hexanone
Synonyms	2-Hexanone; n-butyl methyl ketone; MBK; MNBK.
Uses	Solvent
TLV	25 ppm (skin) (1980 Intended change to 5 ppm).

ANIMAL STUDIES

A. RELEVANT PHARMACOLOGY AND TOXICOLOGY

Peters *et al.* (1981) have identified methyl n-butyl ketone (MBK) and its metabolites, 2,5-hexanedione and pentanone, in rat fetal tissues following maternal inhalation of MBK.

B. ENDOCRINE AND GONADAL EFFECTS

No relevant data found.

C. FERTILITY

No relevant data found.

D. PREGNANCY

Peters *et al.* (1981) exposed pregnant rats to MBK by inhalation to investigate effects on postnatal development and behaviour. Groups of 25 females were exposed to 0, 1000 or 2000 ppm MBK for 6 h/day from day 0 to day 21 of pregnancy. Controls for the 2000 ppm group were pair fed since this level of exposure reduced maternal food consumption. Maternal weight gain was reduced by 10–12% in 1000 and 2000 ppm groups and dams in the 2000 ppm group showed signs of acute intoxication during exposure to MBK with hair loss and muscular weakness.

There were significant reductions in live litter size, pup weight at birth and postnatal growth rate during the first 3 weeks of life in the 2000 ppm group compared with pair-fed controls. Occasional, significant, treatment-related differences were seen in a number of postnatal behavioural tests in both the 1000 and 2000 ppm groups, suggesting, in general, that the young offspring of treated dams were more active than controls and that in old age the treated offspring were less active than controls. It is not known to what extent these changes were a primary effect of MBK and/or its metabolites on the fetus, or were secondary to maternal toxicity. One group exposed to 500 ppm MBK was discarded due to a technical error, so no no-effect level could be determined.

E. MUTAGENICITY

No relevant data found.

F. CARCINOGENICITY

No relevant data found.

HUMAN STUDIES

No relevant data found on any aspect of reproductive toxicity.

SUMMARY AND EVALUATION

EXPERIMENTAL STUDIES

No studies were found on endocrine or gonadal effects or of effects on fertility. One study on postnatal development following maternal inhalation of 1000 or 2000 ppm MBK during pregnancy showed significant reductions in litter size, birth weight and postnatal growth rate at 2000 ppm, a dose which was toxic to the dam. No studies on mutagenicity or carcinogenicity were found.

HUMAN STUDIES

No studies were found on any aspect of reproductive toxicity, mutagenicity or carcinogenicity.

EVALUATION

Due to limited data, no evaluation is possible. Attention is drawn to the lack of data in animals and humans.

Reference

Peters, M. A., Hudson, P. M. and Dixon, R. L. (1981). The effect totigestational exposure to methyl n-butyl ketone has on postnatal development and behaviour. *Ecotoxicology and Environmental Safety* **5**, 291–306.

30. Methyl Chloroform

TECHNICAL DATA

Formula	CH_3CCl_3
CAS registry number	71–55–6
Chemical abstracts name	1,1,1-Trichloroethane
Synonyms	Chloroethane; chlorotene; chlorothene; methyl chloroform; methyltrichloromethane; trichloroethane; α-trichloroethane.
Uses	In cold type metal cleaning, also in cleaning plastic moulds.
TLV	350 ppm

ANIMAL STUDIES

A. RELEVANT PHARMACOLOGY AND TOXICOLOGY

No relevant data found.

B. ENDOCRINE AND GONADAL EFFECTS

No relevant data found.

C. FERTILITY

No relevant data found.

D. PREGNANCY

The teratogenicity of methyl chloroform has been investigated in rats and mice by Schwetz *et al.* (1975). They were exposed to 875 ppm by inhalation for 7 h/day on days 6–15 of pregnancy. Acceptable teratological methods were used, but data was only reported on a per litter basis. The numbers of affected fetuses were not given.

In the mouse experiment, 13 dams were exposed to methyl chloroform and 30 dams served as 0 ppm controls (exposed to filtered air). There was no effect on maternal body weight or liver weight. There were no significant effects on implants/dam, live fetuses/dam, resorptions/dam, fetal body weight or crown-rump length. Soft tissue and skeletal malformations were seen in treated and control groups but there were no significant differences in the incidence of specific malformations on a per litter basis. The numbers of affected fetuses in each group were not given.

In the rat experiment, 23 dams were exposed to methyl chloroform and 30 dams served as 0 ppm controls. There was no effect on maternal body weight but absolute liver weight was significantly increased in exposed dams. Relative liver weight was not significantly increased. There were no significant effects on implants/dam, live fetuses/dam, resorptions/dam, fetal body weight or crown-rump length. Malformations were seen in treated and control groups but there were no significant differences in any specific malformation rates on a per litter basis.

Methyl chloroform does not appear to be teratogenic in rodents at levels two to three times the TLV of 350 ppm.

E. MUTAGENICITY

Methyl chloroform is mutagenic in the Ames test with or without metabolic activation (IARC Monograph Vol. 20, 1979).

F. CARCINOGENICITY

IARC Monograph Vol. 20 (1979) states that available animal evidence on the carcinogenicity of methyl chloroform is inadequate for evaluation.

HUMAN STUDIES

No relevant data on reproductive toxicity available.

SUMMARY AND EVALUATION

EXPERIMENTAL STUDIES

No studies were found on endocrine or gonadal effects or on fertility. One teratogenicity study in mice and rats, in which mean litter data only was reported, found no evidence of embryolethality, fetotoxicity or teratogenicity after inhalation of 875 ppm daily. No other doses were used.

It is mutagenic in bacterial systems with and without activation. There is inadequate evidence to assess carcinogenicity.

HUMAN STUDIES

No studies were found on any aspect of reproductive toxicity, mutagenicity or carcinogenicity, despite its widespread occurrence in the environment.

EVALUATION

No evaluation is possible of the effects on the gonads or fertility. There is limited evidence of lack of teratogenicity in rodents.

Attention is drawn to the absence of human reproductive toxicity data, so no evaluation can be made.

References

Schwetz, B. A., Leong, B. K. J. and Gehring, P. J. (1975). The effect of maternally inhaled trichloroethylene, perchloroethylene, methyl chloroform, and methylene chloride on embryonal and fetal development in mice and rats. *Toxicology and Applied Pharmacology* **32**, 84–96.

IARC Monographs on the Evaluation of the Carcinogenic Risk of Chemicals to Humans: some halogenated hydrocarbons. (1979). Vol. 20, Lyon, France.

31. Methyl Ethyl Ketone

TECHNICAL DATA

Formula	$CH_3COCH_2CH_3$
CAS registry number	78–93–3
Chemical abstracts name	2-Butanone
Synonyms	2-Butanone; ethyl methyl ketone.
Uses	As solvent; in the surface coating industry; manufacture of smokeless powder; colourless synthetic resin.
TLV	200 ppm

ANIMAL STUDIES

A. RELEVANT PHARMACOLOGY AND TOXICOLOGY

No relevant data found.

B. ENDOCRINE AND GONADAL EFFECTS

No relevant data found.

C. FERTILITY

No relevant data found.

D. PREGNANCY

A teratology study of methyl ethyl ketone (MEK) has been carried out by Schwetz *et al.* (1974). Rats were exposed to nominal levels of 1000 or 3000 ppm MEK by inhalation for 7 h/day from days 6–15 of pregnancy. The actual concentrations in the exposure chamber averaged 1126 and 2618 ppm as measured by infra-red spectroscopy. Acceptable teratological methods were used. In 23 rats with litters exposed to 1000 ppm and 21 rats with litters exposed to 3000 ppm there were no effects on implants/dam, live fetuses/dam or resorptions/dam in comparison with 43 air-exposed controls. Fetal body weight and crown-rump length were significantly reduced at 1000 ppm but not at 3000 ppm suggesting a non-treatment-related effect. There was however evidence of a teratogenic effect when the data was analysed on a per litter basis. At 1000 ppm there were no significant differences from controls in the incidence of gross external malformations or soft tissue anomalies but the proportion of litters affected by skeletal anomalies (of any kind) was increased from 58% in controls to 95% at 1000 ppm. When analysed for individual types of skeletal anomaly, there were no significant differences between 1000 ppm and control groups. At 3000 ppm there was a significant increase in gross external malformations. Four fetuses, each from a different litter, were affected, 2 with short jaw and 2 with absent tail and imperforate anus, compared with none in controls. The proportion of litters showing sternebral anomalies was also significantly increased to 43% compared with 11% in the concurrent controls. However, this may be of questionable biological significance since in controls concurrent with the 1000 ppm group, sternebral anomalies were seen in 61% of litters and in the 1000 ppm group in 68% of litters. The overall incidence of skeletal anomalies in the 3000 ppm group, unlike the 1000 ppm group, was not significantly increased. The overall incidence of soft tissue anomalies (s.c. oedema and dilated ureter) was significantly higher at 3000 ppm with 76% of litters affected compared with 51% of litters in controls. In the dams, food consumption was slightly reduced towards the end of the treatment period in the 3000 ppm group but body weight was not affected. There were no signs of liver toxicity or other toxicity in the dams.

In a later experiment, reported in abstract only, from the same group of workers, John *et al.* (1980) exposed rats to 0, 400, 1000 or 3000 ppm MEK by inhalation for 7 h/day on days 6–15 of pregnancy, replicating the experimental design of Schwetz *et al.* (1974). They confirmed an increased incidence of skeletal anomalies indicative of retarded fetal development at 3000 ppm. No gross malformations were mentioned.

Conclusion

From these 2 studies, at 3000 ppm MEK there may be a small increase in major malformations and retarded ossification. Other significant findings at 1000 and 3000 ppm are difficult to evaluate since, on the basis of the data given (by affected litters only), they were not dose-related and controls showed a high variability.

E. MUTAGENICITY

No relevant data found.

F. CARCINOGENICITY

No relevant data found.

HUMAN STUDIES

No relevant data on reproductive toxicity found.

SUMMARY AND EVALUATION

EXPERIMENTAL STUDIES

No studies were found on endocrine or gonadal effects or effects on fertility. There is limited evidence that it is not embryolethal in rats but that it is teratogenic at exposure levels of 3000 ppm, which were non-toxic to the dam during pregnancy, and it increases the incidence of fetal anomalies at 1000 ppm. A no-effect level of 400 ppm is reported.

No data on mutagenicity or carcinogenicity were found.

HUMAN STUDIES

No data on any aspect of reproductive toxicity, mutagenicity or carcinogenicity were found.

EVALUATION

Methyl ethyl ketone may be a low grade teratogen in rats. Attention is drawn to the lack of data on other aspects of reproduction in animals and to the complete lack of data in humans.

References

John, J. A., Pilny, M. K., Kuna, R. A., Deacon, M. M. and Yakel, H. O. (1980). Teratogenic evaluation of methyl ethyl ketone in the rat. *Teratology* **21**, (3), 47A.

Schwetz, B. A., Leong, B. K. J., Gehring, P. B. (1974). Embryo- and fetotoxicity of inhaled carbon tetrachloride, 1,1-dichloroethane and methyl ethyl ketone in rats. *Toxicology and Applied Pharmacology* **28**, 452–464.

32. Nitrogen Dioxide

TECHNICAL DATA

Formula	NO_2
CAS registry number	10102–44–0
Chemical abstracts name	Nitrogen dioxide
Synonyms	None
Uses	Intermediate in nitric and sulphuric acid production. Used in the nitration of organic compounds and explosives, in the manufacture of oxidized cellulose compounds (haemostatic cotton). Has been used to bleach flour.
TLV	5 ppm (1980 Intended change to 3 ppm)

ANIMAL STUDIES

A. RELEVANT PHARMACOLOGY AND TOXICOLOGY

Stupfel *et al.* (1971) have studied possible sex differences in the toxicity of nitrogen dioxide in the mouse. Mice were exposed to 0·1% nitrogen dioxide by inhalation for 2 h 20 min at 110 days of age. At the end of the exposure period 14/21 (67%) of the males were dead and 26/42 (62%) of the females were dead. Forty-eight hours after the end of the exposure all the mice were dead, mostly from pulmonary oedema. There is no evidence of any difference in toxicity when males and females are exposed to high concentrations of nitrogen dioxide.

B. ENDOCRINE AND GONADAL EFFECTS

Females

Shalamberidze and Tsereteli (1971) have studied the effect of inhaled nitrogen dioxide on the oestrous cycle of rats. Cycles were followed for 24 days before exposure in groups of 10 sexually mature rats. They were then exposed to 0·07 ppm (0·126 mg/m^3) or 1·25 ppm (2·36 mg/m^3) for 12 h/day for 3 months. At the end of the exposure, 4 rats/group were killed for pathohistological examination and the rest followed up during a 3-month recovery period. At 0·07 ppm there were no effects on the oestrous cycle or reproductive organs. At 1·25 ppm, mean cycle length progressively increased during exposure from a control length of 5·3 days to 6·4 days after one month, 9·0 days after 2 months and 9·1 days after 3 months. This was due to a 20% increase in the length of oestrous and an 85% increase in the inter-oestrus interval, especially dioestrus, by the third month of exposure. The number of normal cycles/month ("normal" was not defined) decreased from 4·2 in controls to 1·3–1·9 during exposure. During recovery, the mean duration of the cycle and of oestrus returned to control levels by 3 months after the end of exposure, according to the graphs presented in the paper. However, in the text, it is stated that "oestrual indexes" did not return to initial levels until 7 months after the end of exposure. Examination of the rats killed at the end of the exposure period showed circulatory disturbances of varying intensity, such as hyperaemia, stasis, and occasionally haemorrhages, in pituitary, adrenal and thyroid glands, ovaries and uterus. Ovaries showed fewer functionally active follicles and the uterus was depleted of glandular epithelium. Thus, exposure to a level of nitrogen dioxide below the proposed TLV of 3 ppm (currently 5 ppm) has marked, but reversible effects on the oestrous cycle in rats.

Males

No studies found.

C. FERTILITY

Shalamberidze and Tsereteli (1971) studied the effect of exposure to nitrogen dioxide on subsequent reproductive capacity in female rats. Groups of 7 rats were exposed to 0, 0·07 or 1·25 ppm for 12 h/day for 3 months. At the end of the exposure period they were mated with untreated males (2 males/7 females). Outcome in those exposed to 0·07 ppm was not mentioned. At 1·25 ppm, it was reported that there was no effect on the proportion of dams becoming pregnant, though no data is given to support this statement. Litter size at birth was decreased from a mean of 8·0 in controls to 5·1 at 1·25 ppm, and offspring weight was significantly decreased by 20–30% between birth and

12 days of age. Thus exposure to nitrogen dioxide at levels which adversely affect the oestrous cycle (see section B) also impairs reproductive capacity in terms of litter size and offspring weight immediately after cessation of exposure. It is not known whether reproductive capacity, like oestrous cycles, recovers completely with time after exposure.

D. PREGNANCY

Gofmekler *et al.* (1977) exposed rats to 0·43 ppm (0·8 mg/m^3), 0·045 ppm (0·085 mg/m^3), or 0·018 ppm (0·034 mg/m^3) nitrogen dioxide by inhalation, 24 h/day from days 1–21 of pregnancy. Acceptable teratological methods were used but the number of dams in each treatment group was not given. There were no significant, dose-related effects on "fertility", though the latter was not defined. Intrauterine mortality increased in a dose-related manner from 2·3% of total implantation sites in controls to 2·7% at 0·018 ppm, 9·2% at 0·045 ppm, and 10·5% at 0·43 ppm. The latter two rates differ significantly from controls. Stillbirths were also significantly increased from none in controls to 18% at 0·43 ppm. Fetal body weight and fetal liver weight were both decreased in a dose-related manner and differences between controls and treated groups were significant at 0·045 ppm and 0·43 ppm. At the highest dose, 0·43 ppm, body weight was 10% lower than controls and liver weight 27% lower than controls. Reductions in the weight of the fetal heart, lung and kidney in test groups in relation to controls are also mentioned in the text but no further details are given. A dose-related increase in the incidence of s.c. haemorrhages and haematocoeles and "certain development anomalies" (unspecified) was also mentioned but no further information provided. Biochemical studies on tissue ascorbic acid levels, resistance of erythrocytes to acid haemolysis, and toxic peroxide products from the liver and placenta showed some significant changes, but none were clearly dose-related.

Conclusion

This single teratology study suggests nitrogen dioxide may be embryolethal, fetotoxic and teratogenic at exposure levels below the TLV (currently 5 ppm, proposed 3 ppm) and further studies are therefore needed to establish a clear no-effect level.

E. MUTAGENICITY

Chromosome analysis of leukocytes and spermatocytes from male mice exposed to nitrogen dioxide indicate that it was not mutagenic under the test conditions employed. Gooch *et al.* (1977) exposed mice to 0, 0·1, 1·5 or 10 ppm nitrogen dioxide for 6 h and took blood samples for leukocyte culture immediately, one week and 2 weeks after exposure. Spermatocyte preparations were made 8 weeks after exposure. There were no significant increases in chromosome aberrations in leukocytes and no translocations detected in spermatocytes.

F. CARCINOGENICITY

No relevant data found.

HUMAN STUDIES

No relevant data found except for the observation of Goldstein *et al.* (1976) that with use of nitrous oxide anaesthesia in operating theatres there may be oxidation to produce nitric oxide and nitrogen dioxide. They recorded levels of 0·15 ppm nitrogen dioxide 3 m from the operating table with higher peaks occurring in conjunction with more intensive use of energy-releasing devices such as electric cauteries and portable X-ray machines. At the end of surgery levels fell within 30 min to 0·04 ppm. In view of the evidence suggesting a higher risk of spontaneous abortion in female operating personnel and the failure so far to identify which agent(s) are responsible for the increased risk, the possibility that nitrogen dioxide, a much more reactive oxide of nitrogen than nitrous oxide, may play a role should be borne in mind.

SUMMARY AND EVALUATION

EXPERIMENTAL STUDIES

Exposure of rats to 1·25 ppm for 12/h/day for 3 months gradually increased the duration of oestrous cycles, which returned to normal by 3 months after cessation of exposure. Although the proportion of animals becoming pregnant was not reduced, there was a reduction in litter size and offspring weight immediately after cessation of exposure. A limited study showed that at exposure levels down to 0·04 ppm to pregnant rats, embryolethal, fetotoxic and teratogenic effects may be observed. No clear no-effect level was established.

Studies are inadequate to assess the mutagenicity of the substance. No data on carcinogenicity were found.

HUMAN STUDIES

No studies on any aspect of reproductive toxicity, mutagenicity or carcinogenicity were found. The possible role of nitrogen dioxide, produced by oxidation of nitrous oxide used as an anaesthetic, in the reproductive toxicity observed in operating theatre staff should be borne in mind.

EVALUATION

Limited studies have shown that very low levels of nitrogen dioxide, well below the TLV, can disturb the oestrous cycles of rats and can produce embryolethal, fetotoxic and teratogenic effects in rats. Attention is drawn to the need for adequate studies to confirm these effects. Attention is drawn to the lack of any relevant data in humans.

References

Gofmekler, V. A., Brekhman, I. I., Golotin, V. G., Sheparev, A. A., Krivelevich, E. B., Kamynina, L. N., Dobryakova, A. I. and Gonenko, W. A. (1977). The embryotropic action of nitrogen dioxide and a complex of atmospheric pollutants. *Gigiena I Sanitariya* **12**, 22–27.

Goldstein, B. D., Paz, J., Giuffrida, J. G., Palmes, E. D. and Ferrand, E. F. (1976). Atmospheric derivatives of anaesthetic gases as a possible hazard to operating-room personnel. *Lancet* **ii**, 235–237.

Gooch, P. C., Luippold, H. E., Creasia, D. A. and Brewen, J. G. (1977). Observations on mouse chromosomes following nitrogen dioxide inhalation. *Mutation Research* **48**, (1), 117–120.

Shalamberidze, O. P. and Tsereteli, N. T. (1971). Effect of small concentrations of sulfurous gas and nitrogen dioxide on the estrual cycle and the genital function of animals in experiments. *Gigiena I Sanitariya* **36**, (8), 13–17.

Stupfel, M., Bouley, G. and Roussel, A. (1971). Difference of experimental toxicity of several air pollutants related to sex. *Proceedings of the Second International Clean Air Congress*, pp 180–186.

33. Ozone

TECHNICAL DATA

Formula	O_3
CAS registry number	10028–15–6
Chemical abstracts name	Ozone
Synonyms	Triatomic oxygen
Uses	As disinfectant for air and water by virtue of its oxidizing power. For bleaching waxes, textiles, oils. In organic syntheses. Forms ozonides which are sometimes useful oxidizing compounds.
TLV	0·1 ppm

ANIMAL STUDIES

A. RELEVANT PHARMACOLOGY AND TOXICOLOGY

Two studies on the toxicity of ozone have shown no sex differences in the mouse in mortality after exposure to 4 ppm (Stupfel *et al.*, 1971) or 8–12 ppm (Goldstein and Ross, 1973) for several hours, though marked strain differences in susceptibility in the mouse have been noted (Goldstein and Ross, 1973).

B. ENDOCRINE AND GONADAL EFFECTS

The effect of ozone on reproductive organs has only been investigated at relatively low concentrations. Cavender *et al.* (1978) exposed male and female rats and guinea pigs to 0·5 ppm ozone for 6 h/day, 5 days/week for 6 months.

At autopsy, no histological changes were seen in any organs including the prostate, testis, seminal vesicle, ovary and uterus, with the exception of lung lesions in the guinea pig. The effects of exposure to higher concentrations are not known.

C. FERTILITY

No relevant data found.

D. PREGNANCY

In an early study, Kotin and Thomas (1957) investigated the effects of exposure of mice to artificial smog containing 1·25 ppm ozone. Males and females were caged together and exposed continuously to smog, urban atmosphere (0·4 ppm ozone) or ozone-free washed air. Duration of exposure before successful mating was not stated but presumably was only a few days at most. There was a significant reduction in females delivering litters in the smog group (6/20 compared with 13/20 and 14/20 in the other 2 groups). Litter size at first observation was also significantly reduced in the smog group, but the interpretation of this result is unclear since cannibalism of some pups was reported. The true litter size at birth is therefore not known. Postnatally, with continued exposure of pups and lactating mothers to smog, only 4/106 born survived to weaning compared with 60–70% of pups in the other 2 groups.

A series of studies by Brinkman, Lamberts and Veninga have indicated adverse postnatal effects of prenatal exposure to ozone in the mouse. Unfortunately, the methodological information given is very inadequate. Paired male and female mice of 2 different inbred strains, in groups of 17–36, were exposed to 0·1 or 0·2 ppm ozone for 7 h/day 5 days/week for 3 weeks (Brinkman *et al.*, 1964). The timing of exposure in relation to conception is not stated. The mice were allowed to give birth. Average litter size at birth was not significantly reduced in ozone-exposed groups in comparison with air-exposed controls, though in a later paper, Veninga (1967), referring back to their original paper (Brinkman *et al.*, 1964), stated that there was a decrease in litter size mainly due to post-implantation losses. However there was a significant increase in postnatal mortality in the first 3 weeks after birth. In the "grey" strain it rose from 1·6% in controls to 6·8% and 7·5% in 0·1 and 0·2 ppm ozone groups respectively for first litters, and in second litters from 1·9% in controls to 4·9% in the 0·1 ppm groups (no second litters in the 0·2 ppm group). The duration and timing of exposure of parents and second litter offspring is not stated. In the first litters of the C57 black strain postnatal mortality was 9·0% in controls and 34·0% in those exposed to 0·2 ppm (no 0·1 ppm group or second litters).In addition, postnatally-developing anomalies were reported (Veninga, 1967) in offspring in the 0·2 ppm group; an increase in blepharophimosis from 0·6% in controls to 9·6% occurred in the ozone-exposed "grey" strain and from 4·5% to 9·2% in C57 blacks. Unlimited incisor growth increased from 0·9% in controls to 5·4% in C57 blacks exposed to ozone, but the timing and duration of exposure is again unclear; in the text it is stated that exposure was during "embryological development", but in the legend of the photograph of the anomaly, the treatment period is given as during "embryological development and the subsequent 3 weeks after birth".

The effects of ozone exposure of the female during gestation only on prenatal development (Kavlock *et al.*, 1979) or on postnatal development (Kavlock *et al.*, 1980) in the rat has been studied. Groups of 14–37 animals were used and teratological methods were acceptable. Rats were exposed to 0–2 ppm for 72 h continuously on days 6–9 or 9–12 of pregnancy, or for 8 h/day on days 6–15 of pregnancy. The dams were killed for examination of the fetuses on day 19 of pregnancy. Exposure to 1·04 ppm on days 6–9 caused a significant reduction in the average number of implantation sites from 12·9 to 10·7, a non-significant increase in resorptions from 8·1% to 18·5%, and a significant increase in fetal weight, the latter possibly related to the reduction in the number of viable fetuses in the litters. However, exposure to a lower dose of 0·44 ppm on days 6–15 had no effect on implantation or resorption rates. The only increase in anomalies noted in the group exposed to 1·04 ppm on days 6–9 was enlarged renal pelvis affecting 5·8% of fetuses and 20% of the litters compared with none in the concurrent controls. It is not clear why the authors state in their text that there were "no visceral anomalies" since enlarged renal pelvis in fetuses that are not otherwise retarded, and in this case were in fact heavier with more advanced ossification than controls, would normally be regarded as a true teratological effect. However in the groups exposed on days 9–12 of gestation in the concurrent controls (0 ppm), where fetuses were of similar weight to those exposed to 1·04 ppm on days 6–9 of gestation, 6·1% had enlarged renal pelvis, with 2·2%, 0% and 0% of fetuses showing this anomaly in 1·00, 1·26 and 1·49 ppm ozone groups respectively where fetal weights were lower than in controls. Thus the frequency of this anomaly was apparently random with no suggestion of a dose-response relationship.

On days 9–12 of pregnancy groups were exposed to 0, 1·00, 1·26 or 1·49 ppm and 0, 0·64, 0·93 or 1·97 ppm ozone in 2 separate experiments. As expected, there was no effect on implantation rates. There was a significant increase in resorptions to 50·4% and 58·8% in 1·49 and 1·97 ppm groups respectively, compared with 8–13% in all other groups including controls. This was largely due to complete resorption of a number of litters in these 2 treatment groups.

Effects on fetal weight and ossification were variable and significant reductions in fetal weight and delayed ossification seen in the 1·49 ppm group of one experiment were not seen in the 1·97 ppm group of the other experiment. The absence of any statistically significant effect at 1·97 ppm cannot be entirely attributed to the low fetal weight of concurrent controls since fetal weight at 1·97 ppm was higher than at 1·49 ppm. It seems probable that with such high numbers of resorptions in these ozone-exposed groups, effects on survivors are likely to be very variable. There were no significant effects on major malformations or anomalies. This study is notable for the very wide, non-dose-related variations in fetal weight, anomaly and malformation rates including very differing control groups (4 in total) which may be due to examining fetuses very early (day 19) when differences in development rates within groups are greater than if examined just before term.

In additional experiments, fetal heart rate, electrocardiograms, haematocrits and plasma electrolytes, examined on day 20 of gestation after exposure to 1·0–1·2 ppm ozone on days 7–12 or 17–20, were unaltered in comparison to untreated controls.

Exposure to all doses of ozone from 0·44–1·97 ppm caused significant reductions in food intake in comparison with controls together with reductions in water intake. However, it is unlikely that the significant embryoloethality observed at 1·49 and 1·97 ppm after exposure on days 9–12 is secondary to these maternal effects, since food and water intake was only marginally greater in the 1·26 and 0·93 ppm groups and average maternal weight loss was actually greater in these 2 groups than in the 1·49 ppm group. Thus it seems likely that levels above 1·26 ppm are genuinely embryolethal, but not teratogenic. In the one group exposed throughout organogenesis, 0·44 ppm was shown to be a no-effect level.

In a study with the same strain of rats as used in their previous study Kavlock *et al.* (1980) looked at the postnatal effects of continuous exposure to 0, 1·0 or 1·5 ppm ozone on days 9–12 or 17–20 of gestation. At birth litters were reduced to 8 pups and reared by their own mothers. Unlike the mouse study by Brinkman *et al.* (1964) described previously, only one pup out of 22 treated litters died postnatally. A significant, dose-related reduction in body weight was seen after both mid- and late-gestational exposures at 6 days of age, persisting until 15 days in female offspring from those exposed on day 17–20 of pregnancy and until at least 60 days in the males from this group. Those exposed on days 9–12 of gestation showed no significant delays in development of surface righting reflex (9–10 days of age), auditory startle response (12–13 days), or time of eye opening (15–16 days), and no changes in open field behaviour (6–17 days of age). However those exposed to ozone on days 17–20 of gestation were significantly delayed in righting reflex and eye opening by almost a day and showed significant, dose-related reductions in grooming and rearing behaviour in the open field. It is difficult to assess to what extent these maturational delays may be attributed to the observed growth retardation, but the persistence of growth retardation, with 3/21 males in the 1·5 ppm group being severely runted and one dying, suggests a lasting adverse effect of ozone exposure during gestation. In the absence of fostering or cross-fostering experiments it is not possible to say whether this effect is mediated prenatally or postnatally via the mother.

Conclusion

Early studies in the mouse are difficult to evaluate since few or conflicting methodological details are given. However, these reports did suggest there may be adverse effects at levels of 0·1–1·25 ppm, especially postnatally. A single rat study, with good methodology, suggests ozone is not teratogenic but clear increases in embryolethality were seen at 1·5 ppm and possibly reduced fetal weight, though this was not consistently found at levels of 1·5 ppm and above. At 1·0 ppm there was a slight increase in resorptions, and postnatally indications of growth retardation and maturational delays at 1·0 ppm and above. Exposures below 0·5 ppm were without effect in the rat, suggesting that the no-effect level may be somewhere between 0·5 and 1·0 ppm, but further studies are required to confirm or refute this including detailed postnatal examinations.

E. MUTAGENICITY

In vivo studies of the cytogenetic effects of ozone exposure have produced conflicting results. Zelac *et al.* (1971a) report an increase in chromosome aberrations (breaks) in circulating lymphocytes of the Chinese hamster after exposure to 0·2 ppm for 5 h, from which they estimate that permitted levels of ozone exposure (0·1 ppm) would result in break-frequencies orders of magnitude greater than that incurred by permitted levels of radiation exposure (Zelac *et al.*, 1971b). However, Gooch *et al.* (1976) could find no increase in either chromatid- or chromosome-type aberrations in bone marrow samples from Chinese hamsters exposed to 0·23 ppm for 5 h or 5·2 ppm for 6 h, or in circulating leukocytes of mice exposed to 0·15 or 1·21 ppm for 5 h or 0·99 ppm for 2 h. Primary spermatocyte preparations from the same mice 8 weeks after exposure revealed no reciprocal translocations.

Thus the mutagenic effects of ozone remain unclear. The high postnatal mortality observed in mice where both parents were exposed to 0·1 or 0·2 ppm ozone (Brinkman *et al.*, 1964) together with the absence of such an effect in rats where only the dam was exposed during gestation suggest the need for pre-mating exposure studies in the male to be carried out.

F. CARCINOGENICITY

No relevant data found.

HUMAN STUDIES

A. RELEVANT PHARMACOLOGY AND TOXICOLOGY

No relevant data found.

B. ENDOCRINE AND GONADAL EFFECTS

No relevant data found.

C. FERTILITY

No relevant data found.

D. PREGNANCY

No relevant data found.

E. MUTAGENICITY

The high oxidation potential of ozone with production of highly reactive free radicals in the tissues suggests that ozone may pose a genetic hazard (Menzel, 1976; Yao *et al.*, 1978). Brinkman and Lamberts (1958) first drew attention to the possible radiomimetic effects of ozone. Support for this hypothesis comes from experiments showing the sphering of erythrocytes in man after inhalation of 0·2–0·25 ppm ozone, similar to that seen after x-irradiation of red blood cells *in vitro* (Brinkman *et al.*, 1964), and the production of chromatid breaks in KB human cells exposed to 8 ppm ozone *in vitro* for 10 min, equivalent to the frequency of breaks produced in the same cell line by exposure to 200 rad x-irradiation (Fetner, 1962).

Gooch *et al.* (1976) exposed human lymphocytes in culture to ozone at different concentrations between 1 and 14 ppm for varying intervals of 5–90 min either 12 or 36 h after phytohaemagglutinin stimulation. There were significant increases in chromatid deletions at doses of 7·23 ppm and above in the 36 h group, which agrees with the data of Fetner (1962), but the authors of this paper considered this only represented a weak mutagenic effect, since chromatid- rather than chromosome-type aberrations were produced.

Cytogenetic studies of humans exposed to ozone have also been carried out. Merz *et al.* (1975) exposed 6 subjects to 0·5 ppm ozone for 6 h and 10 h and observed an increase in achromatic lesions in lymphocytes after exposure compared with pre-exposure (subjects served as their own controls). The achromatic lesions were interpreted as unrepaired single strand breaks and there were also chromatid deletions. Chromosome-type aberrations were only seen in one individual. Aberrations peaked at 2 weeks after exposure but were still increased 6 weeks after exposure.

However, McKenzie *et al.* (1977) found no evidence of cytogenetic effects in 30 male volunteers inhaling 0·4 ppm ozone for 4 h. Blood samples were taken for lymphocyte culture before exposure, immediately after exposure, and at intervals of 3 days, 2 weeks and 4 weeks after exposure, but no significant increases in any type of aberration were found.

The differences between these 2 *in vivo* studies may be due to the higher exposure level and longer duration of exposure used by Merz *et al.* (1975), but the small number of subjects in that study did not permit any statistical evaluation of the results. However, the suggestion of a cytogenetic effect in that study, together with the evidence from animal *in vivo* studies (see Animal Studies), raises the possibility that ozone may affect cells not directly exposed, and the previously held assumption (see Merz *et al.*, 1975) that anti-oxidant levels in human tissues were high enough to inactivate ozone and prevent damage to cells other than those of the respiratory epithelium directly exposed, may have to be reassessed.

F. CARCINOGENICITY

No relevant data found.

SUMMARY AND EVALUATION

EXPERIMENTAL STUDIES

Exposure of male and female rats and guinea pigs to 0·5 ppm ozone, 6 h daily for 6 months produced no adverse histological effects on the gonads or secondary sex organs. Exposure of mice and rats during pregnancy has shown embryolethal effects and occasional fetal growth retardation at levels around

1·5 ppm and above. No teratogenic effects were observed but postnatal survival and development may be impaired. No adverse effects were seen in rats exposed to levels below 0·5 ppm. Conflicting reports on mutagenicity studies in hamsters do not permit any evaluation. No studies on carcinogenicity were found.

HUMAN STUDIES

No studies were found on endocrine or gonadal effects or of effects of fertility and pregnancy. There are two reports of chromatid breaks in human cells exposed to ozone *in vitro*, and conflicting reports of chromatid damage in persons exposed to 0·4–0·5 ppm for periods of 4–10 h. No data on carcinogenicity were found.

EVALUATION

There is limited evidence that ozone in concentrations over 1·5 ppm may be embryolethal in rodents but is not teratogenic. Attention is drawn to the lack of data on reproductive effects in humans. In view of the known role of reactive oxygen in carcinogenesis in animals, there is need for larger studies on the mutagenicity of ozone since evaluation of the currently available studies is impossible.

References

Brinkman, R. and Lamberts, H. B. (1958). Ozone as a possible radiomimetic gas. *Nature* **181**, 1202–1203.

Brinkman, R., Lamberts, H. B. and Veninga, T. S. (1964). Radiomimetic toxicity of ozonised air. *Lancet* **i**, 133–136.

Cavender, F. L., Singh, B. and Cockerell, B. Y. (1978). Effects in rats and guinea pigs of six-month exposures to sulfuric acid mist, ozone, and their combinations. *Journal of Toxicology and Environmental Health* **4**, (5–6), 845–852.

Fetner, R. H. (1962). Cytology: ozone-induced chromosome breakage in human cell cultures. *Nature* **194**, (4830), 793–794.

Goldstein, B. D. and Ross, S. R. (1973). Susceptibility of inbred mouse strains to ozone. *Archives of Environmental Health* **27**, (6), 412–413.

Gooch, P. C., Creasia, D. A. and Brewen, J. G. (1976).The cytogenic effects of ozone: inhalation and *in vitro* exposures. *Environmental Research* **12**, (2), 188–195.

Kavlock, R., Daston, G. amd Grabowski, C. T. (1979). Studies on the developmental toxicity of ozone. I. Prenatal effects. *Toxicology and Applied Pharmacology* **48**, (1), 19–28.

Kavlock, R. J., Meyer, E. and Grabowski, C. T. (1980). Studies on the developmental toxicity of ozone: postnatal effects. *Toxicology Letters* **5**, 3–9.

Kotin, P. and Thomas, M. (1957). Effects of air contaminants on reproduction and offspring survival in mice. *American Medical Association Archives of Industrial Health* **16**, 411–413.

McKenzie, W. H., Knelson, J. H., Rummo, N. J. and House, D. E. (1977). Cytogenic effects of inhaled ozone in man.*Mutation Research* **48**, (1), 95–102.

Menzel, D. B. (1976). Oxidants and human health. *Journal of Occupational Medicine* **18**, (5), 342–345.

Merz, T., Bender, M. A., Kerr, H. D. and Kulle, T. J. (1975). Observations of aberrations in chromosomes of lymphocytes from human subjects exposed to ozone at a concentration of 0·5 ppm for 6 and 10 hours. *Mutation Research* **31**, (5), 299–302.

Stupfel, M., Romary, F., Magnier, M. and Polianski, J. (1971). Comparative acute toxicity, in male and female mice, of several air pollutants: automobile exhaust gas, nitrogen oxides, sulphur dioxide, ozone, ammonia and carbon dioxide. *Comptes Rendus des Seances Societe de Biologie* **165**, (9), 1869–1872.

Veninga, T. S. (1967). Toxicity of ozone in comparison with ionizing radiation. *Strahlentherapie* **134**, (3), 469–477.

Yao, J. S., Calabrese, E. J. and DiNardi, S. R. (1978). Does ambient ozone pose a serious public health concern as a widespread environmental mutagen? *Medical Hypotheses* **4**, (2), 165–172.

Zelac, R. E., Cromroy, H. L., Bolch, W. E., Dunavant, B. G. and Bevis, H. A. (1971a). Inhaled ozone as a mutagen. 1. Chromosome aberrations induced in Chinese hamster lymphocytes. *Environmental Research* **4**, 262–282.

Zelac, R. E., Cromroy, H. L., Bolch, W. E., Dunavant, B. G. and Bevis, H. A. (1971b). Inhaled ozone as a mutagen. 2. Effect on the frequency of chromosome aberrations observed in irradiated Chinese hamsters. *Environmental Research* **4**, (4), 325–342.

34. Platinum and its Compounds

TECHNICAL DATA

(a) *Platinum*

Formula Pt

CAS registry number 7440–06–4

Chemical abstracts name Platinum

Synonyms None

(b) *Platinum compounds*

Formula	**CAS registry number**	**Chemical abstracts name**
Cl_6H_2Pt	16941–12–1	Platinic chloride
PtI_4	7790–46–7	Platinic iodide
PtO_2	1314–15–4	Platinic oxide
$PtCl_2$	10025–65–7	Platinous chloride
PtI_2	7790–39–8	Platinous iodide

Uses Manufacture of apparatus for industrial and laboratory use, thermocouples, platinum resistance thermometers, acidproof containers, electrodes, etc. Dentistry, jewellery, electroplating. Oxidation catalyst in manufacture of acetic, sulphuric acids and nitric acid from ammonia.

TLV 0·002 mg/m^3 (as platinum).

ANIMAL STUDIES

A. RELEVANT PHARMACOLOGY AND TOXICOLOGY

Moore *et al.* (1975) have investigated the placental transfer of radiolabelled platinum in the rat. ^{191}Pt in saline was injected i.v. to 15 rats on day 18 of pregnancy and they were killed 24 h later. Between injection and sacrifice the dams excreted 18·8% of the dose, which is similar to the amount excreted by adult male rats (19·3%) in the first 24 h after dosing, suggesting there is no difference in metabolism between males and pregnant females. The relative tissue distribution of the platinum 24 h after injection was also similar in males and pregnant females. Radioactive platinum was found in all 60 of the fetuses counted but averaged only 0·01% of the dose/g in whole fetal tissue and 0·05% of the dose/g in fetal liver. Placental levels were relatively high (0·92% of the dose/g). Only the maternal liver (1·44%/g) and maternal kidney (4·22%/g) had higher concentrations than the placenta, suggesting there may be placental binding or accumulation of platinum, limiting the amount transferred to the fetus.

There is no information about platinum transfer in milk, but should it reach the suckling animal, it may persist in the body for a longer period of time than in adults. Moore *et al.* (1975) compared the relative retention of platinum in the body after oral dosing in suckling and adult rats. Twenty-four hours after oral administration of radioactive platinum in saline, whole body retention was higher in 30 g body weight suckling rats (14·7%) than in adult males (7·4%). The authors suggest this difference may be due to a difference in the rate of movement of platinum through the gastro-intestinal tract.

B. ENDOCRINE AND GONADAL EFFECTS

Platinum does penetrate into the testis following i.v. administration but only in low concentrations. Moore *et al.* (1975) found testicular levels peaked 2 days after i.v. administration at 0·27% of the dose/g, which was one third of the blood concentration. By 2 weeks after administration testicular levels were very low at 0·06% of the dose/g.

Fisher *et al.* (1975) have shown that i.p. administration to rats of platinum chloride at doses below the LD_5, equivalent to 5·5 and 11 mg Pt^{4+}/kg, significantly reduced thymidine incorporation into testicular DNA. The lowest dose used, equivalent to 2·8 mg Pt^{4+}/kg, had no significant effect. DNA synthesis, as measured by thymidine incorporation, was also reduced in other tissues (spleen, liver and kidney). If this is a generalized effect of platinum, it may have implications for embryonic and fetal development.

C. FERTILITY

Kraft *et al.* (1978) have reported normal fertility in male rabbits with open-tube gold:platinum (75:25) devices inserted into the vas deferens. Immediately after insertion of the devices, ejaculates with reduced sperm counts and reduced sperm motility and some sperm-free ejaculates were obtained, but sperm count and motility returned to normal within 3 weeks. Artificial insemination with sperm collected from 8 males 117–426 days after insertion of the devices resulted in normal pregnancies with normal numbers of implants in 7/8 cases. Since platinum metal should not release platinum ions, the relevance of this experiment is not clear. However, it has been claimed that pure platinum wire decreases human sperm motility *in vitro* (see human studies).

D. PREGNANCY

Platinum wire inserted directly into the uterus, in common with a number of other metals, prevents implantation of fertilized ova. Chang *et al.* (1970) inserted loops of platinum wire into one horn of rats on day 3 of pregnancy and found an 83% reduction in the number of implantation sites on day 21 compared with the contralateral unoperated horn. Of those blastocysts which did implant in the uterine horn containing the platinum wire, there was no increase in embryonic or fetal death in comparison with the unoperated horn. When a platinum wire was inserted after implantation in the rat (day 6 of pregnancy), Chang and Tatum (1975) found there was no effect on embryonic or fetal survival to term. Similarly, Tobert and Davies (1977) have shown a 37% reduction in the proportion of shed ova implanting in the uterine horns of rabbits containing rectangular pieces of platinum foil.

However, solid platinum wire or foil is considered to be inert and so the adverse effects on implantation are likely to be due to the physical presence of a foreign object in the uterus and the lack of effect on post-implantation development cannot be considered as evidence of safety for soluble platinum. Platinum in the maternal circulation does reach the fetus (Moore *et al.*, 1975), albeit in small amounts, and experiments have yet to be done to evaluate its teratogenic potential. The ability of soluble platinum to reduce DNA synthesis in a number of tissues (Fisher *et al.*, 1975) points to the need for further work.

E. MUTAGENICITY

No relevant data found.

F. CARCINOGENICITY

No relevant data found.

HUMAN STUDIES

A. RELEVANT PHARMACOLOGY AND TOXICOLOGY

No relevant data found.

B. ENDOCRINE AND GONADAL EFFECTS

No relevant data found.

C. FERTILITY

Studies on the effect of platinum metal on human sperm motility have been reported by Kesserü and Leon (1974). Fresh sperm ($>10^8$ per ml) were incubated on glass slides in contact with the test metal strips for periods up to 5 hours. The viability of the sperm was measured and compared with controls incubated for the same period but without the metal strips. Copper caused the greatest effect with almost 100% loss of motility in 4 hours. Silver and zinc were also effective but nickel, platinum and aluminium were only moderately effective. Gold was almost ineffective. For example after 2 and 5 hours' incubation the percentage motilities were, approximately, for copper 10% and 0%, for silver 40% and 7%, for platinum 60% and 30% and for gold 90% and 65%. Approximately 24 samples were tested for each metal. Using 2 metal strips, one of copper and one of platinum, side by side did not modify the effect of the copper. Since platinum ions are not normally released from pure platinum wire, the significance, if any, of the above observations on sperm motility for industrial exposure to platinum and its salts is not known.

D. PREGNANCY

No relevant data found.

E. MUTAGENICITY

No relevant data found.

F. CARCINOGENICITY

No relevant data found.

SUMMARY AND EVALUATION

EXPERIMENTAL STUDIES

Limited placental transfer of platinum occurs but it is concentrated in the placenta. There is no information on transfer in milk, but neonates retain platinum longer than adults. No adverse effect on sperm was observed in rabbits with gold:platinum tubes inserted in the vas deferens. Platinum wire intrauterine devices inhibit fertility but where pregnancy does occur, no adverse effect on the embryo has been observed.

No studies were found on the effects of soluble platinum salts on fertility or pregnancy except that doses of platinum chloride down to 5 mg/kg can reduce DNA synthesis in several tissues including the testis in rats.

No data was found on mutagenicity or carcinogenicity.

HUMAN STUDIES

No studies were found on endocrine or gonadal effects or of effects on fertility, pregnancy, mutagenicity or carcinogenicity.

In vitro tests showed that platinum metal does have a weak toxic effect on sperm.

EVALUATION

There is limited evidence that platinum metal is not toxic *in vivo* to sperm or the developing embryo. Attention is drawn to the lack of information on the effects of platinum salts in animals and humans.

References

Chang, C. C., Tatum, H. J. and Kincl, F. (1970). The effect of intrauterine copper and other metals on implantation in rats and hamsters. *Fertility and Sterility* **21**, (3), 274–278.

Chang, C. C. and Tatum, H. J. (1975). Effect of intrauterine copper wire on resorption of fetuses in rats. *Contraception* **11**, 79–84.

Fisher, R. F., Holbrook, D. J., Leake, H. B. and Brubaker, P. E. (1975). Effect of platinum and palladium salts on thymidine incorporation into DNA of rat tissue. *Environmental Health Perspectives* **12**, 57–62.

Kesserü, E. and Leon, F. (1974). Effect of different solid metals and metallic pairs on human sperm motility. *International Journal of Fertility* **19**, 81–84.

Kraft, L. A., Polidoro, J. P., Culver, R. M. and Hahn, D. W. (1978). Intravas device studies in rabbits: II. Effect on sperm output, fertility and histology of the reproductive tract. *Contraception* **18**, 239–251.

Moore, W. Jr., Hysell, D., Crocker, W. and Stara, J. (1975). Biological fate of a single administration of ^{191}Pt in rats following different routes of exposure. *Environmental Research* **9**, 152–158.

Tobert, A. J. and Davies, D. R. (1977). Effect of copper and platinum intrauterine devices on endometrial morphology and implantation in the rabbit. *Journal of Reproduction and Fertility* **50**, 53–59.

35. Polybrominated Biphenyls

TECHNICAL DATA

Formula

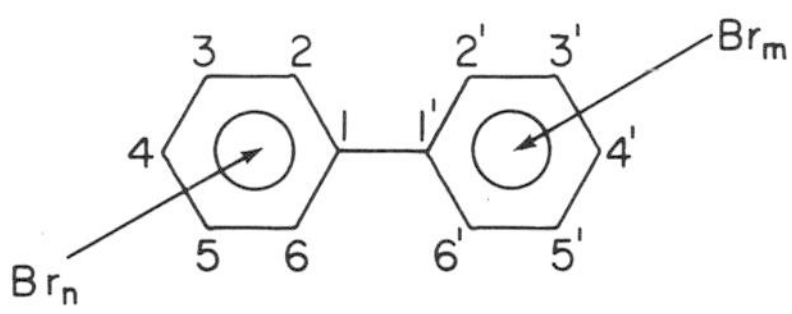

There are 3 compounds which have been commercially produced, hexabromobiphenyl, n + m = 6 ($C_{12}H_4Br_6$); octabromobiphenyl, n + m = 8 ($C_{12}H_2Br_8$); decabromobiphenyl, n + m = 10 ($C_{12}Br_{10}$)

CAS registry numbers

Hexabromobiphenyl (pure chemical) 59080–40–9; Hexabromobiphenyl (technical grade) 36355–01–8; Octabromobiphenyl 27858–07–7; Decabromobiphenyl 13654–09–6.

Chemical abstracts names

2,2′,4,4′,5,5′-hexabromo-1,1′-biphenyl (hexabromobiphenyl, pure chemical); hexabromo-1,1′-biphenyl (hexabromobiphenyl, reagent grade); ar,ar,ar,ar,ar′,ar′,ar′,ar′-octabromo-1,1′-biphenyl (octabromobiphenyl); 2,2′,3,3′,4,4′,5,5′,6,6′-decabromo-1,1′-biphenyl (decabromobiphenyl).

Synonyms

2,2′,4,4′,5,5′-hexabromobiphenyl (hexabromobiphenyl, pure chemical); hexabromodiphenyl (hexabromobiphenyl, reagent grade); octabromodiphenyl (octabromobiphenyl); decabromodiphenyl, perbromobiphenyl (decabromobiphenyl).

Uses (Of hexabromobiphenyl in U.S. all uses discontinued since 1974).
Fire-retardant in acrylonitrile-butadiene-styrene (ABS) plastics, coatings and lacquers and polyurethane foams. Potential uses of PBBs include: synthesis of biphenyl esters; in a modified Würtz synthesis, as colour-activators in light-sensitive compositions; as molecular weight control agents in polybutadiene; as wood preservatives; as voltage stabilizing agents in electrical insulation.

TLV None

ANIMAL STUDIES

A. RELEVANT PHARMACOLOGY AND TOXICOLOGY

The absorption, distribution and metabolism of polybrominated biphenyls (PBBs) in animals, principally cattle and rodents, have been reviewed elsewhere (Di Carlo *et al.*, 1978). The excretion of PBBs is very low (possibly less than 10% of the dose for some compounds); consequently the biological half-life is very long, resulting in accumulation of PBBs with continued intake. Very high concentrations are found in the fat and one important route of excretion is via the fat in breast milk.

PBBs produce a similar spectrum of toxic effects in several species, including reduced food intake and body weight, liver enlargement and a variety of adverse effects on reproduction. Di Carlo *et al.* (1978) have reviewed these effects with a summary of the minimum effective dose of PBBs in the diet in relation to each toxic effect. PBBs are unusual in that toxic effects can appear at quite low doses, yet lethality only appears at high doses. For example the oral LD50 in rats is reported to be as high as 21·5 g/kg (Di Carlo *et al.*, 1978; Sleight and Sanger, 1976).

Placental transfer of PBBs have been shown in the rat and the cow (Di Carlo *et al.*, 1978). Corbett *et al.* (1975) fed mice 1000 ppm in the diet from days 7–18 of pregnancy and found a mean level in three exposed fetuses of 0·53 ppm compared with 0·05 ppm in three control fetuses on day 18 of pregnancy. Beaudoin (1977) gave rats 800 mg/kg PBBs orally by gavage on day 12 of pregnancy. Pooled samples of embryos from four rats taken 24 and 48 h after dosing contained 13 ppm and 6 ppm respectively. Rickert *et al.* (1978) measured placental and fetal levels in rats fed 50 ppm from days 8–21 of pregnancy. On day 21, in treated dams, placental levels were 0·4 ppm (μg/g wet weight tissue) compared with 0·0 in controls, and fetal levels (excluding the liver and gastrointestinal tract) were 1·6 ppm compared with 0·3 ppm in controls. In pups 14 days of age born to dams fed 50 ppm but nursed by controls from delivery, levels (excluding liver and g.i. tract) were 5·4 ppm, suggesting placental transfer in very late pregnancy (day 21–22) may be higher than before.

The same study by Rickert *et al.* (1978) looked at transfer of PBBs in the milk to rat pups born to controls but reared by dams fed 50 ppm in the diet from day 8 of pregnancy to day 14 of lactation or days 1–14 of lactation only. Tissue concentrations at 14 days of age were highly variable, but body levels (excluding liver and gastro-intestinal tract) averaged 133 ppm in the first group and 69 ppm in the second, compared with 0·33 ppm in controls. Liver levels were also high (91 and 68 ppm), especially in comparison with liver levels in the dams that were nursing them (4 and 2·8 ppm). These experiments show that transfer via the milk occurs in substantial quantities and is far more important than *in utero* transfer via the placenta.

B. ENDOCRINE AND GONADAL EFFECTS

Harris *et al.*(1978a) have fed groups of 5 or 6 male rats, 0, 50, 100, 150 and 200 ppm PBBs in the diet for 10 weeks. Weight gain was reduced, but not significantly, at 150 and 200 ppm. Liver weight was increased significantly in all PBB groups, but weights of other organs, including testes and seminal vesicles, were unaffected.

In cattle, Jackson and Halbert (1974) first described testicular atrophy in an 18 month-old bull fed diet contaminated with PBBs for 6 weeks. A semen evaluation showed no spermatozoal motility, with many headless and tail-less spermatozoa. The bull died 3 weeks later and massive liver abscesses were found at autopsy.

Cook *et al.* (1978) examined tissues from four bulls fed a PBB-contaminated diet for an unspecified length of time and then slaughtered. Some testes were normal but most showed reduced or absent spermatozoa with few spermatogenic cells present; the seminiferous epithelium comprised mainly supporting Sertoli cells. The interstitial cells were normal. Other pathological signs were prominent lymphocytic infiltration of liver, kidney, small intestine and lung.

Allen *et al.* (1978) have followed the menstrual cycle in 7 female rhesus monkeys after feeding 0·3 ppm PBB in the diet for 7 months, during which time they ingested an average of 10·4 mg of PBB. Cycles before feeding PBB were normal. Food consumption was unaffected but they lost weight (around 7% of initial body weight), though no other signs of PBB toxicity were evident.

After 6 months, menstrual cycles were lengthened in 4/7 monkeys and the serum progesterone peak was flattened (no quantitative data given). These monkeys were subsequently bred whilst remaining on the diet (see section D for details), and 6 months after weaning of the young serum progesterone levels were still decreased in the four monkeys that had shown menstrual changes before breeding. Serum 17β-oestradiol levels were also measured but the results were not mentioned.

In another experiment, Allen *et al.* (1978) fed an adult male rhesus monkey 300 g daily of a diet containing 25 ppm of PBB. After 25 weeks the monkey died, having consumed slightly over 1 g of PBB and lost 35% of its initial body weight. At autopsy it was found to have alopecia, dry scaly skin, generalized s.c. oedema and marked oedema of the eyelids with loss of eyelashes. Internally it had an enlarged heart, hyperplastic gastroenteritis, severe ulcerative colitis, hypoactive seminiferous tubules, liver hypertrophy, keratinization of hair follicles and sebaceous glands and hyperplasia of bile duct epithelium. Death was attributed to the severe gastrointestinal changes. It is not known if the effect on the seminiferous tubules was a primary effect of PBB, or secondary to the severe PBB-induced illness.

C. PREGNANCY

The effects of exposure to PBBs during pregnancy has been studied in the mouse, rat, cow and monkey.

Rodents

In a study reported in abstract only, Preache *et al.* (1976) gave mice 0, 100 or 200 ppm PBBs in the diet from days 4–16 or 8–16 of pregnancy. The incidence of dead or resorbed fetuses was increased in those fed 200 ppm on days 4–16 of pregnancy and fetal body weight was reduced in those fed 200 ppm on days 8–16 of pregnancy. In other experiments 0, 50 or 100 ppm were fed on days 8–16 of pregnancy or days 1–29 of lactation and postnatal development and behaviour followed in the offspring. In those fed PBBs on days 8–16 of pregnancy, live litter size at birth was reduced at 100 ppm, but there were no significant effects on postnatal mortality, body weight, development of swimming ability or righting reflex, locomotor activity or water-maze escape performance in the tests conducted between 1 and 7 weeks of age. In those fed PBBs during lactation, pup mortality was increased and body weight and locomotor activity decreased at 100 ppm, but not at 50 ppm.

Lucier *et al.* (1978) have given pregnant mice a PBB orally by gavage in doses of 0·3–32 mg/kg/day on days 10–16 of pregnancy. Acceptable teratological methods were used. They noted that no significant fetotoxicity or teratogenicity was seen, but no further details are given. Other groups of 25 mice were given $\frac{1}{2}$ or $\frac{1}{10}$ of the LD50 (not stated) orally by gavage on days 10–16 of pregnancy, and fertility, gestation, viability, survival and lactation indexes were assessed. There were no significant differences between treated and control groups.

Corbett *et al.* (1975) have investigated the teratogenicity of PBBs in groups of 9–16 mice fed 50, 100 or 1000 ppm in the diet from days 7–18 of pregnancy. Acceptable teratological methods were used. Maternal liver weight was significantly increased and abnormal histology (swelling of hepatocytes and focal necrosis) was seen at 1000 ppm. Dams from other treatment groups were not examined. There was no effect on implants/dam or resorptions/dam in comparison with controls, but there was a significant, dose-related decrease in fetal weight, reaching 14% below the control mean in the 1000 ppm group. No abnormalities were seen in control fetuses. At 50 ppm 1/61 had cleft palate, at 100 ppm 3/121 had exencephaly, and at 1000 ppm 2/174 had exencephaly, 4/87 cleft palate and 2/87 hydronephrosis. These incidences for individual abnormalities did not differ significantly from the concurrent controls, but did differ significantly from pooled historical controls. PBB was found in the fetuses (see section A for details).

Corbett *et al.* (1975) also examined the teratogenicity of PBBs in the rat. Groups of 6–12 animals were fed 0, 100 or 1000 ppm PBBs in the diet from days 7–20 of pregnancy. Acceptable teratological methods were used. No information is given about possible maternal toxicity of the doses used. There were no significant effects on implants/dam or resorptions/dam. Mean fetal weight was significantly reduced in a dose-related manner, from 4·23 g in controls, to 3·96 g at 100 ppm and 3·73 g at 1000 ppm. No malformations were seen in any group from a total of 273 fetuses examined.

Aftosmis *et al.* (1972) have also fed PBBs in the diet to rats. Pregnant animals were given 100, 1000 or 10,000 ppm in the diet from days 6–15 of pregnancy. Anasarca was seen in one fetus from each of the two highest dose levels and gastroschisis in another fetus from each of the two highest dose levels. The study is reported in abstract only and no further details are given other than that "no other gross effects were seen in dams or pups".

Harris *et al.* (1978b) have investigated prenatal and postnatal development in the rat following PBB exposure during gestation. In the first experiment, groups of 6–8 rats were given 0·25, 0·5, 1·0, 5·0 or 10·0 mg/day PBBs orally by gavage on days 7–15 of pregnancy. There were 30 control rats. From the average daily food consumption given of 20 g it may be calculated that the top dose of 10 mg is equivalent to 500 ppm in the diet, and from the average day 7 body weight of around 200 g, 10 mg is equivalent to 50 mg/kg. Maternal weight gain was significantly reduced only at the 0·25 mg dose, but maternal liver weight was significantly increased at the three highest doses of 1, 5 and

10 mg. There were no significant effects on implants/dam, live fetuses/dam, resorptions/dam or fetal weight except at 0·25 mg where fetal weight and crown-rump length were significantly reduced, presumably a secondary effect from the random reductions in food intake, water intake and maternal body weight seen in this group. Fetuses were examined for external gross malformations only and none were seen in treated groups, with one in controls.

In their second experiment Harris *et al.* (1978b) gave groups of 8 rats 0 or 10 mg PBBs/day from days 7–15 of pregnancy and allowed the dams to deliver and rear their own litters. There was no effect on litter size or pup weight at birth, but significant reductions in offspring weight were seen in the PBB-exposed group from 3 days of age onwards to the termination of the study at 60 days of age, with male pups more affected than female pups. Postnatal mortality up to weaning was also significantly increased from 1·5% in controls to 14·3% in PBB-exposed offspring and vaginal opening was slightly delayed in PBB-exposed female offspring. In order to differentiate between prenatally mediated effects and postnatally mediated effects, in a third experiment cross-fostering of some pups was carried out. Groups of 8 dams were given 0 or 10 mg of PBBs/day from days 7–15 of pregnancy as before. After littering out, 50% of pups in each control litter were given to PBB-treated dams and 50% of pups from PBB-treated dams given to controls to rear. Measurements of body weight showed the greatest reductions in those born to PBB dams and reared by PBB dams. Pups exposed prenatally to PBBs but reared by controls and control pups reared by PBB dams were of similar weight and intermediate to the PBB pups reared by PBB dams and control pups reared by control dams. There was no control for the fostering procedure itself which may have contributed to the weight reduction in these two intermediate groups, but it seems more likely that PBBs exert effects on growth rate both prenatally and postnatally. Although dosing stopped on day 15 of pregnancy, maternal milk levels of PBBs would still be high during lactation (see section A). Vaginal opening was delayed to a similar degree in all female offspring born to and/or reared by PBB-exposed dams. Pup mortality however ranged from 11–24% and showed no clear treatment related effects.

Wertz and Ficsor (1978) gave groups of 15 rats 0 or 100 mg/kg orally by gavage at 2-day intervals on days 6–16 of pregnancy. A total of 600 mg/kg was given in 6 doses. There were no significant effects on implants/dam, resorptions/dam or fetal weight. Fetuses were examined for external malformations, cleft palate and skeletal abnormalties only. No differences were found between treated and control groups.

Beaudoin (1977) has investigated the teratogenic potential of single high doses of PBBs given on one of days 6–14 of pregnancy in the rat. Acceptable teratological methods were used. Groups of 4–15 rats were given a single dose of 40, 200, 400 or 800 mg/kg PBBs orally by gavage. At doses of 40 or 200 mg/kg all the dams survived. Resorption rates were not increased at 40 mg/kg but were increased in some 200 mg/kg groups, treated on days 6, 8 or 13 of pregnancy. Only two malformed fetuses were seen, one control and one from a 40 mg/kg group, both with absent digits on all four paws. Maternal deaths were seen at 400 and 800 mg/kg, but never exceeded 2/group, with the exception of 800 mg/kg on day 7 when 5/6 dams died. Resorption rates were significantly increased above that in controls in a dose-related manner in all PBB groups given 400 or 800 mg/kg on one of days 6–10 of pregnancy. They were also increased in the 800 mg/kg groups dosed on day 11 or 12, but not on day 13 or 14. Malformations, particularly cleft palate and diaphragmatic hernia were increased in many 400 or 800 mg/kg groups after dosing on all days except day 6 (no survivors) and day 14. In the 400 mg/kg groups 0–11·8% of survivors were malformed and in 800 mg/kg groups 0–60% were malformed. No skeletal malformations were seen and there were no dose-day–related effects on ossification. Fetal and placental weights were unaffected in 40 or 200 mg/kg groups but significant, dose-related reductions in fetal and placental weights were seen in all 400 and 800 mg/kg groups. During the 24–72 h after administration of PBB, dams in all dose groups lost weight and had reduced food and water consumption, but 40 mg/kg groups recovered within 48 h. Higher dose goups showed dose-related reductions in maternal weight gain and all 800 mg/kg groups lost weight between the day of treatment and day 20, when killed. However, pair feeding of an additional group of controls with rats given 800 mg/kg on day 12 had no effect on resorptions, fetal or placental weight. Thus the effects of PBBs seen in this experiment on resorptions, malformations and fetal weight are due to PBBs and not secondary to any effect on food and water intake.

The effects of PBBs on hepatic enzyme activity in preweaning rats have been studied. Dent *et al.* (1978) fed rats 0 or 50 ppm PBBs in the diet from day 8 of pregnancy to day 15 post-partum. Pups were fostered and cross-fostered at birth to separate prenatally mediated effects from postnatally mediated effects. The treatments had no effect on body weight gain in the first and second weeks of life, but at 14 days of age the liver:body weight ratio was significantly increased in all pups exposed prenatally and/or postnatally to PBBs. The activities of hepatic arylhydrocarbon hydroxlyase and epoxide hydratase at 14 days of age were also significantly increased in all PBB-exposed groups and were highest in those born to and reared by PBB-treated dams. The potency of PBBs as enzyme-inducers may be judged from the very small quantities (0·2 μg/g) of PBBs found in the liver of fetuses near term in dams fed 50 ppm in the diet from day 8 of pregnancy, as above (Rickert *et al.*, 1978). Yet pups reared by controls still show significant stimulation at 14 days of age.

Moore *et al.* (1978) have measured liver enzyme levels in pups suckled by dams fed 0, 0·1, 1·0 or 10 ppm PBBs in the diet from days 1–18 of gestation. At 18 days of age, pups showed a dose-related increase in liver:body weight ratio, reaching significant levels in the 10 ppm group. Liver microsomal protein levels in the pups were also increased in a dose-related manner, reaching significant levels at 1·0 and 10 ppm, though the smaller increases seen in this parameter in the experiment of Dent *et al.* (1978) where 50 ppm was fed in the diet, were not significant. The pups suckled by 10 ppm dams showed mixed-type microsomal enzyme induction in the liver, including increased cytochrome P-450, aminopyrine demethylation, benzo(a)pyrene hydroxylation, and UDP-glucuronyl-transferase. Smaller increases were seen in the 1 ppm group and no changes in the 0·1 ppm group. Sleight and Sanger (1976) carried out an ultrastructural examination of the livers from dams and pups in the above experiment. In the pups from the 10 ppm group a variety of ultrastructural changes were seen, especially in the mitochondria, some of which were degenerating. Mitochrondrial changes were also seen to a lesser extent in the pups from the 1 ppm group, but those in the 0·1 ppm group were normal. In both these studies, comparison of enzyme induction and ultrastructural lesions indicated in the lactating dams and their pups show that the pups are more affected than the dams; PBB-induced changes are seen at 1 and 10 ppm in pups but only 10 ppm in the dams. The authors point out however, that because of the small numbers of animals tested at each dietary level (4), 0·1 ppm cannot be taken as an unequivocal no-effect level in the pups.

The enzyme induction with prenatal and/or postnatal exposure to PBBs may be of significance in interactions between PBBs and other drugs or environmental chemicals. The premature induction of mixed-type hepatic enzymes may render the fetus or neonate either more or less susceptible to other agents, depending on whether the developmental toxin is the agent itself or its metabolite.

Cattle

It was the effects of PBBs in cattle, particularly during pregnancy, which first alerted people to the Michigan disaster beginning in 1973, when animal feed was accidentally contaminated with a flame retardant, Firemaster BP-6 (Michigan Chemical Company, U.S.A.), a mixture of polybrominated biphenyls of which the major component is 2,2′,4,4′5,5′-hexabromobiphenyl. The contaminated feed was widely distributed in Michigan for some months before the problem was identified. It resulted in destruction of approximately 30,000 cattle, 6,000 pigs, 1,500 sheep and 1·5 million chickens (Di Carlo *et al.*, 1978). The reports that follow are from veterinary investigators of affected herds and from cattle deliberately fed PBBs in their diet.

Jackson and Halbert (1974) published the first full report on an affected herd. The cows showed anorexia, decreased milk production and lameness. A large number of cows inseminated came back into oestrus within 4–6 weeks. Early embryonic resorption was suspected but could not be confirmed. Further toxic signs developed and cows given the contaminated feed during the last trimester of pregnancy showed delayed parturition of 2–4 weeks. They had large calves, and dystocia due to failure of the pelvic ligaments to relax. The calves were often dead at birth or soon after and milk production was negligible. Autopsy of affected cows that died or were slaughtered showed extensive pathological changes in the liver.

Prewitt *et al.* (1973) reported in field observations of contaminated herds that food consumption and milk production were reduced by 50% and animals with over 20 ppm PBBs in their milk fat suffered dystocia and calves were stillborn or died soon after birth. Newborn calves often had stiff tendons. Metritis and retained placenta were common. Similar symptoms were seen in some cows with only 1 ppm in their milk fat.

Experimental dosing of cattle with PBBs added to the diet has been studied by Moorhead *et al.* (1977, 1978) and by the same group, Durst *et al.* (1978). Groups of 6 heifers were dosed orally with 0, 0·25, 250 or 25,000 mg/day for 60 days, or in the case of the highest dose groups, until moribund, from the time of diagnosis of pregnancy by rectal palpation. In the highest dose group, on 25 g/day (67 mg/kg), abortion occurred in 3/6 heifers after 30, 33 and 39 days of dosing and the remaining 3 were found to contain dead fetuses at autopsy on days 33, 39 and 40 of dosing. These fetuses were oedematous and haemorrhagic. Uterine haemorrhage and necrosis of placental cotyledons were also seen. Many signs of toxicity were also present in this group before death and at autopsy but the ovaries were normal. In the lower dose groups, there were no signs of toxicity and no effects on pregnancy or calving. All the calves survived. Birth weight, weight gain and general health of the calves were normal. Milk production was normal. Following parturition at approximately 220 days after dosing, heifers and calves in the lower dose groups were autopsied and no gross or histopathological damage was seen.

Others have also reported lack of effect of low levels of PBB contamination in the feed. Milk production and calving was normal in herds consuming feed containing an average of 0·09 ppm (Mercer *et al.*, 1976) and in cows with an average fat tissue concentration of 0·3–1·8 ppm (Wastell *et al.*, 1978).

Monkey

Allen *et al.* (1978) fed 7 female rhesus monkeys 0·3 ppm of PBB in the diet for 7 months before breeding, throughout breeding during pregnancy and lactation. Menstrual cycle changes were seen after 6 months on the diet (see section B for details). Controls conceived after 1–3 breedings and delivered normal appearing infants weighing an average of 519 g. PBB-fed monkeys conceived after 1–4 breedings. Two of the 7 PBB-fed monkeys had long implantation bleedings, one aborted a mummified fetus at 146 days' gestation and one gave birth to a stillborn infant at 154 days. The remaining 5 monkeys delivered infants of normal appearance but low birth weight (average 455 g) at 156–165 days' gestation (normal gestation 165 days). Postnatal weight gain up to 16 weeks of age was also depressed in the PBB group. Thus, both menstrual cycle changes and poor outcomes of pregnancy have been observed in females fed PBBs at a dose sufficient to cause weight loss but no other overt signs of PBB toxicity. A number of features of PBB toxicity resemble those of PCB toxicity in the rhesus monkey, including menstrual disorders, low birth weight, alopecia and swollen eyelids (see Polychlorinated Biphenyls, p. 455).

Conclusion

From the limited studies in cattle, it is impossible to separate the effects on pregnancy from those on the general health of the animal. Intrauterine death, stillbirth and high postnatal mortality are seen in cattle fed high doses of PBBs, but early loss of the fetus has only been seen in severely debilitated, moribund animals, and stillbirths and high neonatal mortality may be secondary to the dystocia resulting from failure of the pelvic ligaments to relax. Low levels of feed contamination of <1 ppm appear to be without effect on reproduction. There are no reports of grossly malformed calves. However, the limitations on the amount of experimentation and field observation that can be undertaken in cattle have prevented any systematic observation of reproduction in cattle fed intermediate doses of PBBs to see whether the embryo and fetus are more vulnerable to PBB toxicity than adult tissues.

In rodents, fetotoxic effects (mainly reduced fetal weight) have been seen in the mouse and rat. Though there is no clear agreement about threshold doses at which this effect occurs, in the majority of studies the threshold is around 1000 ppm in the diet, equivalent to about 50 mg/kg. This dose may also affect postnatal development and survival of the pups, partly by a prenatal and partly by a postnatal effect. At doses producing some toxicity in the dams, there may also be an increase in resorptions. Teratogenic effects have not been seen except in rats treated with very high single doses of 400 mg/kg and above. There is evidence, however, that these effects cannot solely be explained by maternal toxicity. Administration postnatally via the milk increases pup mortality and decreases weight gain. It induces hepatic enzyme changes in the pups at maternal doses as low as 1 ppm in the diet, doses which do not affect the maternal liver at all. There is also some evidence that prenatally administered doses below those causing resorption, loss in fetal weight or malformation, nevertheless adversely affect postnatal development in terms of survival, weight gain and vaginal opening in pups, and that these effects are mediated partially in the prenatal period and are not solely due to persistence of PBBs in maternal milk passed to the suckling pups.

A small study in the rhesus monkey has indicated disturbed menstrual function, intrauterine death, low birth weight and poor postnatal growth after feeding PBB in the diet at a level sufficient to cause loss of body weight but no gross signs of PBB toxicity in the mother.

E. MUTAGENICITY

It is not known whether PBBs are mutagenic in bacterial systems. In one mammalian study, groups of 9 mice were given 0, 50 or 500 mg/kg PBBs orally by gavage and killed 12, 24 or 48h later for examination of the bone marrow cells (Wertz and Ficsor, 1978). There were no significant increases in chromosome or chromatid breaks but at both doses at 24 and 48 h, gaps were increased. The genetic significance of gaps is not as yet known.

F. CARCINOGENICITY

IARC Monograph Vol. 18 (1978) reported one study in rats suggesting neoplastic changes in the liver after oral doses of PBBs, but the study was considered to be inadequate.

HUMAN STUDIES

A. RELEVANT PHARMACOLOGY AND TOXICOLOGY

Due to a mix-up in a factory in Michigan producing dairy farm animal food, accidental contamination of the feed occurred in 1973–74 with the polybrominated biphenyl (PBB) compound "Firemaster"—consisting mainly of hexa- and heptabromobiphenyl. This was followed by the illness and death of affected cattle and over 500 farms were quarantined. Approximately 23,000 dairy cattle, 1·6 million chickens and 5 million eggs were destroyed in an attempt to control the spread of contamination. However, contaminated meat, dairy products, poultry and eggs had been consumed for about 9 months before people became aware of the fact, so that widespread dissemination of PBB occurred among the population of Michigan and the majority of residents now have detectable amounts of PBB in their body fat (Dunckel, 1975; Lancet Editorial, 1977; Anderson *et al.*, 1978; DiCarlo *et al.*,

1978). Selikoff and his colleagues of the Mount Sinai School of Medicine were invited by the Michigan State Authorities to conduct comprehensive examinations of exposed Michigan farm residents in 1977 to define the effects of PBB exposure. They reported (Anderson *et al.*, 1978) that compared with a similar population in Wisconsin, the Michigan residents had significantly higher prevalence of skin, neurological and musculo-skeletal symptoms, especially among the younger (16–55 years) age group. Females were more affected neurologically than males. The main neurological symptoms were marked tiredness and fatigue with a striking reduction in both physical and intellectual work capacity. Many of the workers, used to only 6 or 7 hours sleep previously, now required as much as 16–18 hours sleep per day. Although questions were asked about reproductive history, no details were recorded in the report.

The Michigan Department of Public Health, together with the Centre for Disease Control, the FDA, NIH and EPA have established a cohort of 4545 people in Michigan to be examined at regular intervals over several decades to determine the long-term effects of PBB exposure. Four groups are included—quarantined farm residents, farm produce recipients, chemical workers and their families who had been exposed to PBB, and a pilot study control group. In the report on the first 4 years of the investigation (Landrigan *et al.*, 1979), the most frequently reported symptoms were similar to those reported above: i.e. fatigue, headaches, paraesthesia, and joint problems. Serum PBB measurements were made on the majority of subjects and ranged from 0–1900 ppb; 106 values out of 3639 were over 100 ppb, and children under 10 years of age had the highest levels on age group analysis. Males had significantly higher values than females ($P < 10^{-10}$). The highest values were found in the chemical workers and their families (mean 43 ppb), followed by residents of quarantined farms (mean 27 ppb). Comparison of levels obtained from 148 subjects in 1974 and in 1977 showed that levels were generally stable over the 3 years with a mean change of −16 ppb. In 221 subjects, fat samples were also obtained and were on average 363 times higher than the corresponding serum sample.

Analysis of the relationship between prevalence of symptoms and serum PBB surprisingly showed no association; the highest prevalence rates were actually in persons with the lowest serum PBB. A similar surprising result was also reported for neurological symptoms by Valciukas *et al.* (1979).

The presence of halogen-acne has also been reported in 21/1029 subjects studied in Grand Rapids, Michigan (Di Carlo *et al.*, 1978).

Placental Transfer

In a study by Landrigan *et al.* (1979), mentioned above, it was reported that 63 children have been born since 1973 to women exposed to PBB. Fifty-two women were examined at time of delivery and their serum PBB ranged from <1 ppb (limit of detection) to 1150 ppb, with a mean of 26·2 ppb. Cord serum PBB in 58 infants ranged from <1 ppb to 104 ppb, with a mean of 3·2 ppb. The mean maternal:fetal ratio for 13 pairs studied with measurable levels was 7·04 (range 1·5–10·3). This shows that PBB is transferred across the placenta but suggests some degree of barrier as has been demonstrated for PCB.

Transfer in the breast milk

In the study by Landrigan *et al.* (1979) breast milk samples were analysed from 32 women exposed to PBB and the concentrations on a fat basis ranged from 32–93,000 ppb (mean 3614 ppb), with a ratio of milk:serum levels of 122 (range 62–257). A more detailed study was reported by Brilliant *et al.* (1978). They measured the breast milk PBB concentration in 2 areas of Michigan, the upper peninsula (U.P.) which had lower exposure to PBB and the lower peninsula (L.P.) which was more widely contaminated. Two samples of 42 women (U.P.) and 53 women (L.P.) were carefully chosen by a random selection procedure from all deliveries during part of August 1976. Fifty-one (96%) of the 53 U.P. women had detectable PBB levels, and 18 (43%) of the 42 L.P. women had detectable levels. In the U.P. women, the levels on a fat basis were <50 ppb in 16, 50–100 ppb in 17, 100–500 ppb in 15, 500–1000 ppb in 2, and 1200 ppb in one, with a median of 68 ppb. Fifteen of the 18 U.P. levels were <50 ppb. On the basis of this work, the authors estimate that about 8 to 9 million people in the lower peninsula of Michigan would have detectable levels of PBB in their body. A comparison of body fat with milk fat in 10 women showed a high correlation ($r = 0{\cdot}88$) with a ratio of almost exactly one.

B. ENDOCRINE AND GONADAL EFFECTS

As part of the follow-up investigation of the exposed population in the Michigan episode, Rosenman *et al.* (1979) studied seminal fluid of 3 groups of men. Group 1 were 41 farmers and others who had consumed farm produce from contaminated farms. Group 2 were 11 men employed at the chemical company where PBB was manufactured, and Group 3 were 52 graduate students at Michigan University who had not been exposed to PBB. The Group 1 subjects were selected to have no history of thyroid disease, liver disease, renal or urinary tract infection, diabetes, cancer, myocardial infarction or psychiatric illness. These exclusions accounted for 27 of the original 117 contacted, so that some degree of selection took place which may make the sample not entirely typical of all exposed persons. Group 2 was selected in a similar manner; however, in Group 3, men were not excluded for medical reasons, but were all graduate students at Michigan University who were normally resident outside Michigan. They were presumably younger than those in the other groups but no data on age are given. All the subjects in Groups 1 and 2 had PBB present in blood samples (levels not stated) but only one subject in Group 3 had PBB (limit of detection=0·2 ppb). Semen was analysed within 3 hours of collection for motility and count and later a fixed specimen was examined for morphology. Each subject also received a comprehensive physical examination.

No difference was found between the groups in respect of sperm count, motility or morphology and in all groups these were within what would be considered normal ranges. There was no increase in varicocoeles in Groups 1 and 2.

FSH, LH and testosterone were measured in 16 of the exposed subjects and 16 controls but since most FSH and LH results were below the level of detection (not stated) the results are of no value. No details are given of the testosterone values but because of the methodology used the results are valueless. The authors state that there was no correlation between serum PBB level and sperm count or testosterone level.

Criticisms of this study are first, that the survey was carried out 4 years after the initial exposure so that early recoverable effects may have been missed and secondly, that due to exclusions, effects in more severely affected subjects may have been missed. The overall result however is reassuring.

C. FERTILITY

No relevant data found.

D. PREGNANCY

No relevant data found.

E. MUTAGENICITY

No relevant data found.

F. CARCINOGENICITY

IARC Monograph Vol. 18 (1978) reported that no evaluation of the carcinogenicity of PBBs could be made on the basis of the available data.

SUMMARY AND EVALUATION

EXPERIMENTAL STUDIES

PBBs are very fat soluble and marked cumulation in fat occurs. Transplacental transfer occurs in several species studied, but the amount transferred to the neonates via the milk is much greater than that occurring *in utero* via the placenta, and is of greater importance. Cattle fed diets contaminated with unspecified, but toxic, amounts of PBB showed damage to the seminiferous tubules and reduced numbers or absence of sperm, as well as gross pathology in other tissues.

Female monkeys fed diet containing 0·3 ppm PBB showed lengthening of the menstrual cycle in 4 of 7 treated animals after 6 months. There were reduced serum progesterone levels in the affected animals.

Mice and rats given around 1000 ppm in the diet or 50 mg/kg by gavage during pregnancy show reduced fetal weight. In rats given 50 mg/kg by gavage there was reduced postnatal growth and survival, partly mediated prenatally and partly postnatally. At toxic doses embryolethal, but not teratogenic effects have been observed except in rats given very high single doses of 400 mg/kg and above, where teratogenic effects were observed.

In cattle fed toxic amounts of PBB in diets, there is reduced food consumption and reduced milk yield with an increase in resorptions. Gestation may be prolonged and stillbirths and neonatal deaths have been reported though these may be secondary to dystocia which is also produced. Doses of 67 mg/kg have been shown to be toxic during pregnancy and to result in abortions or resorptions in all treated animals. Doses around 1 mg/kg and 0·1 ppm in the diet seem to be non-toxic. Congenital malformations in cattle have not been observed. Limited studies in rhesus monkeys fed 0·3 ppm PBB in the diet suggested an increase in fetal loss, low birth weight and poor postnatal growth. Studies are inadequate to assess the mutagenicity and carcinogenicity of PBB.

HUMAN STUDIES

Studies in people accidentally exposed via the food have shown that PBB crosses the placenta, but some degree of barrier exists and the fetal levels are generally lower than in the mother. Levels in breast milk, however, are about 100 times higher than in plasma and in fact milk is a major excretion pathway for the highly fat soluble PBB.

Limited studies in men with detectable PBB levels in plasma did not show any effect on sperm count motility or morphology. No studies were found on endocrine effects in males or females or on fertility, pregnancy, mutagenicity or carcinogenicity.

EVALUATION

Studies in animals demonstrate the toxicity of low levels of PBB on reproductive cycles and during pregnancy. Embryolethal and fetotoxic effects may be produced with poor postnatal survival. The latter is aggravated by transfer of PBB in milk. A no effect level in primates has not been established. Attention is drawn to the lack of data on PBB in humans, and by analogy with PCBs, information on children exposed to PBB via the milk is required. Data on mutagenicity and carcinogenicity are inadequate for evaluation.

References

Aftosmis, J. C., Dashiell, O. L., Griffith, F. D., Hornberger, C. S., McDonnell, M. M., Sherman, H., Tayfun, F. O. and Waritz, E. I. (1972). Toxicology of brominated biphenyls. II. Skin, eye and inhalation toxicity and an acute test method for evaluating hepatotoxicity and accumulation in body fat.*Toxicology and Applied Pharmacology* **22**, 316–317

Allen, J. R., Lambrecht, L. K. and Barsotti, B. A. (1978). Effects of polybrominated biphenyls in nonhuman primates. *Journal of the American Veterinary Medicine Association* **173**, 1485–1489.

Anderson, H. A., Lilis, R., Selikoff, I. J., Rosenman, K. D., Valciukas, J. A. and Freedman, S. (1978). Unanticipated prevalence of symptoms among dairy farmers in Michigan and Wisconsin. *Environmental Health Perspectives* **23**, 217–226.

Beaudoin, A. R. (1977). Teratogenicity of polybrominated biphenyls in rats. *Environmental Research* **14**, (1), 81–86.

Brilliant, L. B., Van Amburg, G., Isbister, J., Humphrey, H., Wilcox, K., Eyster, J., Bloomer, A. W. and Price, H. (1978). Breast-milk monitoring to measure Michigan's contamination with polybrominated biphenyls. *Lancet* **ii**, 643–646.

Cook, H., Helland, D. R., Vanderweele, B. H. and DeJong, R. J. (1978). Histotoxic effects of polybrominated biphenyls in Michigan dairy cattle. *Environmental Research* **15**, 82–89.

Corbett, T. H., Beaudoin, A. R., Cornell, R. G., Anver, M. R., Schumacher, R., Endres, J. and Szwabowska, M. (1975). Toxicity of polybrominated biphenyls (Firemaster BP-6) in rodents. *Environmental Research* **10**, 390–396.

Dent, J. G., McCormack, K. M., Rickert, D. E., Cagen, S. Z., Melrose, P. and Gibson, J. E. (1978). Mixed function oxidase activities in lactating rats and their offspring following dietary exposure to polybrominated biphenyls. *Toxicology and Applied Pharmacology* **46**, 727–735.

DiCarlo, F. J., Seifter, J. and DeCarlo, V. J. (1978). Assessment of the hazards of polybrominated biphenyls. *Environmental Health Perspectives* **23**, 351–365.

Dunckel, A. E. (1975). An updating on the polybrominated biphenyl disaster in Michigan. *Journal of the American Veterinary Association* **167**, 838–841.

Durst, H. I., Willett, L. B., Schanbacher, F. L. and Moorhead, P. D. (1978). Effects of PBBs on cattle. 1. clinical evaluations and clinical chemistry.*Environmental Health Perspectives* **23**, 83–89.

Harris, S. J., Cecil, H. C. and Bitman, J. (1978a). Effects of feeding a polybrominated biphenyl flame retardant (Firemaster BP-6) to male rats. *Bulletin of Environmental Contamination and Toxicology* **19**, (6), 692–696.

Harris, S. J., Cecil, H. C. Bitman, J. (1978b). Embryotoxic effects of polybrominated biphenyls (PBB) in rats. *Environmental Health Perspectives* **23**, 295–300.

IARC Monographs on the Evaluation of the Carcinogenic Risk of Chemicals to Humans: Polychlorinated biphenyls and polybrominated biphenyls. (1978). Vol. 18, Lyon, France.

Jackson, T. F. and Halbert, F. L. (1974). A toxic syndrome associated with the feeding of polybrominated biphenyl-contaminated protein concentrate to dairy cattle. *Journal of the American Veterinary Medical Association* **165**, 487–489.

Lancet (Editorial). (1977). Polybrominated biphenyls, polychlorinated biphenyls, pentachlorophenyl—and all that. *Lancet* **ii**, 19–21.

Landrigan, P. J., Wilcox, K. R., Silva, J., Humphrey, H. E. B., Kauffman, C. and Heath, C. W. (1979). Cohort study of Michigan residents exposed to polybrominated biphenyls: epidemiologic and immunologic findings. *Annals of the New York Academy of Sciences* **320**, 284–294.

Lucier, G. W., Davis, C. J. and McLachlan, J. A. (1978). Transplacental transfer of the polychlorinated and polybrominated biphenyls. *Developmental Toxicology* **47**, 188–203.

Mercer, H. D., Teske, R. H. and Condon, R. J. (1976). Herd health state of animals exposed to polybrominated biphenyls (PBB). *Journal of Toxicology and Applied Health* **2**, 335–349.

Moore, R. W., Dannan, G. A. and Aust, S. D. (1978). Induction of drug metabolizing enzymes in polybrominated biphenyl-fed lactating rats and their pups. *Environmental Health Perspectives* **23**, 159–165.

Moorhead, P. D., Willet, L. B., Brumm, C. J. and Mercer, H. D. (1977). Pathology of experimentally induced polybrominated biphenyl toxicosis in pregnant heifers. *Journal of the American Veterinary Medical Association* **170**, 307–313.

Moorhead, P. D., Willett, L. B. and Schanbacher, F. L. (1978). Effects of PBB on cattle. II. Gross pathology and histopathology. *Environmental Health Perspectives* **23**, 111–118.

Preache, M. M., Cagen, S. Z. and Gibson, J. E. (1976). Perinatal toxicity in mice following maternal dietary exposure to polybrominated biphenyls. *Toxicology and Applied Pharmacology* **37**, 171.

Prewitt, L. R., Cook, R. M. and Fries, G. F. (1973). Health: polybrominated biphenyl and other health related problems. Field observations of Michigan dairy cattle contaminated with polybrominated biphenyl. *Journal of Dairy Science* **58**, 763–764.

Rickert, D. E., Dent, J. G., Cagan, S. Z., McCormack, K. M., Melrose, P. and Gibson, J. E. (1978). Distribution of polybrominated biphenyls after dietary exposure in pregnant and lactating rats and their offspring. *Environmental Health Perspectives* **23**, 63–66.

Rosenman, K. D., Anderson, H. A., Selikoff, I. J., Wolff, M. S. and Holstein, E. (1979). Spermatogenesis in man exposed to polybrominated biphenyl (PBB). *Fertility and Sterility* **32**, (2), 209–213.

Sleight, S. D. and Sanger, V. L. (1976). Pathologic features of polybrominated biphenyltoxicosis in the rat and guinea pig. *Journal of the American Veterinary Association* **169**, 1231–1235.

Valciukas, J. A., Lilis, R., Anderson, H. A., Wolff, M. S. and Petrocci, M. (1979). The neurotoxicity of polybrominated biphenyls: result of a medical field survey. *Annals of the New York Academy of Sciences* **320**, 337–367.

Wastell, M. E., Moody, D. L. and Plog, J. F. (1978). Effects of polybrominated biphenyl on milk production, reproduction, and health problems in Holstein cows. *Environmental Health Perspectives* **23**, 99–103.

Wertz, G. F. and Ficsor, G. (1978). Cytogenic and teratogenic test of polybrominated biphenyls in rodents. *Environmental Health Perspectives* **23**, 129–132.

36. Polychlorinated Biphenyls

TECHNICAL DATA

Formula

Structural formula of the unsubstituted biphenyl. There are 209 possible isomers.

CAS registry numbers Too numerous to list (see IARC Monograph Vol. 18, 1978).

Chemical abstracts names As above.

Synonyms Chlorinated biphenyl; chorinated diphenyl; chloro-biphenyl; PCB; PCBs; polychlorinated biphenyl; polychlorobiphenyl.

Uses Dielectric in capacitors and transformers; investment casting processes; heat exchange fluid; hydraulic fluid. Have also been used (prior to controls) in plasticizers, surface coatings, inks, adhesives, pesticide extenders, for micro-encapsulation of dyes for carbonless duplicating paper. Have been used in immersion oil for microscopes, as catalyst carrier in polymerization of olefins, in conversion of water-permeable solids to non-permeable states and combined with insecticide to bactericide formulations. Mixtures of PCBs and chlorinated naphthalenes were used to insulate electric wires and cables in mining and shipbuilding industries.

TLV 1 mg/m^3 (skin, 42% chlorine) 0·5 mg/m^3 (skin, 54% chlorine).

ANIMAL STUDIES

A. RELEVANT PHARMACOLOGY AND TOXICOLOGY

There are a wide variety of polychlorinated biphenyls (PCBs). Commercially available PCBs, which are most often used in toxicity experiments, are mixtures of isomers, some of which have been resolved into as many as 50 components (see review by Peakall, 1972). There are 209 possible PCB isomers (Lucier *et al.*, 1978). The major U.S. manufacturer, Monsanto Co., using the trade name Aroclor, has a 4 digit numerical code to describe the chemical composition of each PCB mixture; the first 2 digits represent the molecular type (12—chlorinated biphenyls, 25 and 44—blends of chlorinated biphenyls and chlorinated terphenyls, 54—chlorinated terphenyls), and the last 2 digits represent the approximate weight percentage of chlorine. In this review, wherever possible, the PCB mixture used will be identified using the Monsanto Co. system.

An additional complication in considering the toxicity of PCBs is that contaminants such as dioxins and dibenzofurans may also be present (Gellert, 1978) which can be extremely toxic at low doses. These are oxidation products of PCBs, and whilst some commercial preparations may be relatively free from contaminants at the end of manufacture; subsequent industrial use may encourage oxidation.

In the body, metabolism of PCBs is generally by hydroxylation, through an arene oxide intermediate, followed by faecal excretion (Lucier *et al.*, 1978). However, there are known to be some marked differences between fetal and adult metabolism of PCBs, at least in the rat (Lucier *et al.*, 1978). In adults and newborns, many PCBs are stored in adipose tissue, but certain PCB analogues, such as biphenyls with 1, 2, 4 or 6 chlorine atoms, are not stored and are readily cleared from the body. In fetuses, however, high concentrations of these compounds are found in the fetal intestine, though rapidly cleared followed parturition. It has been suggested that accumulation in the fetal intestine occurs as follows: the PCB is hydroxylated in the maternal compartment, crosses the placenta, is conjugated to glucuronide in the fetal liver, the glucuronide accumulates in the fetal intestine since it cannot cross the placenta, and in the intestine it may be hydrolysed to reform the hydroxylated metabolite, which may be reabsorbed by the circulation and passed back to the fetal liver in a form of enterohepatic circulation. The inability of the fetus to get rid of polar conjugates such as glucuronides through urinary and faecal excretion results in accumulation of PCB metabolites in the fetus which may be of greater or lesser toxicity than the PCBs themselves.

Placental transfer

Placental transfer of PCBs has been shown in a number of species including primates. In the mouse, Török (1975) has studied the distribution of ^{14}C-labelled PCB containing 85% 2,2′-dichlorobiphenyl following maternal i.m. injection, using whole-body autoradiography. Rapid maternal excretion was evident within 30 min of injection. After injection on day 14 of pregnancy fetal uptake was very low on days 14 and 15 but pronounced by day 18. After injection on day 17 of pregnancy, fetal uptake was again pronounced on day 18. The radioactivity (PCB and/or its metabolites) was localised mainly in the fetal intestine but was also seen in kidney and liver.

Masuda *et al.* (1978b) have measured fetal PCB levels in the mouse on day 18 of pregnancy following maternal administration in the diet throughout pregnancy. Kanechlor-500 (Kanegafuchi Chemical Industry Co., Japan), comprising mainly penta- and hexachlorobiphenyls, was fed in the diet at 0·01 (controls), 0·94, 8·4 or 86 ppm from days 1–18 of pregnancy. Regardless of the dietary level of PCBs whole body levels in the fetuses were only 0·1–0·2% of the total maternal intake, showing limited transfer across the placenta.

In the rat, similar limited transfer of PCBs across the placenta to the fetus has been observed. Kato *et al.* (1972) gave radiolabelled ^{3}H-Kanechlor-400, comprising mainly tetra- and pentachlorobiphenyls, orally by gavage to rats in late pregnancy, and measured levels of radioactivity in the placenta, amniotic fluid and fetus 18 h after maternal administration. By 48 h after administration, fetal and placental levels were higher than at 18 h, but on all occasions substantially lower than maternal levels. Takagi *et al.* (1976) gave radiolabelled ^{14}C-PCB, almost identical to Kanechlor-400, orally by gavage twice to rats on days 8 and 15 of pregnancy. On day 18 of pregnancy, 30–44% of the total dose remained in the dam and $<0{\cdot}03\%$ of the maternally retained dose was present in each fetus. Concentrations in individual fetal tissues were found to be highest in skin and placenta (intestine not measured). Curley *et al.* (1973) have found mean PCB levels in the rat fetus of 0·6 or 1·4 ppm following maternal administration of 10 or 50 mg/kg/day respectively of Aroclor 1254, orally on days 7–15 of pregnancy. Baker *et al.* (1977) have similarly noted only a small transfer of PCBs to the fetus (<5 ppm) following administration of 70 ppm Aroclor 1254 in the drinking water (equivalent to around 6·4 mg/kg) before mating and throughout pregnancy in the rat. Mizunoya *et al.* (1974) have shown transfer of PCBs to the fetus following feeding of 10, 50 or 250 ppm Kanechlor-400 in the diet throughout pregnancy in the rat. Concentrations in the whole fetus just before term increased with increasing dose from 0·04–0·64 ppm, but were always lower than maternal blood levels and markedly lower than levels in maternal adipose tissue. Transfer to the fetus in late pregnancy may well be greater; Lucier *et al.* (1978) have shown higher concentrations of mono-, tetra- and hexachlorobiphenyls and/or their metabolites in fetal blood than in maternal blood on day 21 of gestation following maternal administration on day 18. The difference was most marked for the tetrachlorobiphenyl, where the fetal:maternal blood concentration ratio was 5·6.

Placental transfer of PCBs in the rabbit has been shown by Grant *et al.* (1971). Does were dosed orally by gavage with 1, 12·5 or 25 mg/kg/day Aroclor 1254, or 1 or 10 mg/kg/day Aroclor 1221 on days 1–28 of pregnancy and killed at the end of the dosing period. With Aroclor 1254 maternal, placental and fetal levels increased with increasing dose. PCB levels in the whole fetus minus brain, liver, kidney and heart, were undetectable at 1 mg/kg/day, 25 ppm at 12·5 mg/kg/day and 66 ppm at 25 mg/kg/day. With Aroclor 1221 PCBs were undetectable in the fetus after 1 mg/kg/day and with 10 mg/kg/day much lower levels were found in maternal, placental and fetal tissues than after Aroclor 1254; with both Aroclors fetal liver concentrations were higher than maternal liver concentrations, but much lower than maternal adipose tissue concentrations.

Isolated observations of placental transfer of PCBs have been made in the monkey. Allen *et al.* (1974) fed 25 ppm Aroclor 1248 in the diet for 2 months. Three months after returning to normal diet, one monkey conceived, and 5 months later a live infant was born, with tissue PCB levels ranging from 0·01 μg/g in the liver to 27·7 μg/g in the fat. Maternal liver and fat levels were 56·3 and 50·0 μg/g respectively. The placental level was 0·9 μg/g, higher than most fetal tissue levels. Allen and Barsotti (1976) have also measured PCB levels in infants born to monkeys fed on diet containing 2·5 or 5 ppm Aroclor 1248 for 6 months prior to conception and throughout pregnancy. Skin biopsies taken at birth showed PCB levels of 1–4·8 μg/g. One stillborn monkey had tissue PCB levels ranging from 0·5 μg/g in the cerebrum to 99·4 μg/g in the lung. Liver levels were low (2·5 μg/g).

Transfer in the milk

Transfer of PCBs in the milk is generally much higher than placental transfer. In the mouse, Masuda *et al.* (1978b) have shown steadily increasing total amounts of PCBs in 1–5 week old offspring whose mothers were fed on diet containing 0·9 ppm Kanechlor-500 throughout pregnancy and lactation. Total PCBs were as much as 100 times higher in sucklings than in term fetuses from dams fed the same amount in the diet during pregnancy. Mizunoya *et al.* (1974) report similar findings in the rat following administration of 10, 50 or 250 ppm Kanechlor-400 in the diet throughout pregnancy and lactation. At 14 days of age whole body concentrations ranged from 2·4–18·8 ppm and at 28 days of age, individual tissue concentrations were higher in the offspring than in the dams. Baker *et al.* (1977) found up to 20-fold higher PCB concentrations in 10 and 20-day-old rat pups than in term fetuses from dams given 70 ppm Aroclor 1254 in the drinking water throughout pregnancy and lactation.

Similarly, Takagi *et al.* (1976) have shown steadily increasing transfer to the sucklings from 0·1% up to 2% of the dose between one and 25 days of age in rat pups from dams given weekly oral doses of 0·4 mg PCB, similar to Kanechlor-400, during pregnancy and lactation, compared with placental transfer of only 0·03% of the dose in term fetuses. At 25 days of age tissue concentrations in the weanlings were generally higher than in the dams and were particularly high in fat and skin. Skin was the only tissue to show progressively increasing concentrations over the first 25 days of age, whereas, in most other tissues, levels fall from about 10 days of age onwards. By 45 days of age concentrations were similar in the tissue of mothers and offspring.

Curley *et al.* (1973) have shown PCBs in the milk and in 21-day-old weanlings suckled by rats given 10 or 50 mg/kg/day Aroclor 1254 on days 7–15 of pregnancy only. Levels in milk ranged from 16–100 ppm, and, in fetal brain, liver and kidney, from 1–18 ppm, substantially higher than concentrations in term fetuses from such dams.

Lucier *et al.* (1978) have noted a structure-activity relationship for the transfer of PCBs to sucklings in the milk; the greater the chlorine content the greater the transfer.

In the pig, Hansen *et al.* (1975) have shown a similar concentration of PCB residues in tissues of weanlings and their sows fed 20 ppm Aroclor 1242 throughout pregnancy and lactation.

In the monkey, Allen and Barsotti (1976) have noted increased levels of PCBs in the skin, rising from 1–5 ppm at birth to 86–137 ppm by 3 months of age in infants suckling from dams given 2·5 or 5·0 ppm Aroclor 1248 in the diet before mating and throughout pregnancy and lactation. Milk samples from the mothers were found to contain 0·154–0·397 ppm and milk fat 16·4 ppm PCBs. The infants developed clinical signs of PCB intoxication within 2 months of birth.

In extrapolating these studies to humans it should be remembered that different PCBs may produce different effects and that the benzofuran content may vary. Also there is less sub-cutaneous fat in monkey than in human babies, so that storage is less and levels in other tissues may therefore be higher. However, as pointed out later, human milk may contain around 0·1 ppm PCB so that the safety margin is not high.

Conclusion

Placental transfer of a number of PCB mixtures, given by several routes of administration, has been shown in all species examined, viz. mouse, rat, rabbit and monkey. However, with the possible exception of the late fetal period, transfer appears to be limited, partly due to rapid maternal excretion in the faeces and rapid uptake by maternal adipose tissue. Generally, less than 0·2% of the total dose administered to the mother is transferred to the fetuses. There is some evidence that PCBs of differing chlorine content are transferred at different rates across the placenta, generally the higher the chlorine content the greater the transfer.

Transfer to the neonate and infant via the milk is clearly a much more important route than placental transfer, even when dosing occurs during pregnancy only. In the adult, the half-life of PCBs in adipose tissue is very long, and in nursing dams passage of PCBs into the milk fat becomes a major route of excretion, as evidenced by the strikingly lower tissue levels (including fat levels) in nursing rats compared with non-pregnant or pregnant rats given PCBs orally by gavage (Takagi *et al.*, 1976). Thus the potential developmental toxicity of PCBs in the postnatal animal may be much more important than prenatal toxicity. The high affinity of PCBs for skin that has been observed in both fetal and neonatal animals may be of some significance in relation to the skin discolouration observed in human babies exposed to PCBs.

B. ENDOCRINE AND GONADAL EFFECTS

A number of workers have examined reproductive organ weights and testicular function after treatment with PCBs. In the mouse, Sanders and Kirkpatrick (1975) fed groups of 10 males 0, 100, 200 or 400 ppm Aroclor 1254 in the diet for 2 weeks. At the end of that time there was no significant effect on body weight but mean liver weight was significantly increased in all PCB groups. At 400 ppm there was an 18% decrease in testis weight (non-significant), and significant decreases in seminal vesicle weight (by 50%), sperm concentration (by 30%) and total sperm number in the testis (by 40%). Similar but non-significant trends were seen in mice fed 200 or 100 ppm. In a later experiment, Sanders *et al.* (1977) confirmed the absence of any effect on reproductive organ weights in groups of 10 mice fed 50 or 200 ppm for 2 weeks, but sperm concentration/mg of testis was significantly reduced by 13% at 200 ppm. At 50 ppm there was no effect on sperm concentration, though liver weight was significantly increased by this dose. From these experiments, 50 ppm in the diet (equivalent to approximately 6–8 mg/kg body weight/day, assuming daily intake of 5 g of food) would seem to represent a no-effect level for testicular toxicity with short-term feeding.

Orberg and Lundberg (1974) have also confirmed the absence of effect of a similar low dose of PCBs on testicular and seminal vesicle weights with increased liver weight in groups of 10 mice given 0·25 mg Clophen A60 (60% chlorine)/day orally for 28 days. This dose is equivalent to just over 6 mg/kg/day.

PCBs enhance hepatic microsomal enzymes (Orberg and Lundberg, 1974; Derr and Dekker, 1979) and this might be expected to accelerate androgen metabolism, which may account for its effects on the male reproductive organs. In the rat, erythrocyte production is androgen-dependent, and Derr and Dekker (1979) have shown a dose-dependent significant decrease in erythrocytes in male rats given single i.p. injections of 10, 20 or 50 mg/kg of Aroclor 1254, suggesting a decrease in circulating androgen levels. However, PCBs have also been shown to have oestrogenic properties (see later) and these may be partly or wholly responsible for the effects on the male of high doses of PCBs.

Females

Orberg *et al.* (1972) have investigated the effects of PCBs on the oestrous cycle in the mouse. Twelve females were given single i.p. injection of 20 mg/kg Clophen A60 (60% chlorine with some impurities). Cycle length increased from a mean of 5·5 days before injection to 6·8 days for the first cycle after injection, and 6·5 days for the second cycle, returning to normal by the third cycle. Orberg and Kihlstrom (1973) have also observed a prolongation of the cycle from a mean of 6·6 days in vehicle controls to a mean of 8·7 days in 11 females fed 0·025 mg Clophen A60/day in peanut oil for 62 days. This dose corresponds to around 5 ppm in the diet. When subsequently mated, the numbers of implanted ova were reduced in the PCB-treated group (see section C for details).

In the rat, Jonsson *et al.* (1976) have failed to show any increase in oestrous cycle length in groups of 6 females fed 75 or 150 ppm Aroclor 1242 in the diet for 8 or 36 weeks. However, they did observe significant dose-related reductions in plasma progesterone levels at 36 weeks. Oestrogen levels were not studied. Histological examination of the ovaries showed that PCBs, particularly at 150 ppm, produced characteristic changes in the stromal cells (spindling and loose cellular arrangement) and reduced the number of follicles. Reproduction after 36 weeks on the diet was markedly affected in the 75 ppm group and totally inhibited in the 150 ppm group (see section C for details).

Muller *et al.* (1978), however, have produced conflicting evidence about the effect of PCBs on progesterone synthesis. Superovulated rats given an s.c. injection of 20 mg/kg Clophen A30 showed increased progesterone synthesis in ovarian tissue removed and incubated with luteinising hormone in comparison with controls.

PCBs have been shown to affect the menstrual cycle in monkeys with chronic feeding in the diet. Barsotti *et al.* (1976) fed rhesus monkeys 2·5 or 5·0 ppm Aroclor 1248 in the diet. After 2 months on the diet, they began to show clinical signs of PCB toxicity (alopecia, acne, swelling of the eyelids) and progressive weight loss. By 4 months menstrual cycles were disturbed, particularly in the 5 ppm group; cycle length was prolonged by 5–7 days, the duration of menstrual bleeding was increased and some animals showed occasional amenorrhoea. Reproduction was markedly impaired in these monkeys when bred after 7 months on the diet (see section C for details). In another experiment by the same group of workers, Allen *et al.* (1974) reported that menstrual cycles were "regular" in rhesus monkeys fed 25 ppm Aroclor 1248 in the diet for 2 months despite clear signs of PCB intoxication, though it is not clear how closely the cycles were followed and subsequent attempts to breed 3 months after returning to a normal diet had poor outcomes (see section C for details). Muller *et al.* (1978) have made a detailed study of ovulation and hormone levels in PCB-treated rhesus monkeys. Treatment with 4, 16 or 64 mg/kg/day of Clophen A30 (mainly di-, tri- and tetrachlorobiphenyls) given orally by gavage for 28 days had no effect on ovarian histology. Treatment of 4 females with 4 mg/kg/day PCBs throughout one menstrual cycle showed FSH and LH levels were within the normal range, but some animals did not show an LH surge nor a post-ovulatory progesterone peak, suggesting an anovulatory cycle. The majority of oestrogen measurements throughout the cycles were below normal. Laparoscopy showed 2/4 monkeys failed to ovulate and one had a double ovulation, compared with 15/16 single ovulations and one ovulatory failure observed in cycles of controls. It is not known whether the decreased oestrogen levels blocking ovulation are due to decreased ovarian production or increased hepatic metabolism of oestrogens.

PCBs may interfere with oestrogen feedback at the hypothalamic-pituitary level since some experiments have shown PCBs have oestrogenic activity similar to DDT and stilboestrol, which are structurally related to PCBs. Bitman and Cecil (1970) have used the 18 h glycogen response of the immature rat uterus as a measure of oestrogenic activity. In a series of PCBs (Aroclors 1221 up to 1268), compounds containing up to 48% chlorine were active and those containing more chlorine were inactive when injected s.c. Minimum effective doses were 4–8 mg/rat. Gellert (1978) has also shown a significant 24 h uterotropic response in weanling rats injected s.c. with 1000 mg/kg Aroclor 1221, but not following Aroclors 1242, 1254 or 1260. Bitman and Cecil (1970) found Aroclor 1242 did have oestrogenic activity in their more sensitive assay. Comparative measurements suggested Aroclor 1221 had roughly one-millionth of the oestrogenic activity of oestradiol-17β. Aroclor 1221 also induced precocious puberty, persistent vaginal oestrus and premature anovulation in rats treated neonatally, whereas Aroclors 1242, 1254 and 1260 did not (see section D for details).

Komatsu (1972) has also shown significant uterotropic and glycogen responses in immature rats following oral administration of 0·3–0·6 g/kg Kanechlor-400. In mature females PCBs did not increase uterine weight in ovariectomized rats, but did potentiate the effect of oestradiol-17β suggesting that in mature animals PCBs may not have any significant oestrogenic activity by themselves but may potentiate natural oestrogens.

Conclusion

In male mice, sperm counts may be reduced by levels of 100 ppm and above in the diet and reduced testicular and seminal vesicle weights are seen at levels of 400 ppm. Fifty ppm (around 6 mg/kg) would appear to be a no-effect level in the mouse.

In female mice, chronic treatment with doses as low as 0·025 mg/mouse (equivalent to about 0·8 mg/kg or 5 ppm in the diet) prolongs the oestrous cycle, and in the monkey a similar dietary level also prolongs the menstrual cycle. Reductions in progesterone levels in the rat and in oestrogen levels in the monkey have been observed following PCB treatment, with evidence of reduced ovulation or anovulation at doses as low as 4 mg/kg in the monkey.

It is not clear whether increased sex hormone metabolism, decreased sex hormone production, or any intrinsic or potentiating oestrogenic activity of the PCBs, all of which have been observed, are responsible for the adverse effects on the reproductive organs.

C, FERTILITY

PCBs have been shown to have an effect on fertility in the mouse, rat and monkey.

Merson and Kirkpatrick (1976) fed 0 or 200 ppm Aroclor 1254 in the diet to groups of 26–27 pairs of mice for 60 days and recorded reproductive performance during that time. Eight females and one male in the PCB group died between 39 and 57 days after starting on the diet. Six of the 8 females that died were pregnant at the time, but the remaining 18 PCB pairs produced only 9 litters compared with 33 litters produced by 26 control pairs. In controls, 85% had at least one litter and 42% 2 litters, compared with 30% and 4% respectively in the original 27 PCB pairs. Mean litter size at birth was unaffected but none of the offspring born to the PCB pairs survived to weaning. It is not known whether the low litter production was due to male infertility, female infertility or early loss of embryos.

Treatment before mating with much lower doses in the female mouse has been shown to slightly reduce implantation of ova. Orberg and Kihlstrom (1973) showed a significant, 7% reduction in ova implanted in mice given 0·025 mg Clophen A60/day for 62 days, then mated to normal males at the end of the dosing period. This dose is equivalent to around 5 ppm in the diet or 0·8 mg/kg.

Fertility studies have been carried out in the rat but in some studies methodology is poor or reporting of results inadequate. Baker *et al.* (1977) gave male and female rats 70 ppm Aroclor 1254 in the drinking water, equivalent to around 6·4 mg/kg/day, for 9 weeks. In males mated with control females no adverse effects on reproduction were seen, but in the treated females, several died in the seventh week of treatment, and by the ninth week fetal resorption was occurring. The outcome of earlier pregnancies in treated females is not described in detail. Growth rate of the pups from 10 days to 12 weeks of age did not differ significantly from controls, despite transmission of PCBs through the milk, but liver cytochrome P450 and aniline hydroxylase activities were significantly elevated in the 10- and 20-day-old pups, as they were in the exposed adults.

Jonsson *et al.* (1976) gave 75 or 150 ppm Aroclor 1242 to female rats for 36 weeks then placed them with control males. At 75 ppm only 3/5 females mated compared with 7/7 controls, but litter size was unaffected. At 150 ppm none of the 6 females mated. However, numbers in this experiment were small and the females well past their period of peak fertility when placed with the males.

Linder *et al.* (1974) have carried out a comprehensive multigeneration study on groups of 10 or 20 rats exposed to up to 500 ppm PCBs in the diet. The F_0 generation were exposed for 62–67 days before mating for the first time. Exposure was continuous throughout two generations, with 2 litters/generation produced (F_{1a}, F_{1b}, F_{2a}, F_{2b}). In the first experiment rats were fed Aroclor 1254 at 0, 1, 5, 20, 100 or 500 ppm, equivalent to around 0, 0·06, 0·32, 1·5, 7·2 or 37·0 mg/kg/day. At 500 ppm only 4/10 F_0 females produced F_{1a} litters; mean litter size was markedly reduced, 2 litters had no live young, and in the other 2 litters no pups survived beyond 3 days of age. This dose group was discontinued. At 100 ppm litter size at birth was not affected, but survival to weaning was decreased, being 95% and 100% in F_{1a} and F_{1b} control litters compared with 86% and 68% in F_{1a} and F_{1b} 100 ppm litters. Average weaning weight was reduced by 20% and 30% in 100 ppm F_{1a} and F_{1b} litters respectively, in comparison with controls. By the second generation there was a further deterioration in the 100 ppm group; only 7 F_{2a} litters were born from 20 females mated and only 4 F_{2b} litters from 20 females mated. Litter size at birth was significantly reduced. At 20 ppm there was a significant reduction in live litter size at birth in F_{1b}, F_{2a} and F_{2b} litters, but no other adverse effects. At 5 or 1 ppm there were no significant effects on reproduction, but liver:body weight ratios were significantly increased in F_1 and F_2 offspring at 5 ppm and in F_1 offspring at 1 ppm. This effect is probably induced postnatally by PCBs in the milk.

In a second experiment, Linder *et al.* (1974) fed Aroclor 1260 at 0, 5, 20, 100 or 500 ppm, equivalent to around 0, 0·39, 1·5, 7·4 or 37·0 mg/kg/day. At

500 ppm, normal numbers of F_{1a} and F_{1b} litters were born, but live litter size at birth was significantly reduced and survival to weaning was only 35 and 38%, compared with 85 and 99% in F_{1a} and F_{1b} control litters. At levels of 5–100 ppm there were no effects on reproduction, except for an increase in liver:body weight ratios in all PCB-exposed pups at 21 days of age. In both experiments, a portion of the F_0 and F_1 rats were autopsied in detail. Apart from histological changes in the liver, no other pathological or haematological signs of toxicity were observed in rats up to 100 ppm PCBs.

Green *et al.* (1975b) have carried out a dominant lethal test in the rat after administration of Aroclors 1242 and 1254. Triethylenemelamine was used as positive control and produced consistent increases in post-implantation losses. For Aroclor 1242 groups of 10 mature males were given single doses of 625, 1250 or 2500 mg/kg or 5 daily doses of 125 or 250 mg/kg, orally by gavage, and mated with one or 2 untreated females/week for 10–11 weeks. At 1250 and 2500 mg/kg, given as single doses, one or 2 males died and there was body weight loss. At 125 mg/kg × 5, one male died and at 250 mg/kg × 5 there was a mean weight loss. There were no effects on numbers of pregnancies, implants/dam or dead implants/dam for either single or multiple doses. For Aroclor 1254, groups of 10 males were given 5 daily doses of 75, 150 or 300 mg/kg orally by gavage, and mated with untreated females as before. This experiment was replicated once. Other groups of 27–28 males were fed 25 or 100 ppm Aroclor 1254 in the diet for 70 days then each paired for one week with an untreated female. In the multiple dose studies 5/10 males died at 300 mg/kg and a dose related weight loss was seen in all treated groups. In the feeding study only 2 or 3 rats from each group including controls died, but there was weight loss in the 100 ppm group. In the multiple dose study only a few random decreases in implants/dam or dead implants/dam were seen in isolated weeks and none of these changes were replicated. In the 70 day feeding study, there were no effects on implants/dam or dead implants/dam. It is concluded that these compounds have no dominant lethal effects.

Fertility has also been studied in the rhesus monkey following PCB treatment. Allen *et al.* (1974) fed 6 females 25 ppm Aroclor 1248 in the diet for 2 months, during which time they developed severe PCB toxicity and one died. They were removed from the diet and 3 months later were placed with untreated males during their ovulatory period. Three of the 5 females were thought to have conceived, having shown postconceptional bleeding, absence of the subsequent menstrual period and enlarged uterus. However, 2 of these aborted or resorbed the fetuses during the second month of pregnancy. The remaining animal delivered a low-birth weight infant of normal appearance at term. Subsequent attempts to breed the non-pregnant females over the next 5 months failed despite normal menstrual cycles. During this time 6 controls all became pregnant and delivered normal offspring.

The same group of workers have also examined the effects of feeding much lower levels of PCBs over a longer period to female and male monkeys. Barsotti *et al.* (1976) fed 2·5 or 5 ppm Aroclor 1248 in the diet continuously. After 6 months treated females were bred to control males and continued on the PCB diet throughout pregnancy. In the 2·5 ppm group 8/8 became pregnant as determined by HCG assay, but shortly after, 3 of them aborted or resorbed their embryos, and the normal postconceptional bleeding that occurs 17 days after conception was replaced by profuse uterine haemorrhage. In the 5 ppm group, 6/8 became pregnant but the remaining 2 failed to breed on 5 attempts. Of the 6 pregnant animals, 1 resorbed, 3 aborted at 46, 67 and 107 days' gestation, 1 had a still-born and 1 a viable infant. The 6 viable infants born to these 2 groups were normal in appearance except for focal areas of hyperpigmentation of the skin and low birth weight (Allen and Barsotti, 1976).

Barsotti *et al.* (1976) also looked at fertility in 4 male rhesus monkeys fed 5 ppm Aroclor 1248 in the diet. There was no adverse effect on sperm count or breeding performance when mated to control females.

Conclusion

In summary, in single generation studies, adverse effects on fertility are seen in the mouse, rat and monkey, but only at doses causing gross PCB intoxication and death of some of the animals. A single, large dominant lethal study in male rats has shown no effect, even at near-lethal doses where the numbers of spermatogonia are reduced (see section B). In general, the male appears to be relatively resistant to PCB effects on fertility; in the rat and monkey, when males treated with doses of PCBs known to affect female fertility are mated with untreated females, no adverse effects are seen. However, no separate fertility tests on males have been carried out at very high doses which are known to affect male reproductive organ weights as well as sperm counts.

PCBs at non-toxic doses do affect reproduction over several generations. In a single large multigeneration study in the rat, clear effects on reproduction were seen with Aroclor 1254 at 20–100 ppm in the diet, in the absence of signs of gross toxicity. The effects increased with lengthening exposure and successive generations, but no clear adverse effects were seen with a different PCB, Aroclor 1260, up to 100 ppm. Thus, as with other aspects of reproductive toxicity of PCBs, the type of mixture of PCBs used may be important.

In the monkey, it seems likely that the effects of PCBs on fertility or ability to carry to term may be secondary to hormonal disturbances in the menstrual cycle and pregnancy, such as low oestrogen levels (see section B).

D. PREGNANCY

Studies on effects of PCB administration during pregnancy are numerous and so results will be briefly summarized except where unusual effects are seen. The effects of PCBs on avian reproduction (decreased egg production, egg-shell thinning and low hatchability) have been reviewed by Wassermann *et al.* (1979).

Mouse

Treatment during very early pregnancy, before implantation, has adverse effects. Török (1975, 1976) gave 0, 75, 375 or 750 mg/kg/day of 2,2′-dichlorobiphenyl, orally on days 1–3 of pregnancy. The lowest dose was without effect. At 375 mg/kg there was a reduction in mean litter size due to post-implantation mortality, and gestation was prolonged by one day. At 750 mg/kg there was some maternal mortality. In survivors, only 37% were pregnant, and in these, mean litter size was further reduced by decreased implantation of ova as well as post-implantation deaths. Fetal weights were markedly reduced and on day 18 fetal ossification was poor and the lungs immature. In those allowed to go to term, placental weights were increased and gestation prolonged by 3 days, to day 21. Török (1975) also gave 500 mg/kg/day on days 1–6 of pregnancy but no implants, live or dead, were found in 13 females known to have mated. Orberg (1978) gave 0·05 or 0·5 mg/day of 2,4′,5-trichlorobiphenyl or 2,2′,4,4′,5,5′-hexachlorobiphenyl orally on days 1–6 of pregnancy. There was no effect on numbers pregnant, but there was a significant decrease in implants/dam with 0·5 mg doses of both PCBs. The lower doses were without effect.

Treatment during embryogenesis or fetogenesis is without marked effect when fetuses are examined just before term. Török (1975) gave 500 mg/kg/day for 6 days or 750 mg/kg/day for 3 days of 2,2′-dichlorobiphenyl between days 6 and 15 of pregnancy but there was no effect on resorption rates, fetal or placental weights, suggesting that some of the effects seen with administration of the same dose before implantation, described above, may have been due to delayed implantation. Masuda *et al.* (1978b) have also failed to show any adverse effects on prenatal growth, survival or development following addition of 0·94, 8·4 or 86 ppm Kanechlor-500 to the diet on days 1–18 of pregnancy.

Lucier *et al.* (1978) have investigated prenatal and postnatal effects of exposure to a variety of PCBs on days 10–16 of pregnancy. Mice were given orally 0·3–32 mg/kg/day of 3,4,3′,4′-tetrachlorobiphenyl (4-CB) or 2,4,5,2′,4′,5′-hexachlorobiphenyl (6-CB). No significant fetotoxicity or teratogenicity was seen following 6-CB. Fetotoxicity was seen following 16–32 mg/kg/day 4-CB, doses causing no maternal toxicity. Mean total and live litter sizes were reduced (by 40–50% at 32 mg/kg), stillbirths and neonatal deaths were increased, but pups were heavier than controls at birth, presumably due to the smaller litter sizes. At 0·3–10 mg/kg/day, doses below those causing any significant offspring mortality, 4-CB caused a dose-related increase in hydronephrosis and some increase in cryptorchid testes in fetuses examined before term. Fertility in male and female offspring exposed prenatally to 4-CB was not affected in 4 months of breeding but other marked changes did occur postnatally in those exposed to 32 mg/kg/day prenatally. From 2–3 weeks of age up to at least 8 months (the latest age studied), offspring were hyperactive and many showed jerking or rotational movements of the head with episodes of rapid circling (up to 150 turns/min), termed the "spinning syndrome".

More detailed study of the spinning syndrome by the same group of workers (Chou *et al.*, 1979), has shown a slow growth rate in affected mice but not in unaffected litter-mates. Dopaminergic systems are known to be involved in locomotor activity levels and rotational movements, and in spinners the dopamine agonists and antagonists, amphetamine, apomorphine and haloperidol, modify or, in the case of haloperidol, stop spinning altogether. This suggests there is a biochemical lesion of dopaminergic pathways. Detailed study of central nervous system histology and ultrastructure revealed a pathognomonic lesion in affected mice, characterized by longitudinal projections of cylindrical CNS peninsulas in ventral and dorsal nerve roots and to a lesser extent in cranial nerve roots. The lesions were occasionally seen in unaffected litter mates but never in controls. Spinners have also been shown to have impaired forelimb grip strength and difficulty crossing a wire rod, poor visual placement response, and long latencies in a one-way avoidance task; non-spinning litter-mates were also deficient in traversing a wire rod and in avoidance acquisition (Tilson *et al.*, 1979). Whilst cross-fostering studies have not been carried out, it seems likely that the primary lesion is induced prenatally; only very low levels of 4-CB are seen in newborns and by 8 weeks of age no 4-CB can be detected in the tissues following maternal treatment on days 10–16 of gestation. Furthermore, spinning cannot be induced in adults by 4-CB treatment. However, proof of prenatal induction awaits demonstration of the spinning syndrome in offspring fostered at birth to control dams.

Neonatal exposure to PCBs through the milk has been shown to affect subsequent reproductive capacity of males and females. On the day of parturition, Kihlstrom *et al.* (1975) injected dams s.c. with 50 mg/kg Clophen A60 and repeated the injection at weekly intervals throughout 3 weeks of lactation. At sexual maturity male and female offspring of treated dams were mated with other treated or control offspring. When both members of a pair had been exposed to PCBs there was no effect on corpora lutea, pregnancy rate or resorption rate, but there was a significant reduction in implantation rate, suggesting impaired fertilisation or early loss of fertilised ova. If only one member of a pair (male or female) had been exposed to PCBs, there was no reduction in implantation rate.

Rat

In a number of experiments, the effects of PCBs given during organogenesis have been evaluated. Villeneuve *et al.* (1971) gave doses of 0, 6·25, 12·5, 25, 50 or 100 mg/kg/day of Aroclor 1254, orally by gavage, on days 6–15 of pregnancy. Acceptable teratological methods were used. There was no maternal toxicity and no significant embryolethal, fetotoxic or teratogenic effect at any dose level, except for a reduction in fetal weight at 100 mg/kg, which could be accounted for by the larger mean litter size in this dose group compared with controls.

Postnatal effects of prenatal exposure to Aroclor 1254 have also been investigated. Curley *et al.* (1973) gave 0, 10 or 50 mg/kg/day of Aroclor 1254 orally on days 7–15 of pregnancy. There were no effects on live litter size at birth, stillbirths, average litter weight, or survival to weaning. However, after 100 mg/kg/day of Aroclor 1254 orally on days 7–15 of pregnancy, Linder *et al.* (1974) found an increase in stillbirths, high postnatal mortality with only 30% surviving to weaning, and reduced body weight at weaning. They confirmed lack of effects at 10 and 50 mg/kg/day with Aroclor 1254, and showed no effects with 100 mg/kg/day of Aroclor 1260 orally on days 7–15 of pregnancy.

Kato *et al.* (1972) administered 25, 75, 225 or 675 mg/kg/day of Kanechlor-400 orally by gavage throughout pregnancy. In the top 2 dose groups the dams died in mid-pregnancy. At 25 and 75 mg/kg live litter size was unaffected but stillbirths and postnatal deaths were higher than in controls. Postnatal growth rates up to 60 days of age, skeletal radiography and organ histology in the offspring were normal.

Shiota (1976) fed 0, 20, 100 or 500 ppm Kanechlor-300 and Kanechlor-500 in the diet throughout pregnancy. These levels are equivalent to 0·9–1·3 mg/kg (20 ppm), 5·3–7·0 mg/kg (100 ppm) and 23·2–37·7 mg/kg (500 ppm). Acceptable teratological methods were used. Maternal toxicity was seen with 500 ppm Kanechlor-500 only. Implantation, resorption and malformation rates were similar in treated and control groups, but there was a significant reduction in fetal weight at 20 ppm Kanechlor-300 and 500 ppm Kanechlor-300 and Kanechlor-500. In dams allowed to litter out, there were no significant effects on litter size, survival to weaning, body weight up to 6 weeks of age or organ pathology at 6 weeks of age.

Mizunoya *et al.* (1974) fed 0, 10, 50 or 250 ppm of Kanechlor-400 in the diet throughout pregnancy. These levels are equivalent to daily intakes of 0·67 mg/kg (10 ppm), 3·5 mg/kg (50 ppm) and 16·5 mg/kg (250 ppm). No maternal toxicity was observed and there were no significant embryolethal or teratogenic effects, but fetal body weight was significantly reduced in a dose-dependent way at all dose levels. In rats allowed to litter out, litter size at birth was normal but survival to weaning was only 24% at 50 ppm and 8% at 250 ppm compared with 76% in controls. Body weight at 28 days of age was significantly reduced in all PCB groups. At autopsy no gross skeletal anomalies were seen in the offspring but liver and kidney weights were increased and testis weights were markedly reduced in all PCB groups.

Neonatal but not prenatal exposure to some PCBs alters subsequent reproductive function in the rat. Gellert (1978) found 10 mg Aroclor 1221 given s.c. on the second and third days of life induced earlier vaginal opening, persistent vaginal oestrus and anovulation by 6 months of age. At autopsy at 7–8 months of age, body weight and pituitary gland weight was heavier than in controls. Lower doses of 1 mg of Aroclors 1221, 1242, 1254 and 1260 were without effect. Female offspring of dams given 30 mg/kg/day of Aroclors 1221, 1242 and 1260 orally by gavage on days 14–20 of pregnancy did not have any significant increase in the incidence of persistent vaginal oestrus or anovulation at 6 months of age, and male offspring were of normal fertility and showed no decrease in testis weight (Gellert and Wilson, 1979). It is likely, however, that fetal and neonatal exposure to PCBs in this experiment was much lower than in the previous experiment where 10 mg/neonate was given.

Rabbit

Villeneuve *et al.* (1971) gave Aroclor 1254 orally to rabbits throughout pregnancy. At 1 or 10 mg/kg/day there were no signs of maternal toxicity, embryolethal or fetotoxic effects, but at 12·5, 25 and 50 mg/kg/day there was a reduced maternal weight gain or even weight loss and a high incidence of abortions, resorptions and dead fetuses. Results were similar if dosing was started on day 7 rather than day 1. Aroclor 1221, up to 25 mg/kg/day appeared to be without effect.

Pig

Hansen *et al.* (1975) have shown that feeding 20 ppm Aroclor 1242 in the diet to sows throughout pregnancy and lactation results in delivery of an increased number of mummified fetuses and reduced number of live piglets/litter, but has no effect on offspring body weight, organ weight or postnatal mortality rate. Earl *et al.* (1974) fed 1, 10 or 30 mg/kg/day of Aroclor 1254 to miniature pigs from 21 days before breeding and throughout pregnancy and lactation. There was a dose-related decrease in number of pregnancies and live litter size and an increase in postnatal mortality at all doses. In the 10 mg/kg offspring, syndactyly and cleft palates were observed, and in the 30 mg/kg offspring, patent fontanelles and cleft palates were seen.

Dog

Earl *et al.* (1974) gave 0·25, 1·0 or 5·0 mg/kg/day of Aroclor 1254 to bitches throughout pregnancy and lactation. No effects were seen at 0·25 or 1 mg/kg/day, but at 5 mg/kg/day, the number of pregnancies and mean litter size at birth were reduced, while resorptions and postnatal mortality were increased. Enlarged fontanelles, cleft palates and superfluous phalanges were seen in some pups.

Monkey

The outcome of pregnancy in rhesus monkeys fed 2·5 or 5 ppm Aroclor 1248 in their diet for 6 months before breeding and throughout pregnancy and lactation has been described in section C. There was a high incidence of abortion, and in the 6 offspring carried to term a 20% reduction in birth weight and poor postnatal growth up to at least 12 weeks of age. At birth they showed focal areas of hyperpigmentation of the skin, but their general appearance, skeletal development and haematology was normal. After 2 months exposure to PCBs through the mothers' milk, typical signs of PCB intoxication developed and 3 died. The 3 survivors were weaned at 4 months of age and all signs of PCB intoxication receded but hyperpigmentation of the skin of the face remained.

Conclusion

In general, PCBs do not appear to induce gross structural deformities in the offspring, but a fairly consistent picture is seen across the species of low birth weight, high perinatal and postnatal mortality and poor growth rate following prenatal exposure. It should be noted however that excretion of PCB residues in the milk is likely to occur following dosing of the dam during pregnancy only. Exposure during very early pregnancy may interfere with implantation.

In the mouse an unusual effect has been found with prenatal exposure to a tetrachlorobiphenyl, viz. postnatal development of a severe neurological disorder, the spinning syndrome, which may be caused by lesions in dopaminergic pathways. Other unusual effects in the mouse and the rat are impaired reproductive function in offspring exposed neonatally to PCBs.

Teratogenicity has been reported in the mouse (hydronephrosis) following administration of a tetrachlorobiphenyl only, and enlarged fontanelle, cleft palate and abnormal digits following administration of Aroclor 1254 in the mini-pig and the dog. These latter observations are reported by one group in abstract only.

In the monkey, the similarity of low-birth weight and hyperpigmentation of the skin to the effects seen in humans exposed prenatally to PCBs should be noted.

Once again, clear differences in the reproductive toxicities of different PCBs have been shown and it is not possible to give a single no-effect level for all

PCBs. It should be noted, however, that many of the adverse effects on offspring that appear postnatally and some of those seen prenatally, after dosing of the dam during pregnancy, occur in the absence of maternal toxicity.

E. MUTAGENICITY

IARC Monograph Vol. 18 (1978) reported a study showing 4-chlorobiphenyl and Aroclor 1221 were mutagenic in the Ames test with metabolic activation, but Aroclor 1268 and 2,2′,5,5′-tetrachlorobiphenyl were not mutagenic in this system.

Seiler (1977) has shown absence of any effect on the rate of testicular DNA synthesis in male mice given single i.p. injections of 500 mg/kg of Aroclors 1232, 1254, or 1268. Known mutagens or carcinogens cause significant inhibition of DNA synthesis in this test.

Green *et al.* (1975a) have investigated the effect of Aroclors 1242 and 1254 on bone marrow and spermatogonial cells in the rat. Aroclor 1242 was given orally at single doses of 1250, 2500 or 5000 mg/kg, or as a multiple dose of 500 mg/kg/day for 4 days. Aroclor 1254 was given in multiple doses of 75, 150 or 300 mg/kg/day for 5 days. The rats were killed 24 h after the single dose or 24 h after the last dose. Dosing with Aroclor 1242 was lethal to some rats. Dosing with Aroclor 1254 caused less mortality but caused marked weight loss. PCB did not cause any increase in chromosomal aberrations in bone marrow cells or spermatogonia though Aroclor 1242 did produce general mitotic inhibition in spermatogonia at the doses of 5000 mg/kg × 1 and 500 mg/kg × 4. This was not related to general toxicity as the dose of 2500 mg/kg × 1 produced similar toxicity to 500 mg/kg × 4, but there was no mitotic inhibition at 2500 mg/kg.

F. CARCINOGENICITY

IARC Monograph Vol. 18 (1978) reported experimental evidence of a carcinogenic effect of some PCBs in rodents.

HUMAN STUDIES

A. RELEVANT PHARMACOLOGY AND TOXICOLOGY

Since their introduction into industry in 1929, PCBs have been very extensively used in a wide variety of applications in almost every field from paper to pesticides and clothes to space-ships (Peakall, 1972). As a result, widespread contamination of the environment has occurred throughout the world so that PCB has become a constituent of the body of virtually every fish, bird and animal including man (see Wasserman *et al.*, 1979, for an excellent comprehensive review of the tissue levels of PCBs). PCBs tend to accumulate in fat and the average adipose tissue level in Europeans is around 1 ppm with a range from about 0·3–9 ppm, although occasional values in the hundreds of ppm may be found. Few systematic studies have been carried out to examine large population trends but the available evidence suggests that levels are slowly rising despite attempts to control pollution.

Plasma levels in the general population are around 3–30 ppb in European, American and Japanese populations, but occupationally exposed workers may have much higher levels with values up to 1900 ppb being reported and mean levels of 800 ppb being recorded after only one month's exposure in a Japanese electric condenser plant (Wasserman *et al.*, 1979). Symptoms of PCB exposure were common amongst workers occupationally exposed to PCB in 2 U.S. capacitor factories also (Fischbein *et al.*, 1979). During starvation (or "slimming") PCB may be mobilized from fat stores and blood levels may increase up to a thousand-fold.

Breast milk

PCBs are also found in high concentrations in human breast milk with mean levels ranging from 10 ppb in Norway to 100 ppb in Germany and 390 ppb in Poland. The levels in the milk fat average about 1–15 ppm. The 1975 survey by the EPA of pesticide contamination of breast milk (Rogan *et al.*, 1980) showed that of 1038 women sampled, only 9 (1%) had no contamination, 720 (69%) had detectable levels below 50 ppb, and 309 (30%) had levels over 50 ppb on a whole milk basis. Most of the PCB is in the fat in about a 30-fold greater concentration than in whole milk (Rogan *et al.*, 1980). The significance of this may be assessed from calculations provided by Rogan *et al.* (1980). Although the U.S. F.D.A. would take legal action to remove cows' milk from the market at 62·5 ppb of PCB, human milk contains 40–100 ppb as typical levels. A 5 kg infant drinking 700 ml milk at the high end of the PCB range would take in 14 μg/kg PCB which is 14 times the F.D.A. allowable daily intake.

Levels in whole breast milk were measured regularly from 1972–1977 in Osaka, Japan, and showed mean values of 32 to 40 ppb (range 10–240 ppb) which remained steady over the period studied. The levels in milk correlated with the blood levels but were about 10 times higher. There was also an inverse correlation between the amount of PCB in the blood and milk and the number of children, suggesting that the milk was a major route of excretion of PCB for the mother, and a major source of PCB for the baby (Yakushiji *et al.*, 1979). As part of the same series of investigations, it has been found that the blood level of PCB in occupationally exposed women may be 10–100 times that in non-occupationally exposed women. The blood levels in the children of these occupationally exposed women are correspondingly high and both mothers and children have blood levels many times (4–10-fold) higher than that found in patients during the Yusho epidemic (see section D). The high levels in the children seem to be derived from the mother's milk, since the levels are higher if feeding continues longer, and babies fed on artificial milk have much lower levels. When breast feeding persists for more than 3 months, the levels in the baby's blood may actually exceed those in the mother's blood (Kodama and Ota, 1977; Kuwabara *et al.*, 1978, 1979; Yakushiji *et al.*, 1978). Chemical differences have also been recorded in the PCB in blood and milk with duration of lactation (Yakushiji *et al.*, 1978; Yoshida and Nakamura, 1979).

High levels of PCB have also been reported in human milk for occupationally unexposed women in Israel. The level in colostrum was approximately half that found in later milk, due mainly to the lower fat content of colostrum (Miller *et al.*, 1979).

Placental transfer

A detailed comparison of the placental transfer of PCB compared with transfer in the milk was reported by Masuda *et al.* (1978a). They measured PCB levels in blood, milk and maternal tissues and compared these with blood and tissue levels in stillbirths and in babies up to one year of age. The PCB levels in maternal blood were significantly greater than in cord blood ($2{\cdot}5 \pm 0{\cdot}14$ ppb compared with $0{\cdot}61 \pm 0{\cdot}05$, $P < 0{\cdot}001$, $n = 60$ pairs) and the levels were not significantly correlated. Also the tissue levels in stillbirths of greater than 7 months' gestation were only about one-tenth of the levels in the maternal tissues. Both of these factors suggest the existence of some placental barrier between the mother and fetus. However, during lactation, the levels of PCB in the babies' blood increased steadily. In a comparison of blood levels in 42 mothers and babies with ages ranging from 2–12 months, the mean maternal blood level was $1{\cdot}4 \pm 0{\cdot}08$ ppb, and the babies' $2{\cdot}5 \pm 0{\cdot}17$ ppb ($P < 0{\cdot}001$). Maternal whole milk averaged $13 \pm 1{\cdot}2$ ppb and milk fat 350 ± 25 ppb; only the latter value correlated significantly with maternal blood level. These findings suggest that transfer of PCB to the infant via the milk is much more significant in terms of tissue level than transfer through the placenta.

The presence of some degree of placental barrier to PCB is also supported by the report of Nishimura *et al.* (1977) who studied levels of PCB and other organo-chlorine compounds in the tissues of embryos and fetuses obtained from abortions induced for socio-economic reasons. By avoiding specimens from mothers in high risk situations like fishing or living near PCB factories, they hoped to obtain "normal" representative samples of PCB tissue levels. In addition, some samples were obtained from perinatal and adult deaths for comparison.

In 19 embryos (2–3 months' gestation) no PCB was detected (limit of detection not stated but appeared to be about 2 ppb). In all fetal and perinatal samples collected, however, PCB was detected, with a gradual increase in amount as gestation proceeded. The highest concentration was found in the skin and the lowest in the brain. The skin concentration for example, increased from zero in the 2–3 months' embryo, to 57 ± 14 ppb (n = 7) in the 4–7 months' fetus, to 630 ± 60 ppb (n = 4) at term, and 1280 ± 270 (n = 3) in the adult. The results suggest that PCB levels increase in the fetus as the fat levels increase but that cumulation of PCB does not occur in the fetus.

B. ENDOCRINE AND GONADAL EFFECTS

Wassermann *et al.* (1979) refer to 2 reports suggesting endocrine dysfunction in Yusho patients (see section D); alterations in the menstrual cycle were reported in females, and in males, 40% of patients showed elevated urinary androsterone, aetiocholanolone and dehydroepiandrosterone.

C. FERTILITY

No relevant data found.

D. PREGNANCY

The most important poisoning epidemic with PCB occurred in Japan in 1968 where the resulting disease was known as "Yusho" (oil disease) (Kuratsunc *et al.*, 1972). Rice oil became contaminated during manufacture with PCB, Kanechlor-400, which leaked through small holes in a heat exchanger used in the manufacture of the oil. Contamination was of the order of 2000–3000 ppm, but as the heat exchange fluid was not pure PCB, it was contaminated with other toxic chemicals such as benzofurans. However, other substances such as Cu, Ni, Zn, Co, As, Hg and pentachlorophenols were not present. Identification of the precise cause of all the toxic symptoms as being PCB is not therefore possible. In all, about 1057 people were affected with Yusho, with males and females being equally affected and with the majority (90%) being under 50 years of age. Careful investigation revealed that the affected people had consumed a particular brand of oil (K Company rice oil) made on 5th and 6th February 1968, and in one study 64% of persons using this oil were affected. The amount of oil consumed per person averaged 800 ml, so that with the contamination being 2000–3000 ppm, each person was exposed on average to about 2 g of Kanechlor-400, with a minimum dose in affected cases of about 0·5 g.

Thirteen children were born to exposed women, 2 of whom did not have Yusho symptoms but whose husbands did. Two of the children were stillborn, 10 had dark pigmentation of the skin and gums which gradually faded, 9 had conjunctivitis and 8 had neonatal jaundice. Taki *et al.* (1969) reported on 9 of these cases. They found that all of the offspring including the 2 stillbirths had characteristic greyish dark brown staining of the skin, gingiva and nails which faded within several months after birth. All live offspring also had parchment-like desquamation of the skin, all were below the mean weight for gestational age and 5 were defined as "small for gestational age". No characteristic laboratory features were found in the blood picture, serum proteins, serum electrolytes, 17-hydroxy- or 17-keto steroids.

A clear dose-response relationship between oil consumption and severity of the defects in the babies was not established because of the small number affected. The estimated intake of contaminated oil during pregnancy in the women with live affected babies was from 0·3 to 1·4 litres (intake in 4 unknown). One of the mothers with a stillborn baby had consumed 2·6 litres but the intake of the other was unknown. The oil was consumed by some mothers throughout pregnancy and by others only during one trimester but there is insufficient information to state what the relationship was between time of intake and effect on the child.

Four other cases were reported by Funatsu *et al.* (1972) and Yamashita (1977), from poisoned mothers who had consumed 0·6–10 litres of contaminated oil. Two of the mothers had hypertension in pregnancy, one had oedema and one anaemia. The mother of the first case and who had consumed the largest volume of oil, became ill at the 25th week of gestation with malaise, anorexia and chloracne. The baby was born at 36 weeks' gestation and weighed 1800 g which was less than 1·5 S.D. below the mean weight for gestational age. The other mothers had slight or no symptoms; 2 babies were born at 42 weeks' gestation and one at 40 weeks. The clinical signs were similar to those reported above, i.e. dark brown skin pigmentation, parchment-like desquamation, pigmentation of the gingiva, palate and genitalia with gingival hypertrophy in 3 and tooth eruption at birth in 2 cases. There was facial oedema with exophthalmos in 3 of the babies and the fontanelles were wider than usual, with spotted calcification of the parieto-occipital area on X-ray. One baby had hepatomegaly. Slight transient abnormalities of lipid and liver function were noted in the laboratory findings in the first case only, who also had a high protein content in the C.S.F. Skin biopsy showed hyperkeratosis and increased melanin pigment which would account for the brown staining in 3 of the cases. During follow-up of the children for about one year, the skin colour disappeared in all by 5 months, and although all were below mean weight for age, some catch-up did occur in the most severely affected child. No neurological abnormality or mental retardation was observed in any. The abnormal calcification and early tooth eruption suggested some abnormality of calcium metabolism but no clear endocrine abnormality was detected.

Long-term follow-up of children born with the above syndrome has not been reported, though follow-up of 9 children who were born after the Yusho incident and so were exposed to PCB only in the breast milk, revealed "enervation, lack of endurance, hypotonia and apathy" which persisted in 3 of them at least up to 5–6 years of age (Miller, 1977).

However, studies in school children who actually suffered from direct PCB poisoning showed only temporary retardation of growth and by 2 to 3 years later they had caught up with their unaffected classmates (Yoshimura and Ikeda, 1978).

E. MUTAGENICITY

No relevant data available.

F. CARCINOGENICITY

IARC Monograph Vol. 18 (1978) reported that in view of the experimental evidence of carcinogenicity in rodents and epidemiological data in humans suggestive of a relationship between exposure to PCB and the development of malignant melanoma, then, for practical purposes, PCB should be regarded as if it were carcinogenic to humans.

SUMMARY AND EVALUATION

EXPERIMENTAL STUDIES

Limited placental transfer of PCBs has been shown in a number of species including primates. Partly as a result of the enzyme inducing activity of these compounds, metabolism in the fetus may lead to cumulation of metabolites in the fetal tissues. Transfer via the milk is greater than through the placenta in terms of total amount transferred. Milk is a major route of excretion for the mother since the high fat solubility results in low excretion by other routes.

Cumulation of toxic amounts of PCB can occur in the young from this source. High levels of 100 ppm or over can suppress testicular function in mice perhaps related to the oestrogenicity of PCBs. In females, however, lower levels around 5 ppm in the diet can prolong the oestrous cycle in rodents, and the menstrual cycle in monkeys. This may be accompanied by reduced hormone levels and failure of ovulation. Adverse effects on fertility have been observed in males, only at toxic doses, but females are more sensitive to this effect and may show reduced fertility at otherwise non-toxic doses.

Teratogenicity studies have been carried out in a wide range of species. In general PCBs are not teratogenic but a consistent pattern of low birth weight, high peri- and postnatal mortality with poor growth postnatally is observed. Differences exist however between the different PCBs and no overall no-effect levels can be given. Neonatal exposure in rodents, however, has been shown to affect subsequent reproductive function in males and females. Pre- and postnatal exposure in monkeys has been shown to produce a syndrome similar to that seen in humans. Some PCBs are mutagenic *in vitro* with activation, but one comprehensive study on two PCBs in the rat showed absence of dominant lethal activity. Some PCBs are reported to be carcinogenic in mice.

HUMAN STUDIES

PCBs are found in tissues of humans throughout the world and levels are slowly increasing. Levels of around 100 ppb are common in human breast milk, and babies may be exposed to levels exceeding those recommended as the allowable daily intake. In occupationally exposed women the milk levels may be 10 to 100 times higher than in the rest of the population. For the offspring, this source is much more important than the limited amount transferred via the placenta. Some degree of placental barrier exists and cumulation in the fetus only occurs towards the end of pregnancy as the fat in the fetus increases.

Women exposed to very high levels have been reported to have menstrual dysfunction but no studies on fertility were found. In women poisoned with contaminated PCB in cooking oil a disease known as Yusho was produced. Children born to these women had dark greyish-brown staining of the skin, gums and nails which faded slowly. All were underweight and some died. Studies on directly poisoned children showed that the effects were not permanent and "catch-up" occurred by 2–3 years later. No studies on mutagenicity were found. There is evidence suggestive of a relationship between PCB exposure and malignant melanomas and PCBs are regarded as carcinogenic.

EVALUATION

PCBs do not produce structural malformations in animals but do affect fetal and postnatal growth and development. Transfer of large amounts of PCB may occur via milk to young animals resulting in toxic effects. The levels in breast milk which have been shown to produce clinical signs of toxicity in monkey offspring are close to those found in milk of normal "unexposed" women. Even higher levels are found in the milk of exposed women. Evidence in humans largely relates to the Yusho epidemic in which very impure PCB was involved. These results cannot be applied directly to all types of PCB. Attention is drawn to the high milk levels of PCB in exposed women and the need for studies of the effects on these women and on their children.

References

Allen, J. R. and Barsotti, D. A. (1976). The effects of transplacental and mammary movement of PCBs on infant rhesus monkeys. *Toxicology* **6**, 331–340.

Allen, J. R., Carstens, L. A. and Barsotti, D. A. (1974). Residual effects of short-term low-level exposure of nonhuman primates to polychlorinated biphenyls. *Toxicology and Applied Pharmacology* **30**, 440–451.

Baker, F. D., Bush, B., Tumasonis, C. F. and Lo, F. C. (1977). Toxicity and persistence of low-level PCB in adult Wistar rats, fetuses and young. *Archives of Environmental Contamination and Toxicology* **5**, (2), 143–156.

Barsotti, D. A., Marlar, R. J. and Allen, J. R. (1976). Reproductive dysfunction in rhesus monkeys exposed to low levels of polychlorinated biphenyls (Aroclor 1248). *Food and Cosmetic Toxicology* **14**, (2), 99–103.

Bitman, J. and Cecil, H. C. (1970). Estrogenic activity of DDT analogs and polychlorinated biphenyls. *Journal of Agriculture and Food Chemistry* **18**, 1108–1112.

Chou, S. M., Miike, T., Payne, W. M. and Davis, G. J. (1979). Neuropathology of "spinning syndrome" induced by prenatal intoxication with a PCB in mice. *Annals of the New York Academy of Sciences* **320**, 373–395.

Curley, A., Burse, V. W. and Grim, M. E. (1973). Polychlorinated biphenyls: evidence of transplacental passage in the Sherman rat. *Food and Cosmetics Toxicology* **11**, 471–476.

Derr, S. K. and Dekker, J. (1979). Alterations of androgenicity in rats exposed to PCBs (Aroclor 1254). *Bulletin of Environmental Contamination and Toxicology* **21**, 43–45.

Earl, F. L., Couvillion, J. L. and Van Loon, E. J. (1974). The reproductive effects of PCBs in Beagle dogs and miniature swine. *Toxicology and Applied Pharmacology* **29**, 104.

Fischbein, A., Wolff, M. S., Lilis, R., Thornton, J. and Selikoff, I. J. (1979). Clinical findings among PCB-exposed capacitor manufacturing workers. *Annals of the New York Academy of Sciences* **320**, 703–715.

Funatsu, I., Yamashita, F., Tsugawa, S., Funatsu, T., Yoshikane, T. and Hayashi, M. (1972). Polychlorbiphenyls (PCB) induced fetopathy. *Kurume Medical Journal* **19**, (1), 43–51.

Gellert, R. J. (1978). Uterotrophic activity of polychlorinated biphenyls (PCB) and induction of precocious reproductive aging in neonatally treated female rats. *Environmental Research* **16**, (1–3), 123–130.

Gellert, R. J. and Wilson, C. (1979). Reproductive function in rats exposed prenatally to pesticides and polychlorinated biphenyls (PCB). *Environmental Research* **18**, 437–443.

Grant, D. L., Villeneuve, D. C., McCully, K. A. and Phillips, W. E. J. (1971). Placental transfer of polychlorinated biphenyls in the rabbit. *Environmental Physiology* **1**, 61–66.

Green, S., Carr, J. V., Palmer, K. A. and Oswald, E. J. (1975a). Lack of cytogenetic effects in bone marrow and spermatogonial cells in rats treated with polychlorinated biphenyls (Aroclors 1242 and 1254). *Bulletin of Environmental Contamination and Toxicology* **13**, 14–22.

Green, S., Sauro, F. M. and Friedman, L. (1975b). Lack of dominant lethality in rats treated with polychlorinated biphenyls (Aroclors 1242 and 1254). *Food and Cosmetics Toxicology* **13**, 507–510.

Hansen, L. G., Byerley, C. S., Metcalf, R. L. and Bevill, R. F. (1975). Effects of a polychlorinated biphenyl mixture on swine reproduction and tissue residues. *American Journal of Veterinary Research* **36**, (1), 23–26.

IARC Monographs on the Evaluation of the Carcinogenic Risk of Chemicals to Humans: Polychlorinated biphenyls and polybrominated biphenyls (1978). Vol. 18, Lyon, France.

Jonsson, H. T., Keil, J. E., Gaddy, R. G., Loadholt, C. B., Hennigar, G. R. and Walker, E. M. (1976). Prolonged ingestion of commercial DDT and PCB: effects on progesterone levels and reproduction in the mature female rat. *Archives of Environmental Contamination and Toxicology* **3**, 479–490.

Kato, T., Yakushiji, M., Tuda, H., Arima, A., Takahashi, A., Shimomura, M., Miyahara, M., Adachi, M. T., Tashiro, Y., Matsumoto, M., Funatsu, I., Yamashita, F., Ito, Y., Tsugawa, S., Funatsu, T., Yoshikane, T. and Hayashi, M. (1972). Polychlorobiphenyls (PCB) induced fetopathy. *Kurume Medical Journal* **19**, (1), 53–59.

Kihlstrom, J. E., Lundberg, C., Daniellson, P. O. and Sydhoff, J. (1975). Sexual functions of mice neonatally exposed to DDT and PCB. *Environmental Physiology and Biochemistry* **5**, (1), 54–57.

Kodama, H. and Ota, H. (1977). Studies on the transfer of PCB to infants from their mothers. *Japanese Journal of Hygiene* **32**, 567–573.

Komatsu, F. (1972). Estradiol-potentiating action of PCB. *Fukuoka Igaku Zasshi* **63**, (10), 374–377.

Kuratsune, M., Yoshimura, Y., Matsuzaka, J. and Yamagushi, A. (1972). Epidemiologic study on yusho, a poisoning caused by ingestion of rice oil contaminated with a commercial brand of polychlorinated biphenyls. *Environmental Health Perspectives* **1**, (1), 119–128.

Kuwabara, K., Yakushiji, T., Watanabe, I., Yoshida, S., Koyama, K., Kunita, N. and Hara, I. (1978). Relationship between breast feeding and PCB residues in blood of the children whose mothers were occupationally exposed to PCBs. *International Archives of Occupational and Environmental Health* **41**, (3), 189–197.

Kuwabara, K., Yakushiji, T., Watanabe, I., Yoshida, S., Koyama, K. and Kunita, N. (1979). Levels of polychlorinated biphenyls in blood of breast-fed children whose mothers are non-occupationally exposed to PCBs. *Bulletin on Environmental Contamination and Toxicology* **21**, 458–462.

Linder, R. E., Gaines, T. B. and Kimbrough, R. D. (1974). The effect of polychlorinated biphenyls on rat production. *Food and Cosmetics Toxicology* **12**, 63–77.

Lucier, G. M., Davis, C. J. and McLachlan, J. A. (1978). Transplacental transfer of the polychlorinated and polybrominated biphenyls. *Developmental Toxicology* **47**, 188–203.

Masuda, Y., Kagawa, R., Kuroki, H., Kuratsune, M., Yoshimura, T., Taki, I., Kusuda, M., Yamashita, F. and Hayashi, M. (1978a). Transfer of polychlorinated biphenyls from mothers to foetuses and infants. *Food and Cosmetics Toxicology* **16**, (6), 543–546.

Masuda, Y., Kagawa, R., Tokudoma, S. and Kuratsune, M. (1978b). Transfer of polychlorinated biphenyls to the foetuses and offspring of mice. *Food and Cosmetics Toxicology* **16**, (1), 33–37.

Merson, M. H. and Kirkpatrick, R. L. (1976). Reproductive performance of captive white-footed mice fed a PCB. *Bulletin on Environmental Contamination and Toxicology* **16**, (4), 392–398.

Miller, H. J., Cucos, S., Wassermann, D. and Wassermann, M. (1979). Organochlorine insecticides and polychlorinated biphenyls in human milk. *In* "Toxicology and Occupational Medicine" (Ed. W. B. Deichmann), pp. 379–386. Elsevier/North Holland.

Miller, R. W. (1977). Pollutants in breast milk. *Journal of Pediatrics* **90**, (3), 510–511.

Mizunoya, Y., Taniguchi, S., Kusumoto, A., Morita, S., Yamada, A., Baba, T. and Ogaki, S. (1974). Effects of polychlorinated biphenyls on fetuses and offspring in rats. *Journal of Food and Hygiene Society of Japan* **15**, (4), 252–260.

Muller, W. F., Hobson, W., Fuller, G. B., Knauf, W., Coulston, F. and Korte, F. (1978). Endocrine effects of chlorinated hydrocarbons in rhesus monkeys. *Ecotoxicology and Environmental Safety* **2**, 161–172.

Nishimura, H., Shiota, K., Tanimura, T., Mizutani, T., Matsumoto, M. and Ueda, M. (1977). Levels of polychlorinated biphenyls and organochlorine insecticides in human embryos and fetuses. *Paediatrician* **6**, (1), 45–57.

Orberg, J. (1978). *Acta Pharmacologia et Toxicologia* **42**, 323–327.

Orberg, J. and Kihlstrom, J. E. (1973). Effects of long-term feeding of polychlorinated biphenyls (PCB, Clophen A60) on the length of the oestrous cycle and on the frequency of implanted ova in the mouse. *Environmental Research* **6**, 176–179.

Orberg, J. and Lundberg, C. (1974). Some effects of DDT and PCB on the hormonal system in the male mouse. *Environmental Physiology and Biochemistry* **4**, (3), 116–120.

Orberg, J., Johansson, N., Kihlstrom, J. E. and Lundberg, C. (1972). Administration of DDT and PCB. *Ambio* **1**, (4), 148–149.

Peakall, D. B. (1972). Polychlorinated biphenyls: occurrence and biological effects. *Residue Reviews* **44**, 1–21.

Rogan, W. G., Bagniewska, A. and Damstra, T. (1980). Pollutants in breast milk. *New England Journal of Medicine* **302**, (26), 1450–1453.

Sanders, O. T. and Kirkpatrick, R. L. (1975). Effects of a polychlorinated biphenyl (PCB) on sleeping times, plasma corticosteroids, and testicular activities of white-footed mice. *Environmental Physiology and Biochemistry* **5**, (5), 308–313.

Sanders, O. T., Kirkpatrick, R. L. and Scanlon, P. E. (1977). Polychlorinated biphenyls and nutritional restriction: their effects and interactions on endocrine and reproductive characteristics of male white mice. *Toxicology and Applied Pharmacology* **40**, 91–98.

Seiler, J. P. (1977). Inhibitions of testicular DNA synthesis by chemical mutagens and carcinogens. Preliminary results in the validations of a novel short-term test. *Mutation Research* **46**, 305–310.

Shiota, K. (1976). Embryotoxic effects of polychlorinated biphenyls (Kanechlors 300 and 500) in rats. *Okajimas Folia Anatomica Japonica* **53**, 93–104.

Takagi, Y., Otake, T., Kataoka, M., Murata, Y., Aburada, S., Akasaka, S., Hashimoto, K., Uda, H. and Kitaura, T. (1976). Studies on the transfer of (14C) polychlorinated biphenyls from maternal to fetal and suckling rats. *Toxicology and Applied Pharmacology* **38**, 549–558.

Taki, I., Hisanaga, S. and Amagase, Y. (1969). Report on Yusho (chlorobiphenyls poisoning) pregnant women and their fetuses. *Fukuoka Acta Medica* **60**, 471–474.

Tilson, H. A., Davis, G. J., McLachlan, J. A. and Lucier, G. W. (1979). The effects of polychlorinated biphenyls given prenatally on the neurobehavioral development of mice. *Environmental Research* **18**, (2), 466–474.

Török, P. (1975). Effect of 2,2′-dichlorobiphenyl (PCB) on the embryonic development of the NMRI mouse. *Environmental Quality and Safety* **3**, (Supplement), 788–792.

Török, P. (1976). Delayed pregnancy in NMRI mice treated with PCB: 2,2′-dichlorobiphenyl. *Bulletin on Environmental Contamination and Toxicology* **16**, (1), 33–36.

Villeneuve, D. C., Grant, D. L., Khera, K., Clegg, D. J., Baer, H. and Phillips, W. E. J. (1971). The fetotoxicity of a polychlorinated biphenyl mixture (Aroclor 1254) in the rabbit and the rat. *Environmental Physiology* **1**, (2), 67–71.

Wasserman, M., Wasserman, D., Cucos, S. and Miller, H. J. (1979). World PCBs map: storage and effects in man and his biologic environment in the 1970s. *Annals of the New York Academy of Sciences* **320**, 69–124.

Yakushiji, T., Watanabe, I., Kuwabara, K., Yoshida, S., Koyama, K., Hara, I. and Kunita, N. (1978). Long-term studies of the excretion of polychlorinated biphenyls (PCBs) through the mother's milk of an occupationally exposed worker. *Archives of Environmental Contamination and Toxicology* **7**, (4), 493–504.

Yakushiji, T., Watanabe, T., Kuwabara, K., Yoshida, S., Koyama, K. and Kunita, K. (1979). Levels of polychlorinated biphenyls (PCB's) and organochlorine pesticides in human milk and blood collected in Osaka prefecture from 1972 to 1977. *International Archives of Occupational and Environmental Health* **43**, 1–15.

Yamashita, F. (1977). Clinical features of polychlorbiphenyls (PCB)-induced fetopathy. *Paediatrician* **6**, (1), 20–27.

Yoshida, S. and Nakamura, A. (1979). Residual status after parturition of methylsulfone metabolites of polychlorinated biphenyls in the breast milk of a former employee in a capacitor factory. *Bulletin on Environmental Contamination and Toxicology* **21**, (1–2), 111–115.

Yoshimura, T. and Ikeda, M. (1978). Growth of school children with polychlorinated biphenyl poisoning or Yusho. *Environmental Research* **17**, 416–425.

37. Selenium and its Compounds

TECHNICAL DATA

(a) *Selenium*

Formula	Se
CAS registry number	7782–49–2
Chemical abstracts name	Selenium
Synonyms	None

(b) *Selenium compounds*

Formula	**CAS registry number**	**Chemical abstracts name**
H_2SeO_4	7783–08–6	Selenic acid
H_2SeO_3	7783–00–8	Selenious acid
Se_2Br_2	7789–52–8	Selenium bromide
Se_2Cl_2	10025–68–0	Selenium chloride
SeF_6	7783–79–1	Selenium hexafluoride
SeO_2	7446–08–4	Selenium oxide
Br_2OSe	7789–51–7	Selenium oxybromide
Cl_2OSe	7791–23–3	Selenium oxychloride
F_2OSe	7783–43–9	Selenium oxyfluoride
$SeBr_4$	7789–65–3	Selenium tetrabromide
$SeCl_4$	10026–03–6	Selenium tetrachloride
SeF_4	13465–66–2	Selenium tetrafluoride

Uses Ingredient of toning baths in photography; manufacture of ruby/pink/orange/red-coloured glass; metallic base in making electrodes for arc lights, electrical instruments and apparatus, as rectifier in radio and television sets; in selenium photocells, in semiconductor fusion mixtures, selenium cells, telephotographic apparatus; vulcanising agent in rubber-processing; catalyst in Kjeldahl nitrogen-determination method; dehydrogenation of organic compounds.

TLV 0·2 mg/m^3 (as selenium).

ANIMAL STUDIES

A. RELEVANT PHARMACOLOGY AND TOXICOLOGY

Selenium (Se) is a naturally occurring essential trace element and is therefore found in all biological tissues. Elemental Se is relatively non-toxic because of its insolubility but colloidal Se is toxic, and the many different Se-containing compounds have varying toxicities (see Fishbein, 1977, for review). There is some evidence that male rats may be more susceptible to acute and chronic selenite toxicity than female rats (Fishbein, 1977).

Brown and Burk (1972) have shown a sex difference in retention of Se in the rat which further emphasises the sex difference in toxicity. Rats were killed at intervals of up to 10 weeks after i.p. injections of radiolabelled selenious acid (H_2SeO_3). Females showed a higher retention of ^{75}Se in all tissues in comparison with males, except the brain where retention was the same in both sexes.

Change in blood Se levels during treatment with female sex hormones or during normal pregnancy have been investigated in the rat. Behne *et al.* (1976) gave groups of 5 ovariectomized rats oestrone and/or progesterone for 3 weeks and found no change in blood Se levels, but in 5 pregnant rats blood Se levels fell significantly by about 25% between days 10 and 15 of pregnancy and continued to fall thereafter. The cause of this fall is not known, but it may reflect a change in Se metabolism or an increasing fetal requirement for Se.

Pařízek *et al.* (1973) have shown that the toxicity of an organic selenide, dimethylselenide, increases in lactating rats from parturition up to the end of the second week of lactation and decreases during spontaneous weaning or can be abruptly decreased by premature forced weaning of pups. The mechanism of this effect is not known.

Being an essential trace element in most species, it would be remarkable if Se did not cross the placenta to the fetus in most species. Westfall *et al.* (1938) were the first to demonstrate experimentally the passage of Se across the placenta in the cat and the rat. A single pregnant cat was given a dietary supplement of Se-bearing wheat germ at a dose of 0·5 mg Se/kg/day. Twenty days later a dead kitten was born with tissue Se levels of 19–458 μg/100 g, the lowest level being in bone and the highest in hair and liver. Rats were placed on diets containing 8–15 ppm Se as sodium selenite (Na_2SeO_3) or organic Se at early, mid- or late pregnancy. At delivery, pups contained 23–230 μg/100 g tissue, which represented up to 14% of the total maternal intake being present in the fetuses; the lower levels of Se were found in the fetus when inorganic Se was fed and the higher levels when organic Se was fed.

Others have confirmed the placental transfer of Se in the rat. Rosenfeld and Beath (1964) gave low (7·5 μg) or high (2 mg) doses of Se as sodium selenite containing ^{75}Se by injection (route not stated) to rats around day 11–13 of pregnancy. Seven days later ^{75}Se was found in all reproductive tissues and declined in the order placenta, uterus, amniotic fluid and fetus. Placental transfer to the fetus was higher in the low dose than the high dose group, suggesting high doses of Se may have a toxic effect on placental transfer mechanisms.

Pařízek *et al.* (1971) injected sodium selenite containing ^{75}Se s.c. into groups of 5–6 rats on day 19 of pregnancy. Twenty hours later maternal liver contained 6% of the dose, fetuses 3·8% and placentae 1·2%. Twenty-four hours later maternal blood contained 3% of the injected dose and fetal blood 1·5% of the dose, maternal liver 16% of the dose and fetal livers 9% of the dose. Hasegawa and Urakubo (1974) have measured the passage of ^{75}Se into the rat fetus 1 h after i.v. injection of sodium selenite on day 20 of pregnancy. In litters of 6 rats, the fetuses had taken up on average 5% of the total dose, the placentae 1·5% and the ovary and uterus 1·5%. Of the fetal tissues, levels were highest in the liver, adrenal and kidney.

Iijima *et al.* (1978) have similarly shown placental transfer of ^{75}Se injected s.c. as sodium selenite on day 15 of pregnancy in the mouse. Significant radioactivity was found in the placenta and fetus 4 h after the maternal injection, the earliest time point it was measured. Fetal concentrations increased further between 4 h and 8 h after injection, then plateaued around the same concentration as maternal blood between 8 h and 48 h. Maternal blood and brain levels were falling between 4 h and 48 h but fetal levels were not, indicating a fairly long equilibration time for Se transfer across the placenta.

Hidiroglou *et al.* (1969) have measured Se levels in the pregnant ewe fed a low level of Se in the diet (0·024 ppm) or injected i.m. with 6 mg Se 10 days before slaughter at different stages of pregnancy. In those on Se-containing diet, maternal and fetal tissue levels were similar. After injection of Se, both maternal and fetal levels were elevated compared with dietary intake only and maternal levels were up to 3-fold higher than fetal levels in some tissues. In the fetus levels were highest in the kidney, adrenal, spleen and liver.

Pařízek *et al.* (1971) have also shown the passage of Se in the milk to suckling rats. Seven dams were injected s.c. with ^{75}Se as sodium selenite on day 8 of lactation. ^{75}Se could be detected in the milk and 24 h after injection around 10% of the dose was found in the pups (whole litter).

It is worth noting that Se interacts with a number of heavy metals such as cadmium and mercury. The reproductive toxicities in the male and female animals of cadmium and inorganic mercury (see relevant sections) but not organic mercury may be reduced or eliminated, for example, by simultaneous or prior administration of Se (Pařízek *et al.*, 1970). Mercury and Se reciprocally interfere with each other's transfer across the placenta and into the milk; Se decreases mercury transfer and similarly mercury decreases transfer of Se to fetuses and sucklings (Pařízek *et al.*, 1969a, 1969b, 1970, 1971). The mechanisms by which these effects occur are not known but may be related to protein binding of the elements.

Conclusion

These experiments demonstrate placental transfer of Se in the mouse, rat, cat and ewe. Experiments on the rat suggest that transfer across the placenta is substantial within the first hour after maternal administration but full equilibration with maternal blood may take up to 48 h. There is limited evidence that placental transfer and/or fetal retention of organic Se may be greater than that of inorganic Se and there is no evidence of accumulation of inorganic Se in the fetus. Naturally occurring Se is found in the milk of many species and transfer of radiolabelled ^{75}Se in the milk to sucklings in the rat has been demonstrated.

B. ENDOCRINE AND GONADAL EFFECTS

Males

A particular affinity of the testes and epididymides for Se has been demonstrated in the mouse and the rat. Gunn *et al.* (1967) have studied the incorporation of Se into the spermatogenic pathway in mice injected s.c. with radiolabelled ^{75}Se. All tissues examined except the testis and epididymis reached their maximum ^{75}Se concentrations between 1 h and 1 day after injection and had lost the majority of the ^{75}Se by 7 days after injection. Testicular ^{75}Se levels, however, peaked at 7 days, when they contained 2% of the administered dose/g tissue. As testicular levels fell, epididymis levels rose, peaking 2–3 weeks after injection. A similar pattern has been observed in the rat by Brown and Burk (1972) following i.p. injection of ^{75}Se. All tissues except the brain, thymus, testes and epididymides showed a decline in ^{75}Se activity from day 1. (Gunn *et al.* (1967) did not look at brain or thymus in the mouse.) In the rat, brain, thymus and testis levels peaked at 2 weeks and epididymis levels at 4 weeks after injection. At 3 weeks, the testes and epididymides contained 32% of the administered dose of ^{75}Se. On autoradiography, ^{75}Se was found to be localized in the midpiece of the spermatozoa. These findings in the mouse and rat suggest that Se is incorporated at a late stage in the sperm cycle and remains in the spermatozoa as they pass through the reproductive tract.

Freeman and Sangalang (1977) have examined the effects of Se on *in vitro* steroidogenesis in testicular tissue from the grey seal. Se, as selenium dioxide, was added to testicular incubates at a concentration of 0·45 ppm. After 3·5 h incubation, Δ4-androstene-3,17-dione levels were decreased by 82%, dehydroepiandrosterone levels were increased by 263%, 11-ketotestosterone was increased by 501%, but testosterone levels were scarcely altered, showing only a 7% decrease in comparison with controls. The physiological significance of these changes, if any, is not known.

Females

Nobunaga *et al.* (1979) have investigated the effect of Se on mouse oestrous cycles. Mice were given 0, 3 or 6 ppm Se in the drinking water as sodium selenite (0, 11·4 or 22·8 n mol/ml) for 30 days. Water consumption was significantly reduced in a dose-related manner by 20% and 28% in selenite groups but food consumption and body weight were unaffected. There was some evidence of an increase in abnormal cycle lengths in those given 22·8 nmol/ml; in control mice only 6·4% had cycles longer than 4 days but in the high Se group 11·8% had longer cycles. These females were subsequently mated to control males whilst continuing on Se until day 18 of pregnancy. There were no effects on fertility or pregnancy (see sections C and D for details).

C. FERTILITY

Nobunaga *et al.* (1979) have found no effect on fertility of groups of 10–14 female mice fed 3 or 6 ppm Se as sodium selenite in the drinking water for 30 days before mating and during pregnancy. Despite a small increase in the number of abnormal length oestrous cycles in the 6 ppm group, there were no effects on numbers pregnant, implants/dam, live fetuses/dam, resorptions/dam or fetal body weight.

However, Schroeder and Mitchener (1971) have shown an adverse effect of Se at 3 ppm when given for a prolonged period throughout a multigeneration study in the mouse. Mice were given 3 ppm Se as selenate in the drinking water continuously. The Fo generation were given Se from weaning and breeding continued for 3 generations, 5 pairs/generation, each pair breeding up to 6 months of age, often producing 3 litters each. In all generations, the male:female ratio in litters was increased, ranging from 1·30–1·50 compared with 0·94–1·03 in controls. There were also significant progressive increases in the proportions of runts born to Se groups. Two or 3 pairs in each of the F_1, F_2 and F_3 parent generations failed to breed, whereas there were no failures in controls. The F_3 generation showed a further marked deterioration producing only 3 litters from 5 pairs compared with 22 litters in controls, and 16/23 pups in these 3 litters were runts. These findings are compatible with those of Nobunaga *et al.* (1979) who studied one generation only, since marked effects did not appear until later generations.

Rosenfeld and Beath (1954) carried out a 2-generation study in the rat. Five females, given 1·5, 2·5 or 7·5 ppm Se in the drinking water, were bred 5 times during one year, firstly to control males, then subsequently to selenised males. Their offspring were also bred to produce a further generation. At 1·5 ppm there were no effects on reproduction or survival of young. At 2·5 ppm reproduction was normal but second generation females weighed less than controls and reared 50% fewer young than controls. At 7·5 ppm, in the first pregnancies, where Se was given only 5–8 days before parturition and during lactation, normal-sized litters were born but only 13% survived to weaning. After weaning, the dams were continued on Se and mated with males also on 7·5 ppm Se on 5 separate occasions, but failed to produce any young. At this dose rats lost weight and some died. The effects on reproduction were due to the females; if selenised females were mated to control males, no young were produced, but if selenised males were mated to normal females, normal litters with 70% survival to weaning were produced. The young produced by females exposed to 7·5 ppm were runted at birth and unable to suckle (Rosenfeld and Beath, 1964).

In a review of Se toxicity, Rosenfeld and Beath (1964) mention very similar findings from experiments reported by Frank and Potter in the 1930s (original paper not seen by us) on rats fed selenised wheat diets; matings between selenised males and females were infertile, and if one of the pair was normal matings were sometimes fertile but selenised females could not rear their young.

Wahlstrom and Olson (1959) have studied the effect of Se on fertility in the pig. Females were fed 10 ppm Se as sodium selenite in the diet continuously from 8 weeks of age. Signs of toxicity (hair loss) were seen in 2/10 animals. They were mated with a normal male a maximum of 3 times until they conceived and produced 2 litters. The interval from weaning of the first litter to oestrus was increased from 8 days in controls to 13 days in the Se group. Three out of 10 failed to conceive, compared with 1/9 in controls; at autopsy the ovaries of the sterile pigs were cystic or devoid of corpora lutea. Average total litter size (live + stillborn) was not affected but there was a small reduction in mean live litter size and a significant reduction in numbers weaned in first and second litters of Se pigs. There were also significant reductions in birth weight in first litters and weaning weight of first and second litters, and the piglets were less vigorous than controls.

Harr and Muth (1972) in a review of Se poisoning in domestic animals, have also noted a decreased conception rate and increased fetal resorption in cattle, sheep and horses fed diets containing 25–50 ppm Se. These levels also produce other signs of gross toxicity including hair loss, lameness, and degeneration and fibrosis of the heart, liver and kidney.

Conclusion

Short periods of exposure to Se in the diet or drinking water do not appear to affect fertility in the female unless intake is high enough to cause generalized toxicity. However, chronic exposure to otherwise non-toxic doses (3 ppm) in the mouse and rat has been shown to affect fertility and markedly reduce the viability of the young in those managing to reproduce. There is some evidence that male reproduction is not affected by Se, even at toxic doses.

D. PREGNANCY

Evidence that long-term Se intake before mating, during pregnancy and during lactation causes low birth weight, weakness in the offspring and poor postnatal survival in laboratory and domestic animals has been reviewed in section C and will not be considered again here. Other studies on the embryolethal, fetotoxic and teratogenic potential of Se will be reviewed.

Whilst chick embryo studies are not being reviewed in detail, it is worth noting that several studies have shown production of abnormalities of the central nervous system, limbs and eyes, malformations similar to those produced by Se in mammalian species.

In the mouse, Nobunaga *et al.* (1979) have given 0, 3 or 6 ppm Se as sodium selenite in the drinking water for 30 days before mating and throughout pregnancy to groups of 9–14 animals. The mice were killed on day 18 of pregnancy. Acceptable teratological methods were used. Water but not food intake was significantly reduced in a dose related manner but there was no effect on maternal weight gain. There were no significant effects on implants/dam, live fetuses/dam or resorptions/dam, but fetal body weight was significantly reduced by 7% in the 6 ppm Se group. There were no malformations in control or 3 ppm Se groups. In the 6 ppm group 2/88 fetuses were malformed, one with micrognathia and cleft palate and one with cleft palate only. The differences between treated and control groups are not significant. There was however a significant increase in unossified vertebrae in the 6 ppm group, which might be expected from the decrease in fetal weight.

Lee *et al.* (1979) specifically studied cleft palate in the mouse following s.c. injection of Se as sodium selenite. Injection of 3·5 mg/kg/day into 4 dams on days 9–12 of pregnancy resulted in 5·4% cleft palate in the offspring compared with 1·2% in controls, a non-significant increase because the numbers were small. Fetal body weight was not stated for the Se group. Other groups of 7 mice injected with 2 or 3·5 mg/kg/day on days 7–12 of pregnancy showed a dose-related increase in cleft palate from 1·2% in controls to 2·1% at 2 mg/kg/day and 4·6% at 3·5 mg/kg/day, but again these differences are not significant. There was a significant 10% decrease in fetal body weight at 3·5 mg/kg/day.

No conventional teratology studies have been carried out in the rat, though particular aspects of Se developmental toxicity have been studied. Shearer and Hadjimarkos (1973) looked at ^{75}Se retention in developing molar teeth of rat pups whose mothers were given 4 s.c. injections of radio-labelled sodium selenite on days 10, 13, 16 and 19 of pregnancy. At 13 days post-partum, concentrations of ^{75}Se in soft tissues were lower in pups than in mothers but concentrations in hard tissues such as teeth and bone were higher in pups than in mothers and in the developing molar teeth were 9-fold higher than in maternal molars. Most of the ^{75}Se was incorporated into the protein fraction of enamel and dentine and it has been suggested that this interferes with mineralization, thus increasing susceptibility to dental caries. In humans, consumption of increased dietary Se during tooth development increases the prevalence of dental caries.

Se may also be a particular hazard to the developing eye. Ošťádalová *et al.* (1978) gave a single s.c. dose of 0·8–10·3 mg/kg (5–60 μmoles/kg) sodium selenite to male rats at 10 days of age. The highest dose killed all pups within 24 h. In the 1·7–6·8 mg/kg groups there was a significant, dose-related increase in cataracts visible to the naked eye when the pups' eyes opened at 14–16 days of age. Some cataracts were permanent, especially at the higher doses, whilst others were intermittent. At 0·8 mg/kg there were no pup deaths and no cataracts, however at 1·7 mg/kg there were also no deaths but cataracts were seen. Two-month-old males given a single s.c. injection of 3·4 mg/kg had a high mortality but no cataracts were seen in survivors, suggesting the developing eye is peculiarly sensitive to Se toxicity.

In the hamster, Holmberg and Ferm (1969) have failed to produce teratogenic effects with i.v. injection of 2 mg/kg on day 8 of pregnancy. This dose was barely sublethal to the dam yet caused only 6% resorptions and no malformations, which was comparable to controls.

In an early study on the rabbit, Datnow (1928) injected i.v. 3–6 ml/day of a 0·1% suspension of colloidal Se, beginning on day 12, 13 or 14 or pregnancy. Doses of 4–6 ml killed the does within 24–72 h, and at autopsy there were acute congestion and haemorrhage in maternal tissues and the placenta.

However, one doe given 3 ml/day gave birth to a normal litter, suggesting that the effects observed at higher doses were not selective on the reproductive tissues but a generalized effect of colloidal Se on the doe.

In domestic animals, hoof abnormalities have been noted in foals, calves and lambs born to animals grazing on seleniferous pastures (reviewed by Fishbein, 1977). Rosenfeld and Beath (1947, 1964) have reported in detail on malformations in lambs born in seleniferous areas. The eyes and limbs were abnormal and the majority of lambs (85%) died at birth or soon after. Limb deformities in survivors impaired locomotion. The eyes showed varying degrees of deformity. Some had single, large, transparent cysts protruding through the lids and the sclera fused to bone so that rotation of the eye was impossible. Others were microphthalmic with multiple cysts. Colobomas of various structures were common. Lens, cornea and iris were usually abnormal or absent. Histological examination of the eye revealed a bizarre structural arrangement resulting from arrested growth and poor differentiation. Hypoplasia of the reproductive organs was also noted in surviving lambs.

Selenium-metal interactions

In the mouse, Se given as sodium selenite is not highly teratogenic, causing only slight growth retardation and possibly a small increase in cleft palate. However, Se can markedly enhance the embryolethality, growth retardation and cleft palate caused by methylmercury (Lee *et al.*, 1979; Nobunaga *et al.*, 1979). Whilst Se is known to decrease the placental transfer of inorganic mercury (see section A), it is not known what happens in the case of organic mercury.

In the hamster, sodium selenite, which is not teratogenic by itself, markedly reduces or totally prevents the embryolethal and teratogenic effects of cadmium and arsenic salts if injected within 30 min of the teratogen (Holmberg and Ferm, 1969).

Conclusion

In summary prenatal exposure to Se in rodents decreases fetal weight but is not highly teratogenic. However continued exposure postnatally through the milk or acutely via injection markedly reduces postnatal viability and can affect later developing structures such as the eyes and teeth. In domestic animals effects may be more dramatic with joint, hoof and eye abnormalities present at birth, and again a very high postnatal mortality. The effects on the limbs of foals, calves and lambs are very similar to those seen in adult alkali disease, a subacute form of organic selenosis seen in horses, cattle and sheep consuming high Se levels in the diet (Fishbein, 1977). However, the developing eye does seem to be peculiarly sensitive to Se. It is not clear to what extent the high postnatal mortality is secondary to effects on the mother reducing feeding or direct effects of prenatal and/or postnatal exposure. Both may contribute, since in the rat, for example, maternal susceptibility to Se toxicity is markedly increased in the early lactation period and pups also may be weak and runted with a poor sucking response; in domestic animals young may be unable to stand to suckle because of limb deformities and the dams often also show signs of Se toxicity if eating high Se-containing feed.

E. MUTAGENICITY

No relevant data found.

F. CARCINOGENICITY

IARC Monograph Vol. 9 (1975) reported that selenium compounds had been tested in mice and rats by the oral route. Although one experiment in rats produced an increase in liver tumours, the data were insufficient to allow evaluation of the carcinogenicity of selenium compounds.

HUMAN STUDIES

A. RELEVANT PHARMACOLOGY AND TOXICOLOGY

Placental transfer

Selenium, an essential trace metal, is found in the human placenta and fetus. Hadjimarkos *et al.* (1959) first documented levels in placental tissue and cord blood samples from 13 normal deliveries to women living in Oregon in areas not known to be seleniferous. Placental levels ranged from 0·13–0·24 ppm (mean 0·18 ppm) and cord blood levels from 0·07–0·18 ppm (mean 0·12 ppm). Maternal blood levels were not measured.

Baglan *et al.* (1974) measured placental, maternal blood and cord blood levels at delivery in a large number of samples (600–800) obtained from 4 hospitals in Nashville, Tennessee, U.S.A. Mean values of 1·70, 1·10 and 1·04 μg/g dry weight were obtained for placenta, maternal blood and cord blood respectively. Placental, fetal and maternal blood levels were highly correlated. Gestational age at birth did not influence the levels. These results suggest that selenium passes readily across the placenta into the fetus.

Amin *et al.* (1978) have measured serum selenium levels in premature and full term infants. The time of sampling in relation to delivery was not stated. Levels in 65 premature infants averaged $0{\cdot}0899 \pm 0{\cdot}0327$ μg/100 ml compared with levels of 0·0976 ± 0·024 μg/100 ml in 15 full term infants. Sex, weight and gestational age did not influence the levels. The levels reported here are about 10 times higher than those recorded by Hadjimarkos *et al.* (1959).

Robkin *et al.* (1973) have measured selenium levels in fetal liver samples from a total of 46 anencephalics, spontaneous and therapeutic abortuses and premature deliveries. Levels ranged from 2·2–2·9 ppm in dry liver tissue.

Transfer in the breast milk

Hadjimarkos (1970b) was also the first to report on selenium levels in human breast milk. In 1963 he reported levels of 0·021 ppm in samples collected from 15 lactating mothers (original paper not seen by us). Two other small studies reviewed by Shearer and Hadjimarkos (1975) confirmed levels of 0·01–0·02 ppm in human milk. A much larger study by Shearer and Hadjimarkos (1975) of 211 women living in different geographical areas in the U.S.A. found levels ranging from 0·007–0·060 ppm (mean 0·018 ppm). Subjects were aged 17–44 years and were 17–869 days post-partum. The study confirmed that selenium levels in breast milk are influenced by geographic location of residence and the authors suggested that these differences may result from differing intakes of selenium in food in different communities.

Schroeder *et al.* (1970) have recorded a single estimation of 0·24 ppm selenium in breast milk taken from a 52-year-old woman at autopsy, which is very high compared with all other studies. The cause of death was not given, nor is it known if she lived in a seleniferous area.

B. ENDOCRINE AND GONADAL EFFECTS

A passing reference to menstrual disorders has been made by Harr and Muth (1972) who summarized the effects of chronic inorganic selenosis as including follicular skin rash, inflammation of the perivascular lymph channels, loss of hair and nails, haemolytic anaemia and serum bilirubin, leukopenia, increased weight of the spleen, pancreas and liver, fatigue, lasitude and dizziness, and irregular menses. No further details or references are given.

C. FERTILITY

No relevant data found.

D. PREGNANCY

Robertson (1970) reported an unusual cluster of pregnancy problems occurring in one laboratory where there was exposure to selenite-containing powder which was weighed out to prepare bacterial culture medium. In a 5-year period during which 10 women of childbearing age were employed there (6 married, 2 single, 2 no information), 4 certain and one probable pregnancy occurred and all ended in abortion except one which went to term; the infant delivered had bilateral club foot. It was thought that simple clinical factors could possibly have accounted for 2 of these miscarriages. Urinary selenium levels measured in these women towards the end of the 5-year period showed no differences from controls living in the same area. Robertson (1970) also stated that "quite widespread" inquiries at other laboratories carrying out comparable work showed no evidence of similar troubles except in one small unit which employed 10 women over a 5-year period. Nine were single, and of the 3 still handling selenite at the time of inquiry one was married and she had had a miscarriage the year before the inquiry. This single instance of miscarriage could not be regarded as evidence of an abortifacient effect of selenite. The 3, possibly 4, cases of abortion described by Robertson are difficult to evaluate without additional information. Since the appearance of Robertson's report, in a journal with world-wide circulation, no further reports of abortion or teratogenesis in women working with selenium have appeared.

Shamberger (1971) has examined neonatal death rates in different geographical areas, designated high, medium and low selenium States in the U.S.A., using government statistical sources published in 1960. He found neonatal death rates/100,000 live population (mean ± SE) of 720 ± 35, 760 ± 24, and 927 ± 28 in high, medium and low selenium States, the differences between high or medium States and low States being highly significant. These data pointed, if anything, to an inverse relationship between neonatal deaths and selenium. Cowgill (1976), however, has pointed out a very serious error in Shamberger's data; the rates given were not neonatal death rates but rates for all deaths exclusive of those occurring below one year of age. Furthermore, calculation of neonatal death rates per 100,000 live population is unusual, and rates per 1000 live births are more conventionally used. Cowgill calculates, using Shamberger's division of States, that for 1960 neonatal death rates/100,000 live population were 41·76, 46·31 and 50·31 for low, medium and high selenium regions respectively and rates/1000 live births were 18·53, 18·35 and 19·73 for low, medium and high regions respectively. Cowgill has also pointed out that Shamberger has used rather different groupings of States for selenium levels than others have used. Using Cowgill's own division of States neonatal death rates/100,000 live population in 1960 were 21·69, 47·85 and 95·57 for low, medium and high selenium States respectively. Neonatal death rates/1000 live births using the Cowgill division of States ranged from 18·05 to 19·53 in 1960–62 and from 12·22 to 14·73 in 1971–73; in each of these years, the neonatal death rate in the high selenium regions was greater than that in the medium or low selenium regions. Thus, however calculated, all the data point to an association between high selenium areas and increased neonatal death rates. However, Cowgill has pointed out that a number of States are not clear-cut as to the selenium content of forage crops on which the divisions are based. Furthermore, division by States may be insensitive since there may be considerable variability in the extent of seleniferous areas within entire States. No other variables were controlled for and Cowgill (1976) has mentioned a further complication in any data gathered since Shamberger's (1971) publication in that s/he has encountered couples in the low selenium regions taking extra selenium because they thought it might prevent neonatal death. However, the association between selenium and neonatal death suggested by Cowgill's calculations clearly warrants further study.

Jaffé and Vélez (1973) have reported very briefly, in abstract only, that in Venezuela areas of high selenium intake and areas of highest incidence of congenital malformations do not coincide. In one area, Yaracuy, where congenital malformations are rare, the highest level of selenium in urine was 0·38 μg/ml and the authors conclude that selenium intake up to this excretory level would not be teratogenic. The accuracy of recording of congenital malformation rates in Venezuela is not known.

An association has been shown between dietary selenium and prevalence of dental caries in children and it is suggested that selenium consumption during the period of primary tooth formation may be the critical factor (Hadjimarkos *et al.*, 1959; Hadjimarkos, 1970a, 1970b). Thus transfer of selenium across the placenta during gestation and in the breast milk afterwards (see section A) may play a role in the development of dental caries.

A few studies have compared selenium content of the tissues in normal births and in cases of adverse outcome of pregnancy. Robkin *et al.* (1973) have measured fetal liver contents of 7 different elements (Hg, Se, Ag, Co, Cr, Fe, Zn) in cases of anencephalic births, premature births, therapeutic abortions and spontaneous abortions. Whilst significant differences between these 4 groups were obtained for mercury (thought to be due to accumulation of mercury with gestational age) and for zinc (suggesting an association between zinc deficiency and fetal anomalies), for selenium, concentrations ranged from 2·2–2·9 ppm in dry liver tissue and only the anencephalic group (2·9 ppm) differed significantly from the premature group (2·2 ppm). The biological significance, if any, of this observation is not known.

Amin *et al.* (1978) measured serum selenium levels in premature and full term births and in children aged 2–15 years. The mean serum selenium in the premature infants was 0·0899 μg/100 ml which was significantly lower than that in normal children of 0·1076 μg/100 ml but not significantly different from that in full-term infants of 0·0976 μg/100 ml.

Baglan *et al.* (1974) have measured levels of 8 different trace elements (Hg, Pb, Cd, Se, Rb, Zn, Fe, Co) in maternal and fetal blood and placenta at delivery in cases of normal and abnormal outcome of pregnancy. They compared the normal:abnormal ratio for each element for each tissue in 14 different types of abnormality (3 categories of neonatal deaths, 4 categories of postnatal illness and 7 categories of congenital malformation). The number of cases in each category ranged from 5–53. In the majority of cases (83%) the ratios were between 0·80 and 1·25, but no details were given on those lying outside this range and the authors imply that the outliers were randomly distributed. The largest category was respiratory disease (53 cases) and detailed results for these have been published separately (Brill *et al.*, 1974). Ratios of respiratory disease subjects: normals for selenium were 0·91, 0·95 and 0·99 for placenta, maternal blood and fetal blood respectively, suggesting selenium does not play any significant role in that problem.

E. MUTAGENICITY

In vitro studies reviewed by Ray and Altenburg (1978) and Ray *et al.* (1978) have produced conflicting results (original papers not seen by us). One study has shown that sodium selenite at a concentration of 1×10^{-5} M inhibits cell division in human lymphocyte cultures, whilst in another mitotic figures have been observed with sodium selenite concentrations of $2{\cdot}6 \times 10^{-4}$ M. Another study has shown unscheduled DNA synthesis in human fibroblasts cultured with sodium selenite "activated" by crude liver extract. Ray and Altenburg (1978) have shown induction of sister-chromatid exchange (SCE) in whole human blood cultures by sodium selenite concentrations of $7{\cdot}9 \times 10^{-6}$ M and above. However, with purified human lymphocyte cultures, sodium selenite up to toxic levels did not increase SCE frequency above control levels. Addition of red blood cells or red blood cell lysate to purified lymphocytes cultured with sodium selenite resulted in SCE frequencies comparable to those in sodium selenite-exposed whole blood cultures, suggesting that chemical modification of sodium selenite is required for induction of cytogenetic abnormalities. These results are in accord with those on unscheduled DNA synthesis discussed above.

F. CARCINOGENICITY

IARC Monograph Vol. 9 (1975) stated that the available data at that time provided no suggestion that selenium is carcinogenic in humans.

SUMMARY AND EVALUATION

EXPERIMENTAL STUDIES

Both organic and inorganic selenium cross the placenta readily, and are also present in breast milk. The testes and epididymis show a high affinity for selenium and it is incorporated into the mid-piece of the sperm. Although brief exposure to otherwise non-toxic doses does not appear to affect fertility, chronic exposure of mice and rats to levels of 2·5–3 ppm in the diet reduce fertility of females and cause reduced birth weight and high postnatal mortality in offspring. Similar effects with toxic levels have been reported in farm animals. Limited studies suggest that it has a low degree of teratogenicity in rodents although adequate studies in rats have not been reported. However, malformations, particularly of the eye and limbs, have been reported in farm animals fed on high selenium diets.

No studies on mutagenicity were found and the data on carcinogenicity is insufficient for evaluation. No reports of transplacental carcinogenicity were found.

HUMAN STUDIES

Selenium readily crosses the placenta and the fetal and maternal blood levels at term are very similar, with some cumulation in the placenta. It is also found in breast milk in amounts varying with site of residence, but an average concentration is around 0·02 ppm. There are no adequate data on endocrine or gonadal effects or of effects on fertility. There are no adequate studies on the effects of occupational exposure to selenium on the outcome of pregnancy although an unconfirmed association with abortions has been suggested. Several studies have failed to demonstrate high selenium levels in malformed offspring or in neonatal deaths. The evidence on mutagenicity is inadequate to assess its effect in human cells *in vitro* or *in vivo*. Available data provides no evidence that it is carcinogenic in humans.

EVALUATION

There is adequate evidence for an antifertility effect following chronic exposure in animals. There is limited evidence that it is teratogenic in animals. Attention is drawn to the lack of data on reproductive effects in humans following occupational exposure. Data on mutagenicity and carcinogenicity are inadequate for evaluation.

References

Amin, S., Chen, S. Y., Castro-Magana, M., Maddaiah, V. T. and Collipp, P. J. (1978). Selenium in premature infants. *Federation Proceedings* **37**, (3), 758.

Baglan, R. J., Brill, A. B., Schulert, A., Wilson, D., Larsen, K., Dyer, N., Mansour, M., Schaffner, W., Hoffman, L. and Davies, J. (1974). Utility of placental tissue as an indicator of trace element exposure to adult and fetus. *Environmental Research* **8**, (1), 64–70.

Behne, D., Elger, W., Schmelzer, W. and Witte, M. (1976). Effects of sex hormones and pregnancy on the selenium metabolism. *Bioinorganic Chemistry* **5**, (3), 199–202.

Brill, A. B., Baglan, R. J., Fleet, W., Schaffner, W. and Schulert, A. (1974). A network to determine causality between abnormal trace element levels in congenital defects. *Proceedings—Annual NSF Trace Contamination Conference* (1st 1973), pp. 522–527.

Brown, D. G. and Burk, R. F. (1972). Selenium retention in tissue and sperm of rats fed a torula yeast diet. *Federation Proceedings* **31**, (2), 692.

Cowgill, U. M. (1976). Selenium and neonatal death. *Lancet* **i**, 816–817.

Datnow, M. M. (1928). An experimental investigation concerning toxic abortion produced by chemical agents. *Journal of Obstetrics and Gynaecology of the British Commonwealth* **35**, 693–724.

Fishbein, L. (1977). Toxicology of selenium and tellurium. *Advances in Modern Toxicology* **2**, 191–240.

Freeman, H. C. and Sangalang, G. B. (1977). A study of the effects of methyl mercury, cadmium, arsenic, selenium and a PCB (Aroclor 1254) on adrenal and testicular steroidogenesis *in vitro*, by the gray seal Halichoerus grypus. *Archives of Environmental Contamination and Toxicology* **5**, 369–383.

Gunn, S. A., Gould, T. C. and Anderson, W. A. D. (1967). Incorporation of Selenium into spermatogenic pathway in mice. *Proceedings of the Society for Experimental Biology and Medicine* **124**, (4), 1260–1263.

Hadjimarkos, D. M. (1970a). Selenium. (Letter) *Lancet* **i**, 721.

Hadjimarkos, D. M. (1970b). Selenium in man. (Letter) *New Zealand Medical Journal* **71**, 205–206.

Hadjimarkos, D. M., Bonhorst, C. W. and Mattice, J. J. (1959). The selenium concentration in placental tissue and fetal cord blood. *Journal of Paediatrics* **54**, 296–298.

Harr, J. R. and Muth, D. H. (1972). Selenium poisoning in domestic animals and its relationship to man. *Clinical Toxicology* **5**, (2), 175–186.

Hasegawa, A. and Urakubo, G. (1974). Hygienic chemical studies on selenium compounds. III. Distribution of sodium selenite in pregnant rat and fetus. *Journal of Hygienic Chemistry* **20**, (6), 341–343.

Hidiroglou, M., Hoffman, I. and Jenkins, K. J. (1969). Selenium distribution and radiotocopherol metabolism in the pregnant ewe and fetal lamb. *Canadian Journal of Physiology and Pharmacology* **47**, (11), 953–962.

Holmberg, R. E. and Ferm, V. H. (1969). Interrelationships of selenium, cadmium and arsenic in mammalian teratogenesis. *Archives of Environmental Health* **18**, 873–877.

IARC Monographs on the Evaluation of the Carcinogenic Risk of Chemicals to Humans: Some aziridines, N-, S- and O- mustards and selenium (1975). Vol. 9, Lyon, France.

Iijima, S., Tohyama, C., Chiung-chen, L. and Matsumoto, N. (1978). Placental transfer and body distribution of methylmercury and selenium. *Toxicology and Applied Pharmacology* **44**, 143–146.

Jaffé, W. G. and Vélez, B. F. (1973). Selenium intake and malformations in humans. *Archivos Latinamericanos de Nutricion* **23**, (4), 515–517.

Lee, M., Chan, K. K.-S., Sairenji, E. and Niikuni, T. (1979). Effects of sodium selenite on methylmercury-induced cleft palate in the mouse. *Environmental Research* **19**, 39–48.

Nobunaga, T., Satoh, H. and Suzuki, T. (1979). Effects of sodium selenite on methylmercury embryotoxicity and teratogenicity in mice. *Toxicology and Applied Pharmacology* **47**, 79–88.

Oštádalova, I., Babický, A. and Obenberger, J. (1978). Cataract induced by administration of a single dose of sodium selenite to suckling rats. *Experientia* **34**, (2), 222–223.

Pařízek, J., Babický, A., Oštádalová, I., Kalouskova, J. and Pavlik, I. (1969b). The effect of selenium compounds on the cross-placental passage of 203 Hg. Atomic Energy Commission Conference—690501 **17**, 137–143.

Pařízek, J., Benes, I., Oštádalová, I., Babický, A., Benes, J. and Pitha, J. (1969a). The effects of selenium on the toxicity and metabolism of cadmium and some other metals. *In* "Mineral Metabolism in Paediatrics", a Glaxo Symposium. (Eds, Barltrop, D. and Burland, W. L.), Chapter 8, pp. 117–134. Blackwell Scientific Publications, Oxford and Edinburgh.

Pařízek, J., Oštádolová, I., Kalouskova, J., Babický, A., Pavlik, L. and Bibr, S. (1971). Effect of mercuric compounds on the maternal transmission of selenium in the pregnant and lactating rat. *Journal of Reproduction and Fertility* **25**, 157–170.

Pařízek, J., Oštádalová, I., Kalouskova, J., Babický, A. and Benes, J. (1970). Metabolic principles of the reproductive function and its development. Effects of various trace elements from the viewpoint of physiology and pathophysiology of multiplying. *Ceskoslovenska Gynekologie* **35**, (3), 140–142.

Pařízek, J., Kalouskova, J., Babický, A. and Benes, J. (1973). Lactation and methylated metabolites of selenium. *Physiologia Bohemoslovaca* **22**, (4), 422.

Ray, J. H. and Altenburg, L. C. (1978). Sister-chromatid exchange induction by sodium selenite: dependence on the presence of red blood cells or red blood cell lysate. *Mutation Research* **54**, 343–354.

Ray, J. H., Altenburg, L. C. and Jacobs, M. M. (1978). Effect of sodium selenite and methyl methanesulfonate on N-hydroxy-2-acetylaminofluorene co-exposure on sister-chromatid exchange production in human whole blood cultures. *Mutation Research* **57**, 359–368.

Robertson, D. S. F. (1970). Selenium—a possible teratogen? (Letter) *Lancet* **i**, 518–519.

Robkin, M. A., Swenson, D. R. and Sheperd, T. H. (1973). Trace metal concentrations in human fetal livers. *Transactions—American Nuclear Society* **17**, 97–98.

Rosenfeld, I. and Beath, O. A. (1947). Congenital malformations of eyes of sheep. *Journal of Agricultural Research* **75**, 93–103.

Rosenfeld, I. and Beath, O. A. (1954). Effect of selenium on reproduction in rats. *Proceedings of the Society for Experimental Biology and Medicine* **87**, 295–297.

Rosenfeld, I. and Beath, O. A. (1964). The effect of selenium on reproduction and congenital malformations. *In* "Selenium, Geobotany, Biochemistry, Toxicity and Nutrition". (Authors, Rosenfeld, I. and Beath, O. A.), pp. 198–208. Academic Press, London.

Schroeder, H. A. and Mitchener, M. (1971). Toxic effects of trace elements on the reproduction of mice and rats. *Archives of Environmental Health* **23**, 102–106.

Schroeder, H. A., Frost, D. V. and Balassa, J. J. (1970). Essential trace elements in man: selenium. *Journal of Chronic Diseases* **23**, 227–243.

Shamberger, R. J. (1971). Is selenium a teratogen? *Lancet* **ii**, 1316.

Shearer, T. R. and Hadjimarkos, D. M. (1973). Comparative distribution of 75 Se in the hard and soft tissues of mother rats and their pups. *Journal of Nutrition* **103**, (4), 553–559.

Shearer, T. R. and Hadjimarkos, D. M. (1975). Geographic distribution of selenium in human milk. *Archives of Environmental Health* **30**, (5), 230–233.

Wahlstrom, R. C. and Olson, O. E. (1959). The effect of selenium on reproduction in swine. *Journal of Animal Science* **18**, 141–145.

Westfall, B. B., Stohlman, E. F. and Smith, M. I. (1938). The placental transmission of selenium. *Journal of Pharmacology and Experimental Therapeutics* **64**, 55–57.

38. Styrene

TECHNICAL DATA

Formula $C_6H_5CH{=}CH_2$

CAS registry number 100–42–5

Chemical abstracts name Ethenylbenzene

Synonyms Cinnamene; phenethylene; phenylethene; phenylethylene; styrol; styrole; styrolene; vinylbenzene; vinylbenzol.

Uses Manufacture of plastics; synthetic rubber; resins; insulator.

TLV 100 ppm (1980 Intended change to 50 ppm).

ANIMAL STUDIES

A. RELEVANT PHARMACOLOGY AND TOXICOLOGY

The absorption, distribution and metabolism of styrene in the rat have been extensively studied. The elimination of styrene following either inhalation, i.v. administration, or oral administration in aqueous solutions is similar, and follows a dose-dependent, two-compartment mathematical model (Withey, 1978). Styrene has a very high fat solubility and it is the fat which comprises the peripheral compartment in the two-compartment model for uptake, distribution and clearance of styrene, the other compartment being the blood (Ramsey and Young, 1978). With inhalation exposures, at least up to 80 ppm, the pharmacokinetic profiles for absorption and elimination of styrene in the rat and the human are very similar (Ramsey and Young, 1978). In both species, styrene is cleared mainly by metabolism at a rate directly proportional to its blood concentration, and styrene does not accumulate with repeated exposures until uptake saturates this metabolic clearance mechanism, which in the rat occurs above exposures of 200 ppm (Ramsey and Young, 1978). Toxicity may therefore considerably increase above this level. In both the rat and the human, styrene is first metabolised in the liver to styrene oxide by microsomal oxidation (Harkonen, 1978). Styrene oxide, an epoxide, is biologically reactive and can bind to macromolecules including DNA and RNA. It is the formation of this epoxide intermediate which gives cause for concern about possible mutagenicity and carcinogenicity (see sections E and F).

B. ENDOCRINE AND GONADAL EFFECTS

Izyumova (1972) has looked at the effect of styrene exposure by inhalation on oestrous cycles in the rat. Groups of 20 females with regular cycles were exposed to 0, 1·18 ppm (5 mg/m^3) or 11·8 ppm (50 mg/m^3) for 4 months followed by a "recovery" period in which there was no exposure to styrene. The daily duration of exposure was not stated. Signs of general toxicity were evident in both groups exposed to styrene; leukocytes were significantly increased after 3 months' exposure to 11·8 ppm and after 4 months' exposure to 1·18 ppm and remained elevated during the first month of the recovery period. Urinary hippuric acid content decreased after 4 months' exposure to 11·8 ppm, suggesting liver toxicity, and body weight also decreased in this group. Variable increases in the length of the oestrous cycle occurred in exposed females. After one month, cycle length was significantly increased to 5·3 days in the 11·8 ppm group compared with 4·2 days in controls. After 2 and 3 months there were no differences but by the end of the fourth month the cycle averaged 5·8 days in the 11·8 ppm group, 5·3 days in the 1·18 ppm group and 4·0 days in controls. These effects were even more pronounced after one month of the recovery period; cycles averaged 7·0 days in the 11·8 ppm group, 5·5 days in the 1·18 ppm group and 4·7 days in controls. The lengthening of the cycles was due to significant increases in the duration of oestrus, which, at the time of greatest disturbance (the "recovery" phase) was 5·5, 3·4 and 1·4 days in 11·8, 1·18 and 0 ppm groups respectively. Abnormally short cycles were also seen during the "recovery" phase. These animals were not followed beyond one month post-exposure, so it is not known if the cycles returned to normal.

In a further study of the same experimental design from the same group of workers, Zlobina *et al.* (1975) exposed rats to 1·18 ppm and a lower concentration of 0·23 ppm (1·0 mg/m^3) styrene by inhalation for 4 months. Changes in the oestrous cycle in the 1·18 ppm groups were similar to the previous study (Izyumova, 1972) and a tendency to prolonged oestrus was also seen in the 0·23 ppm group but the difference in this group was only significant in the recovery phase where duration of oestrus was 3·4, 2·7 and 1·4 days in 1·18, 0·23 and 0 ppm groups respectively. One difference between this and the previous study was that general signs of toxicity were more evident in the 1·18 ppm group; in this study, body weight, oxygen consumption and urinary hippuric acid content were all affected, whereas in the previous study these changes were only seen at 11·8 ppm.

The mechanism of the oestrous cycle changes were also investigated by Zlobina *et al.* (1975). Pituitary extracts taken from females exposed to 0, 0·23 or 1·18 ppm for 4 months were injected into female infant mice; the weight of the uterus and ovaries were lower in those injected with extracts from styrene-exposed rats compared with those injected with extracts from controls.

Conclusion

Chronic exposure to styrene by inhalation in the rat appears to alter gonadotrophic function and disturb oestrous cycles, at levels around or just below those causing overt toxicity.

C. FERTILITY

A 3-generation reproduction study in the rat has been carried out on behalf of the Manufacturing Chemists Association, U.S.A. (1979). Male and female rats were given styrene in the drinking water at concentrations of 0, 125 and 250 ppm. At least 10 males and 20 females (Fo generation) from each group were mated to produce the F1 generation. These were mated within their respective dose groups to produce the F2 generation and these in turn mated to produce the F3 generation. Dosing was continued throughout. The following indices were determined for each group of each generation: fertility, total pups born, mean litter size, pup survival and body weight from birth to weaning, sex ratio, liver and kidney weights, and cytogenetic evaluation of bone marrow cells. In addition, gross autopsy, including organ weight, of F1 and F2 parents, and histopathology of weanling livers and kidneys, and tissues of representative F1 and F2 parents, was carried out. No adverse effects of exposure to styrene in the drinking water were seen.

Fabry *et al.* (1978) have carried out a dominant lethal test in mice of styrene oxide, the major metabolite of styrene. Groups of approximately 17 males were injected with styrene oxide at 0 or 250 mg/kg i.p. (A dose of 500 mg/kg killed all mice within hours, 250 mg/kg killed few). After injection each male was caged with 3 untreated females which were replaced with fresh females each week for 3 weeks. The females were killed 17 days after caging with the male, and the numbers pregnant, corpora lutea, implantations, live and dead fetuses were counted. There were no significant differences between treated and control groups in any of these indices. Thus a single 250 mg/kg dose of styrene oxide has no effect on fertility and no dominant lethal effects at post-meiotic stages of the sperm cycle. Premeiotic stages were not studied as mating was discontinued after the third week.

D. PREGNANCY

The embryolethality and teratogenicity of styrene has been evaluated in a number of species, but the methodology employed in some studies was poor.

Ponomarkov and Tomatis (1978) have given 3 different strains of mouse styrene on day 17 of pregnancy. A single dose of 300 mg/kg orally by gavage in C57BL mice had no effect on litter size or pre-weaning mortality. A dose of 1350 mg/kg orally by gavage in 020 or BD IV mice had no effect on litter size, but preweaning mortality was increased from 22% in controls to 43% in treated 020 mice and from 2·5% in controls to 10% in treated BD IV mice.

Kankaanpää *et al.* (1980) have exposed mice and Chinese hamsters to styrene by inhalation. Groups of 15 mice were exposed to 0 or 250 ppm for 6 h/day from days 6–16 of pregnancy. There were no significant effects on implants/dam or live fetuses/dam, but resorption rate was significantly increased from 18·2% in controls to 26·9% at 250 ppm. Fetuses were examined externally for malformations, then decapitated and the head examined for cleft palate, and the decapitated trunks examined for skeletal defects. There was no examination of internal soft tissue malformations nor skull bone defects. One control fetus was malformed (exteriorisation of the liver) and 3 treated fetuses were malformed (rib fusion, extra ribs). This difference is not significant. Exposure of mice to high concentrations of 500 and 750 ppm caused a dose-related increase in maternal toxicity and resorptions; at 500 ppm 2/6 dams died and the resorption rate was 47% in the 4 remaining pregnancies, and at 750 ppm 3/5 dams died and the remaining 2 had 95% resorptions.

Kankaapää *et al.* (1980) exposed Chinese hamsters to 300, 500, 750 or 1000 ppm for 6 h/day from days 6–18 of pregnancy. The numbers of litters/group were 15 (controls), 2 (300 ppm), 3 (500 ppm), 5 (750 ppm), and 7 (1000 ppm). There were no significant effects on implants/dam, live fetuses/dam or resorptions/dam up to 750 ppm. At 1000 ppm, however, 66% of implants were resorbed compared with 26% in controls. Examination of the fetuses covered external appearance and skeletal structure of the trunk and limbs only. No malformations were found in any group.

No information on maternal weight gain in pregnancy or fetal body weight at term was given for either species, but the authors state that Chinese hamsters tolerate styrene well and that the embryotoxicity observed at 250 ppm in the mouse and 1000 ppm in the Chinese hamster is not solely due to maternal toxicity. Due to inadequate teratological methods, the teratogenic potential of styrene in these species cannot be evaluated from this study.

Ragule (1974) has investigated prenatal and postnatal mortality following exposure to 0·35 ppm (1·5 mg/m^3), 1·18 ppm (5 mg/m^3) or 11·8 ppm (50 mg/m^3) by inhalation in the rat. The daily duration of exposure is not stated (possibly continuous). In the first experiment rats were exposed to 0 (15 animals), 1·18 (23 animals) or 11·8 ppm (23 animals) for the whole of pregnancy. It is not clear whether some rats were killed before term and some allowed to litter out or whether all were allowed to litter out. From the results reported, the former would appear to be the case. In those exposed to 11·8 ppm pre-implantation losses were increased to 20·7% from 3·6% in controls, and total embryomortality (not defined) to 25·2% compared with 15·5% in controls. The number of stillbirths was significantly increased from 0 in controls to 0·2 in 1·18 and 11·8 ppm groups; however, the text does not explain what these figures refer to—presumably they are litter means. Similarly, postnatal deaths in the second week of life were significantly increased from 0 in controls to 0·6 at 1·18 ppm and 1·7 at 11·8 ppm. The text also stated that no abnormalities in "embryonic development" were seen using the Wilson slicing technique but it is not stated whether the material examined was obtained before term by Caesarian section or postnatally.

In Ragule's second experiment groups of 20 rats were exposed to 0, 0·35 or 1·18 ppm throughout gestation or for the first third of pregnancy. All females were killed on day 21. Pre-implantation deaths were significantly increased in all groups exposed to styrene (no details given). Post-implantation losses (resorptions/dam) were significantly increased from 0·0 in controls to 0·2 at 0·35 ppm and 1·3 at 1·18 ppm, in those exposed throughout gestation. In those exposed during the first third of pregnancy, it was significantly increased from 0·0 in controls to 0·7 at 1·18 ppm. Total embryonic mortality (not defined) was not significantly increased in those exposed to 0·35 ppm for the first third of or the whole of pregnancy. Fetal size and weight was significantly reduced in those exposed to 1·18 ppm throughout gestation but not in those exposed during the first third of pregnancy and not in either of the 0·35 ppm groups. Results of toxicity studies on the dams, described in the methods, were not given, and there was no mention of examination of fetuses for malformations in this second study.

In summary, these experiments indicate a clear increase in prenatal mortality (principally pre-implantation losses) and a possible increase in postnatal mortality following exposure to 11·8 ppm throughout gestation but equivocal effects after exposure to 1·18 and 0·35 ppm throughout gestation. In the 1·18 ppm groups, common to both experiments, effects on pre-implantation and post-implantation losses were not replicated; in the first experiment they were not significantly different from controls and in the second they were. The absence of any pre-implantation losses, resorptions, stillbirths or postnatal deaths in the 35 control animals used in these experiments is remarkably unusual. Until the reliability of this control data can be established, the small increases in prenatal and postnatal mortality seen in some 0·35 ppm and 1·18 ppm groups cannot be taken as proof of styrene's toxicity at these levels.

Vergieva *et al.* (1979) have reported absence of any significant effects in the rat after exposure of animals between days 2 and 21 of pregnancy to 47 ppm (200 mg/m^3) or between days 2 and 16 of pregnancy to 165 ppm (700 mg/m^3) for 4 h/day, 5 days/week. The numbers of pre-implantation losses, post-implantation losses and malformations were recorded in some dams killed just before term. In others, allowed to litter out, postnatal survival, weight gain, liver function and behaviour were assessed. No significant differences between treated and control groups were found, except for raised haemoglobin and red blood cell counts in both mothers and offspring one month after birth.

Murray *et al.* (1978) have studied the teratogenic potential of styrene in the rat and the rabbit. Acceptable teratological methods were used. Groups of 29–39 rats were exposed to 0, 300 or 600 ppm of styrene by inhalation for 7 h/day, or given 0, 180 or 300 mg/kg/day orally by gavage in 2 daily divided doses, on days 6–15 of pregnancy. In the 300 ppm group one dam died and was found to be aborting on day 20 of pregnancy and one dam delivered her litter early on day 21, but no deaths or early deliveries occurred in the control, 600 ppm or orally dosed groups. Maternal weight gain was significantly reduced in all styrene-treated groups on days 6–9 of pregnancy, but not thereafter. Food consumption at this time was reduced in treated groups and water consumption was increased in 300 and 600 ppm groups on days 9–20 of pregnancy. There were no significant, dose-related effects on implants/dam, live fetuses/dam, resorptions/dam, fetal body weight, or malformations. Gross external, soft tissue and skeletal abnormalities were seen in treated and control groups, but only skeletal variants (e.g. lumbar spurs, delayed ossification) occurred in styrene-exposed litters at an incidence significantly greater than controls: however, the incidence was within the range seen in historical controls.

In the rabbit study (Murray *et al.*, 1978) groups of 20 does were exposed to 0, 300 or 600 ppm styrene by inhalation for 7 h/day on days 6–18 of pregnancy. There were no maternal deaths and one control doe and one 600 ppm doe delivered prematurely. There were no significant effects on maternal weight gain, implants/doe, live fetuses/doe, resorptions/doe or fetal body weight. No major malformations were found but there was a significant increase in the skeletal variant of unossified fifth sternebra at 600 ppm compared with concurrent controls. However the incidence was within the range seen in historical controls.

In summary, these experiments showed no effects in the rabbit at doses not toxic to the mother, or in the rat at the same doses which were toxic to the mother, except for an increase in the frequency of skeletal variants.

Conclusion

At doses not toxic to the mother, substantial increases in resorption rate have been seen in the mouse at 250 ppm and the Chinese hamster at 1000 ppm, but not in the rat or rabbit, with exposure during embryogenesis. With exposure commencing on day 1 of pregnancy, one study has found increased pre-implantation losses in rats exposed to 11·8 ppm, but another study using 47 and 165 ppm found no effect. At maternally toxic doses there was a clear increase in resorption rate in the mouse but not in the rat. In the one study where adequate teratological methods were used, no increases in gross malformations were seen in the rat or the rabbit exposed to 300 or 600 ppm by inhalation or after 180 or 300 mg/kg orally in the rat. Skeletal variants were increased in the rat after 300 or 600 ppm and in the rabbit after 600 ppm, but increases were within historical control ranges. There was no effect on fetal weight. Thus styrene may be embryolethal at high doses in animals particularly resistant to the general toxic effects of styrene, but it does not appear to be teratogenic on the limited data available.

E. MUTAGENICITY

Styrene is mutagenic in the Ames test with metabolic activation (IARC Monograph Vol. 19, 1979). Cytogenicity tests on mouse cells have been carried out using styrene and styrene oxide. Černá and Kypěnová (1977) gave single or repeated injections over 5 consecutive days of styrene i.p. at a dose of $\frac{1}{2}$ LD50. Analysis of bone marrow cells taken 6, 24 or 48 h after the last injection showed no increase in chromosomal aberrations in comparison with controls. Fabry *et al.* (1978) gave a single i.p. injection of 250 mg/kg styrene oxide to mice and took samples of bone marrow cells, polychromatic erythrocytes (micronucleus test) and spermatocytes. In a total of 757 bone marrow cells taken at invervals of 1, 2, 6 and 13 days after injection, only one chromatid break was seen. Erythrocytes taken 30 h after injection had no significant increase in micronuclei compared with controls. Spermatocytes taken 11 weeks after injection showed no increase in reciprocal translocations in pre-meiotic cells. These same males showed no increase in post-meiotic dominant lethal mutations (see section C for details). However, mating after injection in the dominant lethal test only lasted for 3 weeks, and the 11-week gap between injection and sampling of the spermatocytes together with the short sperm cycle in the mouse of around 5 weeks would mean that effects on late spermatogonia and early spermatocytes would be missed. Whilst an effect as specific as this would be unusual, it cannot be ruled out.

Detoxification of a potential mutagen such as styrene oxide depends on the activity of microsomal epoxide hydrase (EH) and glutathione-S-transferase (GSH-S-T). The possible importance of such detoxification reactions in the testis have been investigated by Mukhtar *et al.* (1978). In the rat, testicular GSH-S-T activity has reached 50% of the adult level by 6 days of age and is 3–4 times higher than hepatic GSH-S-T activity. EH activity in liver and testes is low prepubertally but increases dramatically at puberty and has reached maximum by 45 days of age. In adult rat testes, GSH-S-T and EH activities are twice as high in germ cells as in interstitial cells. Thus the germ cells may be relatively protected from styrene oxide toxicity.

De Raat (1978) has investigated the potential of styrene and styrene oxide to induce sister chromatid exchanges (SCE) in Chinese hamster ovary cells *in vitro*. Styrene oxide was a potent inducer of SCE. Styrene itself did not increase SCE unless a metabolic activation system was added (rat liver homogenate, S9 fraction) together with an inhibitor of epoxide hydrases, suggesting sufficient styrene oxide could be generated under these circumstances to induce SCE.

F. CARCINOGENICITY

IARC Monograph Vol. 19 (1979) reported a study showing styrene was carcinogenic in the mouse but not in the rat following oral administration.

HUMAN STUDIES

A. RELEVANT PHARMACOLOGY AND TOXICOLOGY

No relevant data found.

B. ENDOCRINE AND GONADAL EFFECTS

Pokrovskii (1967) quotes results of an early investigation carried out by his institute on over 200 women exposed continually to styrene in a concentration of 20–128 mg/m^3 (i.e. about 5–30 ppm). During their first year of exposure 21% had disturbances of the menstrual cycle but the incidence declined with duration of exposure though some individuals developed more serious symptoms. No further details or any control values are given.

Zlobina *et al.* (1975) studied a group of 110 women involved in polystyrene processing in the Zhilevskiy Plastics plant, which is described as using very modern machinery and methods so that the women workers were exposed to very low concentration of styrene (unspecified) close to the MAC (MAC in Czechoslovakia is 200 mg/m^3 = 48 ppm). The women however spend about half of the working time in cabins maintained at 37–38°C. Investigations consisted of questionnaires, medical records and detailed gynaecological examinations. The experimental group of 110 women was compared with a control group of 231 women workers from plant management and the childrens' group who had had no previous exposure to industrial chemicals. The 2 groups were matched for age, education, income, number of children and a number of other social factors. Analysis of non-genital disease showed a higher incidence of gastro-intestinal disease in the experimental group.

The results of the gynaecological examination showed no significant difference between the groups with respect to inflammatory disease of the vagina or cervix, infertility or benign tumours. There was a significantly higher incidence in the experimental group however of inflammatory disease of the uterus and tubes (12·7% versus 4·7%) and of menstrual disorders (29% versus 9%), mainly of irregularity of rhythm and hypermenstrual syndrome, especially in the older (30–40 year) age group. Ten of the women with menstrual dysfunction were examined in more detail by an unclear method (possibly smears) and 7 showed moderate to severe oestrogen insufficiency. From comparison with studies carried out by the authors on rats, they suggest that the menstrual changes in women exposed to the MAC level of styrene may be related to changes in pituitary function.

A group of 25 male workers in a synthetic rubber plant at an unspecified site (probably the Netherlands) and who were exposed to low (unmeasured) levels of styrene, were compared with 28 unexposed technical and administrative staff of the same plant (Wink, 1972). Urine levels were measured of 17-oxogenic steroids (mainly of adrenal origin) and 17-oxosteroids (of adrenal and testicular origin). Only the mean ± S.D. values for the group were given: 17-oxogenic steroids 783 ± 398 μg/hour and 649 ± 230 μg/hour for exposed and controls respectively. Neither of these differences are significant ($P > 0{\cdot}05$). The overall methodology was felt by the authors to be inadequate but of sufficient interest to warrant further study.

C. FERTILITY

No relevant data found.

D. PREGNANCY

Zlobina *et al.* (1975) studied reproductive histories in 67 women exposed to low levels of styrene in a polystyrene fabrication plant compared with an unexposed control group of 70 women from the management side of the same plant. Number of pregnancies, births, induced and spontaneous abortions were recorded and no significant differences were found between the groups (no details given of numbers). Toxicosis was reported more frequently in the first half of pregnancy in the exposed women (49% versus 19%), and nephropathy (no definition) was observed more frequently in the exposed group in the second half of pregnancy (10·4% versus 1·4%).

No large epidemiological studies on the possible teratogenicity of styrene have been carried out. However, Holmberg (1977) published an interesting report of a study in Finland in which all mothers of children with reported C.N.S. defects during 1976–77 were interviewed, along with a control chosen as the mother whose delivery immediately preceded the affected birth in the clinic. The interviewer asked about exposure to noxious influences at work. In all, 43 case mothers were interviewed and 2 of them worked in the reinforced plastics industry and were exposed to styrene, polyester resin, organic peroxides and acetone. The exposure was verified by visits to the factories, but no measurements taken. One mother had bronchitis in the third month of pregnancy and received penicillin, the other mother had contractions in the second month and was treated with isoxuprine for one week. Both worked during most of their pregnancies. From the fact that at that time about 250 women of childbearing age were employed in the reinforced plastics industry and the national annual fertility rate was 65 per 1000, 16 births would be expected per year or 12 births during the 9 month period of study. Since the rate of anencephaly and hydrocephalus was 0·5 per 1000, the observation of 2 such births in 12 is 300 times the expected rate. Such coincidences can and do, of course, occur by chance and no conclusion can be drawn from this study. There is not even clear evidence that the women were in fact exposed to styrene at the critical time for induction of the defects. However, the author felt the cases worth reporting.

In a report of the continuation of this study over 2 years (Holmberg, 1979) a total of 120 cases of C.N.S. defects and their controls were studied. One further case exposed to styrene was included but she was an insulin-dependent diabetic who would be expected to have an increased risk of a malformed child. There was however a significant difference ($P < 0{\cdot}01$) in the number of case mothers who were exposed to "organic solvents" in the first trimester (14/120) compared with controls (3/120). Twelve of the case mothers were exposed at work and 2 at home from use in handicrafts; the 3 controls were exposed at work. It is difficult to assess the significance of this report because of the wide variety of "organic solvents" involved—acetone, alcohol, benzene, ethylene oxide, ether, petrol, styrene, white spirit, toluene, xylene, etc., each appearing usually in only one or 2 cases with white spirit being the commonest—present in 4 cases. The larger Russian study referred to above (Zlobina *et al.* 1975) made no mention of malformations in the 67 pregnancies in which the mothers were exposed to low levels of styrene, though if there had been a high incidence of C.N.S. defects it would seem likely to have been reported.

E. MUTAGENICITY

A number of studies have demonstrated that styrene and styrene oxide are mutagenic to human lymphocytes *in vitro* (Linnainmaa *et al.*, 1978a, 1978b; Fabry *et al.*, 1978). It has been convincingly demonstrated that there is an increase in chromosomal damage, mostly breaks, in workers exposed to high environmental levels of styrene even for short periods of a few months (Meretoja *et al.*, 1977, 1978; Bardodej, 1978; Fleig and Thiess, 1978). However, in styrene and polystyrene production plants where the styrene is produced and kept in sealed containers, and the environmental contamination is very low, then no increase in chromosomal damage may be found in workers even after many years of exposure (Thiess and Fleig, 1978).

F. CARCINOGENICITY

IARC Monograph Vol. 19 (1979) stated that no case reports or epidemiological studies on carcinogenicity in humans were available for evaluation.

SUMMARY AND EVALUATION

EXPERIMENTAL STUDIES

Styrene is highly fat soluble and although no experimental studies have been found, it would be expected to cross the placenta and into milk. Limited studies in rats have shown that inhalation of around 1 ppm can alter gonadotrophic function and increase the oestrous phase of the cycles without causing other signs of toxicity. A multigeneration study, in which styrene was administered to rats in drinking water up to 250 ppm, failed to show any adverse effects on reproduction. No dominant lethal activity or adverse effect on fertility was seen in a limited study in mice injected i.p. with 250 mg/kg styrene oxide. Teratological studies have been carried out in mice, rats, hamsters and rabbits and some conflicting results have been obtained. Embryolethal effects have been reported in mice and hamsters at doses not toxic to the dams, but not in rats and rabbits. Satisfactory studies in rats and rabbits exposed to up to 600 ppm by inhalation or 300 mg/kg orally in rats showed no embryolethality or teratogenicity. Styrene is mutagenic with activation, *in vitro* but not *in vivo*. It is carcinogenic in mice but not in rats.

HUMAN STUDIES

There is limited evidence that exposure of women to around 30 ppm styrene may induce menstrual cycle irregularities possibly due to suppressed oestrogen levels. No studies on fertility were found in males. No effects on numbers of pregnancies were reported in one study of women workers. An increase in toxic signs in early pregnancy was reported however. There are no adequate reports of teratogenic effects. Chromosomal damage has been reported in workers exposed to high concentrations of styrene even for short periods of a few months. These effects are not seen even after many years if the levels of exposure are low. No studies on carcinogenicity were found.

EVALUATION

Although some effect on oestrous cycles has been reported in rats, most adequate studies have shown that exposure even to moderately toxic levels does not have an adverse effect on fertility or reproduction. Limited studies have shown that it is not teratogenic in animals.

Human data is inadequate for evaluation. Studies on menstrual cycles in exposed women are required to confirm or deny the reported effects. Attention is drawn to the lack of adequate human data.

References

Bardodej, Z. (1978). Styrene, its metabolism and the evaluation of hazards in industry. *Scandinavian Journal of Work and Environmental Health* **4**, (Supplement 2), 95–103.

Černá, M. and Kypěnová, H. (1977). Mutagenic activity of chloroethylenes analysed by screening system tests. *Mutation Research* **46**, (3), 214–215.

De Raat, W. K. (1978). Induction of sister chromatid exchanges by styrene and its presumed metabolite styrene oxide in the presence of rat liver homogenate. *Chemical-Biological Interactions* **20**, (2), 163–170.

Fabry, L., Léonard, A. and Roberfroid, M. (1978). Mutagenicity tests with styrene oxide in mammals. *Mutation Research* **51**, (3), 377–381.

Fleig, I. and Thiess, A. M. (1978). Mutagenicity study of workers employed in the styrene and polystyrene processing and manufacturing industry. *Scandinavian Journal of Work and Environmental Health* **4**, (Supplement 2), 254–258.

Harkonen, H. (1978). Styrene, its experimental and clinical toxicology: a review. *Scandinavian Journal of Work and Environmental Health* **4**, (Supplement 2), 104–113.

Holmberg, P. C. (1977). Central nervous defects in two children of mothers exposed to chemicals in the reinforced plastics industry. Chance or causal relation? *Scandinavian Journal of Work and Environmental Health* **3**, (4), 212–214.

Holmberg, P. C. (1979). Central nervous system defects in children born to mothers exposed to organic solvents during pregnancy. *Lancet* **ii**, 177–179.

IARC Monographs on the Evaluation of the Carcinogenic Risk of Chemicals to Humans: Some monomers, plastics and synthetic elastomers and acrolein (1979). Vol. 19, Lyon, France.

Izyumova, A. S. (1972). The action of small concentrations of styrol on the sexual function of albino rats. *Gigiena I Sanitariya* **37**, (4), 29–30.

Kankaanpää, J. T. J., Elovaara, E., Hemminki, K. and Vainio, H. (1980). The effect of maternally inhaled styrene on embryonal and foetal development in mice and Chinese hamsters. *Acta Pharmacologia et Toxicologia* **47**, (2), 127–129.

Linnainmaa, K., Meretoja, T., Sorsa, M. and Vainio, H. (1978a). Cytogenic effects of styrene and styrene oxide. *Mutation Research* **58**, (2/3), 277–286.

Linnainmaa, K., Meretoja, T., Sorsa, M. and Vainio, H. (1978b). Cytogenic effects of styrene and styrene oxide on human lymphocytes and Allim cepa. *Scandinavian Journal of Work and Environmental Health* **4**, (Supplement 2), 156–162.

Manufacturing Chemists Association, Washington, D.C., U.S.A. (1979). Toxicological study on styrene incorporated in drinking water of rats for two years in conjunction with a three-generation reproduction study.

Meretoja, T., Jarventaus, H., Sorsa, M. and Vainio, H. (1978). Chromosome aberrations in lymphocytes of workers exposed to styrene. *Scandinavian Journal of Work and Environmental Health* **4**, (Supplement 2), 259–264.

Meretoja, T., Vainio, H., Sorsa, M. and Harkonen, H. (1977). Occupational styrene exposure and chromosomal aberrations. *Mutation Research* **56**, 193–197.

Mukhtar, H., Lee, I. P., Foureman, G. L. and Bend, J. R. (1978). Epoxide metabolizing enzyme activities in rat testes: postnatal development and relative activity in interstitial and spermatogenic cell compartments. *Chemical-Biological Interactions* **22**, (2–3), 153–165.

Murray, F. J., John, J. A., Balmer, M. F. and Schwetz, B. A. (1978). Teratologic evaluation of styrene given to rats and rabbits by inhalation or by gavage. *Toxicology* **11**, 335–343.

Pokrovskii, V. A. (1967). Peculiarities of the effect produced by some organic poisons on the female organism. *Gigiena Truda I Professional 'Nye Zabolevaniya* **11**, (2), 17–20.

Ponomarkov, V. and Tomatis, L. (1978). Effects of long-term oral administration of styrene to mice and rats. *Scandinavian Journal of Work and Environmental Health* **4**, (Supplement 2), 127–135.

Ragule, N. Y. (1974). Embryotropic action of styrene. *Gigiena I Sanitariya* (11), 85–86.

Ramsey, J. C. and Young, J. D. (1978). Pharmacokinetics of inhaled styrene in rats and humans. *Scandinavian Journal of Work and Environmental Health* **4**, (Supplement 2), 84–91.

Thiess, A. M. and Fleig, I. (1978). Chromosome investigations on workers exposed to styrene/polystyrene. *Journal of Occupational Medicine* **20**, (11), 747–749.

Vergieva, T., Zaikov, H. and Palatovv, S. (1979). A study on the embryotoxic action of Styrol. *Khigiena i Zdraveopazvane* **22**, (1), 39–43.
Wink, A. (1972). Effect of long-term exposure to low levels of toxic substances on urinary excretion of 17-oxogenic steroids and 17-oxosteroids. *Annals of Occupational Hygiene* **15**, 211–215.
Withey, J. R. (1978). The toxicology of styrene monomer and its pharmacokinetics and distribution in the rat. *Scandinavian Journal of Work and Environmental Health* **4**, (Supplement 2), 31–40.
Zlobina, N. S., Izyumova, A. S. and Ragule, N. Y. (1975). The effect of low styrene concentrations on the specific functions of the female organism. *Gigiena Truda I Professional 'Nye Zabolevaniya* (12), 21–25.

39. Tellurium and its Compounds

TECHNICAL DATA

(a) *Tellurium*

Formula Te

CAS registry number 13494–80–9

Chemical abstracts name Tellurium

Synonyms aurum paradoxum; metallum problematum

(b) *Tellurium compounds*

Formula	CAS registry number	Chemical abstracts name
$Te(OH)_6$	7803–68–1	Telluric (VI) acid
$TeBr_2$	7789–54–0	Tellurium dibromide
$TcCl_2$	10025–71–5	Tellurium dichloride
TeO_2	7446–07–3	Tellurium dioxide
TeF_6	7783–80–4	Tellurium hexafluoride
$TcBr_4$	10031–27–3	Tellurium tetrabromide
$TeCl_4$	10026–07–0	Tellurium tetrachloride
TeI_4	7790–48–9	Tellurium tetraiodide
H_2TeO_3	10049–23–7	Tellurous acid

Uses Colouring agent in chinaware, porcelains, enamels, glass; reagent in producing black finish on silverware; manufacture of special alloys with marked electrical resistance; semiconductor research.

TLV 0·1 mg/m^3 (as tellurium).

ANIMAL STUDIES

A. RELEVANT PHARMACOLOGY AND TOXICOLOGY

Metallic tellurium is insoluble, poorly absorbed and not very toxic when given orally, but in contact with water it forms tellurous acid which is easily absorbed in the intestine. Other tellurium salts are also soluble and toxic (Agnew *et al.*, 1968).

Placental transfer of tellurium has been demonstrated by a number of workers, and penetration into the fetal brain has been studied in some detail since prenatal exposure specifically induces hydrocephalus in the offspring whereas exposure of the adult does not (see section D).

Agnew *et al.* (1968) were the first to show placental transfer to tellurium. They gave i.v. injections of tellurous acid containing radioactive tellurium to pregnant rats, 2 or 3 days before term. Maternal and fetal/newborn blood and tissue levels were measured at 4 h and 1 week after the maternal injection. By 4 h, small amounts of radioactivity were detected in fetal plasma and brain, and slightly larger amounts in the fetal liver and kidney. However, uptake into the fetal brain was 5–10-fold higher than uptake into maternal brain, relative to their surrounding plasma levels. At 1 week, neonatal levels were much higher than the fetal levels at 4 h.

Duckett and Ellem (1971) also injected rats i.v. with radioactive tellurium as tellurous acid on days 12–20 of pregnancy and studied its penetration and distribution in the fetus by whole body radioactivity counts and radioautographs of body sections. Tellurium penetrated into the fetal choroid plexus vessels within 1–2 min of injection into the mother. Between 1 and 30 min after injection, the concentration of tellurium was 1–5% of that in the placenta, suggesting rather slow placental transfer. The slow transfer is perhaps not surprising since in the adult (and fetus) it is rapidly bound to plasma and red blood cell proteins (Agnew and Cheng, 1971), thus only limited amounts of unbound tellurium are available for transfer. The binding may also account for its very slow elimination from adults and fetuses (Agnew *et al.*, 1968). Agnew and Cheng (1971) have also suggested that binding to protein may detoxify tellurium.

Duckett and Ellem (1971) observed tellurium in the fetal telencephalon, the site of origin of the postnatal hydrocephalus, at 12 and 15 days' gestation. They speculated that it reaches the telencephalic parenchyma by passing from the blood vessels inside the choroid plexus, through the epithelial layer of the choroid plexus into the ventricle and thence through the germinal layer into the telencephalic parenchyma, there being no internal vasculature at this stage. By 15 days' gestation, when there is an internal vasculature, tellurium is found throughout the telencephalon within 2 min of maternal injection, presumably penetrating the parenchyma directly from the blood vessels. It is also found in the parenchyma of all other fetal organs but apparently exerts its major teratogenic effect on the telencephalon.

Further study of the distribution of radioactive tellurium in the rat fetus at different stages of gestation has been carried out by Agnew (1972). Rats were injected i.p. with tellurous acid on one of days 7–11, 14, 15, 17 or 20 and the fetuses removed 24 h after the maternal injection. Radioactivity counts indicated that passage of tellurium into the embryo and fetus decreased with advancing gestation. At 8–11 days, whole embryo:maternal blood ratios were around 0·3 but by days 12–21 averaged only 0·16. Placental tellurium levels on days 12–21 were similar to those of maternal blood which is not surprising in view of its tight binding to blood proteins. The distribution of tellurium within the embryo and fetus was studied by radioautography. At 9–11 days' gestation, tellurium was concentrated in the periphery of the yolk sac cavity, but could also be seen in the neural tube cells. By days 12–15, there was preferential deposition in the fetal liver. By day 18, high uptake into the choroid plexus and low uptake into the rest of the brain was particularly striking. The author noted that penetration into the fetal CNS decreased with increasing gestational age, findings which may be relevant to the time for maximal sensitivity to tellurium-induced hydrocephalus on days 9–10 (see section D).

Conclusion

Placental transfer of tellurium given as tellurous acid has been shown in rats, with high uptake into the fetal brain, the main teratogenic target for tellurium (see section D). However, placental transfer is slow, probably due to binding of tellurium to red blood cell proteins in the maternal circulation.

B. ENDOCRINE AND GONADAL EFFECTS

No relevant data found.

C. FERTILITY

No relevant data found.

D. PREGNANCY

Garro and Pentschew (1964) were the first workers to report that prenatal exposure to tellurium caused postnatal hydrocephalus. Long-Evans strain rats were fed diets containing 500–2500 ppm tellurium throughout pregnancy and switched back onto normal diet 3–5 days before delivery or immediately after delivery. Hydrocephalus developed in "over 200" of the offspring (the number of dams in each group was not stated). At 2500 ppm, 100% of the offspring developed hydrocephalus, at 1250 ppm 60–90% developed hydrocephalus and at 500 ppm a lower, unspecified proportion developed hydrocephalus and not all members of the litter were affected. At birth the offspring were smaller than controls (no data given) and the hydrocephalus could be demonstrated within 2 h of birth, reaching a maximum at 3 weeks of age with 99% lethality within one month. The pathogenesis of the hydrocephalus was obscure, since they could find no obstructive lesions or malformations of the ventricular system. Others have confirmed the effects of tellurium in the diet in rats, albeit finding a lower incidence of hydrocephalus than Garro and Pentschew. Agnew *et al.* (1968) found that 1250 or 2500 ppm in the diet throughout pregnancy (4 dams per group) failed to produce hydrocephalus in the Wistar rat, but 3300 ppm did. In 10 treated litters, 36/77 offspring developed hydrocephalus. Two of the litters had no affected pups, other litters a variable number. Anatomical studies confirmed that it was an internal communicating type of hydrocephalus.

Duckett (1971) fed 3000 ppm metallic tellurium in the diet throughout pregnancy in the Wistar rat, resulting in 20/24 litters developing hydrocephalus (100% affected in these 20 litters) and 30/237 offspring being stillborn. No control data were given. At 3 days of age, 179/237 were hydrocephalic and 66% of the affected pups did not survive beyond 10 days. Whilst confirming that the hydrocephalus began as a communicating, non-obstructive type, Duckett noted that within about 5 days it had converted into the obstructive type, with closure of the sub-arachnoid space due to increasing pressure of CSF and/or closure of the cerebral aqueduct. Duckett (1976) has also reported early changes in the fetal brain after feeding 3000 ppm in the diet throughout pregnancy. At 13 and 15 days' gestation fetuses from treated dams were similar to controls except for morphological abnormalities in the ependymal layer of the telencephalon; there was absence of the normally abundant microvilli and the mitochondria were greatly reduced in number, some small with distorted cristae.

Two studies have delineated the susceptible period during gestation for induction of hydrocephalus in the offspring. Duckett *et al.* (1971) fed tellurium in the diet at 2500 ppm on days 1–9, 10–15 or 16–21 of pregnancy (20 rats per group). Hydrocephalic offspring were only seen after prenatal exposure on days 10–15 of pregnancy; 12/20 litters had affected individuals with an average of 5/9 pups affected. Feeding 2500 ppm for one day only on one of days 10–15 failed to produce hydrocephalus. However, Agnew and

Curry (1972) did obtain hydrocephalus after treatment on single days, giving tellurium by i.m. injection (13 mg/kg). Injecting on one of days 7–13, hydrocephalus was seen after treatment on day 9 (19% of offspring affected) or day 10 (31% affected). With treatment on other days, hydrocephalus was only seen in one pup treated on day 7 and in one control pup. They suggested that tellurium is better absorbed parenterally than orally and so single parenteral administrations are sufficient to cause hydrocephalus.

Studies on species other than the rat have been few. Garro and Pentschew (1964) reported a pilot experiment on 3 pregnant rabbits injected with metallic tellurium (time, dose and route not stated), in which 12/16 offspring which survived had "definite disturbance of equilibrium with ataxia" for about 3 months. These neurological symptoms subsided and disappeared in all but one animal. James *et al.* (1966) gave potassium tellurate to 4 pregnant ewes. They were given 2 mg/kg/day, orally from day 1 of pregnancy, for 45–151 days. All 4 lambs were normal at birth. However, they were unable to detect any tellurium in the tissues of ewes or lambs after birth.

Conclusion

In none of the studies on tellurium have malformations other than hydrocephalus been mentioned, though some studies specifically noted the absence of any other abnormalities. However, since in all the studies to date dams were allowed to litter out, grossly abnormal pups may have been eaten at birth by the dams. These studies therefore are not adequate evidence of lack of any other teratogenic effects at hydrocephalus-inducing doses or lower doses. One study reported an incidence of stillbirths, but in the absence of control data the significance of this is difficult to evaluate. However, clearly the telencephalon is the major target organ for tellurium damage. Although the defect is not obvious until after birth there is evidence from the timed insult experiments and early fetal brain changes that the primary lesion(s) are induced prenatally. However, it is also possible that continued postnatal exposure may contribute to the severity of the lesion. Tellurium is only cleared very slowly from the body due to its tight binding to blood proteins and could be passed across to the offspring in the milk for some time after removal of tellurium from the dam's diet. These studies on tellurium in the rat illustrate the importance of postnatal evaluation of prenatal exposure to compounds, since conventional teratological examination of near-term fetuses would almost certainly have failed to detect any adverse effects of tellurium on the brain.

E. MUTAGENICITY

No relevant data found.

F. CARCINOGENICITY

No relevant data found.

HUMAN STUDIES

A. RELEVANT PHARMACOLOGY AND TOXICOLOGY

No relevant data found.

B. ENDOCRINE AND GONADAL EFFECTS

No relevant data found.

C. FERTILITY

No relevant data found.

D. PREGNANCY

No relevant data found.

E. MUTAGENICITY

Paton and Allison (1972) have studied the effect of addition of tellurium salts to human lymphocyte cultures *in vitro*. Ammonium tellurate or sodium tellurite was added in doses sufficient to cause toxicity, manifested by a marked reduction in mitotic index. Sub-toxic doses were then added to cultured lymphocytes for 48 h and these were then examined for chromosome breaks. Ammonium tellurate, at $2{\cdot}4 \times 10^{-7}$ M concentration, resulted in 13% of cells having breaks compared with 2% in untreated controls ($P < 0{\cdot}05$). Sodium tellurite, at a concentration of $1{\cdot}2 \times 10^{-8}$ M, caused a small but non-significant increase in the frequency of breaks to 8%. Thus there is evidence that tellurium salts can cause chromosome damage to human cells in culture.

F. CARCINOGENICITY

No relevant data found.

SUMMARY AND EVALUATION

EXPERIMENTAL STUDIES

Tellurium has been shown to cross the placenta in rats with high uptake into the brain and liver of the fetus. Due to binding to red cells in the maternal circulation equilibration between the mother and fetus is very slow. No studies were found on endocrine or gonadal effects or of effects on fertility. When fed in the diet at levels around 2500 ppm (about 120 mg/kg body weight) to rats, a very high incidence of hydrocephalus is produced in the offspring. In one study effects were also observed at dietary levels of 500 ppm, so a no-effect level is not clearly established. Studies in other species are inadequate to assess teratogenicity.

No studies were found on mutagenicity or carcinogenicity.

HUMAN STUDIES

No studies were found on endocrine or gonadal effects or of effects on fertility or pregnancy. There is limited evidence that tellurium can cause chromosome damage to lymphocytes *in vitro*. No studies on mutagenicity *in vivo* were found nor studies on carcinogenicity.

EVALUATION

There is sufficient evidence that tellurium is teratogenic in rats and a no-effect level has not been established. Attention is drawn to the high teratogenic potential in the absence of embryolethal effects in rodents, and to the lack of any relevant human data on reproductive toxicity. Attention is drawn to the lack of data on mutagenicity and carcinogenicity.

References

Agnew, W. F. (1972). Transplacental uptake of 127 m Tellurium studied by whole-body autoradiography. *Teratology* **6**, 331–338.

Agnew, W. F. and Cheng, J. T. (1971). Protein-binding of Tellurium-127 m by maternal and fetal tissues of the rat. *Toxicology and Applied Pharmacology* **20**, 346–356.

Agnew, W. F. and Curry, E. (1972). Period of teratogenic vulnerability of rat embryo to induction of hydrocephalus by tellurium. *Experientia* **28**, (12), 1444–1445.

Agnew, W. F., Fauvre, F. M. and Pudenz, P. H. (1968). Tellurium hydrocephalus: distribution of tellurium-127 m between maternal, fetal and neonatal tissues of the rat. *Experimental Neurology* **21**, 120–132.

Duckett, S. (1971). The morphology of tellurium-induced hydrocephalus. *Experimental Neurology* **31**, 1–16.

Duckett, S. (1976). Fetal encephalopathy following ingestion of tellurium. *Experientia* **26**, (11), 1239–1241.

Duckett, S. and Ellem, K. A. D. (1971). Localization of tellurium in fetal tissues, particularly brain. *Experimental Neurology* **32**, 49–57.

Duckett, S., Sandler, A. and Scott, T. (1971). The target period during fetal life for the production of tellurium hydrocephalus. *Experientia* **27**, (9), 1064–1065.

Garro, F. and Pentschew, A. (1964). Neonatal hydrocephalus in the offspring of rats fed during pregnancy non-toxic amounts of tellurium. *Archiv fur Psychiatrie und Nervenkrankheiten* **206**, 272–280.

James, L. F., Lazav, V. A. and Binns, W. (1966). Effects of sublethal doses of certain minerals on pregnant ewes and fetal development. *American Journal of Veterinary Research* **27**, (116), 132–135.

Paton, G. R. and Allison, A. C. (1972). Chromosome damage in human cell cultures induced by metal salts. *Mutation Research* **16**, (3), 332–336.

40. Tetrachloroethylene

TECHNICAL DATA

Formula	$Cl_2C{=}CCl_2$
CAS registry number	127–18–4
Chemical abstracts name	Tetrachloroethylene
Synonyms	Carbon bichloride; carbon dichloride; ethylene tetrachloride; per; perc; perchlor; perchlorethylene; perchloroethylene; perk; tetrachlorethylene; 1,1′,2,2′-tetrachloroethylene.
Uses	Dry cleaning; degreasing metals; solvent.
TLV	100 ppm (skin) (1980 Intended change to 50 ppm).

ANIMAL STUDIES

A. RELEVANT PHARMACOLOGY AND TOXICOLOGY

In rodents, the major metabolite of tetrachloroethylene is trichloroacetic acid, comprising 70–90% of urinary metabolites (Ikeda and Imamura, 1973).

B. ENDOCRINE AND GONADAL EFFECTS

In the rat administration of compounds which inhibit drug-metabolizing enzymes inhibits the metabolism of oestrogens. Tetrachloroethylene is a less potent inhibitor of drug-metabolising enzymes than, for instance, carbon tetrachloride, but it does have a limited capacity to do so (Levin *et al.*, 1970). However, in experiments where 1·2 ml/kg of tetrachloroethylene was given 24 h before administration of oestrone-6,7-H^3, there was no potentiation of the uterotropic action of the oestrone or any increase in the concentration of tritiated oestrone in the uterus, whereas there was potentiation with carbon tetrachloride (Levin *et al.*, 1970). It therefore seems unlikely that tetrachloroethylene alters the rate of metabolism of oestrogens.

C. FERTILITY

No relevant data found.

D. PREGNANCY

Schwetz *et al.* (1975) from the Dow Chemical Company, U.S.A., have exposed rats and mice to 300 ppm tetrachloroethylene for 7 h/day on days 6–15 of pregnancy. The dams were killed just before term and the fetuses examined by acceptable teratological methods but results are given on a per litter basis only. The number of treated animals in each case was 17 and the number of controls (air-exposed) 30 for both rat and mouse studies.

Effects of tetrachloroethylene on the dams varied between species. In the mouse, relative liver weight was significantly increased and the absolute liver weight increased, but not significantly so, with no effect on maternal body weight. In the rat there was a non-significant decrease in absolute and relative liver weights and a significant 4–5% decrease in mean body weight. Food consumption was unaffected.

Effects on the embryo and fetus also differed. In the mouse there was no effect on implantation sites, live fetuses or resorption rates, but mean fetal weight was significantly reduced, 59% of litters containing runts (weight less than 3 standard deviations below the mean) compared with 38% of control litters. Whereas in the rat, the resorption rate was significantly increased from 4% in controls to 9% in the exposed group, whilst fetal body weight was unaffected (mean actually slightly higher than controls).

In the mouse, examination for anomalies revealed an increase in delayed ossification of the skull bones (significant) and of the sternebrae (non-significant), as might be expected from the fetal weight data. There were also significant increases in the incidence of split sternebrae and subcutaneous oedema. No gross malformations were found. In the rat, gross malformations (short tail) were reported but the incidence did not differ significantly from that in controls. There were no other significant differences in soft tissue or skeletal abnormalities.

The results of this study are difficult to assess, partly because no indication of the numbers of fetuses affected within affected litters is given and partly because of the uncertain nature of the "subcutaneous oedema" reported. Exposure to tetrachloroethylene and the concurrent controls were part of a large study on four different solvents; the incidence of subcutaneous oedema in the mouse ranged from 8–59% of litters affected, which seems very high, and whilst the incidence in the tetrachloroethylene group was highest at 59%, it was as high as 45% in non-concurrent controls (27% in concurrent controls). In the rat, the incidence of this particular anomaly also varied enormously between groups from 0% (tetrachloroethylene group) to 28% (trichloroethylene group). It is therefore important to know how strict were the criteria for designation of "subcutaneous oedema" and in particular, whether the designation was made before or after fixing, subcutaneous oedema being a common fixative artefact.

However, the retardation of growth and ossification and the increased incidence of split sternebrae in fetal mice exposed to tetrachloroethylene were clear, unequivocal effects and, in the absence of any effect on maternal body weight, suggest that tetrachloroethylene has some fetotoxicity in the mouse at a level which also exhibits some maternal hepatotoxicity, but has no effect in the rat, where there is no hepatotoxicity at 300 ppm.

The results of a behavioural teratology study in the rat by Nelson *et al.* (1980) on behalf of NIOSH have been reported. Rats were exposed to 0 or 900 ppm tetrachloroethylene for 7 h/day on days 7–13 or 14–20 of pregnancy (9–16 rats per group). The dams were affected by this level, showing reduced food consumption and lower weight gain during exposure, but histopathological examination of the maternal liver and kidney in dams sacrificed on day 21 of pregnancy revealed no abnormalities.

Postnatally, offspring were tested for olfaction, neuromuscular ability, exploratory and circadian activity, aversive and appetitive learning. There was evidence of impaired neuromuscular ability; offspring from dams exposed on days 7–13 were poorer than controls in ascent of a wire mesh screen during the second week of life and were poorer than controls on a rotorod test on one of the 3 days tested in the fourth week of life. Offspring from dams exposed on days 14–20 performed less well in ascent of a wire mesh screen. However, the latter group were consistently superior to controls on the rotorod later in development. Both exposed groups were generally more active in open field tests than controls but only those exposed on days 14–20 of gestation differed significantly from controls. Biochemical analyses of whole brain neurotransmitter levels showed no effects in newborns but significant reductions in acetylcholine levels at 21 days of age in both exposed groups of offspring and reduced dopamine levels at 21 days of age in those from dams exposed on days 7–13. There were no significant differences between exposed and control groups on any other of the tests. Exposure of offspring to 100 ppm on days 14–20 of gestation showed no significant differences from controls on any of the above behavioural tests (Nelson *et al.*, 1980). It was not stated whether neurotransmitter levels were measured in this low-dose group.

Conclusion

In view of these results suggesting some fetotoxicity in the mouse but not the rat at 300 ppm and postnatal effects in the rat at 900 ppm but not 100 ppm, there is a need for further studies at low levels between 900 and 100 ppm to establish a more accurate no-effect-level.

E. MUTAGENICITY

Černá and Kypěnová (1977) have reported absence of mutagenicity in bacteria *in vitro* and no cytogenetic effects on mouse bone marrow cells after either a single i.p. injection ($\frac{1}{2}$ LD50 — actual dose not stated) or 5 consecutive daily injections (each $\frac{1}{6}$ LD50) in animals killed 6, 24 or 48 h after the last injection.

F. CARCINOGENICITY

IARC Monograph Vol. 20 (1979) reported there is limited evidence that tetrachloroethylene is carcinogenic in mice.

HUMAN STUDIES

A. RELEVANT PHARMACOLOGY AND TOXICOLOGY

The biological half-life of tetrachloroethylene in occupationally exposed workers has been studied by Ikeda and Imamura (1973). They measured the urinary excretion of tetrachloroethylene and its metabolites as total trichloro-compounds (the major metabolite is trichloroacetic acid) over the weekend when the workers were not exposed. In 9 men the half-life was $123 \pm 23{\cdot}5$ hours and in 4 women it was $190 \pm 32{\cdot}9$ hours. The difference between the sexes was considered to be unreliable since with such a long half-life (weighted mean = 144 hours i.e. 6 days) only a 20% decrease in metabolites was measured over the 3-day test period, resulting in a wide variation in results.

Tetrachloroethylene is widely distributed throughout the body and passes into breast milk. This may result in damage to the baby. Bagnell and Ellenberger (1977) reported a case of obstructive jaundice in a 6-week-old baby probably due to exposure to tetrachloroethylene. The baby, born at 36 weeks' gestation, weighed 2480 g and was otherwise healthy and not jaundiced. Likewise no abnormalities were detected at routine examination at 5 weeks. However at 6 weeks the baby became jaundiced and had hepatomegaly and direct reacting hyperbilirubinaemia with raised serum enzymes. The father worked in a dry cleaning establishment and frequently suffered signs of toxic exposure to solvents. The mother regularly visited the firm to have lunch with her husband and occasionally had mild dizzy spells after these brief exposures. Measurement of the mother's blood 2 hours after a lunch-time exposure showed a level of tetrachloroethylene of 0·3 mg/100 ml and her breast milk level one hour after the visit was 1·0 mg/100 ml. Without further exposure the milk level fell to 0·3 mg/100 ml. No chlorinated hydrocarbons were detected in her urine. Breast feeding of the baby was discontinued, her condition rapidly improved and by 11 days the serum total bilirubin had fallen from 8·4 mg/100 ml to 1·7 mg/100 ml and the serum enzymes were normal. The baby remained normal during a 2-year follow-up. Liver function tests on the parents were normal despite blood levels of 3 mg/100 ml tetrachloroethylene in the father. Whether babies are much more sensitive to the hepatotoxic effects of tetrachloroethylene or whether some other toxic interaction was involved in this case is not known. More information is required.

B. ENDOCRINE AND GONADAL EFFECTS

No relevant data found.

C. FERTILITY

No relevant data found.

D. PREGNANCY

No relevant data found.

E. MUTAGENICITY

No relevant data found.

F. CARCINOGENICITY

IARC Monograph Vol. 20 (1979) stated that at that time no case reports or epidemiological studies were available for evaluation. Blair *et al.* (1979) from the National Cancer Institute, U.S.A., have carried out a mortality study of 330 former laundry and dry-cleaning workers and demonstrated a significant ($P < 0{\cdot}05$) increase in malignant neoplasms, primarily due to an excess of lung and cervical cancer. The authors emphasize the need for larger studies to confirm or deny this result.

SUMMARY AND EVALUATION

EXPERIMENTAL STUDIES

No studies were found on endocrine or gonadal effects or effects on fertility. There is one study in pregnant mice and rats exposed to 300 ppm during embryogenesis. No adverse effects were observed except for a decreased fetal weight with retarded ossification in the mice. Abnormal postnatal development of rats exposed to 900 ppm but not 100 ppm during pregnancy has also been reported.

It was not found to be mutagenic *in vitro* or *in vivo* in one study but there is limited evidence that it is carcinogenic in mice.

HUMAN STUDIES

Tetrachloroethylene is present in breast milk and one case has been reported of jaundice and liver damage in a baby whose mother was exposed to tetrachloroethylene in a dry cleaning shop and had a milk content of 1·0 mg/100 ml. No other data on reproductive effects were found. There is one report of an increase in cancer incidence in people formerly working in the dry cleaning industry where tetrachloroethylene (as well as other solvents) is used.

EVALUATION

Available data both in animals and humans are inadequate for evaluation. Because of exposure of the general population to tetrachloroethylene used in dry cleaning, attention is drawn to the lack of adequate data.

References

Bagnell, P. C. and Ellenberger, H. A. (1977). Obstructive jaundice due to a chlorinated hydrocarbon in breast milk. *Canadian Medical Association Journal* **117**, 1047–1048.

Blair, A., Decoufle, P. and Grauman, D. (1979). Causes of death among laundry and dry cleaning workers. *American Journal of Public Health* **69**, 508–511.

Černá, M. and Kypěnová, H. (1977). Mutagenic activity of chloroethylenes analysed by screening system tests. *Mutation Research* **46**, (3), 214–215.

IARC Monographs on the Evaluation of the Carcinogenic Risk of Chemicals to Humans: Some halogenated hydrocarbons (1979). Vol. 20, Lyon, France.

Ikeda, M. and Imamura, T. (1973). Biological half-life of trichloroethylene and tetrachloroethylene in human subjects. *International Archiv fur Arbeitsmedizin* **31**, (3), 209–224.

Levin, W., Welch, R. M. and Conney, A. H. (1970). Effect of carbon tetrachloride and other inhibitors of drug metabolism on the metabolism and action of estradiol-17β and estrone in the rat. *Journal of Pharmacology and Experimental Therapeutics* **173**, 247–255.

Nelson, B. K., Taylor, B. J., Setzer, J. V. and Hornung, R. W. (1980). Behavioural teratology of perchloroethylene in rats. *Journal of Environmental Pathology and Toxicology* **3**, 233–250.

Schwetz, B. A., Leong, B. M. J. and Gehring, B. J. (1975). The effect of maternally inhaled trichloroethylene, perchloroethylene, methyl chloroform and methylene chloride on embryonal and fetal development in mice and rats. *Toxicology and Applied Pharmacology* **32**, 84–96.

41. Thallium and its Compounds

TECHNICAL DATA

(a) *Thallium*

Formula Tl

CAS registry number 7440–28–0

Chemical abstracts name Thallium

Synonyms None

(b) *Thallium compounds*

Formula	CAS registry number	Chemical abstracts name
$TL(CH_3COO)$	563–68–8	Thallium acetate
TLBr	7789–40–4	Thallium bromide
TL_2CO_3	6533–73–9	Thallium carbonate
$TlCl_2$	7791–12–0	Thallium chloride
TLF	7789–27–7	Thallium fluoride
TLOH	12026–06–1	Thallium hydroxide
TLI	7790–30–9	Thallium iodide
$TLNO_3$	10102–45–1	Thallium nitrate
TL_2O	1314–12–1	Thallium oxide
TL_2SeO_4	7446–22–2	Thallium selenate
TL_2O_3	1314–32–5	Thallium sesquioxide
TL_2SO_4	7446–18–6	Thallium sulphate
TL_2S	1314–97–2	Thallium sulphide
TLF_3	7783–57–5	Thallium trifluoride

Uses Salts used as rodent poison; semiconductor research; as alloy with mercury for switches and closures operating at subzero temperatures.

TLV 0·1 mg/m^3 (as thallium) (skin).

ANIMAL STUDIES

A. RELEVANT PHARMACOLOGY AND TOXICOLOGY

Several workers have studied the placental transfer of thallium in rodents with different routes of administration. Di Nucci *et al.* (1979) gave a single 25 mg/kg dose of thallium sulphate orally to rats on day 13 of pregnancy and measured maternal, fetal and placental levels 72 h later. Thallium did cross the placenta in appreciable quantities as shown by the maternal:fetal ratio of concentrations in the liver and brain of 0·5 and 0·64 respectively. Levels in the placenta were high, but, in the amniotic fluid were low.

Maternal:fetal ratios (tissues unspecified) of a similar order of magnitude were reported by Gibson *et al.* (1967) following subcutaneous injection of thallium sulphate on day 17 of pregnancy in the mouse or day 18 of pregnancy in the rat. The dams were killed at intervals between 1 h and 24 h after injection. The maternal:fetal ratios at equilibrium conditions were 0·46 in the mouse (8 h) and 0·84 in the rat (16 h). The biological half-life in both species was estimated as 24 h.

However, in a later study, Gibson and Becker (1970) report only very limited placental transfer following intra-arterial infusion of thallium sulphate on day 20 of pregnancy in the rat. Doses ranging from 0·2–6·4 mg/min/kg were infused, the highest dose resulting in some maternal deaths, and maternal blood levels were compared with levels in the whole fetus. By 32 min after the start of the infusion, whole fetus levels were increased but were approximately thirty-fold lower than maternal blood levels, a difference which they did not think could be accounted for by the sequestering of thallium in maternal erythrocytes. Approximately two-thirds of blood thallium is sequestered in this way and thus not available for placental transfer. However, since in their earlier study steady-state equilibrium was not reached for 16 h after s.c. injection in the rat on day 18 of pregnancy, it could be that in this experiment observations were terminated too early at 32 min, before equilibrium was reached. According to their data, between 16 and 32 min, the last 2 sampling points, fetal thallium levels were certainly still rising sharply. Thus transfer of thallium to the fetus might still be substantial in late pregnancy, albeit taking a long time to reach equilibrium.

Placental transfer of thallium has been demonstrated in the cat (Fitzek and Henning, 1976). In a report of a single case of thallium intoxication leading to abortion in a pregnant cat, concentrations 4 days after ingestion of thallium were 11·7 μg/g for the eviscerated fetus compared with tissue concentrations ranging from 1·5–67·7 μg/g in the adult female. Maternal blood concentration was 10·8 μg/g and that of the fetus 11·4 μg/g. The concentration in the fetal heart and lung were particularly high at 51·9 μg/g compared with 16–29 μg/g in the dam. Clearly there is substantial placental transfer of thallium in the cat and the authors suggest that the high concentration in the fetal heart and lungs may have been lethal and precipitated abortion. However, the dose ingested caused death of the dam after 5 days; thus the abortion may have been secondary to the maternal toxicity.

Conclusion

Placental transfer of thallium has been shown in the mouse, rat and cat. Transfer is not rapid, but with equilibration over time, fairly substantial quantities of thallium may be transferred to the fetus.

B. ENDOCRINE AND GONADAL EFFECTS

No relevant data found.

C. FERTILITY

No relevant data found.

D. PREGNANCY

Gibson and Becker (1970) have investigated the embryotoxicity and teratogenicity of thallium in the rat. Thallium sulphate was given i.p. on days 8–10 at 2·5 mg/kg or days 12–14 at 2·5 or 10 mg/kg to normal diet or potassium-deficient diet rats. Potassium administration promotes urinary excretion of thallium and reduces its toxicity in the rat. In this experiment, after administration of 10 mg/kg thallium sulphate on days 12–14 to potassium-deficient rats, 5/5 died, suggesting that potassium deficiency does enhance thallium toxicity in the adult. Both dose levels caused some maternal toxicity (diarrhoea, lethargy, irritability and hair loss). Acceptable teratological methods were used. Thallium treatment had no effect on resorption rates, but significantly reduced fetal body weights by 9–14% in a dose-related manner in normal diet rats at both dosing periods. In rats on a potassium deficient diet, fetal body weight was low in controls and not reduced further by thallium.

On teratological examination, there was a significant increase in hydronephrosis in normal diet rats after treatment with 2·5 mg/kg on days 12–14 (47% compared with 16% in controls), but at 10 mg/kg on days 12–14 the incidence was identical to that of controls (16%), suggesting that the former finding may be due to chance. The incidence of missing or unossified vertebral bodies was also significantly increased after dosing on days 12–14 in normal diet rats, but the frequency was not dose-related. Non-ossification of phalanges was also significantly increased in thallium-treated potassium-deficient rats, compared with potassium-deficient controls. This anomaly was not seen in any of the normal diet groups. However, this was the only indication that thallium may be more fetotoxic in potassium-deficient rats.

In view of the ability of thallium to cause achondroplasia in the chick embryo, Nogami and Terashima (1973) have made a special study of the effect of thallium on bone morphogenesis in the neonatal rat. Rats were injected i.p. with 20 or 40 mg/kg at 6 and 9 days of age. Histological examination showed severe hypoplasia in the columnar cartilage of the long bone and a defective calcifying zone. There was evidence of inhibition of mucopolysaccharide synthesis, incorporation of radiolabelled sulphur into cartilage mucopolysaccharides being only half that of controls. The study is reported in abstract only and no indication of the numbers of rats used is given.

The single case of abortion in a cat ingesting an unknown amount of thallium has been discussed in section A.

Conclusion

One study in the rat has shown thallium is fetotoxic, causing reduced body weight and increased missing vertebral bodies, but only doses causing some maternal toxicity have been tested. The data on teratogenicity is equivocal, since hydronephrosis was seen at the low dose (2·5 mg/kg i.p.) but not at the high dose (10 mg/kg i.p.), with no difference in resorption rate between these 2 groups. However, it should be noted that thallium has been shown to concentrate in the neonatal kidney of the rat and mouse (Gibson *et al.*, 1967) and so particular care should be taken in future studies to establish whether or not thallium affects fetal kidney development.

E. MUTAGENICITY

No relevant data found.

F. CARCINOGENICITY

No relevant data found.

HUMAN STUDIES

A. RELEVANT PHARMACOLOGY AND TOXICOLOGY

There is evidence from a few case reports of thallium toxicity in newborns where the mother is known to have ingested thallium (see section D) that thallium does cross the placenta. In a single case report by Stevens and Barbier (1976) of a pregnant woman still breast-feeding her previous child, who had ingested thallium early in pregnancy, it was reported that thallium could not be found in the breast milk around an estimated 95 days after poisoning occurred, whilst detectable levels of 20 μg thallium/24 h in maternal urine were still found at this time. By 100 days after poisoning all traces of thallium had disappeared from maternal urine and faeces.

B. ENDOCRINE AND GONADAL EFFECTS

No relevant data found.

C. FERTILITY

No relevant data found.

D. PREGNANCY

Karkos (1970) reported that thallium compounds have been widely used to perform illegal abortions, but no further information was given.

In the rarely reported cases of thallium poisoning during pregnancy, it has been noted that the fetus may suffer from thallium toxicity with patches of alopecia, a typical sign of poisoning, on the baby's scalp (Di Nucci *et al.*, 1979).

Stevens and Barbier (1976) have reviewed 20 cases of thallium poisoning during pregnancy which have appeared in the literature between 1931 and 1976, involving accidental poisoning, administration in attempted suicide or administration to attempt to procure an abortion. In 6 cases thallium exposure was during the first trimester of pregnancy but outcome of pregnancy is only reported in 2 of these cases where there had been accidental chronic poisoning; birth was at 40 weeks in both cases with rather low birth weights of 2800 g and 3100 g. The babies were symptomless and congenital abnormalities were not mentioned. In the 12 cases where poisoning had occurred between 20 and 42 weeks of gestation and the outcome of the pregnancy was reported, premature birth (36–37 weeks) was seen and low birthweight was common (mean 2890 g). Of the 9 babies born at 40 weeks in which birth weight was recorded, 4 weighed less than 2800 g. Rashes on the baby were also seen in a few cases and alopecia on the baby's scalp in 2 cases. Eight of the babies were noted as symptomless. In some cases the estimated or known ingested dose was given and they ranged from 0·15–1·20 g. In the 2 cases of alopecia, where the babies had clearly been affected *in utero*, ingestion of 0·15 g at 28 weeks had occurred in one case and ingestion of 0·80 g at 28 weeks in the other. Delivery was also premature in both cases with a birth weight of 2310 g in one case (weight unrecorded in the other). In none of the cases where thallium was taken in an attempt to procure abortion, at doses of 0·05–1·00 g where stated, did abortion actually occur, but in one case of serious maternal intoxication with ingestion of 1·20 g at 42 weeks' gestation the bady died 5 days after birth.

One other single case-report of thallium poisoning during pregnancy has been located. Johnson (1960) recorded the case of a multiparous woman aged 20 who was admitted to hospital at 28 weeks' gestation, having drunk the greater part of a bottle of thallium-containing rodenticide "Thall-Rat" 2–3 weeks previously. She continued to have serious symptoms of poisoning and eventually delivered a live female infant at around 38 weeks weighing 2800 g. The baby was vigorous and normal except for several patches of alopecia on the scalp. Samples of placenta, cord blood and baby's urine were examined for thallium but none was found. Maternal urine still contained small amounts at this time (0·15 mg/l) and so lactation was suppressed and the baby was not breast-fed. Mother and baby were discharged one month after delivery, the baby then weighing 3090 g. However, the baby was readmitted at 10 weeks of age, weighing 3230 g, for failure to thrive. Her condition was otherwise normal. The baby was discharged 2 weeks later weighing 3910 g.

From these case reports it would seem that thallium does have the potential to affect the fetus, producing alopecia, as in adults, and possibly growth retardation. There are however no reports to date of affected offspring where the mother has not also shown clinical signs of poisoning.

E. MUTAGENICITY

No relevant data found.

F. CARCINOGENICITY

No relevant data found.

SUMMARY AND EVALUATION

EXPERIMENTAL STUDIES

Placental transfer of thallium has been shown to occur in rodents and cats with equilibration between maternal and fetal levels taking several hours.

No studies were found on endocrine or gonadal effects or effects on fertility. One study in the rat has shown that thallium, in maternally toxic doses of 2·5 and 10 mg/kg i.p., is fetotoxic and retards development but is not teratogenic. No studies on mutagenicity or carcinogenicity were found.

HUMAN STUDIES

Thallium crosses the placenta in humans but one study suggested that it does not appear in milk. No studies were found on endocrine or gonadal effects or of effects on fertility. Although reported to be abortifacient, doses around 1 g may produce severe toxic effects in the mother but do not cause abortion. Toxic effects on the fetus may result in growth retardation and alopecia, as in adults. Malformations have not been reported. No studies on mutagenicity or carcinogenicity were found.

EVALUATION

Data in animals are inadequate for evaluation. In humans, limited data suggests that thallium in high doses in pregnancy may reduce birth weight but is not teratogenic. Attention is drawn to the lack of adequate data on the reproductive toxicity of thallium in animals and humans, and to the lack of mutagenicity and carcinogenicity data.

References

Di Nucci, A., Ferrini, B., Gregotti, C., Richelmi, P. and Manzo, L. (1979). Placental transfer of thallium and its modification by Prussian Blue. *I.R.C.S. Medical Science: Drug Metabolism and Toxicology; Environmental Biology and Medicine; Nervous System; Pharmacology; Physiology: Social and Occupational Medicine* **7**, 272.

Fitzek, A. and Henning, A. (1976). Verteilung von Thallium im Organismus einer traechtigen Hauskatze. *Deutsche Tieraerztliche Wochenschrift* **83**, (2), 66–68.

Gibson, J. E. and Becker, B. A. (1970). Placental transfer, embryotoxicity and teratogenicity of thallium sulphate in normal and potassium-deficient rats. *Toxicology and Applied Pharmacology* **16**, 120–132.

Gibson, J. E., Sigsestad, C. P. and Becker, B. A. (1967). Placental transport and distribution of thallium-204 sulfate in newborn rats and mice. *Toxicology and Applied Pharmacology* **10**, 408.

Johnson, W. (1960). A case of thallium poisoning during pregnancy. *The Medical Journal of Australia* **2**, 540–542.
Karkos, J. (1970). Intoxication caused by thallium compounds. *Polski Tygodnik Lekarski* **25**, (11), 413–416.
Nogami, H. and Terashima, Y. (1973). Thallium-induced achondroplasia in the rat. *Teratology* **8**, (1), 101–102.
Stevens, W. J. and Barbier, F. (1976). Thalliumintoxicatie Gedurende de Zwangerschap. *Acta Clinica Belgica* **31**, (4), 188–193.

42. Toluene

TECHNICAL DATA

Formula	$C_6H_5CH_3$
CAS registry number	108–88–3
Chemical abstract name	Methylbenzene
Synonyms	Toluol, methyl benzene.
Uses	In manufacture of benzoic acid, benzaldehyde, explosives, dyes and many other organic compounds; also as a solvent in the extraction of various principles from plants.
TLV	100 ppm (skin)

ANIMAL STUDIES

A. RELEVANT PHARMACOLOGY AND TOXICOLOGY

The absorption, distribution, metabolism and elimination of toluene following different routes of administration have been reviewed by Cohr and Stokholm (1979); following absorption some (up to 50%) is exhaled unchanged, and the major proportion is oxidized by the hepatic microsomal enzyme system to benzoic acid and conjugated with glycine to form hippuric acid or with glucuronic acid to form benzoylglucuronide and excreted in the urine. Small quantities may be oxidized to phenols, o-cresol and p-cresol.

There are no reports on placental transfer studies with toluene, but in view of its low molecular weight and lipid solubility it is likely that it is readily transferred across the placenta.

B. ENDOCRINE AND GONADAL EFFECTS

No relevant data found.

C. FERTILITY

No relevant data found.

D. PREGNANCY

Euler (1967) exposed mice to a mixture of toluene and trichloroethylene similar to that which has been used in the soling of shoes. The mixture comprised 32 ppm (120 mg/m^3) toluene and 64 ppm (340 mg/m^3) trichloroethylene, equivalent to inhaling 157 mg/kg toluene and 406 mg/kg trichloroethylene in the mice. They inhaled the mixture for 10 days before mating, or during part or the whole of pregnancy. Differences were noted between treated and control groups in pregnancy rates, length of pregnancy, damaged embryos, birth weights and neonatal mortality, but the direction and magnitude of these differences is not stated. No groups were exposed to toluene alone.

Nawrot and Staples (1979) have given mice 0·3, 0·5 or 1·0 ml toluene/kg orally by gavage on days 6–15 of pregnancy, or 1·0 ml/kg on days 12–15 of pregnancy. There was no maternal toxicity except a decrease in maternal weight gain in those dosed on days 12–15. There was a significant increase in embryolethality at all 3 dose levels and a significant reduction in fetal weight in the 0·5 and 1·0 ml/kg groups after dosing on days 6–15. Those dosed with 1·0 ml/kg on days 6–15 had a significant increase in numbers of fetuses with cleft palate which was not simply due to general growth retardation. Treatment on days 12–15 only had no adverse effects on the offspring. The study is reported in abstract only and no further details are given.

Comprehensive teratological investigations on inhaled toluene in mice and rats have been carried out by Hudák and co-workers (Hudák *et al.*, 1977; Hudák and Ungváry, 1978). Acceptable teratological methods were used. Mice were exposed to 0, 133 or 399 ppm (500 or 1500 mg/m^3) toluene for 24 h/day on days 6–13 of pregnancy. In the high dose group all 15 exposed dams died within the first 24 h of exposure. No maternal deaths occurred in the 11 mice exposed to 133 ppm, and there were no effects on implants/dam, live fetuses/dam, dead and resorbed fetuses/dam, malformations or anomaly rates, but fetal weight was significantly reduced by 10% in comparison with controls. It is not stated whether 133 ppm had any effect on maternal weight gain (Hudák and Ungváry, 1978).

Hudák and Ungváry (1978) exposed rats to 266 ppm (1000 mg/m^3) toluene for 8 h/day on days 1–21 of pregnancy, or to 399 ppm (1500 mg/m^3) toluene for 24 h/day on days 1–8 or 9–14 of pregnancy. Groups of 9–19 rats were used. In the 399 ppm groups, 5/9 died during exposure on days 1–8 and 2/19 during exposure on days 9–14, but maternal weight gain in survivors was unaffected. There were no signs of maternal toxicity at 266 ppm. There were no significant effects in toluene-exposed groups on implants/dam, live fetuses/dam, dead or resorbed fetuses/dam or malformation rates. Fetal body weight was significantly reduced by 13% in those exposed to 266 ppm throughout pregnancy, but not in the 399 ppm groups exposed in early or mid-pregnancy. There was a significant increase in retarded ossification in the 266 ppm groups exposed throughout pregnancy and in the 399 ppm group exposed on days 1–8 of pregnancy. In those exposed to 399 ppm on days 9–14 of pregnancy there were significant increases in fused and extra ribs in the fetuses.

Hudák *et al.* (1977) have also exposed rats to higher concentrations of toluene. Groups of 9–21 rats were exposed to 1600 ppm (600 mg/m^3) toluene by inhalation for 24 h/day on days 1–8, 7–14, 9–14 or 9–21 of pregnancy. Twenty-eight air-exposed rats served as controls. Some maternal mortality was seen in all toluene-exposed groups (up to 33%) and maternal weight gain was reduced in all toluene-exposed groups but only significantly in those exposed on days 9–14 of pregnancy. Live fetuses/dam were significantly reduced only in those exposed on days 7–14 of pregnancy, where 17% of implants were dead or resorbed. Otherwise there were no significant effects on implants/dam, live fetuses/dam, dead or resorbed fetuses/dam or malformation rates. Fetal weight was significantly reduced by around 12% in those exposed on days 1–8 or 7–14 and by 20% in those exposed on days 9–21. Placental weight was also significantly reduced in those exposed on days 9–21 of pregnancy. Significant increases in retarded ossification were seen in all toluene-exposed groups and significant increases in skeletal anomalies of the ribs and sternebrae were seen in those exposed to toluene on days 7–14 or 9–14 of pregnancy.

Conclusion

In similarity with benzene, toluene does not appear to be teratogenic. It is fetotoxic, causing a reduction in fetal weight in mice and rats and retarded ossification and some increase in skeletal anomalies in rats, at doses that are below those toxic to the dam as well as at toxic doses. Embryolethality has also been seen with inhalation of very high concentrations lethal to some of the dams, or following oral administration of non-toxic doses.

E. MUTAGENICITY

Toluene does not appear to have been tested in bacterial mutagenicity testing systems. Lyapkalo (1973) has investigated the effects of toluene on dividing bone marrow cells; rats were injected s.c. with 1 g toluene/kg/day for 12 days. Chromosome gaps and breaks were seen in 12% of cells compared with 57% in benzene treated rats and 4% in untreated controls. Dobrokhotov (1972) showed that injections of 0·8 g toluene/kg/day induced a similar frequency of aberrations in bone marrow cells from rats as 0·2 g/kg/day of benzene. Exposure of rats to toluene by inhalation, at a concentration of 163 ppm (610 mg/m^3) for 4 months, has also been shown to induce bone marrow cell chromosome aberrations, which are still increased in frequency one month after the end of the exposure period (Dobrokhotov and Enikeev, 1977).

In both these experiments by Dobrokhotov, combination of benzene and toluene exposure was not synergistic, only additive in their effect on bone marrow cells, and it can be seen that toluene is less mutagenic than benzene.

F. CARCINOGENICITY

No relevant data found.

HUMAN STUDIES

A. RELEVANT PHARMACOLOGY AND TOXICOLOGY

The biological half-time for hippuric acid (the major metabolite of toluene) in urine has been quoted as 74 min for women and 117 min for men (reviewed by Cohr and Stokholm, 1979).

No studies have been found on placental transfer of toluene.

B. ENDOCRINE AND GONADAL EFFECTS

Menstrual function has been studied in workers exposed to toluene. The study of Michon (1965) showing prolonged and heavy bleeding in women exposed to benzene, toluene and xylene at levels stated not to have exceeded the maximum permissible levels (31 ppm benzene, 67 ppm toluene, 58 ppm xylene) has been discussed in section B of Benzene. In this group, the disturbances seem most likely to have been caused by the benzene exposure.

Others, however, have reported effects in women exposed to toluene and other chemicals not including benzene.

Syrovadko *et al.* (1973) have investigated the health of women working in the manufacture of electrical insulating materials who were exposed to the vapour of white spirit containing 16% toluene and xylene, used for dissolving and thinning the resins and varnishes that are used. The concentrations in the workplace were said to fluctuate between 35 and 95 ppm for the 2 aromatic hydrocarbons. A total of 168 exposed women and 201 controls, working in the factory offices and not exposed, were examined by a therapist, a neuropathologist and a gynaecologist. The age range of the women was as follows: under 26 years, 5·9% of exposed, 10·3% of controls; 26–40 years, 58·8% of exposed, 57·6% of controls; over 40 years, 34·9% of exposed, 21·3% of controls. Length of service for the majority in both groups was 6–15 years. A number of health complaints were reported in both groups. In exposed workers there were significant decreases ($P<0{\cdot}01$) in haemoglobin levels and total red blood cell counts in comparison with controls. The overall incidence of gynaecological disease in the 2 groups was similar, but prolapse of the uterus and vaginal walls were found significantly more often in exposed workers (8·9%) than in the controls (0·5%, $P<0{\cdot}01$). Menstrual function was studied in women up to 40 years old. Of 127 exposed to white spirit menstrual disturbances were found in 23·3% compared with 15·7% in 172 controls ($P<0{\cdot}05$). Of those with menstrual disturbances, polyhypermenorrhoea (16·5% in exposed, 10·4% in controls) and dysmenorrhoea (32·2% in exposed, 26·6% in controls) were the most common. No underlying gynaecological disease could be found in these women to explain the disturbances observed. Some women also noticed changes in menstrual function after coming to work in the industry (increased blood loss, pain, alterations in cycle length); the incidence of this change was 15·4% in the exposed group compared with 7·9% in controls ($P<0{\cdot}05$).

Whilst significant disturbances of the menstrual cycle and alterations in haemoglobin, which could be related to the increased menstrual bleeding, have been reported in this study, it is not clear what chemicals besides toluene and xylene these workers might also have been exposed to. The study was carried out on women working in sections where petroleum white spirit was used. However, in another study on women engaged in the production of electrical insulating materials (enamel-coated wires), Syrovadko and Malysheva (1977) reported a higher incidence of similar menstrual problems in women exposed to synthetic di-electric varnishes with polyvinylacetol or polyester bases containing the solvents phenyl chloride, ethylcellosolv and tricresol. It is not known if the women in the first study, exposed to white spirit, were also exposed to these other varnishes during the course of their work, but in a later paper Syrovadko (1977), referring to their earlier work, attributes the effects seen to the "combined effect of various solvents (toluene, xylene, white spirit, and others) and sometimes coupled with other substances" and states that they have not dealt separately with the varnishes or the solvents used in the varnishes. Thus it is likely that the women in the study just considered were exposed to a number of chemicals besides toluene.

In the later study (Syrovadko, 1977), however, the possible effects of toluene are more clearly delineated. Women engaged in the production of varnished cloth and mica insulating materials, using organo-silicone varnishes containing up to 70% toluene, were studied. In addition to toluene, small amounts of silica dust (up to 10 mg/m^3) are released into the air and carbon monoxide may also be released in small amounts during furnace drying. Monomeric organo-silicone compounds were not detected in the air. Toluene concentrations in the air sampled at a number of different points in the operatives' working area varied from 13–120 ppm with a mean of around 55 ppm. There was also direct contact with toluene through the skin of the hands and forearms particularly when varnish was applied by hand, though skin absorption of toluene is poor compared with inhalational absorption. A total of 140 women workers exposed to toluene for 5–20 years were compared with 201 controls working in the office of the same factory. Disorders of the nervous system, cardiovascular system and peripheral blood were found more frequently in exposed women than in controls. As in the previous study on women exposed to white spirit containing toluene (Syrovadko *et al.*, 1973), a significantly higher incidence of prolapse of the uterus and vaginal walls was found in the women exposed to toluene in this study (6·5% compared with 0·5% in controls, $P < 0{\cdot}05$). The authors suggest that this problem may be due to the body position required at work. Menstrual disturbances were found in 40·7% of the exposed women, compared with 15·7% in the controls ($P < 0.01$). Polyhypermenorrhoea (18·3% in the exposed group, 4·2% in controls) and irregular cycles (5·9% in the exposed group, 1·1% in controls) were the commonest disturbances found.

Whilst these studies of menstrual function in women working in the production of electrical insulating materials suggest that toluene may be related to menstrual disturbances, there are a number of difficulties in interpretation of the data which must be taken into account. Firstly, it seems probable that these 3 separate studies from the same group of workers all relate to the same factory and much of the data may be reporting on the same women several times over; the size of the control group and the incidence of menstrual disturbances in controls is identical in 2 of the papers (Syrovadko *et al.*, 1973; Syrovadko, 1977). Secondly, the background of the control group (office workers in the same factory) may well be quite different in terms of nutritional status, socioeconomic status, etc. than the shop floor operatives in the exposed group and these factors may well affect gynaecological function. Thirdly, it is very likely that many in the exposed groups were exposed to a number of chemicals and the relative contributions of these, including toluene, to the gynaecological problems observed is impossible to evaluate.

A single case of impotence has been reported by Takeuchi *et al.* (1972) in a worker exposed to organic solvents (mainly toluene) in the paints industry. The worker was exposed to concentrations estimated to be as high as several hundred to over 1000 ppm of toluene at times, in a small poorly ventilated area. He complained of dizziness, headache, tinnitus, insomnia, slight fever, poor appetite, loss of weight and cramp in the lower extremities as well as impotence. Clinical examination revealed hypofunction of the hypothalamo-pituitary-adrenal system, paraesthesia on one side, continuous slight fever, slight orthostatism, and abnormal EEG. Another paints worker had similar symptoms but impotence was not mentioned. In view of the severe signs of toxicity in the first worker the reported impotence may well be secondary to the general malaise or to specific effects on the nervous system. No other reports on the effects of toluene on males have been found.

C. FERTILITY

See observation of Syrovadko (1977) in section D.

D. PREGNANCY

A few case reports of malformations in association with toluene exposure have appeared. Euler (1967) has reported 2 cases of multiple malformations where the deformities were similar in children born to women who worked in shoemaking and were exposed to toluene and trichloroethylene, used as a soling solution. The average concentration of toluene in the air was 298 ppm (1·12 mg/l) and of trichloroethylene 230 ppm (1·22 mg/l). No further details of these cases were given.

Toutant and Lippmann (1979) have reported a single case of outcome of pregnancy in a woman addicted to solvents (primarily toluene). The woman, aged 20 years, had a 14-year history of daily heavy solvent abuse, and a 3-year history of alcohol intake of about a six-pack of beer weekly. On admission to hospital she had ataxia, tremors, mild diffuse sensory deficits, short-term memory loss, blunted affect, and poor intellectual functioning compatible with severe solvent and/or alcohol abuse. The male child, born at term, was at the 10th centile for weight and the 5th centile for head size. It was microcephalic, with a flat nasal bridge, hypoplastic mandible, short palpebral fissures, mildly low-set ears, pronounced sacral dimple, sloping forehead and inco-ordination of arm movements, with unusual angulation of the left shoulder and elbow. There was a poor sucking reflex and movements were jerky at 2–4 days of age, though this improved spontaneously. No joint or muscular abnormalities were found at physical examination or X-ray. The authors of this report point out the similarities between this case and fetal alcohol syndrome and suggest that there may be an analogous "fetal solvents syndrome" or that excessive solvent intake may enhance the toxicity of alcohol.

The only study of the outcome of pregnancy in a substantial number of women exposed to toluene is by Syrovadko (1977). The details of this study on women working in production of electrical insulating materials, using organo-silicone varnishes containing up to 70% toluene, have already been described in section B. Toluene exposure averaged 55 ppm (range 13–120 ppm). The factory had its own maternity section where the women had their deliveries. Records of labour and newborns were examined for 133 women in contact with toluene and for 201 controls from the factory offices. There was no detectable effect on fertility; in the exposed group, records showed a mean pregnancy rate of 3·2/worker, compared with 2·6/worker in controls. There were no significant differences between exposed and control groups in the course of pregnancy, duration of labour, blood loss during labour, perinatal mortality or adverse effects on the new born. Average birth weights did not differ significantly (exposed group 3432 ± 34 g, control group 3518 ± 28 g) but there were twice as many babies of low birth weight (2500–3000 g) in the exposed group as in the controls (20% compared with 9%, $P < 0{\cdot}05$). There was no indication of excessive bleeding problems post-partum, as has been found with benzene poisoning in pregnancy, but the possible effect on birth weight warrants further investigation.

In the study of Holmberg (1979) on central nervous system defects in children born to mothers exposed to organic solvents during pregnancy (discussed in detail in section D of Styrene), 3 of the cases were exposed to toluene, or toluene in combination with other solvents; in one case with hydranencephaly which died 24 days after birth, there was exposure to toluene, xylene, white spirit and methyl ethyl ketone from rubber products manufacture, and a previous child had also died from brain injury, though it is not stated whether there was also exposure to organic solvents at that time; in the second case with multiple abnormalities of hydrocephaly, agenesis of the corpus callosum, pulmonary hypoplasia and diaphragmatic hernia, which died 2 h after birth, there was exposure to toluene through metal products manufacture; in the third case of lumbar meningomyelocoele, which survived, there was exposure to toluene and white spirit from building. The difficulties in interpretation of this study have already been discussed (see section D Benzene and Styrene).

E. MUTAGENICITY

Forni *et al.* (1971) have examined peripheral lymphocytes from 34 male workers at a rotogravure plant, exposed to benzene then toluene, or toluene alone. The toluene contained traces of xylene. The results were compared with those from 34 healthy male controls matched for age with no history of exposure to benzene or its homologues. Persons with exposure to occupational or therapeutic X-irradiation, recent viral diseases or vaccinations were excluded, but a few cases and controls had a history of diagnostic X-rays. In all but one case, 100 metaphases/person were examined. In the 10 workers exposed to benzene then toluene, there was a significant increase in chromosome aberrations (stable and unstable) in comparison with controls or the group exposed to toluene only; 8/10 of these benzene-exposed cases had a history of slight anaemia, leukopenia or severe benzene haemopathy. Of the 24 workers exposed to toluene only for 3–15 years (mean 9·75 years), the incidence of aberrations (unstable changes and calculated breaks) was slightly higher than controls, but the differences were not statistically significant; 7/24 of the toluene-exposed group had a history of slight anaemia, moderate thrombocytopenia or moderate leukopenia.

Funes-Cravioto *et al.* (1977) studied the incidence of chromosome aberrations in cultured lymphocytes from 73 workers in chemical laboratories and the printing industry. They found a significantly increased incidence (approximately 2-fold) of chromatid and isochromatid breaks when compared with 49 controls. A similar increased incidence was also observed in 14 children aged 4–11 years of 11 women laboratory workers who had worked during pregnancy. There was also an increased incidence of sister-chromatid exchange in 12 technicians and in the 4 children of 2 of the female technicians who had worked during pregnancy. The technicians came from 8 different laboratories but all were exposed to one or more of chloroform, toluene, benzene, cyclohexane, diethyl ether, isooctane, methanol, toluene or xylene, with chloroform, benzene, and toluene being most common, though the atmospheric concentration of these solvents was not measured in most instances. In a group of 34 of the subjects there was a correlation between the frequency of chromosome breaks and duration of exposure. There was no correlation between exposed mothers and their children, with sex or smoking habits. The subjects and controls in this study were not carefully matched and it is impossible to state that the chromosome aberrations were a direct result of exposure to organic solvents but this was a common factor in all the working environments studied. The biological significance of the changes observed is unknown as far as the health of the workers is concerned.

Mäki-Paakkanen *et al.* (1980) have also studied the incidence of chromosome aberrations and sister-chromatid exchange (SCE) in peripheral blood lymphocytes from 32 male rotogravure workers with daily exposure to toluene. Exposure to toluene ranged from 5–35 years (mean 14 years) and exposure levels were calculated as 7–112 ppm. Benzene contamination averaged 0·006% and did not exceed 0·05%. Results were compared with 14 male subjects of similar mean age (34 years) working in a research institute. Information on previous occupational history, recent viral infections, diagnostic X-irradiation and smoking habits was obtained for all exposed and control subjects. A total of 100 metaphases/subject were studied for chromosome aberrations and 30 harlequin-stained metaphases/person for SCEs. There were no significant differences in aberrations of the chromosomal or chromatid types, or in gaps or in SCEs between control and exposed groups, though in both groups significant increases in the frequency of SCE was seen in smokers compared with non-smokers. In view of this result and that of Forni *et al.* (1971) described previously, where exposure to toluene was the main chemical exposure, it seems unlikely that toluene has any cytogenetic effect and that the effects observed by Funes-Cravioto *et al.* (1977) are more likely to be due to other chemicals to which their study group was also exposed.

Gerner-Smidt and Friedrich (1978) have studied the frequency of SCE and chromosomal aberrations in human lymphocytes exposed *in vitro* to benzene, toluene or xylene. Unexpectedly, benzene did not have any cytogenetic effects and the authors attribute this to the possibility that it is a metabolite of benzene, rather than benzene itself, which is mutagenic. The 2 highest concentrations of toluene (1520 and 152 μg/ml) caused significant cell growth inhibition, but no increases in the frequency of chromosomal aberrations or SCE were detected. Xylene had a similar effect to toluene. Thus there is indication from this *in vitro* study that toluene had no cytogenetic effects.

F. CARCINOGENICITY

No relevant data found.

SUMMARY AND EVALUATION

EXPERIMENTAL STUDIES

No studies were found on endocrine or gonadal effects or on effects on fertility. Teratogenicity studies have been carried out in mice and rats exposed orally and by inhalation. It is not teratogenic but is fetotoxic causing reduction in fetal weight in mice and rats. Retarded ossification with increased skeletal anomalies have been reported in rats at doses non-toxic to the dams. Limited studies have shown mutagenic activity *in vivo*. No studies were found on carcinogenicity.

HUMAN STUDIES

Limited studies have suggested that women exposed to toluene may have an increase in menstrual disorders, usually increased bleeding and lengthening of the cycle. These women, however, were usually exposed to other solvents as well so that the role of toluene is uncertain. One study has suggested that toluene exposure does not reduce fertility but that fetal growth may be retarded. Studies *in vitro* and *in vivo* have suggested that toluene is not mutagenic. No studies on carcinogenicity were found.

EVALUATION

Limited studies suggest that toluene is fetotoxic but not teratogenic at doses sub-toxic to the dam. The data in humans are inadequate for evaluation but the similarity of effects reported on fetal growth to those observed in animals draws attention to the need for further studies of occupationally exposed women. Attention is drawn to the lack of adequate data on endocrine and gonadal function and effects on the menstrual cycle. Toluene does not appear to be a potent mutagen but the available data are inadequate for evaluation. Attention is drawn to the lack of carcinogenicity data.

References

Cohr, K. H. and Stokholm, J. (1979). Toluene. A Toxicological review. *Scandinavian Journal of Work and Environmental Health* **5**, (2), 71–90.

Dobrokhotov, B. (1972). Mutagenic effect of benzene and toluene under experimental conditions. *Gigiena I Sanitariya* **37**, (10), 36–39.

Dobrokhotov, B. and Enikeev, M. I. (1977). Mutagenic action of benzene, toluene and a mixture of these hydrocarbons in a chronic experiment. *Gigiena i sanitariya* (1), 32–34.

Euler, H. H. (1967). Animal experimental studies of an industrial noxa. *Archiv fur Gynakologie* **204**, (2), 258–259.

Forni, A., Pacifico, E. and Limonta, A. (1971). Chromosome studies in workers exposed to benzene or toluene or both. *Archives of Environmental Health* **22**, 373–378.

Funes-Cravioto, F., Kolmodin-Hedman, B., Lindsten, J., Nordenskjold, M., Zapata-Gayon, C., Lambert, B., Norberg, E., Olin, R. and Swenson, A. (1977). Chromosome aberrations and sister-chromatid exchange in workers in chemical laboratories and a rotoprinting factory and in children of women laboratory workers. *Lancet* **ii**, 322–325.

Gerner-Smidt, P. and Friedrich, U. (1978). The mutagenic effect of benzene, toluene and xylene studied by the SCE technique. *Mutation Research* **58**, (2/3), 313–316.

Holmberg, P. C. (1979). Central-nervous-system defects in children born to mothers exposed to organic solvents during pregnancy. *Lancet* **ii**, 177–179.

Hudák, A., Rodics, K., Stuber, I. and Ungváry, G. (1977). Effects of toluene inhalation on pregnant CFY rats and their offspring. *Munkavedelem* **23**, (1–3 Suppl.), 25–30.

Hudák, A. and Ungváry, G. (1978). Embryotoxic effects of benzene, and its methyl derivatives: toluene, xylene. *Toxicology* **11**, 55–63.

Lyapkalo, A. A. (1973). Genetic activity of benzene and toluene. *Gigiena Truda i Professional'nye Zabolevaniya* **17**, (3), 24–28.

Mäki-Paakkanen, J., Husgafvel-Pursiainen, K., Kalliomäki, P.-L., Tuominen, J. and Sorsa, M. (1980). Toluene-exposed workers and chromosome aberrations. *Journal of Toxicology and Environmental Health* **6**, (4), 775–781.

Michon, S. (1965). Disturbances of menstruation in women working in an atmosphere polluted with aromatic hydrocarbons. *Polski Tygodnik Lekarski* **20**, 1648–1649.

Nawrot, P. S. and Staples, R. E. (1979). Embryofetal toxicity and teratogenicity of benzene and toluene in the mouse. *Teratology* **19**, (2), 41A.

Syrovadko, O. N. (1977). Working conditions and health status of women handling organosilicon varnishes containing toluene. *Gigiena Truda I Professional 'Nye Zabolevaniya*, (12), 15–19.

Syrovadko, O. N. and Malysheva, Z. V. (1977). Work conditions and their influence on some specific functions of women engaged in the manufacture of enamel-insulated wires. *Gigiena Truda I Professional 'nye Zabolevaniya* (4), 25–28.

Syrovadko, O. N., Skornin, V. F., Pronkova, E. N., Sorkina, N. S., Izyumova, A. S., Gribova, I. A. and Popova, A. F. (1973). Effect of working conditions on the health status and some specific functions of women handling white spirit. *Gigiena Truda I Professional'Nye Zabolevaniya* **17**, (6), 5–8.

Takeuchi, I., Nichizaki, T., Takagi, S. and Mabuchi, C. (1972). Diencephalic syndrome in two workers exposed to mainly toluene vapour. *Japanese Journal of Industrial Health* **14**, 563–581.

Toutant, C. and Lippman, S. (1979). Fetal solvents syndrome. *Lancet* **i**, 1356.

43. Toluene-2,4-Diisocyanate

TECHNICAL DATA

Formula	CH_3 (benzene ring with NCO at positions 2 and 4)
CAS registry number	584–84–9
Chemical abstract name	2,4 diisocyanato-1-methylbenzene
Synonyms	TDI; 2,4-diisocyanatotoluene; isocyanic acid; 4-methyl-meta-phenylene ester; 4-methyl-meta-phenylene diisocyanate; 4-methyl-meta-phenylene isocyanate; 2,4-TDI; toluene 2,4-diisocyanate; 2,4-tolylene diisocyanate.
Uses	In the manufacture of polyurethane foams and other elastomers.
TLV	0·02 ppm (1980 Intended change to 0·005 ppm).

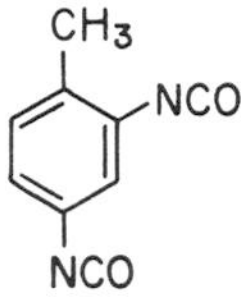

ANIMAL STUDIES

No relevant data found.

HUMAN STUDIES

No relevant data found except for the study below.

Le Quesne *et al.* (1976) reported on a group of firemen who were heavily exposed to toluene di-isocyanate (TDI) while fighting a fire in a factory where polyurethane foam was manufactured. During the course of the fire a total of

4500 litres of TDI leaked from 2 storage tanks and the men were exposed intermittently over 8 h to TDI in the air and some of them by direct contact with TDI which soaked their clothing and equipment. Other chemicals were also used at the plant but with the massive leakage of TDI it was felt that their symptoms were most likely to be due to that chemical. During and after the fire 31/35 men complained of respiratory symptoms and 16/35 of gastrointestinal symptoms. In 23 cases, the men complained of neurological symptoms such as difficulty in concentrating, poor memory, headache, irritability or depression. In 5 of these cases there had been acute onset of euphoria, ataxia and loss of consciousness. Amongst the various neurological abnormalities observed up to 3 weeks after the fire, there were 2 complaints of impotence for 2 weeks. One of the cases was one of the 5 men who suffered from loss of consciousness during the fire and he still showed signs of ataxia and had an abnormal EEG at 3 weeks with persistent neurological symptoms including prominent depression up to 4 years after the fire. In the other case, there was confusion in the first 3 weeks and ataxia and abnormal EEG at 3 weeks with persistent memory difficulties up to 4 years after the fire. Of the 23 complaining of neurological effects, 18 were re-examined 4 years after the fire and 13 were found to be still clinically affected with difficulty in concentration, irritability and depression. Psychometric testing also confirmed a selective memory deficit in long-term recall in those still affected. Thus, from the spectrum of effects observed it seems likely that the reported temporary impotence in 2 of the exposed individuals was probably secondary to neurological impairment following heavy exposure to TDI.

SUMMARY AND EVALUATION

EXPERIMENTAL STUDIES

No relevant studies were found.

HUMAN STUDIES

No relevant studies were found except for a report of transient impotence in 2 grossly exposed men who demonstrated numerous other toxic signs.

EVALUATION

Available data is inadequate for evaluation. Attention is drawn to the lack of any animal or human data.

Reference

Le Quesne, P. M., Axford, A. T., McKerrow, C. B. and Jones, A. P. (1976). Neurological complications after a single severe exposure to toluene di-isocyanate. *British Journal of Industrial Medicine* **33**, 72–78.

44. o-Toluidine

TECHNICAL DATA

Formula	NH_2 / CH_3 (structural formula)
CAS registry number	95–53–4
Chemical abstracts name	2-methylbenzenamine
Synonyms	2-aminotoluene; o-methylaniline; ortho-Aminotoluene; 1-methyl-2-aminobenzene; 2-methylaniline; 1-amino-2-methylbenzene; 2-amino-1-methylbenzene; 2-methyl-1-aminobenzene; ortho-methylbenzenamine; 2-toluidine; orthotolylamine.
Uses	Manufacture of various dyes; printing textiles blue-black; making various colours fast to acids; dye intermediate.
TLV	5 ppm (1980 intended change to 2 ppm).

ANIMAL STUDIES

A. RELEVANT PHARMACOLOGY AND TOXICOLOGY

No relevant data found.

B. ENDOCRINE AND GONADAL EFFECTS

No relevant data found.

C. FERTILTIY

No relevant data found.

D. PREGNANCY

No relevant data found.

E. MUTAGENICITY

No relevant data found.

F. CARCINOGENICITY

IARC Monographs Vol. 16 (1978) reports that tumours have been found after administration of o-toluidine by various routes in animals, but the studies are inadequately reported to allow proper evaluation of its carcinogenic potential.

One study relevant to the transplacental carcinogenic potential of o-toluidine has been reported. Shabad (1969) injected o-toluidine s.c. into pregnant mice at a dose of 2 mg/mouse every 4–5 days of pregnancy. Just before term, fetal lung and kidney tissue was explanted into cultures. Cultures from treated dams showed longer life times, stimulated proliferation, hyperplasia and focal nodules in comparison with explants from controls. A number of other known carcinogens in adults behaved similarly when injected into pregnant mice. This work suggests o-toluidine may be a potential transplacental carcinogen, but further information is needed before any firm conclusion may be drawn.

HUMAN STUDIES

No relevant data found on any aspect of reproduction. IARC Monograph Vol. 16 (1978) states that available epidemiological evidence on the carcinogenicity of o-toluidine are inadequate and do not allow any firm conclusions to be drawn.

SUMMARY AND EVALUATION

EXPERIMENTAL STUDIES

No studies were found on endocrine or gonadal effects or of effects on fertility, pregnancy or mutagenicity. Studies are inadequate to assess its carcinogenicity in animals. One study reported that organ cultures of embryonic tissues taken from treated mice showed changes which were similar to those produced by some other known carcinogens. This suggests that it may act as a transplacental carcinogen.

HUMAN STUDIES

No relevant studies were found.

EVALUATION

No evaluation is possible.

Attention is drawn to the lack of data on reproductive effects in animals and humans.

References

IARC Monographs on the Evaluation of the Carcinogenic Risk of Chemicals to Humans: Some aromatic amines and related nitro compounds—hair dyes, colouring agents and miscellaneous industrial chemicals (1978). Vol. 16, Lyon, France.

Shabad, L. M. (1969). Transplacental effects of blastomogenic substances and some further studies on organ cultures. *Arzneimittel Forschung* **19**, (7), 1044–1046.

45. Trichloroethylene

TECHNICAL DATA

Formula	$CCl_2{=}CHCl$
CAS registry number	79–01–6
Chemical abstracts name	Trichloroethene
Synonyms	Ethinyl trichloride; trichloroethene, Trilene.
Uses	Solvent for fats, waxes, resins, oils, rubber, paints and varnishes. Solvent for cellulose esters and ethers. Used for solvent extraction in many industries. In degreasing, in dry cleaning. In the manufacture of organic chemicals, pharmaceuticals, such as chloroacetic acid.
TLV	100 ppm (1980 Intended change to 50 ppm).

ANIMAL STUDIES

A. RELEVANT PHARMACOLOGY AND TOXICOLOGY

Ikeda and Imamura (1973) have found no sex differences in the rat in the half-life of urinary metabolites of trichloroethylene after either inhalation exposure (50–250 ppm) or i.p. injection (1·5 g/kg). Possible sex differences in toxicity have not been studied.

The rapid passage of trichloroethylene across the placenta into the fetus was shown as long ago as 1949. Helliwell and Hutton (1949, 1950), using sheep and goats in the last month of pregnancy, showed that inhaled trichloroethylene passed into the fetal circulation very quickly and by 5–10 minutes concentrations in the fetal and maternal blood were similar. In the sheep the concentration of trichloroethylene was consistently higher by about 19% in the fetal circulation (umbilical vein) than in the maternal circulation (carotid artery) after about 15 minutes inhalation of vapour, across a range of vapour concentrations. In the goat, peak fetal concentrations were similar to maternal concentrations.

B. ENDOCRINE AND GONADAL EFFECTS

No relevant data found.

C. FERTILITY

Trichloroethylene has been assessed for dominant lethality in the mouse. Slacik-Erben *et al.* (1980) exposed male mice to 0, 50, 202 or 450 ppm for 24 h, with 50 mice per dose level. Each male was then mated with a new untreated female every 4 days, altogether 12 times. There were no biologically significant effects on pregnancy rates, pre- or post-implantation losses at any dose level, any variation being within the range of controls.

Effects of trichloroethylene on female fertility have not been investigated in any detail. Dorfmueller *et al.* (1979) have reported absence of effects on fertility or mating success after exposure to 1800 ppm trichloroethylene for 3 weeks in female rats. This was a pilot study and no further details are given.

D. PREGNANCY

The teratogenic potential of trichloroethylene has been studied in rodents. In an early study published in 1936, Taylor reported that 9 female rats exposed to 500 ppm (0·05%) trichloroethylene for 6 h/day, 5 days/week for 6 months did not show "any disfunction of the sex organs" and all gave birth to healthy litters but no further methodological details or results were given. Healy and Wilcox (1978) exposed rats to 100 ppm for 4 h/day, 7 days/week from day 6–20 of pregnancy. They reported a significant reduction in fetal weight and a significant increase in resorptions in the exposed group. The study is reported in abstract only and no further details are given. The fetuses were examined for abnormalities but no results (negative or positive) were given.

Schwetz *et al.* (1975) exposed rats to 0 ppm (30 animals) or 300 ppm (18 animals) trichloroethylene for 7 h/day on days 6–15 of pregnancy. Acceptable teratological methods were used. Slight maternal toxicity was evident as a 4–5% reduction in maternal body weight in the trichloroethylene group in comparison with controls during and/or following exposure, but there was no effect on relative or absolute liver weights on day 21 of pregnancy. There were no significant effects on implantation sites, live litter size, resorptions, fetal weight or abnormalities. No gross malformations were found in the trichloroethylene-exposed group. The incidences of soft tissue and skeletal anomalies were reported as affected litters only. There was a high incidence of subcutaneous oedema in both treated and control groups, 28% and 17% of litters respectively being affected. However, this may not be a true anomaly (for discussion see Tetrachloroethylene, section D). As the number of fetuses with anomalies is not given, the possible teratogenicity of trichloroethylene cannot be fully evaluated from this study, but clearly at 300 ppm in the rat they found no gross effects on growth or development.

Dorfmueller *et al.* (1979) investigated prenatal and postnatal development in the rat after exposure to a high concentration of 1800 ppm trichloroethylene. The design of their experiment incorporated longer exposures than conventionally used in teratogenicity testing, since it has been shown in human studies that the blood levels of the toxic metabolite, trichloroethanol, are higher following sub-acute exposure than after acute exposure, whilst levels of trichloroethylene are similar. Rats were exposed to trichloroethylene before mating for an average of 22 days and/or exposed on days 1–20 of pregnancy. Daily exposure periods were for 6 h/day, 5 days/week in the pre-mating period and 6 h/day, 7 days/week during pregnancy. Each treatment group comprised 30 rats, 15 of which were killed on day 21 of pregnancy for teratological examination and the remaining 15 allowed to litter out for postnatal evaluation. Fetuses were examined by conventional teratological methods, but only 68–80% of fetuses (8/litter) were examined in each treatment group.

There were no signs of maternal toxicity, and weight gain during pregnancy, relative and absolute liver weights and serum enzyme levels (indicative of kidney or liver damage) were all unaffected. (1800 ppm is subnarcotic but had been shown to cause histopathologic lesions in adult male rats exposed for 4 weeks (Taylor, 1936).) There were no effects on implantation sites/litter, litter size, resorption rates or fetal body weight in any treatment group. The overall incidence of skeletal anomalies, principally incomplete ossification of the sternum, and the incidence of displaced right ovary were significantly increased in the group exposed during gestation only in comparison with filtered air-exposed controls, suggesting slight developmental delay in this group. However, mean fetal body weights were similar in this group (gestation exposure only) and controls. Furthermore, in the group exposed before mating as well as during gestation, skeletal and soft tissue anomaly rates were actually lower than in filtered air controls. This overall picture suggests that the slight increase in anomalies detected in the group exposed during gestation only may not be of biological significance.

In the postnatal part of the study by Dorfmueller *et al.* (1979), growth rates up to 100 days of age and activity in a novel environment at 10, 20 and 100 days of age were assessed. There was a significant reduction in body weight from 20 days of age onwards in offspring from dams exposed before mating only or before mating and during pregnancy, compared with those exposed during pregnancy only or controls exposed to filtered air. Apart from this effect of premating exposure there were no other significant differences.

In the mouse, Schwetz *et al.* (1975) found no adverse effects from exposure to 300 ppm. Twelve mice were exposed for 7 h/day from days 6–15 of pregnancy and the results compared with those from 30 controls exposed to filtered air only. Acceptable teratological methods were used, but, as in their rat study discussed previously, teratological data is reported on a per litter basis only. Unlike in rats there was no reduction in maternal weight gain as a result of trichloroethylene exposure. Relative and absolute maternal liver weights were also unaffected. There were no significant effects on implantation sites/litter, live litter size, resorption rate, fetal body weight, gross soft tissue or skeletal abnormalities.

Euler (1967) has investigated the effects of exposure to a combination of toluene (32 ppm) and trichloroethylene (64 ppm) in female mice. This combination has been used in the soling of shoes. Mice were exposed at varying times; for 10 days before mating, or from fertilization to implantation, or during organogenesis, or shortly before birth, or during the whole of pregnancy. A total of 368 females were used in exposed and control groups but no further breakdown of group sizes was given. He reported that he found no malformations, but the mice were allowed to litter out so abnormal offspring may have been destroyed by the dam at birth. He reported there were differences in pregnancy rates, length of gestation, birth weights and neonatal mortality between treated and control groups. However, no numerical data were given nor details of the outcome in the different treatment groups. In view of the paucity of the data presented and the possible contribution of toluene to the adverse effects observed, it is impossible to assess the real effect of trichloroethylene in these experiments.

Conclusion

In summary, data from the one study of Healy and Wilcox (1978) showing low levels of trichloroethylene exposure (100 ppm) during pregnancy in the rat affect fetal weight and intrauterine mortality adversely is difficult to evaluate since the numerical data have never been published in a full study. Schwetz *et al.* (1975) did not find any adverse effects in rats or mice from exposure to 300 ppm during organogenesis (days 6–15). However, Healy and Wilcox exposed rats through to late pregnancy (days 6–20) and exposure to toxic agents late in pregnancy when the fetus is growing rapidly is much more likely to affect fetal weight than earlier exposures where catch-up growth is possible in later stages after exposure has ceased. However, Dorfmueller *et al.* (1979) found no effect on fetal body weight or intrauterine mortality rate from exposure on days 1–20 of pregnancy in the rat at higher doses (1800 ppm instead of 100 ppm) and for longer periods (6 h/day instead of 4 h/day). It seems very unlikely that exposure to lower doses would be more fetotoxic than exposure to higher doses. However, Dorfmueller *et al.* (1979) did find some adverse effects on minor anomalies from gestational exposure only and on postnatal growth rates from pre-mating exposure only at 1800 ppm. Further work is necessary on levels between 300 and 1800 ppm to establish a no-effect level.

E. MUTAGENICITY

Trichloroethylene is mutagenic in the Ames test (Simmon, 1977), but it has been suggested that contamination of trichloroethylene with epichlorohydrin may be largely responsible for this positive finding (Biles *et al.* 1978).

Černá and Kypěnová (1977) could detect no mutagenic effect on mouse bone marrow cells after single i.p. injection of $\frac{1}{2}$ LD50 trichloroethylene (actual dose not stated) or 5 consecutive daily injections (each injection $\frac{1}{6}$ LD50) in animals killed 6, 24 and 48 h after the last injection. The study was reported in abstract only.

White *et al.* (1979) found no significant effect on sister chromatid exchange in Chinese hamster ovary cells *in vitro* exposed to trichloroethylene for 24 h (initial concentration equivalent to the maximum acceptable concentration in humans—level not given).

F. CARCINOGENICITY

IARC Monograph Vol. 20 (1979) reported that there was limited evidence that trichloroethylene is carcinogenic in mice.

HUMAN STUDIES

A. RELEVANT PHARMACOLOGY AND TOXICOLOGY

The biological half-life of trichloroethylene in occupationally exposed workers was studied by Ikeda and Imamura (1973). They measured the urinary excretion of trichloroethylene metabolites by measuring total trichlorocompounds, trichloroethanol and trichloroacetic acid over the weekend when the workers were not exposed. In all 24 men and 6 women were studied who had been exposed to trichloroethylene concentrations at work of the order of 5–200 ppm for up to 8 hours per day. The mean half-life was found to be 41 h (range 26–51 h) with no relationship between daily exposure and half-life. No difference was found between men and women. An experimental study of respiratory uptake and excretion of trichloroethylene by 5 male and 5 female Japanese students exposed to 252–380 ppm for 2–7 h showed that there was no sex difference in rate of uptake and equilibration. However, men excreted trichloroethylene significantly ($P < 0{\cdot}05$) more rapidly than women. The difference, however, seemed small and unlikely to be of practical significance though the method of calculation used by the authors was unclear (Nomiyama and Nomiyama, 1974).

Placental transfer

Trichloroethylene passes rapidly through the placenta into the fetus. In a study of maternal and fetal blood levels taken at delivery under trichloroethylene and nitrous oxide anaesthesia, Laham (1970) found a ratio of about 1 between maternal venous (arm vein) blood and umbilical venous blood in a total of 10 patients after about 10 to 20 min exposure. In 3 patients the fetal levels were greater than the maternal levels. The author suggested that this may be due to metabolism of the trichloroethylene in the mother but not in the fetus, but this was not studied.

B. ENDOCRINE AND GONADAL EFFECTS

No systematic studies have been reported on endocrine or gonadal effects of trichloroethylene except for a briefly reported study by Wink (1972). He analysed 4 h urine samples from 14 male workers exposed for periods from a few months to many years to trichloroethylene. All subjects excreted trichloroacetic acid, giving evidence of actual exposure, but no levels of exposure were measured. Their results were compared with 14 unexposed controls from the same factory approximately matched for workload, age (mean 42 years), social environment and sleep activity pattern. No difference was found in mean excretion of 17-oxogenic steroids (mainly from the adrenal) or 17-oxosteroids (partly adrenal and partly testicular in origin). Wide variations exist in the urinary levels of these metabolites, however, and the significance of this observation is doubtful.

There are 2 individual case reports which are relevant. Sagawa *et al.* (1973) described a case of a woman of 20 years of age who was exposed accidentally at work to a very high concentration of trichloroethylene vapour, probably several thousand ppm, sufficient to cause unconsciousness lasting 2 h. She developed very widespread neurological symptoms suggestive of a transverse lesion of the spinal cord at about the level of T2. She did not menstruate for several months following the accident and by one year later she menstruated only irregularly and her basal body temperature suggested lack of ovulation. No other investigations were carried out to study this in detail.

The second case report was by Saihan *et al.* (1978) of a 42 year old man who developed impotence, gynaecomastia, peripheral neuropathy, lymphadenopathy, scleroderma, malabsorption and Raynaud's phenomenon following prolonged exposure to trichloroethylene at work. On the basis of the similarity of his symptoms to those which have been reported in other workers exposed to the chemically similar compounds vinyl chloride and tetrachloroethylene, the authors suggest that his symptoms may have been due to trichloroethylene exposure. Various other possibilities are discussed however, and no conclusion about the role of trichloroethylene can be reached.

C. FERTILITY

No relevant data found.

D. PREGNANCY

Trichloroethylene has been used in the past as an anaesthetic in obstetrics but has been superseded by less toxic compounds. It is still used in obstetrics for its analgesic potency but it may be somewhat more hazardous than other available gas mixtures and may aggravate the normal acidosis and hypoxia of the second stage of labour (Phillips and Macdonald, 1971; Huff, 1971; Aviado *et al.*, 1976). The use of trichloroethylene as an anaesthetic and analgesic however raises matters not of relevance for this review.

E. MUTAGENICITY

Konietzko *et al.* (1978) performed chromosome analyses of cultured lymphocytes from 28 workers aged 23–67 years (mean 42) who had been employed on degreasing using trichloroethylene for 1–21 years. Nine of the men had abnormally high rates of hypodiploid cells with otherwise normal karyotypes. In these 9 cases, the trichloroethylene concentration but not the duration of exposure was greater than in the others. In a brief report of another study (or possibly extension of the same study) Konietzko (1979) also reported an increase in chromosomal aberrations in workers exposed to trichloroethylene and stated that the effect was related to the intensity but not duration of exposure.

F. CARCINOGENICITY

IARC Monograph Vol. 20 (1979) stated that there were no case reports available and the one small epidemiological study showing no significant excess of cancer was considered inadequate for assessment. For a later study on laundry and dry-cleaning workers see section F, Tetrachloroethylene.

SUMMARY AND EVALUATION

EXPERIMENTAL STUDIES

Trichloroethylene rapidly crosses the placenta and equilibrates in the fetus in sheep and goats. Exposure of male mice to up to 450 ppm for 24 h had no effect on fertility and did not induce dominant lethal mutations. Exposure of rats during pregnancy at up to 1800 ppm showed no embryolethal or teratogenic effects though fetal and postnatal growth were sometimes slightly retarded. No teratogenic or other adverse effects were observed in pregnant mice or rats up to 300 ppm. Data on mutagenicity are conflicting possibly due to contamination of some samples with epichlorohydrin. There is limited evidence that it is carcinogenic in mice.

HUMAN STUDIES

Trichloroethylene readily passes across the placenta and equilibrates in the fetus. No systematic studies of its effects on fertility or gonadal function in males or females were found. No studies on occupational exposure in pregnancy were found. There is limited evidence that exposure to high concentrations may cause chromosome damage. One small epidemiological study showed no significant excess of cancer.

EVALUATION

There is limited evidence from animal studies that trichloroethylene is not embryolethal or teratogenic at concentrations up to 1800 ppm. There is limited evidence that it is carcinogenic in mice. Data in humans are inadequate for assessment. Attention is drawn to the lack of data on fertility in animals and to the lack of data in humans of reproductive effects. There is limited evidence that it may be mutagenic in humans.

References

Aviado, D. M., Simaan, J. A., Zakhari, S. and Ulsamer, A. G. (1976). Methyl chloroform and trichloroethylene in the environment. Solvents in the Environment Series, (Ed. Goldberg, L.). CRC Press, Cleveland, Ohio.

Biles, R. W., Connor, T. H., Trieff, N. M. and Legator, M. S. (1978). The influence of contaminants on the mutagenic activity of dibromochloropropane (DBCP). *Journal of Environmental Pathology and Toxicology* **2**, (2), 301–312.

Černá, M. and Kypěnová, H. (1977). Mutagenic activity of chloroethylenes analysed by screening system tests. *Mutation Research* **46**, (3), 214–215.

Dorfmueller, M. A., Henne, S. P., York, R. G., Bornschein, R. L. and Manson, J. M. (1979). Evaluation of teratogenicity and behavioral toxicity with inhalation exposure of maternal rats to trichloroethylene. *Toxicology* **14**, 153–166.

Euler, H. H. (1967). Animal experimental studies of an industrial noxa. *Archiv fur Gynakologie* **204**, (2), 258–259.

Healy, T. E. J. and Wilcox, A. (1978). Chronic exposures of rats to inhalational anaesthetic agents. *Journal of Physiology* **276**, 24P–25P.

Helliwell, P. J. and Hutton, A. M. (1949). Analgesia in obstetrics. *Anaesthesia* **4**, 18–21.

Helliwell, P. J. and Hutton, A. M. (1950). Trichloroethylene anaesthesia. 1. Distribution in the foetal and maternal circulation of pregnant sheep and goats. *Anaesthesia* **5**, 4–13.

Huff, J. E. (1971). New evidence on the old problems of trichloroethylene. *Industrial Medicine* **40**, (8), 25–33.

IARC Monographs on the Evaluation of the Carcinogenic Risk of Chemicals to Humans; Some halogenated hydrocarbons (1979). Vol. 20, Lyon, France.

Ikeda, M. and Imamura, T. (1973). Biological half-life of trichloroethylene and tetrachloroethylene in human subjects. *Internationale Archiv fur Arbeitsmedizin* **31**, (3), 209–224.

Konietzko, H. (1979). Trichloroethylene, health hazards in occupational medicine. *Fortschritte der Medizin* **97**, (14), 671–674.

Konietzko, H., Haberlandt, W., Heilbronner, H., Reill, G. and Weichardt, H. (1978). Chromosome studies on trichloroethylene workers. *Archives of Toxicology* **40**, 201–206.

Laham, S. (1970). Studies on placental transfer. *Industrial Medicine* **39**, (1), 46–49.

Nomiyama, K. and Nomiyama, H. (1974). Respiratory retention, uptake and excretion of organic solvents in man. Benzene, toluene, n-hexane, trichloroethylene, acetone, ethyl acetate and ethyl alcohol. *International Archiv fur Arbeitsmedizin* **32**, (1/2), 75–83.

Phillips, T. J. and Macdonald, R. R. (1971). Comparative effect of pethidine, trichloroethylene and entonox on fetal and neonatal acid-base and $_{p}O_2$. *British Medical Journal* **3**, 558–559.

Sagawa, K., Nishitani, H., Kawai, H., Kuge, Y. and Ikeda, M. (1973). Transverse lesion of spinal cord after accidental exposure to trichloroethylene. *Internationale Archiv fur Arbeitsmedizin* **31**, (4), 257–264.

Saihan, E. M., Burton, J. L. and Heaton, K. W. (1978). A new syndrome with pigmentation, scleroderma, gynaecomastia, Raynaud's phenomenon and peripheral neuropathy. *British Journal of Dermatology* **99**, 437–440.

Schwetz, B. A., Leong, B. K. J. and Gehring, P. J. (1975). The effect of maternally inhaled trichloroethylene, perchloroethylene, methyl chloroform, and methylene chloride on embryonal and fetal development in mice and rats. *Toxicology and Applied Pharmacology* **32**, 84–96.

Simmon, V. F. (1977). Structural correlations of carcinogenic and mutagenic alkyl halides. *In* "Structural Correlates of Carcinogenisis and Mutagenesis" (Eds. Asher, I. M. and Zerros, C.) pp. 163–171. FDA Office of Science.
Slacik-Erben, R., Roll, R., Franke, G. and Uehleke, H. (1980). Trichloroethylene vapours do not produce dominant lethal mutations in male mice. *Archives of Toxicology* **45**, (1), 37–44.
Taylor, H. (1936). Experiments on the physiological properties of trichloroethylene. *Journal of Industrial Hygiene and Toxicology* **18**, 175–193.
White, A. E., Takehise, S., Eger, E. I., Wolff, S. and Stevens, W. C. (1979). Sister chromatid exchanges induced by inhaled anaesthetics. *Anaesthesiology* **50**, 426–430.
Wink, A. (1972). Effect of long-term exposure to low levels of toxic substances on urinary excretion of 17-oxogenic steroids and 17-oxosteroids. *Annals of Occupational Hygiene* **15**, 211–215.

46. Vinyl Chloride

TECHNICAL DATA

Formula	$CH_2{=}CHCl$
CAS registry number	75–01–4
Chemical abstracts name	Chloroethylene
Synonyms	Chlorethene; chlorethylene; chloroethene; ethylene monochloride; monochloroethene; monochloroethylene.
Uses	Plastics industry; refrigerant; in organic syntheses; production of vinyl chloride resins, methyl chloroform; component of propellant mixtures.
TLV	5 ppm

ANIMAL STUDIES

A. RELEVANT PHARMACOLOGY AND TOXICOLOGY

Elimination of vinyl chloride monomer (VCM) from the body is very rapid; Feron *et al.* (1975) found over 90% of a dose of 300 mg/kg VCM, given orally by gavage or by i.p. injection, was recovered from exhaled gases within 4 h of administration. In a sub-acute study, where groups of 15 male and female weanling rats were given 30, 100 or 300 mg/kg/day VCM by gavage for 6 days/week for 13 weeks, Feron *et al.* (1975) found no sex differences in toxicity in terms of organ weights and histology, haematological parameters or liver toxicity.

Ungváry *et al.* (1978) have shown placental transfer of maternally inhaled VCM. Groups of 3 rats were exposed to 0, 2000, 7000 or 12,000 ppm (0, 5500, 18,000 or 33,000 mg/m^3) for 2·5 h on day 18 of pregnancy, then killed. Levels in maternal blood averaged 19·0–48·4 μg/ml in VCM-exposed groups, levels in fetal blood 12·8–30·5 μg/ml and in amniotic fluid 4·3–13·5 μg/ml, showing substantial transfer of VCM to the fetus during continuous maternal exposure to relatively high concentrations. In view of the lipophilic nature of VCM this substantial transfer is not surprising, but since there is rapid excretion of VCM when given acutely as a single dose, placental transfer following administration by gavage or injection is likely to be much lower than with continuous inhalation.

B. ENDOCRINE AND GONADAL EFFECTS

No relevant data found.

C. FERTILITY

Absence of dominant lethal effects has been shown in mice and rats. Anderson *et al.* (1977) exposed groups of 20 male mice to 0, 3000, 10,000 or 30,000 ppm VCM by inhalation for 6 h/day for 5 days and then mated them with 2 untreated females/week for 8 weeks. Survival was significantly reduced to 45% in the highest dose group. There were no significant effects on numbers mating, numbers pregnant, pre- or post-implantation losses except for a reduction in total implants/female in week 4 of mating in the highest dose group. However, this latter finding was due largely to a small number of implants in one female and is not therefore likely to be of any biological significance. Treatment with positive control substances, cyclophosphamide or ethyl methane-sulphonate, showed clear dominant lethal effects.

Short *et al.* (1977) exposed groups of 12 male rats to 0, 50, 250 or 1000 ppm VCM by inhalation for 6 h/day, 5 days/week for 11 weeks. During the eleventh week of exposure, each male was housed between exposures with 2 untreated females for 7 successive evenings or until mating with both females had occurred. There was a significant reduction in the number of males in the 1000 ppm group that mated with 2 females (8/12 compared with 12/12 in controls). Two of the males in the 1000 ppm group did not mate at all, whereas in all other groups every male mated at least once. At both 250 and 1000 ppm the ratio of pregnant to mated females was significantly reduced from 24/24 in controls to 16/23 at 250 ppm and 14/18 at 1000 ppm. However, there were no significant effects on total implants/dam or dead implants/dam in those that were pregnant in any group. The authors also mention that in a chronic study in their laboratory, no effects on the testes or accessory organs were found with exposure of male rats to 250 or 1000 ppm VCM for 9–12 months, though carcinomas of the liver and lung were seen.

Conclusion
Dominant lethal effects have not been observed in mice and rats exposed to clearly carcinogenic or near lethal levels of VCM by inhalation. However, in the rat study, findings indicative of reduced mating performance, infertile matings and/or early losses of fertilised ova have been seen with sub-acute exposure to 250 ppm. There have been no studies of the effect of VCM on female fertility.

D. PREGNANCY

Teratology studies on inhaled VCM have been carried out in the mouse, rat and rabbit. John *et al.* (1977) exposed all 3 species to VCM during organogenesis in a study on behalf of the Manufacturing Chemists Association, U.S.A. Acceptable teratological methods were used. Groups of 27–37 mice were exposed to 50 or 500 ppm for 7 h/day on days 6–15 of pregnancy, each with concurrent 0 ppm control groups. At 500 ppm there was some evidence of maternal toxicity; food consumption, weight gain and liver weight were all significantly reduced and 5/29 animals in this group died. There were no deaths or signs of maternal toxicity in the 50 ppm group. There were significant decreases in total implants/dam and mean fetal weight and a significant increase in resorption rate in the 500 ppm group in comparison with concurrent controls. However, it should be noted that there was considerable variation between the 2 control groups and differences between the 500 ppm VCM group and the other control group concurrent with the 50 ppm VCM group were not significant. There were no significant effects on malformation or anomaly rates, except for an increase in unfused sternebrae and delayed ossification of the sternebrae and skull in the 500 ppm group.

John *et al.* (1977) exposed groups of 17–33 rats to 500 or 2500 ppm VCM for 7 h/day on days 6–15 of pregnancy, each with concurrent 0 ppm control groups. Maternal weight gain was significantly reduced in the 500 ppm group in comparison with concurrent controls, but was similar to that in the 0 ppm group concurrent with the 2500 ppm group. It was not reduced in the 2500 ppm group. The significant difference observed in the 500 ppm group is probably due to the low body weight of concurrent controls in early pregnancy which was made up during the course of pregnancy. Absolute and relative liver weights were increased in the 2500 ppm group and one of the dams in this group died. There were sporadic significant differences in outcome of pregnancies between VCM and control groups, but, apart from an increase in dilated ureter in fetuses from the 2500 ppm group, none of the changes were dose-related and are therefore unlikely to be treatment-related effects.

John *et al.* (1977) also exposed groups of 7–20 rabbits to 500 or 2500 ppm

VCM for 7 h/day on days 6–18 of pregnancy, each with concurrent 0 ppm control groups. One doe in the 2500 ppm group died. Weight gain and food consumption were highly variable in VCM and control groups. A significant decrease in food consumption in the 500 ppm group in relation to concurrent controls, but not in the 2500 ppm group, is probably of no biological significance. Likewise, significant decreases in implantation sites/dam and live fetuses/dam in the 500 ppm group are most probably the consequence of the significant decrease in corpora lutea/dam in this group and of no biological importance. There was also a significant increase in delayed ossification of the sternebrae at 500 ppm but not at 2500 ppm.

Ungváry *et al.* (1978) have confirmed the absence of teratogenicity of VCM in the rat. They exposed groups of 13–28 rats to 0 or 1500 ppm VCM (4000 mg/m^3) for 24 h/day on days 1–9, 8–14 or 14–21 of pregnancy. Acceptable teratological methods were used. There was no maternal mortality and no significant reduction in weight gain except in those exposed in the third week of pregnancy. Maternal liver:body weight ratio was significantly increased in those exposed in the first or second but not the third week of pregnancy. No histological changes were seen in maternal livers at autopsy. There were no effects on live fetuses/dam, dead fetuses/dam, fetal weight, malformation or anomaly rates due to VCM, but there was a significant increase in resorption rate from 3·4% in untreated controls to 5·5% in those exposed on days 1–9 of pregnancy.

Mirkova *et al.* (1978), however, claim to have found significant embryolethality, teratogenicity and fetotoxicity following exposure to a level as low as 2·5 ppm (6·15 mg/m^3) continuously throughout gestation in the rat. Adequate numbers of rats (40 treated and control) and acceptable teratological methods were used. Results however are reported in qualitative terms only with no significance levels or without control comparisons. Embryomortality in the VCM group was doubled in comparison with controls and fetal weight was reduced, but no further information is given. There was an 8-fold rise in "anomalies of a general nature (haematoma)" in comparison with controls. Teratogenic effects were also seen affecting the brain, blood vessel walls and ossification of the sternum; VCM exposed fetuses had 2·5% encephalocoele, 54% hydrocephalus with intracerebral haematomata, 14% isolated haematomata, and 3% additional ossification centres in the sternum. No control abnormality rates are given. Retarded brain development may be mistaken for true internal hydrocephalus; however, the occurrence of such a high incidence of intracerebral haematomas is an unusual finding and cannot be dismissed.

Mirkova *et al.* (1978) also studied postnatal development of offspring born to rats exposed to 2·5 ppm VCM throughout pregnancy. Postnatal weight gain and survival were unaffected but some change in liver function was evident from increased barbiturate-induced sleeping time and changes in biliary excretion at 1–2 months of age.

Bingham *et al.* (1979) have noted low birth weights in pups born to rats exposed to 600 or 6000 ppm VCM for 4 h/day on days 9–21 of pregnancy in comparison with controls, but more detailed information on postnatal development in these animals is not yet available.

Conclusion

Two separate groups of workers, using doses of 500–2500 ppm VCM, have shown absence of teratogenicity and fetotoxicity in the rat, and one of these groups has shown absence of teratogenicity in the rabbit at 500–2500 ppm and in the mouse at 50–500 ppm. The highest doses were toxic to the dam in all 3 species. There was a suggestion of a small increase (around a doubling) in embryomortality following exposure to 1500 ppm VCM in the rat in early pregnancy (days 1–9), but no increased embryomortality was seen in the mouse, rat or rabbit if exposure was confined to the period of organogenesis. One group of workers claimed to have observed a doubling in embryomortality, a high incidence of cerebral malformations and fetotoxicity with exposure to only 2·5 ppm throughout pregnancy. The study was poorly reported and in view of the large difference in dose level between this and other negative studies, these results await confirmation.

Reports of studies to date on postnatal development after prenatal VCM exposure are inadequate for proper assessment, with the exception of a transplacental carcinogenicity study (see section F for details) which suggests that *in utero* exposure to VCM may induce a wider variety of tumours more readily than adult exposure. Tumours have been seen in offspring exposed prenatally to 6000 ppm VCM but not in their exposed mothers. It is not known whether, as with adult carcinogens, there is no threshold level for tumour induction for transplacental carcinogens.

E. MUTAGENICITY

VCM is mutagenic in yeast cells in the host-mediated assay (Loprieno *et al.*, 1976) and in bacteria in the Ames test after metabolic activation by liver enzymes (Bartsch and Montesano, 1975). VCM without metabolic activation is mutagenic in the Ames test but it is not clear whether this may be due to non-enzymatic breakdown products or to VCM *per se* (Bartsch and Montesano, 1975; Simmon, 1977). The major VCM metabolites formed *in vitro* by hepatic microsomal enzyme preparations from mice, rats and humans are chloroethylene oxide (an epoxide) and chloroacetaldehyde; these are clearly mutagenic in bacterial systems (Bartsch and Montesano, 1975), and other potential metabolites of VCM, such as the monomer, dimer and trimer hydrates of chloroacetaldehyde, are also Ames-positive (Laumbach *et al.*, 1977). The comparative metabolism of VCM *in vivo* is not known.

F. CARCINOGENICITY

IARC Monograph Vol. 19 (1979) reported studies showing that vinyl chloride is carcinogenic in mice, rats and hamsters following oral or inhalational administration.

VCM, an adult carcinogen in animals and humans, has been shown to be a transplacental carcinogen in the rat. Maltoni (1976) exposed groups of 30 rats to 6000 or 10,000 ppm for 4 h/day on days 12–18 of pregnancy. By the end of the experiment 143 weeks later, 3 of the breeding females in the 10,000 ppm group had developed tumours (angioma or angiosarcoma), and none in the 6000 ppm group. In their offspring, 6/32 animals from the 6000 ppm group and 8/54 animals from the 10,000 ppm group had tumours of various types (including angiosarcoma) and sites; the earliest tumours developed at 22–24 weeks of age (Maltoni and Lefemine, 1974).

HUMAN STUDIES

A. RELEVANT PHARMACOLOGY AND TOXICOLOGY

No relevant data found.

B. ENDOCRINE AND GONADAL EFFECTS

Walker (1976) has recorded loss of libido as one of the presenting symptoms in men exposed to high levels (unspecified) of vinyl chloride monomer (VCM) on at least one occasion. She examined a total of 37 men aged 26–59 years (average age 40 years) who had been employed at a polyvinyl chloride (PVC) manufacturing plant for 9 months to 5½ years (average 2 years 8 months). Thirty had at some time been reactor operators. Four were maintenance men, 2 worked as "baggers" and 1 was a warehouseman. Presenting symptoms in order of frequency included excessive fatigue, cold hands, aches in bones, dyspnoea, paraesthesia, cold feet, aches in muscles, impaired grip and loss of libido in 13/37 cases. Walker (1975) has elsewhere described the men as suffering from impotence, but no further details have been given. Clinically the men showed signs of Raynaud's phenomenon, severe in some cases, and circulatory changes which may account for some of the symptoms such as dyspnoea, pains in the limbs, paraesthesia and fatigue. It is not known if such changes might also account for the reported loss of libido or potency.

C. FERTILITY

No relevant data found.

D. PREGNANCY

Selikoff, in a personal communication to Infante (1976) first observed stillbirth and miscarriage rates that were thought to be high in the wives of VCM workers. He studied 2 plants and found rates of 140/1000 pregnancies in one plant and 72/1000 pregnancies in the other. Comparison with registered rates for stillbirth and miscarriage in the state of Georgia showed that the rates observed in wives of VCM workers were 2–4 times higher than those for Georgia as a whole. However, reliability of ascertainment in both cases and Georgia registry data is not known.

Infante (1976) has studied congenital malformation rates in 3 Ohio, U.S.A. communities that have PVC production facilities: Painesville, Ashtabula and Avon Lake, with populations of 12,000–24,000. Data on specific congenital malformations in Ohio residents have been recorded on birth certificates since 1968. For the entire State, the malformation rate/1000 live births was 10·14 for the years 1970–1973. Rates for these years combined in the 3 study populations were 17·37 (Ashtabula), 18·10 (Painesville) and 20·33 (Avon Lake), significantly higher than expected from the State rate ($P<0·01$). Comparison of malformation rates in the study populations compared to those in the balance of the counties in which they were located also showed a significantly higher rate than expected in 2 out of the 3 study populations and if data from all 3 populations and the balance of the counties was combined then the difference was highly significant ($P<0·001$). Comparison of rates in the 3 study cities with rates in 10 other cities surrounding the index cities showed lower malformation rates in 8 of them (2·06–12·05/1000 live births). The 2 non-index cities with high rates were Geneva (25·4/1000) located 12 miles from Ashtabula, and North Ridgeville (27·3/1000) located 8 miles from Avon Lake. The authors determined that race, maternal age and reporting from different hospitals could not account for the high rates observed in the 3 study populations. Combining the data on malformations from the 3 study areas there appeared to be a significant excess risk for defects of the central nervous system (CNS), upper alimentary tract, genital organs and club foot.

The relative risk of CNS malformations amongst live and stillbirths was increased in Ashtabula (1·95) and Painesville (5·80) but not in Avon Lake (0·00). Painesville has 2 PVC plants and the other 2 areas one each, but vinyl chloride levels in the 3 study areas were not monitored and the authors of the report stressed that these preliminary findings do not link PVC production with the increases in congenital malformations but indicate the need for further study of possible contributing factors.

Edmonds *et al.* (1975), using data collected through the U.S. Public Health Service Center for Disease Control's hospital-based birth defects monitoring programme, studied CNS malformation rates in 2 hospitals located in cities with PVC plants, in Pennsylvania and in Painesville, Ohio. White infants born in 1970–1974 only were included. An increase, primarily in spina bifida and anencephaly, was noted in Painesville but not in Pennsylvania in comparison with rates for each State as a whole. Anencephaly rates/10,000 births were 14·1 in Painesville compared with 5·7 for Ohio as a whole and for spina bifida 21·2 in Painesville compared with 8·9 in Ohio as a whole. However, the rates are based on a total of only 15 cases of anencephaly and spina bifida in Painesville in 1970–1974. The 15 cases were also compared with 30 controls (the first normal white infant born before or after each case) to compare parents' occupation and residence at the time of the infant's birth. None of the parents of the 15 cases had ever worked at the PVC plants in Painesville but 2 fathers of controls had worked at one of the plants. None of the parents of cases or controls lived within 2 miles of the plant and a significantly larger proportion of control mothers than case mothers worked (including housewives) within a 10-mile radius of the PVC plant. Thus, although this study confirmed an increase in CNS malformations in Painesville no direct association with PVC production could be shown.

Edmonds *et al.* (1978) have carried out another study in Kanawha County. Of the 40 PVC polymerisation plants in the U.S., 17 were located in counties which in 1974 had at least one hospital participating in the Center for Disease Control's birth defects monitoring programme. Ten were excluded because data were available on fewer than 50% of the births in the county. Of the remaining 7 counties, 2 had CNS malformation rates significantly higher than national rates in 1970–1974. They were Painesville, Ohio and Kanawha County, West Virginia. A detailed epidemiological investigation was therefore undertaken in Kanawha County. All infants born with a CNS defect in 1970–1974 whose parents were resident in Kanawha County at the time of birth were identified. Controls were taken as the first normal infants born to parents resident in Kanawha County whose birth certificates preceded or followed each case in the records of the West Virginia State Department of Vital Statistics. Cases and controls were then matched for month of birth, race, paternal education and maternal age. A total of 47 cases of CNS malformations were identified, giving an overall rate for 1970–1974 of 28·8/10,000 births, but the yearly rates declined dramatically from 40·6 in 1970, 42·9 in 1971, 37·6 in 1972, 16·3 in 1973 to 3·2 in 1974. Families of 46 infants with defects and 46 matched controls were interviewed. Two fathers of cases and 2 fathers of controls were employed at the PVC plant at the time of conception and fathers of 3 other controls had worked briefly in the plant on a contract basis. None of the case or control mothers had ever worked at the plant. There were no significant differences between case and control parents in either distance of place of residence from the plant or distance of place of work (residence if housewife or unemployed). However, it was noted that the 9 case families living within 3 miles of the plant had a different residential distribution (mostly to the north-east) than control families (mostly to the south). For this study data on air pollution with VCM was available. From 1967–1973 annual mean emissions ranged from 235–270 lb/h, declining to 180 lb/h in 1974 and 76 lb/h in 1975. Estimates of abnormal emissions available from 1970 onwards declined steadily from 28 in 1970, 18 in 1971, 12 in 1972, 5 in 1973 and 2 in 1974, to 0 in 1975. The largest known single emission produced atmospheric VCM levels of 0·1–0·2 ppm to the north-east of the plant. This study provides no support for a relationship between parental occupation in PVC manufacture and CNS malformations, though the numbers actually employed at the plant in the total sample are too small to draw any firm conclusions. The decline in VCM emissions alongside the decline in CNS malformation rates between 1970 and 1974, however, is striking and whilst the greatest decrease in malformation rates occurred in 1973, preceding the marked decline in overall VCM emissions in 1974, the decrease in malformation rates does parallel more closely the estimates of abnormally high emissions. So whilst the study does not provide any clear evidence of an association between atmospheric VCM and CNS malformations, it does not permit such an association to be ruled out. The authors of this study have pointed out, however, that there are 7 major chemical plants in the Kanawha River Valley, emitting an estimated 52,457 tons a year of over 100 different organic compounds including VCM. Thus to implicate VCM alone would be difficult.

Infante *et al.* (1976a) have studied the outcome of pregnancy in wives of 95 VCM polymerization workers. They were compared with 2 control groups of 158 wives of PVC fabrication workers or rubber workers, who were known to have little or no VCM exposure, respectively. Data on paternal age, pregnancy outcome, and estimated time of conception for each pregnancy were ascertained by interview of the male workers and wives were not interviewed. Age-adjusted fetal death rates for pregnancies occurring prior to exposure were not significantly different at 6·1% for the VCM-exposed group and 6·9% for controls, but for pregnancies occurring after exposure they were

15·8% in the VCM-exposed group compared with 8·8% in controls ($P<0{\cdot}05$). Mean paternal age at conception was similar for each group before or after exposure but the majority of fetal deaths in the VCM group were from the younger-aged husbands; in those aged 30 years or older fetal mortality rates were 13·0% and 12·0% in VCM and control groups respectively, whilst in those aged less than 30 years, rates were 20·0% and 5·3% in VCM and control groups respectively. It is possible that younger employees had higher VCM exposures, the older workers in more senior jobs being less exposed. Comparison of fetal death rates with the VCM group before (6·1%) and after exposure (15·8%) was also significantly different ($P<0{\cdot}02$) whereas the comparison within controls (6·9% versus 8·8%) was not. The trend to higher fetal death rates after VCM exposure was still maintained when wives with one, more than 2 or more than 3 abortions were successively eliminated. The authors considered that the effects observed were unlikely to be due to direct exposure to VCM since VCM is highly volatile and unlikely to be carried home, for example, on clothing by the father. The effects are more likely to be due to damage to the paternal germ cells from VCM exposure.

A number of criticisms have been made of this study including the use of a questionnaire and the low response rates (62–77% of those selected for interview) and the misleading method of age-adjustment (Paddle, 1976), though the latter criticism has been rebutted to a certain extent (Infante *et al.* 1976b). Buffler (1979) has also pointed out that there is lack of information on maternal age, parity, socio-economic status and dose and timing of exposure of the husband in relation to each pregnancy, and there is unreliability of husband's recall, particularly of early spontaneous abortions, and possibly response bias since the workers were aware of some health effects of VCM. Buffler (1979) has described the methodology of a more rigorous study on over 200 VCM exposed workers where wives are being interviewed too to collect data on reproductive history. The results of this study are not available at this time.

In summary, 3 studies of communities living close to PVC plants suggest there may be an association between such a location and an increased risk of malformation, particularly of the CNS. However, none of the studies produced clear-cut association and other uncontrolled variables, including other industrial pollutants, may account for the differences observed. A single study of VCM-exposed workers showing an increase in fetal death rates in their wives is more convincing but had a number of methodological problems, and further more rigorous studies of PVC workers are required before any definite conclusions may be reached.

E. MUTAGENICITY

There have been a number of studies of chromosome aberrations in lymphocytes of workers exposed to VCM, some showing an increased frequency and some showing no increase in comparison with controls.

Funes-Cravioto *et al.* (1975) found a mean frequency of 9·52% cytogenetically abnormal cells in cultured lymphocytes from 7 workers exposed to VCM for 9–29 years, compared with 1·94% in 3 controls. VCM levels in the plant in the weeks before collection of blood samples were estimated to be 20–30 ppm. However, there was considerable heterogeneity, 2 VCM workers not differing significantly from controls. Only one case showed any symptoms of vinyl chloride disease; he had slight thrombocytopenia and α_1-trypsin deficiency and had the highest chromosome aberration rate in the group (18%).

Ducatman *et al.* (1975) have also found a significantly higher incidence of unstable chromosome aberrations (fragments, dicentrics and rings) in lymphocytes from 11 VCM polymerization workers compared with 10 from the same factory but not knowingly exposed to VCM. Exposure data was not available, but it was assumed levels exceeded 500 ppm from time to time, based on reports of odour, dizziness and headaches. However, there were no significant differences between exposed and control groups in breaks, gaps or stable chromosome changes. Furthermore, the groups were not matched for age; the exposed group averaged 40 years of age, and controls 27 years. It is possible that this age difference might account for the increase in frequency of unstable chromosome changes.

Purchase *et al.* (1975, 1978) have published preliminary and full data on a larger study of 81 VCM-exposed workers employed in PVC manufacture as autoclave workers, maintenance workers and workers associated with VCM manufacture. Exposure averaged 6–15 years in the different sub-groups and exposure levels for autoclave workers (the highest exposed group) were estimated as 300–400 ppm in 1960–1970, 15 ppm in mid-1973 and 5 ppm in 1975. Blood samples for lymphocyte culture were collected in mid-1974. In the 24 controls (19 on site, 5 off site), an average of 1·08% of cells were abnormal compared with the various exposed groups where averages ranged from 1·40% in laboratory workers and managers to 3·18% in autoclave operators. The means for the sub-groups were significantly higher than controls in the case of VC maintenance workers (2·43%), VC operators (2·43%) and autoclave operators (3·18%). Chromosome aberrations were correlated with overall exposure levels, length of employment, with a history of exposure to excursion levels in the year prior to sampling and with smoking habits, but not with liver function tests.

Szentesi *et al.* (1976) have studied chromosome aberrations in lymphocytes from 45 PVC workers exposed to VCM for 1–12 years (mean age 27 years), 44 industrial controls working in other chemical plants (mean age 44 years) and

49 normal controls with no occupational exposure to chemicals (mean age 29 years). There were significant increases in chromatid-type aberrations and in unstable chromosome-type aberrations in PVC workers compared with either of the control groups and aberrations were correlated with length of exposure.

Kučerová (1976) has published a small study on 9 workers with long-term exposure to VCM at 500 ppm or more ranging from 8–16 years. Blood samples for lymphocyte culture were taken twice, 8 months apart. There was considerable heterogeneity, some workers having aberration rates close to that of controls (1·2%) and other having much higher rates (3–11%). Furthermore workers with a high aberration rate in one sample did not necessarily have a high aberration rate in the other. The authors attributed this to irregular exposure due to the cyclic character of the production process. The overall aberration rate in the exposed group was 3·0% at the first sampling and 2·6% at the second. These same workers were studied again on a third occasion, 2 years after the first sampling (Kučerová *et al.*, 1979) and the aberration rate averaged 5·2% compared with 1·8% in 8 age-matched controls. It was confirmed that there was considerable variability within exposed individuals at the 3 sampling points. They also analysed for sister-chromatid exchange (SCE) and found a significant increase from 9·41 SCE/cell in controls to 13·80 SCE/cell in the exposed group. Mean exposure rates were stated in this paper to be 20–150 ppm VCM.

Hansteen *et al.* (1978) have also found differences in a group of workers sampled twice 2–2·5 years apart. A total of 39 PVC workers were studied, 14 chosen at random, 13 because they had been heavily exposed to VCM and 12 who had shown clinical abnormalities in an earlier health screen but were normal at the time of cytogenetic analysis, with average length of employment 10·3 years, 13·7 years and 16·5 years respectively. Blood samples were first taken in 1974 when air concentrations of VCM at the plant were estimated to be around 80 ppm. Prior to this levels were estimated as 2000 ppm in 1950–1954, 1000 ppm in 1955–1959, 500 ppm in 1960–1967 and 100 ppm in 1968–1972. Results were compared with 16 controls not connected with the PVC plant. In the first investigation, the mean frequency of chromosome breakage was 3·41% in the exposed groups and 1·79% in controls ($P<0{\cdot}025$). In the 3 subgroups exposed to VCM it was highest (3·97%) in the heavily exposed workers. At the repeat study, there was no significant difference between exposed and control groups in either frequency of breakage or sister-chromatid exchange (SCE). This decrease in breakage frequency in the exposed group in 1977 was attributed to the marked reduction in VCM exposure occurring from 1974 onwards; in 1974 levels were decreased to 25 ppm and then to 1 ppm from 1975 onwards. The results on SCE analysis do not agree with those of Kučerová *et al.* (1979), but recent exposure levels in the latter study were much higher.

Fleig and Thiess (1978) have studied aberration rates in 10 workers exposed to VCM but showing no symptoms and in 20 workers showing symptoms of VCM induced illness including one case with angiosarcoma. Exposure levels were not known. Results were compared with 20 age-matched controls working in the same factory but not exposed to VCM. The frequency of aberrations (including gaps) was 5·5% in controls, 7·5% in exposed workers without symptoms and 11·2% in exposed workers with symptoms. In the angiosarcoma case the rate was 16·6% but he had received polychemotherapy 9 months before cytogenetic analysis and it is not known if the aberrations were due partly to drug treatment as well as VCM exposure.

There are, however, a number of negative studies on chromosome aberrations in VCM-exposed workers. Fleig and Thiess (1974) in their first study found no increase in aberrations in a group of 10 PVC workers compared with 4 controls (range 0–5% in both groups). Picciano *et al.* (1977) could also find no increase in aberrations in a large group of 209 workers employed for up to 28 years (mean 4 years) in VCM production. Results were compared with pre-employment examinations of 295 prospective employees with no known history of exposure to clastogenic agents. The mean age of the VCM-exposed group was 39·5 years compared with 25·1 years in controls, which, if anything, would bias results in the direction of positive findings in the exposed group. The aberration frequency averaged 3·7% in VCM workers and 4·5% in controls. When the exposed groups were broken down into subgroups on the basis of exposure levels (<1 ppm, 1–5 ppm and >5 ppm), the aberration rate in those exposed to >5 ppm was almost identical to that in controls. The authors suggest that their negative findings may be due to the relatively low exposures in their workers compared with that in other positive studies.

Heath *et al.* (1977) have also found no increase in chromosome breaks in VCM-exposed workers compared with controls from other industries. Mean frequency of breaks was 6·7% in 14 workers exposed to high VCM levels (not specified), 7·8% in 4 men exposed to lower VCM levels and 5·9% in 17 industrial controls working in rubber tyre manufacture. However, all 3 of these groups differed significantly from a group of 4 male controls not occupationally exposed to chemicals, where the aberration rate was 3·6%. The negative results in this study may reflect the small sample size and possible inappropriateness of industry controls who may also have been exposed to clastogenic agents.

Koizumi *et al.* (1979) have also shown no significant difference in chromosome aberrations between 15 workers exposed to VCM for 6–24 years (mean 11·5 years) and 15 controls, fairly closely matched for age.

In summary, there have been 7 positive studies and 4 negative studies on VCM-exposed workers, but the balance of evidence would seem to indicate that chromosome aberrations are related to level of exposure and duration of exposure. With a history of average exposures above 20 ppm and intermittent exposure to higher excursion levels most studies have shown an increase in the frequency of chromosome aberrations. It is notable that 3/4 negative studies were published after 1976 when exposure levels in most plants would be considerably lower than in previous years. The fourth negative study had very small sample sizes and the same authors subsequently published a positive study on larger groups of workers.

F. CARCINOGENICITY

IARC Monograph Vol. 19 (1979) states that vinyl chloride is a human carcinogen and its target organs are liver, brain, lung and haemolymphopoietic system.

SUMMARY AND EVALUATION

EXPERIMENTAL DATA

Vinyl chloride rapidly crosses the placenta and equilibrates in the fetus. No studies on endocrine or gonadal effects were found. Exposure of male mice up to 30,000 ppm and rats to up to 1000 ppm did not produce any evidence of dominant lethal mutations and only a transient effect on fertility was observed in rats at the highest toxic doses. No studies on female fertility were found. Studies in mice, rats and rabbits exposed to up to 2500 ppm during pregnancy showed no adverse effects. One unconfirmed study in rats, however, did report embryolethal and teratogenic effects from exposure as low as 2·5 ppm during pregnancy. Studies on postnatal survival are insufficient for analysis. Vinyl chloride is mutagenic in a variety of *in vitro* systems with activation. It is carcinogenic in mice, rats and hamsters and is a transplacental carcinogen in rats. Exposure of pregnant rats to 6000 ppm produced no tumours in the dams when assessed 143 weeks later but did produce various tumours including angiosarcomas in 6 of 32 offspring, the earliest of which developed in less than 6 months.

HUMAN STUDIES

Among the symptoms experienced by men exposed to vinyl chloride occupationally, impotence and loss of libido have been reported commonly. No studies on fertility were found. Three studies of communities living near

PVC plants have suggested that there may be a higher incidence of CNS defects in children at these sites than expected. None of these studies were conclusive, however, and usually many other industrial chemicals could also have been involved. One study showed an increased fetal death rate in the wives of exposed workers. More rigorous studies are needed to examine these claims and also to define if the effect is on the pregnant woman or is mediated via the sperm of exposed men. Mutagenicity studies on exposed workers have produced conflicting results but several good studies have shown increases in chromosomal abnormalities related to duration and extent of exposure. Where exposure was greater than 20 ppm most studies showed positive results. It is a human carcinogen with target organs of liver, brain, lung and haemo-lymphopoietic system.

EVALUATION

Data on endocrines, gonads and fertility are inadequate for evaluation. Limited studies in animals have shown that it is not teratogenic or embryotoxic at otherwise non-toxic doses. It is a transplacental carcinogen and the fetus may be more susceptible than the dam but this requires confirmation. Data on its teratogenic potential in humans are inadequate for evaluation but attention is drawn to the need for further studies to evaluate its embryolethal and teratogenic effects by studies in both exposed women and men. It is a human carcinogen but there are no data on its transplacental carcinogenic potential in humans.

References

Anderson, D., Hodge, M. C. E. and Purchase, I. F. H. (1977). Dominant lethal studies with the halogenated olefins vinyl chloride and vinylidene dichloride in male CD-1 mice. *Environmental Health Perspectives* **21**, 71–78.

Bartsch, H. and Montesano, R. (1975). Mutagenic and carcinogenic effects of vinyl chloride. *Mutation Research* **32**, 93–114.

Bingham, E., Warkany, J. and Radike, M. (1979). Teratological effects of vinyl chloride and ethanol in rats. Annual Report of Program 1978–1979, pp. 140–143. Center for the Study of the Human Environment, Department of Environmental Health, Kettering Laboratory, University of Cincinnati, U.S.A.

Buffler, P. A. (1979). Some problems involved in recognising teratogens used in industry. *Contributions to Epidemiology and Biostatistics* **1**, 118–137.

Ducatman, A., Hirschhorn, K. and Selikoff, I. J. (1975). Vinyl chloride exposure and human chromosome aberrations. *Mutation Research* **31**, (3), 163–168.

Edmonds, L. D., Falk, H. and Nissim, J. E. (1975). Congenital malformations and vinyl chloride (letter). *Lancet* **ii**, 1098.

Edmonds, L. D., Anderson, C. E., Flynt, J. W. and James, L. M. (1978). Congenital central nervous system malformations and vinyl chloride monomer exposure: A community study. *Teratology* **17**, 137–142.

Feron, V. J., Speek, A. J., Willems, M. I., Battum, D. and DeGroot, A. P. (1975). Observations on the oral administration and toxicity of vinyl chloride in rats. *Food and Cosmetics Toxicology* **13**, (6), 633–638.

Fleig, I. and Thiess, A. M. (1974). Chromosomen-Untersuchung bei Vinylchlorid-Exposition. *Arbeitsmedizin, Sozialmedizin, Praeventivmedizin* **9**, 280–283.

Fleig, I. and Thiess, A. M. (1978). Mutagenicity of vinyl chloride. External chromosome studies on persons with and without VC illness, and on VC exposed animals. *Journal of Occupational Medicine* **20**, (8), 557–561.

Funcs-Cravioto, F., Lambcrt, B., Lindstcn, J., Ehrcnbcrg, L., Natarajan, A. T. and Osterman-Golkar, S. (1975). Chromosome aberrations in workers exposed to vinyl chloride. *Lancet* **i**, 459.

Hansteen, I., Hillestad, L., Thiis-Evensen, E. and Heldaas, S. S. (1978). Effects of vinyl chloride in man: a cytogenic follow-up study. *Mutation Research* **51**, (2), 271–278.

Heath, C. W., Dumont, C. R., Gamble, J. and Waxweiler, R. J. (1977). Chromosomal damage in men occupationally exposed to vinyl chloride monomer and other chemicals. *Environmental Research* **14**, 68–72.

IARC Monographs on the Evaluation of the Carcinogenic Risk of Chemicals to Humans: Some monomers, plastics and synthetic elastomers and acrolein (1979). Vol. 19, Lyon, France.

Infante, P. F. (1976). Oncogenic and mutagenic risks in communities with polyvinyl chloride production facilities. *Annals of the New York Academy of Sciences* **271**, 49–57.

Infante, P. F., McMichael, A. J., Wagoner, J. K., Waxweiler, R. J. and Falk, H. (1976a). Genetic risks of vinyl chloride. *Lancet* **i**, 734–735.

Infante, P. F., Wagoner, J. K., McMichael, A. J., Waxweiler, R. J. and Falk, H. (1976b). Genetic risks of vinyl chloride (letter). *Lancet* **i**, 1289–1290.

John, J. A., Smith, F. A., Leong, B. K. J. and Schwetz, B. A. (1977). The effects of maternally inhaled vinyl chloride on embryonal and fetal development in mice, rats and rabbits. *Toxicology and Applied Pharmacology* **39**, 497–513.

Koizumi, A., Dobashi, Y. and Tachibana, Y. (1979). Chromosome changes induced by industrial chemicals. *Japanese Journal of Industrial Health* **21**, (1), 3–10.

Kučerová, M. (1976). Cytogenic analysis of human chromosomes and its value for the estimation of genetic risk. *Mutation Research* **41**, (1), 123–130.

Kučerová, M., Polivkova, Z. and Batora, J. (1979). Comparative evaluation of the frequency of chromosomal aberrations and the SCE numbers in peripheral lymphocytes of workers occupationally exposed to vinyl chloride monomer. *Mutation Research* **67**, 97–100.

Laumbach, A. D., Lee, S., Wong, J. and Streips, U. N. (1977). Studies on the mutagenicity of vinyl chloride metabolites and related chemicals. *Detection and Prevention of Cancer (Proceedings of the 3rd International Symposium)* **1**, (1), 155–170.

Loprieno, N., Barale, R., Baroncelli, S., Bauer, C., Bronzetti, G., Cammellini, A., Cercignani, G., Corsi, C., Gervasi, G., Leporini, C., Nieri, R., Rossi, A., Stretti, G. and Turchi, G. (1976). Evaluation of the genetic effects induced by vinyl chloride monomer (VCM) under mammalian metabolic activation: studies *in vitro* and *in vivo*. *Mutation Research* **40**, (2), 85–96.

Maltoni, C. (1976). Occupational chemical carcinogenesis: new facts, priorities and perspectives. IARC Scientific Publications **13**, 127–149.

Maltoni, C. and Lefemine, G. (1974). Carcinogenicity bioassays of vinyl chloride I. Research plan and early results. *Environmental Research* **7**, 387–405.

Mirkova, E., Mihailova, A. and Nosko, M. (1978). Embryotoxic and teratogenic action of vinyl chloride. *Khigiena i Zdraveopazvane* **23**, (5), 440–443.

Paddle, G. M. (1976). Genetic risks of vinyl chloride (letter). *Lancet* **i**, 1079.

Picciano, D. J., Flake, R. E., Gay, P. C. and Killian, D. J. (1977). Vinyl chloride cytogenetics. *Journal of Occupational Medicine* **19**, (8), 527–530.

Purchase, I. H. F., Richardson, C. R. and Anderson, D. (1975). Chromosomal and dominant lethal effects of vinyl chloride (letter). *Lancet* **ii**, 410–411.

Purchase, I. H. F., Richardson, C. R., Anderson, D., Paddle, G. M. and Adams, W. G. (1978). Chromosomal analyses in vinyl chloride-exposed workers. *Mutation Research* **57**, (3), 325–334.

Short, R. D., Minor, J. L., Winston, J. M. and Lee, C.-C. (1977). A dominant lethal study in male rats after repeated exposures to vinyl chloride or vinylidene chloride. *Journal of Toxicology* **3**, 965–968.

Simmon, V. F. (1977). Structural correlations of carcinogenic and mutagenic alkyl halides. *In* "Structural Correlates of Carcinogenesis and Mutagenesis" (Eds. Asher, I. M. and Zerros, C.), pp. 163–171. FDA Office of Science.

Szentesi, I., Hornyak, E., Ungváry, G., Czeizel, A., Bognor, Z. and Trimar, M. (1976). High rate of chromosomal aberration in PVC workers. *Mutation Research* **37**, (2/3), 313–316.

Ungváry, G., Hudák, A., Tatrai, E., Lorincz, M. and Folly, G. (1978). Effects of vinyl chloride exposure alone and in combination with Trypan Blue—applied systematically during all thirds of pregnancy on the fetuses of CFY rats. *Toxicology* **11**, 45–54.

Walker, A. E. (1975). A preliminary report of a vascular abnormality occurring in men engaged in the manufacture of polyvinyl chloride. *British Journal of Dermatology* **93**, 22–23.

Walker, A. E. (1976). Clinical aspects of vinyl chloride disease: skin. *Proceedings of the Royal Society of Medicine* **69**, 286–289.

47. Vinylidene Chloride

TECHNICAL DATA

Formula	$CH_2{=}CCl_2$
CAS registry number	75–35–4
Chemical abstracts name	1,1-Dichloroethene; 1,1-dichloroethylene.
Synonyms	Asym-dichloroethylene
Uses	Intermediate in production of "vinylidene polymer plastics".
TLV	10 ppm

ANIMAL STUDIES

A. RELEVANT PHARMACOLOGY AND TOXICOLOGY

Andersen and Jenkins (1977) have examined sex differences in the toxicity of vinylidene chloride in the rat. All doses were given orally by gavage and hepatotoxicity estimated by measuring plasma transaminase levels 24 h after dosing. Females were less susceptible than males, the threshold dose for hepatotoxicity being around 100 mg/kg in females compared with around 50 mg/kg in males. However, with effective doses the time course of the hepatotoxic effect, peaking at 24 h after dosing, was similar in males and females. These experiments were carried out on fasted rats and both Andersen and Jenkins (1977) and McKenna *et al.* (1978) have shown enhanced hepatotoxicity of vinylidene chloride when given to fasted rats compared with fed rats. This may be of relevance in the interpretation of experiments on reproductive function, where the doses given are high enough to diminish food intake.

The explanation of the sex difference in toxicity observed by Andersen and Jenkins (1977) may be related to the greater microsomal oxidation of compounds by males than females if vinylidene chloride is metabolised to a more toxic compound. Other data presented in their paper and that of Norris (1977) is consistent with the hypothesis of formation of a toxic metabolite by microsomal oxidation. Norris (1977) has also obtained preliminary data showing that the production of reactive metabolite(s) from vinylidene chloride is greater in the mouse than in the rat, and the mouse is known to be more susceptible to its toxic effects than the rat or man.

B. ENDOCRINE AND GONADAL EFFECTS

No relevant data found.

C. FERTILITY

Norris (1977) reported on a 3 generation reproduction study carried out on behalf of the Manufacturing Chemists Association, U.S.A., in which both male and female rats were exposed to vinylidene chloride through the drinking water. Groups of 10 males and 20 females (treated) or 15 males and 30 females (controls) were given drinking water containing 0, 60, 100 or 200 ppm (mg/l). Treatment began in the Fo generation at 6–7 weeks of age and they were mated at 90 days of age to produce the F1a generation. Because of reduced fertility of Fo females in all groups, they were mated again to produce the F1b litters, from which a single mating produced the F2 generation, and from these in turn, 3 matings produced the F3a, F3b and F3c generations. Dosing was continuous throughout the study. There was a slight effect on pup survival in the F2 generation but Norris states it was "non-compound related". There was a marked effect on pup survival at all doses in the F3a litters but it was not seen in the F1a, F1b, F3b or F3c litters. There were no effects on litter size, sex ratio at birth and weaning, growth and survival of neonates (other than those mentioned above), toxicity prior to mating, fertility, length of gestation, delivery of live litters, gross or microscopical appearance of tissues and organs from dams and pups. No numerical data on these aspects of reproduction are presented in the paper; however, there appear to be no gross effects on reproduction when dosing is continued through 3 generations. The decreased survival of F3a litters may be a chance finding, since F3b and F3c litters were unaffected.

Short *et al.* (1977) have carried out a dominant lethal study in rats exposed to vinylidene chloride by inhalation. Males were exposed to 55 ppm for 6 h/day, 5 days/week for 11 weeks. During the eleventh week of exposure they were housed overnight for 7 successive evenings or until the male mated with 2 untreated females, with exposure to vinylidene chloride continuing during the daytime. On day 13 of pregnancy the females were killed, corpora lutea counted and the contents of the uterus examined. In controls 12/12 mated with 2 females and in the 55 ppm vinylidene chloride group 9/11 mated with 2 females and 2/11 with one female. These differences are not significant. Every treated male produced at least one litter with one or more viable implants, but only 13/20 females that mated with treated males were pregnant compared with 24/24 in control matings. There were no significant effects on implants/dam, implants/corpus luteum, viable/total implants or distribution of dead implants. This study indicates a significant increase in infertile matings or in total pre-implantation loss in some females. The latter is unlikely since there was no evidence of pre-implantation losses in pregnant females. There is no evidence of any dominant lethal effects from post-implantation loss rates.

Anderson *et al.* (1977) have carried out a dominant lethal study in the mouse. Groups of 20 males were first mated to establish fertility and then exposed to 10, 30, 50 or 75 ppm vinylidene chloride by inhalation for 6 h/day for 5 days (10 and 30 ppm), 2 days (50 ppm) or 1 day (75 ppm). At 10 ppm all survived, at 30 ppm 18/20 survived, at 50 ppm 8/20 survived and at 75 ppm 2/20 survived. In controls, exposed to air only, 50/50 survived. At the end of the exposure period those surviving in the 10, 30 and 50 ppm groups were placed with 2 fresh females/week for 5 days/week for 8 weeks. The females were killed 13 (week 0 matings) or 15 (week 1–8 matings) days after first placing with the males and examined for pregnancies. In the control, 10 and 30 ppm groups mating success in week 0 was 100% and in weeks 1–8 ranged from 82–100%, but was generally slightly higher in vinylidene chloride-exposed groups than in controls. In the 50 ppm group mating success in week 0 of those surviving vinylidene chloride exposure was significantly reduced to 38%, and was significantly lower than controls in each of the subsequent 8 weeks, varying from 43–86%. In control, 10 and 30 ppm groups over 70% of females that were mated became pregnant, whereas in the 50 ppm group only 30–50% of those mated became pregnant, the reduction being significant in weeks 0–6. However, since pre-exposure fertility in the 8 mice surviving exposure to 50 ppm was low (because of poor survival non-proven males had to be included in the experimental group) it is not possible to ascertain from this experiment whether vinylidene chloride had any additional effect itself on fertility. With the exception of a positive control group given cyclophosphamide there were no significant effects on total implants/dam or dead implants/dam, indicating that there were no significant pre-implantation losses or dominant lethal effects.

Conclusion

Given the slight loss in fertility in male rats exposed to 55 ppm by inhalation and possible loss in fertility in male mice exposed to 50 ppm by inhalation, one might expect to have also seen effects in the rat multigeneration study where 200 ppm was given in the drinking water, since it has been estimated that the daily intake from this route of administration is equivalent to the daily intake from 7 h exposure to 120 ppm by inhalation (Murray *et al.*, 1979). However, 200 ppm vinylidene chloride in the drinking water has no effect on food consumption or weight gain (Norris, 1977; Murray *et al.*, 1979), whereas inhalation of vinylidene chloride affects food consumption and weight gain, certainly at 80 ppm (Murray *et al.*, 1979), and possibly at levels as low as 25 ppm (Norris, 1977). Since the toxicity of vinylidene chloride is enhanced in fasted animals (see section A for details) the threshold for reproductive toxic effects may be considerably lower in animals exposed by inhalation than in those exposed by ingestion.

No dominant lethal effects have been detected in rats or mice.

D. PREGNANCY

Short *et al.* (1977) have carried out a very comprehensive study on the prenatal and postnatal effects of exposure to vinylidene chloride by inhalation in the mouse and the rat. The LC50 in pregnancy was estimated as around 80 ppm for mice and 460 ppm for rats. Acceptable teratological methods were used.

In the first mouse experiment, groups of 15–23 animals were exposed to 15, 30, 57, 144 or 300 ppm for 23 h/day on days 6–16 of pregnancy, with 65 controls exposed to 0 ppm. There was also a concurrent food restricted control group. Maternal weight gain during exposure of those carrying to term was significantly reduced at 30 ppm, but not at 15 or 57 ppm. At 144 and 300 ppm all dams lost their pregnancies or died before term. At 57 ppm only 5/21 exposed females were pregnant at term and at 30 ppm only 2/19 were pregnant. Implants/dam in these 2 groups were also reduced from 11·1 in controls to 4·0 at 30 ppm and 6·8 at 57 ppm and all the implants were resorbed early in pregnancy. In those exposed to 15 ppm there were no significant differences in comparison with 0 ppm controls in pregnancy rate, implants/dam, live fetuses/dam, resorptions/dam or fetal weight. In the 15 ppm group sporadic malformations occurred including hydrocephalus, occluded nasal passages, microphthalmia, small liver and hydronephrosis in a total of 73 fetuses from 15 litters. No abnormalities were seen in 0 ppm controls or food restricted controls. However, the differences between 0 and 15 ppm groups for specific malformations were not significant. Retarded ossification of the incus and sternebrae was also seen.

Because of the huge losses from resorptions at levels of 30 ppm and above, further groups of mice were exposed to 0, 41, 54 or 74 ppm for 23 h/day on fewer days of gestation, all treatments ending on day 15 of pregnancy, in order to assess better the teratogenic potential of vinylidene chloride. Even with short exposures maternal weight gain was affected at all doses used. With exposures beginning on day 10, there was a similar outcome to the first experiment, viz. increased resorptions and malformations such as hydrocephalus in comparison with 0 ppm controls. However, in both these mouse experiments, with the exception of increased hydrocephalus, similar effects were also seen in mice not exposed to vinylidene chloride but food restricted to a level similar to that seen in vinylidene chloride exposed dams. Thus effects on resorptions and malformations, with the possible exception of hydrocephalus, could not be attributed directly to vinylidene chloride, but were probably secondary to the maternal toxicity induced.

In their first rat study (Short *et al.*, 1977), groups of 18–20 animals were exposed to 15, 57, 300 or 449 ppm for 23 h/day on days 6–16 of pregnancy, with 58 controls exposed to 0 ppm. There was also a concurrent food-restricted control group. Maternal weight increased in controls on days 6–16 of pregnancy but showed dose-related decreases in all treated groups, from 15 ppm upwards. Partial post-exposure recovery of weight was seen in 15, 57 and 300 ppm groups but not in the 449 ppm group. The proportion of dams carrying to term was significantly decreased in a dose-related manner in 57, 300 and 449 ppm groups. Of those carrying to term, implants/dam were not affected but early resorptions were significantly increased from 2% in controls to 49% at 57 ppm and 64% at 449 ppm (300 ppm not affected) largely due to 6 dams in each group with complete resorptions. Live fetuses/dam were correspondingly reduced in these 2 groups. Fetal weight was reduced in a dose-related manner and the reductions were significant in 57, 300 and 449 ppm groups. Malformations were seen in all groups and hydrocephalus was significantly increased in a dose-related way from 2·5% in controls to 7·3% at 15 ppm, 15·1% at 57 ppm and 33·3% at 300 ppm. Retarded ossification was seen in all exposed groups. Food-restricted controls showed reduced fetal weight and retarded ossification but no significant increase in resorption rate or in the frequency of hydrocephalus.

It would seem from these mouse and rat experiments that many of the adverse effects of vinylidene chloride exposure on the embryo and fetus are secondary to maternal toxicity and in particular the reduction in food intake in exposed dams. One reason for such severe reductions may be that the food became contaminated with vinylidene chloride during the 23 h exposures. Fresh food was provided once daily. However, an increased frequency of hydrocephalus in the mouse and rat and increased resorptions in the rat could not be explained by reduced food intake, though other aspects of maternal toxicity, rather than a direct effect of vinylidene chloride may be responsible for these effects. Further work on doses non-toxic to the dam (below 15 ppm) are required.

Short *et al.* (1977) also exposed groups of rats to 0, 56 or 283 ppm for

23 h/day on days 8–20 of pregnancy and followed postnatal development of the pups. They assessed litter size, weight gain, righting, auditory startle, bar holding and visual placing reflexes, general physical maturation, swimming and locomotor development. In both exposed groups there was significant retardation of development of the surface righting reflex, lower weight gain and later incisor eruption. However, no other parameters were affected and the effect on the body weight had disappeared by 21 days of age. Thus the postnatal effects of prenatal vinylidene chloride exposure appear to be minimal.

Murray *et al.* (1979) carried out a teratology study in rats and rabbits on behalf of the Manufacturing Chemists Association, U.S.A. Acceptable teratological methods were used. Groups of 18–47 rats were exposed to 0, 20, 80 or 160 ppm vinylidene chloride for 7 h/day by inhalation or to 0 or 200 ppm in the drinking water on days 6–15 of pregnancy. Those exposed to 200 ppm in the drinking water ingested approximately 40 mg/kg/day vinylidene chloride, which the authors suggest is equivalent to a single 7 h inhalation exposure of 120 ppm. There were no deaths in any group but some maternal toxicity was evident from significant reductions in maternal weight gain during the early part of treatment and reduced food consumption in dams exposed to 80 or 160 ppm by inhalation. Water intake was significantly increased in all groups inhaling vinylidene chloride. No signs of maternal toxicity were seen in those given vinylidene chloride in the drinking water. There were no significant effects on implants/dam, live fetuses/dam, resorptions/dam or fetal body weight in any of the treated groups. Malformations were seen in treated and control groups and there was a significant increase in delayed ossification of vertebrae at 160 ppm and significant increases in delayed ossification of the skull and in wavy ribs at both 80 and 160 ppm. There was no significant difference in overall major malformation rates calculated after exclusion of the skeletal anomalies mentioned above. There were no significant effects on malformation or anomaly rates in those given vinylidene chloride in the drinking water.

In the rabbit study (Murray *et al.*, 1979) groups of 16–22 does were exposed to 0, 80 or 160 ppm by inhalation for 7 h/day on days 6–18 of pregnancy. One doe exposed to 80 ppm and 2 does exposed to 160 ppm died, but the causes of death were not those that would be associated with vinylidene chloride toxicity. Maternal toxicity was evident, however, from significantly increased maternal weight loss during the treatment period in does exposed to 160 ppm and significantly increased post-exposure weight gains at both 80 and 160 ppm. There was no effect on implants/dam, but live fetuses/dam were reduced to a mean of 6 at 160 ppm compared with a control mean of 8, and resorptions/dam were significantly increased to a mean of 2·7 at 160 ppm compared with a control mean of 0·3. Fetal body weight and fetal malformations did not differ significantly between treated and control groups, but skeletal variants did; at 160 ppm there was a significant increase in thirteenth pairs of ribs and a decrease in delayed ossification of the fifth sternebra.

The results of this study on rats and rabbits show that vinylidene chloride exposure does not cause major malformations even at doses which are toxic to the dam, but it is embryolethal at 160 ppm in the rabbit and causes wavy ribs and delayed ossification in the rat at 80 and 160 ppm. However, maternal toxicity was also evident at these doses and it is not clear to what extent the effects on the embryo and fetus may be secondary to those on the mother. In the rabbit study the authors mention that the occurrence of resorptions in the litters correlated well with individual maternal weight loss, suggesting the effect was secondary to maternal toxicity. It should also be remembered that the general toxicity of vinylidene chloride is enhanced in fasted animals. However, it is unusual to see effects on the embryo and fetus such as death, wavy ribs and delayed ossification, in the absence of reduced fetal body weight, ascribed to maternal toxicity alone. A question therefore remains as to whether vinylidene chloride may be having a direct effect on the embryo and fetus and further studies are needed to clarify this point.

Conclusion

General vinylidene chloride toxicity decreases in the order mouse-rat-rabbit for any given exposure level and severity of effects on the embryo and fetus generally mirrors this pattern. It is clear that much of the embryolethality, fetotoxicity and teratogenicity of vinylidene chloride exposure during pregnancy is secondary to maternal toxicity, which sets up a vicious circle of reduced food intake, which in turn increases the toxicity of vinylidene chloride. However some effects on the embryo and fetus could not be explained by reduced food intake alone, though they could be secondary to other aspects of maternal toxicity. Studies employing doses which are not toxic to the dam are required. There have been no such studies to date.

E. MUTAGENICITY

Vinylidene chloride is reported to be mutagenic in the Ames test with metabolic activation (Simmon, 1977, IARC Monograph Vol. 19, 1979). This is probably due to its metabolism to a reactive epoxide, 1,1-dichloroethylene oxide (Bardodej, 1976).

Norris (1977) reported on a cytogenetic study carried out in rats on behalf of the Manufacturing Chemists Association, U.S.A. Rats were exposed for 6 h/day, 5 days/week for 6 months to 0, 25 or 75 ppm vinylidene chloride by inhalation. No chromosomal aberrations were seen in bone marrow cell cultures from control or treated rats. No further details were given.

F. CARCINOGENICITY

IARC Monograph Vol. 19 (1979) reports on studies showing vinylidene chloride produces malignant tumours in mice and rats, some of the tumours being similar to those produced by vinyl chloride; however, assessment is difficult since some of the evidence came from studies still in progress.

HUMAN STUDIES

No relevant data found on any aspects of reproductive toxicity.

F. CARCINOGENICITY

IARC Monograph Vol. 19 (1979) stated that the single epidemiological study available at that time reported no tumours were associated with vinylidene chloride exposure, but that the data were not adequate to permit the assessment of human carcinogenicity.

SUMMARY AND EVALUATION

EXPERIMENTAL STUDIES

No studies were found on endocrine or gonadal effects. Slight reductions in fertility of male mice and rats were observed following inhalation exposure to 50 ppm. No adverse effects were observed however in a rat multigeneration study with up to 200 ppm in drinking water. No dominant lethal effects have been observed in mice and rats.

Teratogenicity studies in mice, rats and rabbits have shown no increase in major malformations with the exception of hydrocephalus in some studies although marked embryolethality and fetotoxicity with increase in various anomalies have been observed. In all of these studies maternal toxicity was observed and it is impossible to define to what extent the embryotoxicity is secondary to this maternal toxicity and reduced food intake. It is mutagenic in bacterial tests but not *in vovo* in one study. It is carcinogenic in mice and rats.

HUMAN STUDIES

No relevant data were found. A single epidemiological study did not show evidence of carcinogenicity.

EVALUATION

There is evidence that it is embryolethal and fetotoxic in several species. The data are inadequate to assess whether these effects would be observed at doses non-toxic to the dams. No data are available in humans on reproductive effects and the data on carcinogenicity is inadequate for evaluation.

Attention is drawn to the lack of data at low levels of exposure for establishing a no-effect level in animals and to the lack of data in humans.

References

Andersen, M. E. and Jenkins, L. J. Jr. (1977). Oral toxicity of 1,1-dichloroethylene in the rat: effects of sex, age and fasting. *Environmental Health Perspectives* **21**, 157–163.

Anderson, D., Hodge, M. C. E. and Purchase, I. F. H. (1977). Dominant lethal studies with the halogenated olefins vinyl chloride and vinylidene dichloride in male CD-1 mice. *Environmental Health Perspectives* **21**, 71–78.

Bardodej, Z. (1976). Metabolic studies and the evaluation of genetic risk from the viewpoint of industrial toxicology. *Mutation Research* **41**, 7–14.

IARC Monographs on the Evaluation of the Carcinogenic Risk of Chemicals to Humans: Some monomers, plastics and synthetic elastomers and acrolein (1979). Vol. 19, Lyon, France.

McKenna, J. A., Zempel, J. A., Madrid, E. O., Braun, W. H. and Gehring, P. J. (1978). Metabolism and pharmacokinetic profile of vinylidene chloride in rats following oral administration. *Toxicology and Applied Pharmacology* **45**, 821–835.

Murray, F. J., Nitschke, K. D., Rampy, L. W. and Schwetz, B. A. (1979). Embryotoxicity and fetotoxicity of inhaled or ingested vinylidene chloride in rats and rabbits. *Toxicology and Applied Pharmacology* **49**, 189–192.

Norris, J. M. (1977). Toxicological and pharmacokinetic studies on inhaled and ingested vinylidene chloride in laboratory animals. *Pap. Synth. Conf. (Prepr.)*, pp. 45–50.

Short, R. D., Minor, J. L., Peters, P., Winston, J. M., Ferguson, B., Unger, T., Sawyer, M. and Lee, C. C. (1977). Toxicity studies of selected chemicals. Task II. The developmental toxicity of vinylidene chloride inhaled by rats and mice during gestation. EPA/560/6–77–022.

Simmon, V. F. (1977). Structural correlations of carcinogenic and mutagenic alkyl halides. *In* "Structural Correlates of Carcinogenesis and Mutagenesis" (Eds. Asher, I. M. and Zerros, C.), pp. 163–171. FDA Office of Science.

48. Xylene

TECHNICAL DATA

Formula

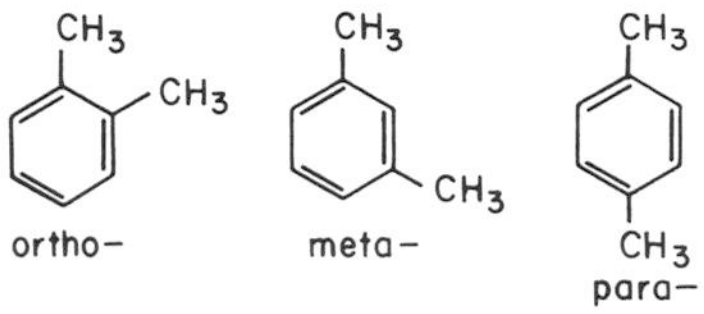

ortho- | meta- | para-

(ortho-: $C_6H_4(CH_3)_2$ with CH_3 groups at 1,2; meta-: 1,3; para-: 1,4)

CAS registry number 1330–20–7

Chemical abstracts name Dimethylbenzene

Synonyms Xylol

Uses Solvent; raw material for production of benzoic acid, phthalic anhydride, isophthalic and terephthalic acids and their dimethyl esters used in manufacture of polyester fibres; manufacture of dyes and other organics; sterilizing catgut; with Canada balsam as oil-immersion in microscopy; cleaning agent in microscopy.

TLV 100 ppm (skin)

ANIMAL STUDIES

A. RELEVANT PHARMACOLOGY AND TOXICOLOGY

Xylene occurs in 3 isomeric forms, ortho-, meta- and para-xylene, depending on the substitution positions of the 2 methyl groups on the benzene ring. Commercial xylene is a mixture of the 3 isomers, generally with m-xylene predominating, but it may also contain substantial amounts of other contaminants such as ethyl benzene. The acute toxicities of the 3 isomers differ (Ungváry *et al.*, 1979).

The metabolism of xylene has been summarized by Dean (1978). Relatively little xylene is exhaled unchanged, in contrast to benzene and toluene. Metabolism is by oxidation of one of the methyl groups in meta- and para-xylene, forming toluic acids which are conjugated with glucuronic acid and excreted in the urine as toluric acids. Ortho-xylene is almost completely oxidized and conjugated to form o-tolylglucuronic acid. There may be some hydroxylation of the benzene nucleus to form xylenols excreted unchanged or as conjugates.

Jenkins *et al.* (1971) have shown a sex difference in toxicity of mineral spirits containing 18–20% xylene as the main aromatic fraction, in the guinea pig. Animals were exposed to around 900 mg/m^3 of mineral spirits by inhalation for 90 days. Twice as many males as females died, but it is not known whether the toxicity was due primarily to the xylene constituent.

Placental transfer of xylene has been shown in the mouse. Nawrot *et al.* (1980) gave radiolabelled m-xylene by gavage to mice on day 12 or 15 of pregnancy and killed them 2, 6·5 or 24 h after dosing. Highest radioactivity levels in maternal liver and fetal tissue were seen 2 h after dosing, and by 24 h very little remained. At least 95% of the radioactivity in the fetuses was due to metabolites rather than m-xylene itself.

B. ENDOCRINE AND GONADAL EFFECTS

No relevant data found.

C. FERTILITY

No relevant data found.

D. PREGNANCY

Effects of xylene on pregnancy in the rat have been investigated. Teslina (1974) has given groups of 32 rats s.c. injections of xylene in doses of 0·15 g/kg (1/50 LD50) or 0·4 g/kg (1/20 LD50) on days 1–10 or 1–18 of pregnancy. Dams were killed on the last day of injection. Signs of maternal toxicity (reduced weight gain, kidney and haematologic changes) were seen in all dose groups. Of those given 0·4 g/kg/day on days 1–18, 5 rats died. After dosing on day 1–10 of pregnancy, pre-implantation losses of 58% and 38% were seen in 0·4 and 0·15 g/kg groups respectively. After dosing on days 1–18 of pregnancy, pre- and post-implantation losses totalled 69% in the 0·4 g/kg group and there was a reduction in fetal body weight of survivors at both dose levels.

Krotov and Chebotar (1972) have exposed rats to p-xylene by inhalation. Twenty-nine rats were exposed to 115 ppm (500 mg/m^3) for 24 h/day from days 1–20 of pregnancy. In xylene-exposed rats there were significant increases in pre-implantation losses of 32% compared with 11% in controls, and post-implantation losses of 39% compared with 5% in controls. No teratogenic effects were observed but no details of this aspect of the study are given.

Hudák and Ungváry (1978) have exposed 20 rats to 230 ppm (1000 mg/m^3) xylene by inhalation for 24 h/day on days 9–14 of pregnancy. Twenty-six air-exposed animals served as controls. Acceptable teratological methods were used. Xylene caused no maternal deaths and maternal weight gain was normal. There were no effects on implants/dam, live fetuses/dam, dead or resorbed fetuses/dam or fetal weight. Two fetuses had agnathia, a non-significant increase in malformations, but this abnormality was not seen in any of the other 7 groups of solvent-exposed or control groups of rats in this study. There was a significant increase in skeletal anomalies (fused ribs, extra ribs) in xylene-exposed fetuses.

The xylene used in the above experiment was a mixture of 10% o-xylene, 50% m-xylene, 20% p-xylene and 20% ethyl benzene. Ungváry *et al.* (1979) have also investigated the teratogenicity of the pure isomers when inhaled. Details of the work on o- and m-xylene are not available in English but some information has been given by Ungváry *et al.* (1979). Both isomers were toxic to the dams, causing death of some animals exposed to m-xylene, reduced food intake in those exposed to o-xylene and reduced weight gain and increased liver weight in both m- and o-xylene-exposed dams. Neither isomer was teratogenic even at maternally toxic doses, but fetotoxicity was seen with both isomers; skeletal anomalies were increased, as in treatment with the mixture of isomers (Hudák and Ungváry, 1978), except that the effects of each isomer were not as great as that of the mixture. Ortho-xylene did not affect the incidence of extra ribs but m-xylene in high concentrations did increase it.

Detailed results on p-xylene are available (Ungváry *et al.*, 1979). Groups of 20 rats were exposed to 0, 35, 350 or 700 ppm (0, 150, 1500 or 3000 mg/m^3) p-xylene for 24 h/day on days 7–14 of pregnancy. Acceptable teratological methods were used. No maternal deaths occurred, but food consumption in the 700 ppm group was markedly reduced during exposure, being only about 20% of the control intake on days 9 and 10 of pregnancy. However, overall maternal weight gain in this group was not significantly affected, presumably because of the rebound increase in food intake seen after treatment stopped on day 14. No weight, histological or histochemical changes were found in the maternal livers. There were no significant effects on implants/dam, but 32% of rats in the p-xylene groups that mated had no implants compared with 10% in controls. As implantation occurs around the time of the start of treatment (day 7) this may indicate increased pre-implantation losses. In the 700 ppm group, 7/20 dams had complete resorptions compared with none in any of the other groups. Thus, average live litter size was significantly decreased and post-implantation losses were significantly increased from 4% in controls to 69% in the 700 ppm group. There were no significant effects on live fetuses/dam or dead and resorbed fetuses/dam in the 35 and 350 ppm groups. Placental weight was significantly reduced in all p-xylene exposed groups and fetal weight was reduced in a dose-related manner, but only reached a significant level, with a 12% reduction, in the 700 ppm group. There were no significant effects on the malformation rates. Agnathia, seen in their previous experiment with a mixture of xylene isomers, was not seen at all. Retarded ossification was seen in 31, 38 and 57% of fetuses in 35, 350 and 700 ppm groups, compared with 14% in controls, a significant increase in all 3 groups. A significant increase in the frequency of extra ribs was also seen in the 700 ppm group. Five randomly selected fetuses from each group were examined for organ histology and no pathology was found, but histochemical studies showed delayed enzyme development in the kidneys of fetuses in the 700 ppm group.

In the course of an experiment on an insecticide preparation, Rumsey *et al.* (1969) have immersed groups of 9–10 rats once on day 6, 9 or 12 of gestation in a mixture of xylene and emulsifier (alkylphenoxy polyethoxyethanol). There was no effect on pregnancy rate, live litter size at birth, average numbers weaned or weaning weight after these single immersions.

Conclusion

It can be seen that, in common with benzene and toluene, neither xylene as a mixture nor any of its isomers separately are teratogenic. However, with dosing in early pregnancy xylene caused pre-implantation losses and this is probably due to the p-xylene component. Xylene mixture and the isomers o-xylene and m-xylene cause significant fetotoxicity in terms of increased skeletal anomalies at doses below those toxic to the dam, as well as at maternally toxic doses. Para-xylene, however, at maternally toxic and sub-toxic doses, causes significant embryolethality and is fetotoxic in terms of reduced body weight, retarded ossification and kidney development, and increased incidence of extra ribs. There are marked differences in maternal toxicity of the isomers. Para-xylene would seem to be a particular problem in that it is the least maternally toxic and the most embryo- and fetotoxic of the 3 isomers.

E. MUTAGENICITY

No relevant data found.

F. CARCINOGENICITY

No relevant data found.

HUMAN STUDIES

A. RELEVANT PHARMACOLOGY AND TOXICOLOGY

No relevant data found.

B. ENDOCRINE AND GONADAL FUNCTION

Michon (1965) reported menstrual disturbances in women working in a factory producing leather and rubber shoes who were exposed to benzene, toluene and xylene (see Benzene section B for details). However, of the 3 solvents, it is likely that benzene was the most probable cause of the increased intensity and duration of bleeding.

Syrovadko *et al.* (1973) have investigated gynaecological disorders and menstrual function in women working in the manufacture of electrical insulating materials exposed to white spirit containing up to 16% of aromatic hydrocarbons, toluene and xylene (see Toluene section B for details). It is not possible to ascertain, however, which of the various chemicals they were exposed to, if any, might be the cause of the observed increase in menstrual disorders (hyper-menorrhoea, dysmenorrhoea).

C. FERTILITY

No relevant data found.

D. PREGNANCY

Holmberg (1979) has published a case-control study of children with central nervous system defects taken from the Finnish Register of Congenital Malformations (see section D of Styrene for details). Significantly more case than control mothers had been exposed to organic solvents during the first trimester of pregnancy. Of the 14 cases, one had been exposed to xylene, toluene, white spirit and methyl ethyl ketone in rubber products manufacturing. The child had hydrancephaly and died 24 days after birth. A previous child born to this woman also had brain injury and died at 4 years of age but it is not known if she was exposed to solvents at that time. Holmberg suggests that this history of predisposition and parental age were more likely to be causally related to the defect than solvents exposure. Three other cases were exposed to white spirit which may have contained xylene, and one control was exposed to xylene. This study provides only very tentative evidence that solvents may be causally related to CNS malformations and further evidence is required before any conclusions may be drawn.

Kučera (1968) has investigated the incidence of spinal malformations in Czechoslovakia from 1959–1966. In over 1·5 million live and stillbirths, 20,000 were malformed. There were 9 cases of caudal regression syndrome and in 5/9 of these cases the mothers were exposed to fat solvents during pregnancy. In one of these cases, xylene was the solvent involved. However, with further data added subsequently, making a total of 155 cases, Kučera has found the association between caudal regression syndrome and exposure to fat solvents much less strong; only 9% of mothers with babies with caudal regression syndrome were exposed to organic solvents in pregnancy. (T. Shepard reporting to the American Teratology Society, Michigan, 1978, after a personal communication from Kučera.)

E. MUTAGENICITY

Gerner-Smidt and Friedrich (1978) have exposed human lymphocytes *in vitro* to xylene at concentrations of 15·2, 152 and 1520 μg/ml and found growth inhibition at the highest concentration, but no increase in sister-chromatid exchange or structural chromosome aberrations.

Funes-Cravioto *et al.* (1977) studied the incidence of chromosome aberrations in cultured lymphocytes from 73 workers in chemical laboratories and the printing industry. They found a significantly increased incidence (approximately 2-fold) of chromatid and isochromatid breaks when compared with 49 controls. A similarly increased incidence was also observed in 14 children age 4–11 years of 11 women laboratory workers who had worked during pregnancy. There was also an increased incidence of sister-chromatid exchange (SCE) in 12 technicians and in the 4 children of 2 of the female technicians who had worked during pregnancy. The technicians came from 8 different laboratories but all were exposed to one or more of chloroform, toluene, benzene, cyclohexane, diethyl ether, isooctane, methanol, toluene or xylene, with chloroform, benzene and toluene being most common, though the atmospheric concentrations of these solvents was not measured in most instances. In a group of 34 of the subjects there was a correlation between the frequency of chromosome breaks and duration of exposure. There was no correlation between exposed mothers and their children, with sex or smoking habits. The subjects and controls in this study were not carefully matched and it is impossible to state that the chromosome aberrations were a direct result of exposure to organic solvents but this was a common factor in all the working environments studied. The biological significance of the changes observed is unknown as far as the health of the workers is concerned.

F. CARCINOGENICITY

No relevant data found.

SUMMARY AND EVALUATION

EXPERIMENTAL STUDIES

Xylene crosses the placenta in mice and may be metabolised in the fetus. No studies were found on endocrine or gonadal effects or of effects on fertility. Several teratology studies in rats have shown that it is embryolethal and fetotoxic at doses not toxic to the dams. P-xylene has the least maternal toxicity but the most embryo and fetal toxicity causing reduced fetal weight and retarded development. None of the isomers are teratogenic.

No studies on mutagenicity or carcinogenicity were found.

HUMAN STUDIES

No studies on endocrine or gonadal function or on fertility relating unequivocally to xylene were found. Although studies implicating solvent exposure as potential teratogens and mutagens have been published, none clearly implicate xylene. No studies on carcinogenesis were found.

EVALUATION

There is limited evidence that xylene may be embryolethal and fetotoxic in rats and no no-effect level has been established, but it is not teratogenic. Other data are inadequate for evaluation. Attention is drawn to the lack of data on fertility, mutagenicity and carcinogenicity in animals and of any adequate reproductive or other relevant data in humans.

References

Dean, B. J. (1978). Genetic toxicology of benzene, toluene, xylenes and phenols. *Mutation Research* **47**, (2), 75–97.

Funes-Cravioto, F., Kolmodin-Hedman, B., Lindsten, J., Nordenskjold, M., Zapata-Gayon, C., Lambert, B., Norberg, E., Olin, R. and Swenson, A. (1977). Chromosome aberrations and sister-chromatid exchange in workers in chemical laboratories and a rotoprinting factory and in children of women laboratory workers. *Lancet* **ii**, 322–325.

Gerner-Smidt, P. and Friedrich, U. (1978). The mutagenic effect of benzene, toluene and xylene studied by the SCE technique. *Mutation Research* **58**, (2/3), 313–316.

Holmberg, P. C. (1979). Central-nervous-system defects in children born to mothers exposed to organic solvents during pregnancy. *Lancet* **ii**, 177–179.

Hudák, A. and Ungváry, G. (1978). Embryotoxic effects of benzene, and its methyl derivatives: toluene and xylene. *Toxicology* **11**, 55–63.

Jenkins, L. J., Coon, R. A., Lyon, J. P. and Siegel, J. (1971). Effect on experimental animals of long-term inhalation exposure to mineral spirits. II. Dietary, sex and strain influences in guinea pigs. *Toxicology and Applied Pharmacology* **18**, 53–59.

Krotov, Y. A. and Chebotar, N. A. (1972). A study of embryotoxic and teratogenic action of some industrial substances formed during production of dimethylterephthalate. *Gigiena Truda I Professional 'Nye Zabolevaniya* **16**, 40–43.

Kučera, J. (1968). Exposure to fat solvents: a possible cause of sacral agenesis in man. *Journal of Pediatrics* **72**, 857–859.

Michon, S. (1965). Disturbances of menstruation in women working in an atmosphere polluted with aromatic hydrocarbons. *Polski Tygodnik Lekarski* **20**, 1648–1649.

Nawrot, P. S., Albro, P. W. and Staples, R. E. (1980). Distribution and excretion of ^{14}C-m-xylene in pregnant mice. *Teratology* **21**, (3), 58A.

Rumsey, T. S., Cabell, C. A. and Bond, J. (1969). Effect of an organic phosphorous systemic insecticide on reproductive performance in rats. *American Journal of Veterinary Research* **30**, 2209–2214.

Syrovadko, O. N., Skornin, V. F., Pronkova, E. N., Sorkina, N. S., Izyumova, A. S., Gribova, I. A. and Popova, A. F. (1973). Effect of working conditions on the health status and some specific functions of women handling white spirit. *Gigiena Truda I Professional 'Nye Zabolevaniya* **17**, (6), 5–8.

Teslina, O. V. (1974). Study of permeability of the placenta to iodine-131 on exposure to the action of xylene. Experimental study. *Akusherstvo I Ginekologiya Moskva* (7), 63–64.

Ungváry, G., Tatrai, E., Hudák, A., Barcza, G. and Lorincz, M. (1979). Study on the embryotoxic effect of para-xylene. *Egeszsegtudomany* **23**, (2), 152–158.

Index

C

N

O

V

W

X

Y

Z